Algal Bioremediation

Lakhan Kumar • Kaustubha Mohanty
Irem Deniz • Fazlurrahman Khan
Yasha Hasija
Editors

Algal Bioremediation

Sustainable Solutions, Challenges, and Future Prospects

Springer

Editors
Lakhan Kumar
Biological Science & Engineering
Maulana Azad National Institute of Technology
Bhopal, Madhya Pradesh, India

Irem Deniz
Bioengineering
Manisa Celal Bayar University
Muradiye-Yunusemre, Manisa, Türkiye

Yasha Hasija
Biotechnology
Delhi Technological University
Delhi, Delhi, India

Kaustubha Mohanty
Chemical Engineering
Indian Institute of Technology Guwahati
Guwahati, Assam, India

Fazlurrahman Khan
Ocean and Fisheries Development International Cooperation Institute
Pukyong National University
Busan, Korea (Republic of)

ISBN 978-981-95-8792-6 ISBN 978-981-95-8793-3 (eBook)
https://doi.org/10.1007/978-981-95-8793-3

This Springer imprint is published by the registered company Springer Nature Singapore Pte Ltd.
The registered company address is: 152 Beach Road, #21-01/04 Gateway East, Singapore 189721, Singapore

Preface

The world population has experienced exponential growth and improved living standards over the last two centuries, driven by the advent of modern technologies and their widespread adoption by the public. It has accelerated industrialization, increased mass public movement toward urban centers, and increased the exploitation of natural resources, without adequately addressing the associated dangers. The most affected is the environment, whether soil, water, or air. Climate change is one of the most pressing challenges of our time. The level of carbon dioxide in our atmosphere has risen to almost double the pre-industrial level. The presence of lethal chemicals in the biosphere has attracted worldwide attention, prompting efforts to remediate them to protect public health and the environment. In other words, environmental sustainability has become one of the defining imperatives of the twenty-first century.

In order to tackle environmental pollution, several physicochemical techniques-based strategies have been successfully developed and employed, but the associated cost, economic and environmental, and the requirement of additional treatment in most of the treatment strategies have limited their use and necessitated the development of holistic and eco-friendly methods. Bioremediation, the use of biological entities and derived products to degrade and remove environmental pollutants, offers a novel, scalable, and environmentally benign solution. In this book, we have focused on providing comprehensive information on the potential of using algal diversity as a bioremediation agent for environmental pollutants.

Algae diversity includes cyanobacteria, microalgae, and macroalgae. Recent scientific endeavors have reported on the largely successful remediation of various pollutants, including heavy metals, dyes, pharmaceuticals and active ingredients, cosmetics, pesticides, and hydrocarbons, as well as several other emerging pollutants using algae. In addition to removing pollutants, algal systems can further enhance the Circular Bioeconomy. The conversion of algal biomass through methods such as pyrolysis, hydrothermal liquefaction, and gasification creates opportunities to pair environmental remediation strategies with bioenergy generation and the further synthesis of bioproducts. Newer innovations in genomics, metagenomics, and systems biology also help in the development, improvement, and scaling up of algal-based bioremediation strategies. Algae possess remarkable and diverse metabolic pathways and mechanisms that enable them to remediate various pollutants via biosorption, bioaccumulation, enzymatic and redox transformations, and eventual degradation and metabolic assimilation. Because they can grow in diverse environments and require fewer resources than terrestrial plants, they have become an attractive candidate for engineered treatment systems.

Our book, *Algal Bioremediation: Sustainable Solutions, Challenges, and Future Prospects*, was conceived to provide foundational information on pollutants and their remediation using algae, integrating modern biotechnological advancements into algal systems to improve bioremediation efficiency and further their integration into circular bioeconomic models for resource recovery. It further presents insights into pollutant transport into the algal cell and its intracellular fate, as well as the metabolic pathways that process these pollutants. By linking mechanistic biology with system-level optimization, the volume aims to provide a comprehensive and cohesive technical foundation for advancing algae-based remediation technologies for environmental pollutants.

Bhopal, Madhya Pradesh, India — Lakhan Kumar
Guwahati, Assam, India — Kaustubha Mohanty
Manisa, Türkiye — Irem Deniz
Busan, Republic of Korea — Fazlurrahman Khan
Delhi, India — Yasha Hasija

Contents

Editors and Contributors

About the Editors

Lakhan Kumar works as an Assistant Professor at Maulana Azad National Institute of Technology, Bhopal, India. He completed his BTech in Biotechnology from Dr. B.R. Ambedkar National Institute of Technology, Jalandhar. He obtained his MTech in Industrial Biotechnology and PhD in Algal Biotechnology from Delhi Technological University, Delhi, where he investigated the application of microalgae for biodiesel production, accumulation, and enhancement of biochemicals of industrial significance, as well as phycoremediation, synthesis of biochar, and nanoparticles for environmental remediation. He has more than eight years of academic and research experience. He has been awarded the Research Excellence Award by Delhi Technological University, Delhi. He has actively participated in Training, Conferences, Workshops, and Seminars on recent trends in biobased resource recovery, bioremediation, nanobiotechnology, and biofuels. He has published over 50 peer-reviewed articles, in addition to 7 books on Algal Biofuels, Biorefinery, and Bioremediation. He is a reviewer for several reputable journals and a member of a society focused on Environmental and Social Development. He enjoys mentoring and inspiring young and aspiring biotechnologists through seminars, training, and outreach programs.

Kaustubha Mohanty obtained his PhD degree in Chemical Engineering from the Indian Institute of Technology, Kharagpur, and is currently a Professor and Head of the Chemical Engineering department at the Indian Institute of Technology, Guwahati. His key research areas are biofuels, biological wastewater treatment, membrane technology, microalgae biorefinery, biomass pyrolysis, and the water-energy nexus. He has published more than 220 research papers in peer-reviewed journals. He is Chief Editor of the *Journal of Chemistry* (Taylor & Francis), Associate Editor of *The Journal of Institution of Engineers* (India) Series: E (Springer), and Editorial board member of *Renewable Energy* (Elsevier), *ACS ES&T Water*, *Journal of Analytical and Applied Pyrolysis* (Elsevier), *Biomass*

Conversion & Biorefinery (Springer), and a few other journals. He is a Fellow of the Royal Society of Chemistry, UK, a Fellow of the International Association of Advanced Materials, Sweden, a Fellow of the Biotech Research Society of India, a Fellow of the Institution of Engineers (India), and a Fellow of the Indian Institute of Chemical Engineers.

Irem Deniz currently serves as an Associate Professor in the Department of Bioengineering at Manisa Celal Bayar University/Turkey. Her research interests include, but is not limited to, bioprocess, enzyme technology, scale-up, bioreactors, gasification, biochemical engineering, bioconversion of agricultural raw and waste commodities into value-added products, bioenergy/biofuels, microalgae, novel bioreactors, and downstream processing. She has published over 30 articles in SCI-indexed journals, 8 chapters, and edited 3 international books. She is an Editorial Board Member of the *Biochemical Engineering Journal* (Elsevier, SCI IF:3.226) and a member of the International Bioprocess Association (IFIBiop, IBA).

Fazlurrahman Khan is an Assistant Professor at the Ocean and Fisheries Development International Cooperation Institute, Pukyong National University (PKNU) in Busan. His academic journey began with a Master of Science in Biotechnology from Madurai Kamaraj University, India, followed by a PhD in Microbiology from Jawaharlal Nehru University. His research is at the forefront of microbial pathogenesis. His work explores the mechanisms of biofilm formation on both biotic and abiotic surfaces, identifying natural and synthetic molecules that inhibit the biofilm and virulence properties of pathogens, as well as the molecular interactions between fungal and bacterial pathogens. He has made substantial contributions to the field, authoring over 200 research and review papers. His scholarly work is widely recognized, and he serves on the editorial boards of several prestigious journals, including *Scientific Reports*, *AMB Express*, *Microbial Pathogenesis*, and *BMC Microbiology*. Additionally, he has contributed as a Guest Editor for *Microbial Pathogenesis*, *Foods*, *JovE*, *Antibiotics*, and *Marine Drugs*.

Yasha Hasija is currently a Professor and Head of the Biotechnology Department at Delhi Technological University. She has over 15 years of experience in teaching and research, spanning Bioinformatics, Diseases, Genetics, Omics, and Translational Biotechnology. She has dedicated her career to advancing biotechnology through teaching, research, and leadership. She has published over 150 research articles and review papers in esteemed national and international journals, with her work being cited 2,004 times, holding an h-index of 20, and an i10-index of 40. She serves on the Editorial Board of numerous international journals and has made significant contributions to Biotechnology and Bioinformatics as an author and editor of notable books. Her contributions have been recognized with several prestigious awards, including the Government of India's Department of Science and Technology Award for attending the Nobel Laureates' meeting in Lindau, Germany, and the Human Gene Nomenclature Award at the Human Genome Meeting in Montpellier, France. She has delivered over 100 talks as a speaker and resource person at various workshops, conferences, and seminars at both national and international levels.

Contributors

Ruchika Agarwal Department of Environmental Science, School of Earth Sciences, Central University of Rajasthan, Ajmer, Rajasthan, India

Edita Baltrėnaitė-Gedienė Institute of Environmental Protection, Vilnius Gediminas Technical University, VILNIUS TECH, Vilnius, Lithuania

Priyadarshini Banerjee Department of Pharmaceutical Sciences and Technology, Birla Institute of Technology - Mesra, Ranchi, India

Crisóstomo Barajas-Ferreira Research Center for Sustainable Development in Industry and Energy, Program of Chemical Engineering, Universidad Industrial de Santander, Bucaramanga, Colombia

Andres Fernando Barajas-Solano Department of Environmental Sciences, Universidad Francisco de Paula Santander, Cúcuta, Colombia

Gurunathan Baskar Department of Biotechnology, St. Joseph's College of Engineering, Chennai, India

Prakash Binnal Department of Chemical Engineering, Siddaganga Institute of Technology, Tumakuru, Karnataka, India

Katarzyna Chojnacka Department of Advanced Material Technologies, Wroclaw University of Science and Technology, Wroclaw, Lower Silesia, Poland

Jefferson E. Contreras-Ropero Research Center for Sustainable Development in Industry and Energy, Program of Chemical Engineering, Universidad Industrial de Santander, Bucaramanga, Colombia

Ana Julia de Lima Grutzmacher Bioprocess Intensification Group, Federal University of Santa Maria, UFSM, Santa Maria, Rio Grande do Sul, Brazil

Mariany Costa Deprá Bioprocess Intensification Group, Federal University of Santa Maria, UFSM, Santa Maria, Rio Grande do Sul, Brazil

Jayabrata Dhar Department of Mechanical Engineering, National Institute of Technology Durgapur, Durgapur, India

Rosangela Rodrigues Dias Bioprocess Intensification Group, Federal University of Santa Maria, UFSM, Santa Maria, Rio Grande do Sul, Brazil

Puja Dokania Department of Biotechnology and Medical Engineering, National Institute of Technology, Rourkela, Odisha, India

Darissa Alves Dutra Bioprocess Intensification Group, Federal University of Santa Maria, UFSM, Santa Maria, Rio Grande do Sul, Brazil

Susmita Dutta Department of Chemical Engineering, National Institute of Technology Durgapur, Durgapur, India

Janet B. García-Martínez Department of Environmental Sciences, Universidad Francisco de Paula Santander, Cúcuta, Colombia

Lira Gaysina Department of Bioecology and Biological Education, M. Akmullah Bashkir State Pedagogical University, Ufa, Russia

Kartik Chandra Ghanta Department of Chemical Engineering, National Institute of Technology Durgapur, Durgapur, India

Eduardo Jacob-Lopes Bioprocess Intensification Group, Federal University of Santa Maria, UFSM, Santa Maria, Rio Grande do Sul, Brazil

Eliana Marcela Jiménez-Bambague School of School of Natural Resources and the Environment, Universidad del Valle, Ciudad Universitaria Meléndez, Cali, Colombia

Viatcheslav Kafarov Research Center for Sustainable Development in Industry and Energy, Program of Chemical Engineering, Universidad Industrial de Santander, Bucaramanga, Colombia

Fazlurrahman Khan Marine Integrated Biomedical Technology Center, The National Key Research Institutes in Universities, Pukyong National University, Busan, Republic of Korea
Ocean and Fisheries Development International Cooperation Institute, Pukyong National University, Busan, Republic of Korea

Taehyeong Kim Department of Applied Biosciences, Kyungpook National University, Daegu, Republic of Korea

Khushi Kumari Department of Biotechnology, Dr B R Ambedkar National Institute of Technology, Jalandhar, India

Monika Kumari Department of Pharmaceutical Sciences and Technology, Birla Institute of Technology - Mesra, Ranchi, India

Eduarda Funari Machado Bioprocess Intensification Group, Federal University of Santa Maria, UFSM, Santa Maria, Rio Grande do Sul, Brazil

Richard Luan Silva Machado Bioprocess Intensification Group, Federal University of Santa Maria, UFSM, Santa Maria, Rio Grande do Sul, Brazil

Fiderman Machuca-Martínez School of School of Natural Resources and the Environment, Universidad del Valle, Ciudad Universitaria Meléndez, Cali, Colombia

Carlos Arturo Madera-Parra School of School of Natural Resources and the Environment, Universidad del Valle, Ciudad Universitaria Meléndez, Cali, Colombia

Jogeswar Mahanta Department of Biotechnology and Medical Engineering, National Institute of Technology, Rourkela, Odisha, India

Muhilan Mahendhiran Department of Agri Business Management, Faculty of Agriculture, Vivekananda Global University, Jaipur, Rajasthan, India

Sanhita Maity Amity Institute of Applied Sciences, Amity University Jharkhand, Ranchi, Jharkhand, India

Arun Kumar Mani Department of Chemistry and Biosciences, Srinivasa Ramanujan Centre, SASTRA Deemed University, Kumbakonam, Tamil Nadu, India

Simran Maratha Department of Environmental Science, School of Earth Sciences, Central University of Rajasthan, Ajmer, Rajasthan, India

K. M. Meera Sheriffa Begum Department of Chemical Engineering, National Institute of Technology, Tiruchirappalli, Tamil Nadu, India

Bikash Kumar Mondal Department of Chemical Engineering, National Institute of Technology Durgapur, Durgapur, India

Ishita Mukherjee Department of Chemistry, Birla Institute of Technology Mesra, Ranchi, Jharkhand, India

Anant Nag Department of Pharmaceutical Sciences and Technology, Birla Institute of Technology - Mesra, Ranchi, India

Rakhya Ranjan Nanda Department of Biotechnology, Dr B R Ambedkar National Institute of Technology, Jalandhar, India

Vishal Kumar Parida Amity School of Engineering and Technology, Amity University Jharkhand, Ranchi, Jharkhand, India

Sana Parveen Department of Environmental Science, School of Earth Sciences, Central University of Rajasthan, Ajmer, Rajasthan, India

Shailesh Kumar Patidar Department of Environmental Science, School of Earth Sciences, Central University of Rajasthan, Ajmer, Rajasthan, India

Priyadarsani Patra Department of Biotechnology and Medical Engineering, National Institute of Technology, Rourkela, Odisha, India

Arpita Patro Department of Biotechnology and Medical Engineering, National Institute of Technology, Rourkela, Odisha, India

Anirban Pradhan Department of Chemistry, Birla Institute of Technology Mesra, Ranchi, Jharkhand, India

Kishanta Kumar Pradhan Department of Pharmaceutical Sciences and Technology, Birla Institute of Technology - Mesra, Ranchi, India

Edgar Omar Rueda Puente Departamento de Agricultura y Ganadería, Universidad de Sonora, Hermosillo, Sonora, México

M. Ramya Department of Biotechnology, St. Joseph's College of Engineering, Chennai, India

Prabhaharan Renganathan Department of Bioecology and Biological Education, M. Akmullah Bashkir State Pedagogical University, Ufa, Russia

Winston Franz Ríos-Ruiz Laboratorio de Microbiología Agrícola "Raúl Ríos Reátegui", Departamento Académico Agrosilvopastoril, Facultad de Ciencias Agrarias, Universidad Nacional de San Martín, Tarapoto, Peru

Prangya Ranjan Rout Department of Biotechnology, Dr B R Ambedkar National Institute of Technology, Jalandhar, India

Balaram Sahoo Department of Biotechnology and Medical Engineering, National Institute of Technology, Rourkela, Odisha, India

Satadal Sahoo Department of Chemistry, Birla Institute of Technology Mesra, Ranchi, Jharkhand, India

Rojalini Samanta Department of Pharmacy, Usha Martin University, Ranchi, Jharkhand, India

Angana Sarkar Department of Biotechnology and Medical Engineering, National Institute of Technology, Rourkela, Odisha, India

Arnab Sau Department of Chemical Engineering, National Institute of Technology Durgapur, Durgapur, India

Adriane Terezinha Schneider Bioprocess Intensification Group, Federal University of Santa Maria, UFSM, Santa Maria, Rio Grande do Sul, Brazil

Suvetha Selvam Department of Chemistry and Biosciences, Srinivasa Ramanujan Centre, SASTRA Deemed University, Kumbakonam, Tamil Nadu, India

Sri Meenakshi Selvaraju Department of Chemistry and Biosciences, Srinivasa Ramanujan Centre, SASTRA Deemed University, Kumbakonam, Tamil Nadu, India

Jaya Sharma Department of Biotechnology, Dr B R Ambedkar National Institute of Technology, Jalandhar, India

Dawid Skrzypczak Department of Advanced Material Technologies, Wroclaw University of Science and Technology, Wroclaw, Lower Silesia, Poland

Poojasri Sowndarajan Department of Chemistry and Biosciences, Srinivasa Ramanujan Centre, SASTRA Deemed University, Kumbakonam, Tamil Nadu, India

B. R. Sreelekhmy Division of Environmental Biotechnology, Department of Biosciences, Rajagiri College of Social Sciences (Autonomous), Kochi, India

Nazia Tabassum Marine Integrated Biomedical Technology Center, The National Key Research Institutes in Universities, Pukyong National University, Busan, Republic of Korea

Rafał Taf Department of Advanced Material Technologies, Wroclaw University of Science and Technology, Wroclaw, Lower Silesia, Poland

Sabeela Beevi Ummalyma Division of Environmental Biotechnology, Department of Biosciences, Rajagiri College of Social Sciences (Autonomous), Kochi, India

Kaushal Kant Verma Department of Pharmaceutical Sciences and Technology, Birla Institute of Technology - Mesra, Ranchi, India

Leila Queiroz Zepka Bioprocess Intensification Group, Federal University of Santa Maria, UFSM, Santa Maria, Rio Grande do Sul, Brazil

Antonio Zuorro Department of Chemical Engineering, Materials, and Environment, Sapienza University, Rome, Italy

1 Harnessing Microalgal Systems for Sustainable Pollution Management: Mechanisms, Innovations, Bioreactor Technologies, and Future Perspectives

Rakhya Ranjan Nanda, Jaya Sharma, Khushi Kumari, and Prangya Ranjan Rout

Abstract

Industrial, agricultural, and urban pollutants pose a significant threat to both ecological and human health. Traditional remediation methods are sometimes effective, but they are often limited by restrictive pricing, complex operational procedures, and high energy requirements. Additionally, these methods can generate secondary pollutants, thereby compromising their sustainability. Algal bioremediation, also known as phycoremediation, leverages the natural capabilities of microalgae and cyanobacteria for remediation of pollutants. It offers a sustainable and multifunctional option for removing and detoxifying various environmental pollutants, including heavy metals, nutrients, and emerging organic pollutants. This study explains the principles and mechanisms of algal biosorption, bioaccumulation, enzymatic degradation, and phycoremediation. It also highlights the combined roles of extracellular polymeric substances and algal-bacterial groups. Additionally, it examines the operational factors and bioreactor technologies involved, highlighting recent advancements in process improvement and the challenges associated with large-scale use. Real-world case studies demonstrate the ecological effectiveness and cost benefits of algal systems, showing success in removing pollutants, recovering resources, and integrating circular bioeconomy practices. Although the current factors include scale-up limitations, biofouling, and environmental inconsistency, the combination of genetic engineering, artificial intelligence-controlled, and intelligent bioreactor setups offers potential solutions to improv-

R. R. Nanda · J. Sharma · K. Kumari · P. R. Rout (✉)
Department of Biotechnology, Dr B R Ambedkar National Institute of Technology, Jalandhar, India
e-mail: routpr@nitj.ac.in

L. Kumar et al. (eds.), *Algal Bioremediation*,
https://doi.org/10.1007/978-981-95-8793-3_1

ing the algal bioremediation process. The findings of our study recommend the creation of policy frameworks, industrial partnerships, and research alliances to harness the full potential of algae-based remediation for environmental stewardship and sustainability.

Keywords

Algal Bioremediation · Remediation · Environmental Pollutants · Phycoremediation · Bioreactor Technologies · Pollution Control

1.1 Introduction

Environmental pollution refers to an undesirable alteration of the natural environment, which may be physical, chemical, or biological, primarily resulting from anthropogenic activities and leading to adverse changes in the quality of air, water, and soil. In the twenty-first century, rapid industrialization, urban expansion, intensified agriculture, and unsustainable consumption patterns have led to an unprecedented increase in the diversity and complexity of environmental contaminants. When introduced into terrestrial, aquatic, and atmospheric systems, these pollutants disrupt the ecological balance and pose substantial risks to both public health and biodiversity. The major categories of these environmental pollutants include heavy metals (e.g., cadmium, lead, arsenic, mercury), synthetic organic compounds (e.g., dyes, polycyclic aromatic hydrocarbons (PAHs), endocrine-disrupting chemicals, pesticides), pharmaceuticals residues, excess nutrients (notably nitrogen and phosphorus), and emerging pollutants such as microplastics, pharmaceuticals, personal care products, pesticides, hormones, flame retardants, and nanomaterials (Rout et al., 2021a, b). Aquatic ecosystems are highly vulnerable due to direct exposure to waste from both direct and indirect sources. The non-biodegradable materials, e.g., heavy metals and xenobiotic compounds, are concentrated at higher levels of the toxic pyramid, and result in long-term, toxic effects, including endocrine disruption, increased cancer risk, and genetic damage of both the wildlife and human populations (Sharma et al., 2018; Dudeja et al., 2025). Moreover, changes in climate and altered hydrological patterns amplify the impact of pollutants by altering the environmental behavior and fate of pollutants, for instance, enhancing the volatility and solubility of certain compounds, thereby intensifying their mobility and harm potential. This provides insight into the necessity of developing and implementing robust pollution control strategies that are both environmentally compatible and effective in the long term.

Traditional physicochemical remediation techniques, such as chemical precipitation, membrane filtration, incineration, ion exchange, activated carbon adsorption, and advanced oxidation processes (AOPs), have been widely applied for contaminant removal. Although these techniques can be effective under specific conditions, these approaches often suffer from high capital and operational costs, intensive energy requirements, generation of secondary pollutants, and poor adaptability to

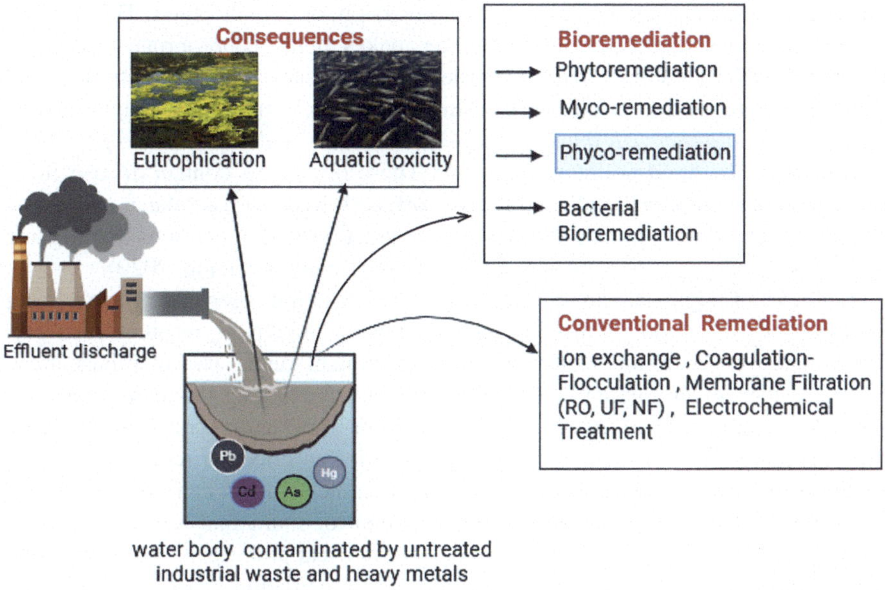

Fig. 1.1 Comparison between bioremediation and conventional methods for wastewater treatment

complex contaminant mixtures. Most importantly, they generally lack the ecological compatibility necessary for long-term environmental recovery and regeneration. In contrast, bioremediation offers a promising and ecologically viable alternative, which are defined as use of biological systems, i.e., microorganisms, vegetation, or their enzymes to neutralize, breakdown, or remove contaminants from polluted media, and it provides a cost-efficient, sustainable, and less invasive method for environment purification, a schematic of traditional and bioremediation strategies are shown in Fig. 1.1 (Ayilara & Babalola, 2023). The concept of bioremediation involves fostering ecological resilience by restoring microbial balance and facilitating natural biochemical cycles. Techniques can be tailored to specific environments and pollutants/contaminants, enabling the treatment of a diverse array of pollutants under both in situ and ex situ conditions. However, bioremediation efficiency depends on several factors, including the nature of the contaminant, bioavailability, ecological conditions (e.g., pH, temperature, and redox potential), and the metabolic capabilities of the biological agents employed.

Among the biological systems used in bioremediation, microalgae and macroalgae have garnered significant attention, owing to their remarkable versatility, adaptability, and environmental relevance. These photosynthetic microorganisms thrive in aquatic and semi-aquatic habitats, even under extreme stressful conditions characterized by high salinity, metal toxicity, and nutrient load (Ahmad & Ashraf, 2024). Phycoremediation, also known as algal bioremediation, is the exploitation of the inherent physicochemical characteristics of algae to remove pollutants in contaminated waters. Algae can remove a wide range of contaminants by either biosorption, bioaccumulation, enzymatic conversion, or complexation. This growth, accompanied by sunlight and carbon dioxide, makes them an appropriate wastewater treatment (WWT) method that simultaneously generates biomass, nutrients, and captures carbon (Rawat et al., 2010). Through research, many microalgal genera, such as *Chlorella, Scenedesmus, Spirulina, Anabaena*, and *Nannochloropsis*, have been found to be good pollutant removers. These organisms contain diverse functional groups in their cell walls, including carboxyl, hydroxyl, sulphate, and amine groups, which contribute to a high level of interaction with metal ions and organic pollutants, resulting in passive and active uptake (Leong & Chang, 2020).

The use of algae as an environmental remediation agent has far-reaching consequences in various industries, with wastewater treatment, resource recovery, and bioenergy generation being the most prominent ones. The pharmaceutical, tanning, paper, metal plating, and textile industries are among the many industries that release industrial effluents, which are often persistently contaminated with chemicals. Algal-based treatment systems can offer an effective remediation route for these effluents. Conventional wastewater treatment plants can also be significantly relieved by algal consortia in the treatment of municipal sewage, which is highly characterized by a significant amount of nutrient and organic loads (Olguín, 2012). Additionally, biomass produced after the remediation process serves as an excellent feedstock for biofuels, biofertilizers, bioplastics, and high-value bioactive molecules, thereby creating a closed-loop biorefining structure that aligns with the principles of the circular economy and is sustainable (Santos et al., 2025). This chapter provides a comprehensive and detailed exploration of algal bioremediation, emphasizing fundamental biological processes and real-world applications. The essentials of the mechanism of pollutant uptake and the pathways involved in contaminant elimination are outlined. The chapter further discusses the methods of bioremediation, including biosorption, bioaccumulation, biodegradation, and phycoremediation, and sheds light on algal species that exhibit outstanding remediation capacity. This is further addressed through process optimization strategies, including bioreactor design, operational conditions, and scalability issues, as discussed in the corresponding case studies and real-life applications within various environmental contexts. This chapter then concludes by summarizing the key findings and their broader implications for sustainable environmental management and resource recovery.

1.2 Principles of Algal Bioremediation

Algal bioremediation is a complex interplay of physicochemical interactions, metabolic mechanisms, and environmental adaptability. This section will provide a detailed analysis of the fundamental principles of algal bioremediation, including the mechanisms of pollutant uptake, metabolic processes, and regulatory mechanisms that underpin contaminant removal. Extracellular polymeric substances (EPS) role and influence of environmental parameters are also taken into consideration to develop a comprehensive view of algal remediation dynamics.

1.2.1 Pollutant Uptake Mechanism

Algae employ both active and passive processes to remove the contaminants from the surroundings. These include diverse mechanisms such as biosorption, bioaccumulation, ion exchange, and surface complexation, which collectively contribute to immobilization or internalization of diverse pollutants. Biosorption is a passive, metabolism-independent technique that involves the rapid attachment of contaminants, especially heavy metals and dyes, to algal cell surfaces. This interaction occurs via functional groups, including hydroxyl, carboxyl, amino, and phosphate moieties, on the algal cell wall, making biosorption particularly effective at the early stages of contaminant sequestration. Biosorption efficiency is highly dependent on pH, temperature, ionic strength, and biomass composition (Ciobanu et al., 2024). Bioaccumulation, on the other hand, is an active, energy-dependent process in which the living algal cell assimilates the pollutant through active transport or endocytosis. The contaminants that have been internalized are stored in vacuoles, attached to intracellular ligands (e.g., phytochelatins (PCs), metallothioneins (MTs)), or metabolized. This process is especially important for long-term pollutants that cannot attach to the surface and must undergo intracellular remediation. Algae are also well known to excrete extracellular polymeric substances (EPS), which increase the affinity of hydrophobic organic pollutants, such as polycyclic aromatic hydrocarbons (PAHs) and synthetic dyes (Dudeja et al., 2025; Diankristanti & Ng, 2024). Ion exchange and surface complexation mechanisms also contribute to metal removal. Cell walls of many algae are rich in uronic acids and polysaccharides, which induce a negatively charged site for electrostatic interactions of metal cations (e.g., Pb^{2+}, Cd^{2+}, Cu^{2+}). Whereas ion exchange processes substitute lighter cations (e.g., Ca^{2+}, Mg^{2+}) with toxic metals, which in turn remove the latter from solution (Sarma et al., 2024). Depending upon the algal species, pollutant properties, and environmental conditions, the dominance and efficiency of each mechanism may vary.

1.2.2 Algal Metabolism in Pollutant Removal

The metabolic activity of algae plays a critical role in the transformation, degradation, and detoxification of pollutants. The process is driven by a network of enzymes that support phototrophic energy production and adaptive stress responses. Nitrogen and phosphorus removal is facilitated primarily by assimilation into algal biomass and microbial interactions in mixed cultures. Nitrogenous compounds, such as ammonia and nitrate, are incorporated into amino acids and nucleic acids. Phosphorus is utilized in ATP synthesis, nucleic acid production, and the phosphate is used for membrane structures (Popa et al., 2025). Organic pollutants include pesticides, pharmaceutical residues, and phenolic compounds, which are metabolized with the help of enzymes, such as peroxidases, laccases, monooxygenases, and reductases. The enzymes mediate hydroxylation, demethylation, and deamination reactions, which in turn reduce the toxicity of the pollutant while increasing its solubility

(Touliabah et al., 2022). Certain algal species, such as *Chlorella minutissima*, are capable of redox transformations (i.e., Cr(VI) to Cr(III), after which 96.5% of Cr(III) is removed from the niche), intracellular compartmentalization of metals, and heavy metal binding to chelating proteins. Algal species, when exposed to high levels of heavy metals, often upregulate enzymes responsible for antioxidant activity, such as superoxide dismutase and glutathione reductase, and can mitigate reactive oxygen species (ROS)-induced cellular damage (Chakravorty et al., 2024). Although the literature supports that *Chlorella, Spirulina, and Anabaena can tolerate high concentrations of heavy metals*. The toxicity levels vary according to type of heavy metal, for instance, *Chlorella vulgaris* can tolerate as high as 2172 mmol/kg of cobalt (Co), 1917 mmol/kg of copper (Cu), and 1175 mmol/kg of cadmium (Cd), and *Spirulina platensis* can adsorb up to 1754 mmol/kg for Cu, 1359 mmol/kg for Co, and 639 mmol/kg for Cd; however, the growth conditions for *S. platensis* are stringent (Phiri & Oh, 2024). Meanwhile, *Anabaena* sp. PCC7120, when exposed to 100 μM Cd for 48 hrs, caused acute toxicity, but the recovery was possible with physiological damage (Srivastava et al., 2020). Another study mentions the tolerance for *Anabaena variabilis* sp. MEGCH1 to be in the range of 10–30 μM for Zn^{2+}, making them tolerant enough to perform algal bioremediation (Diengdoh et al., 2023). Facilitated by photosynthesis-generated ROS (i.e., singlet oxygen, hydrogen peroxide) also contribute to the breakdown of pollutants, especially aromatic hydrocarbons and dyes. This type of mechanism is unique to photoautotrophs and underscores the multifaceted bioremediation potential of algal species (Li et al., 2024). An overview of algal mechanisms involving pollutant removal, illustrating carbon fixation, phosphorus assimilation and storage, and detoxification or sequestration of heavy metals, is shown in Fig. 1.2.

1.2.3 Role of Extracellular Polymeric Substances (EPS)

Extracellular polymeric substances (EPS), high-molecular-weight compounds that algae secrete, are composed mainly of polysaccharides, proteins, lipids, and nucleic acids. They secrete a hydrated matrix surrounding the cells and play multiple roles in bioremediation. The EPS matrix functions as a platform to bind pollutants, especially hydrophobic compounds and metals. Functional groups that comprise EPS, such as uronic acids and thiol groups, exhibit a high affinity for a diverse range of contaminants, while increasing retention time and facilitating microbial degradation (Chen et al., 2015). One of the most significant roles of EPS is in metal binding and detoxification. The matrix contains a variety of functional groups, including hydroxyl, carboxyl, phosphate, thiol, and uronic acid residues, that exhibit a strong affinity for metal cations, namely Pb^{2+}, Cd^{2+}, Cu^{2+}, and Hg^{2+}. Complexation, electrostatic attraction, and ion exchange occur in these groups, which allows extracellular polymer substances (EPS) to entrap metals and slow down their migration in the niche or the environment. EPS converts the freely circulating metal ions into stable and nontoxic complexes through chelation, which can be later removed or metabolized by the algal cells. Accordingly, the fact that EPS is a

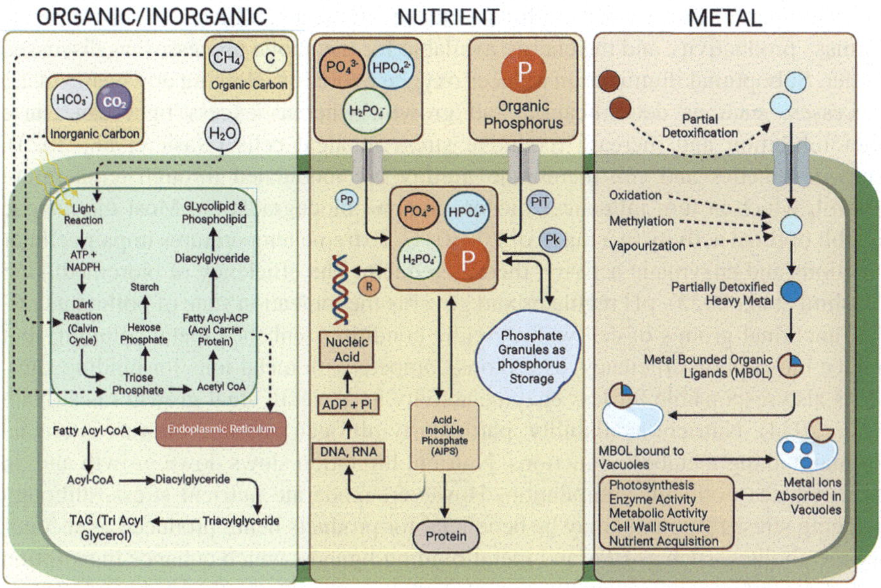

Fig. 1.2 Integrated pathways of algal-mediated pollutant removal depicting conversion of carbon sources, nutrient recovery via phosphorus accumulation, and detoxification of heavy metals through binding and compartmentalization (PiT—Pi Transferase, Pk—Phosphate kinase, R—Ribonucleases, Pp—Phosphatase)

central element of biosorption-based metal removal and a significant part of the total detoxification capacity of algal systems warrants further discussion (Yadav et al., 2020). The other purpose of EPS is that it acts as a protective layer, shielding algal cells against adverse environmental conditions and thereby contributing to their survival in highly polluted waters. EPS is able to fix the toxicants and inhibit membrane destruction. EPS enables biofilm formation and synergistic interactions among other microorganisms in complex microbial communities, thereby coordinating pollutant degradation (Xiao & Zheng, 2016). Additionally, EPS could influence the process of metal speciation, thereby affecting the rates of metal mobility and bioavailability in an aqueous environment. EPS-mediated chelation has the potential to convert metal ions in their free state into metal complexes, thereby decreasing acute toxicity and facilitating further detoxification.

1.2.4 Influence of Environmental Factors on Algal Bioremediation

Environmental factors, including light intensity, photoperiod, temperature, pH, nutrient availability, and contaminant concentration, significantly influence the efficacy of algal bioremediation. These parameters affect algal multiplication, photosynthetic functioning, enzyme activity, and the rate of pollutant uptake, all of which determine the total rate and efficiency of contaminant removal. Light intensity and photoperiod directly affect photosynthesis efficiency, which is responsible for biomass productivity and the energy available for metabolic processes, as discussed earlier. Suboptimal illumination reduces oxygen evolution, slowing down enzymatic processes, such as detoxification and growth, whereas excess light can cause photoinhibition and increase oxidative stress in algal cells (Nasir et al., 2023). Enzyme kinetics and cell membrane fluidity are modulated through temperature control, which in turn influences biosorption and biodegradation. Most microalgae exhibit optimal activity in a range of 20–30 °C. Extreme temperatures impair cellular functions and enzymatic activity, thereby reducing the efficiency of bioremediation (Hashmi et al., 2023). pH regulates and governs the ionization state of pollutants and the functional groups of cell walls. Acidic conditions enhance metal solubility but reduce biosorption efficiency, as protons compete with metal ions for binding sites. pH is also responsible for less enzyme activity and overall algal growth rates (Nath et al., 2024). Nutrient availability, particularly nitrogen and phosphorus, is crucial for maintaining metabolic functions. Nutrient limitation slows down growth and, in turn, reduces pollutant assimilation. However, moderate nutrient stress, although inducing stress responses, may be beneficial for products being produced as secondary metabolites, such as EPS and metal-binding ligands, which enhance biosorption and stress tolerance. Concentrations of contaminants play a dual role; low levels induce adaptive metabolism and may induce tolerance, while high levels can be highly toxic and may inhibit photosynthesis, respiration, and cell division. Hence, bioremediation systems must include optimization standards for thresholds of tolerance and characteristics of pollutants (Hashmi et al., 2023).

1.3 Methods of Algal Bioremediation

Microalgae are small, unicellular or simple multicellular photosynthetic organisms that live in marine or freshwater environments. Their unique metabolic functions in remediating various pollutants, including heavy metals, organic contaminants, and excess nutrients, play a crucial role in bioremediation (Ali et al., 2024). The methods of microalgal bioremediation include biosorption, bioaccumulation, and biodegradation. Biosorption and bioaccumulation involve microalgae taking up pollutants through a specific cellular process such as passive adsorption onto the cell wall, active transport across the cell membrane, ion exchange, complexation with functional groups (e.g., hydroxyl, carboxyl, and amino groups), and intracellular sequestration into vacuoles or binding with metal-binding proteins like metallothioneins and phytochelatins, whereas biodegradation is an enzymatic degradation of pollutants. Wastewater treatment (WWT) usually happens in three stages: preliminary, secondary, and tertiary. In the preliminary stage, screening and sedimentation remove large solids and debris. The second stage, biological oxidation, is mainly completed with aerobic bacteria that degrade organic matter and ammonia. In the microalgae-based treatment, there is a relaxation of focus on bacteria as microalgae utilize nitrogen and phosphorus nutrients to grow and reduce biological oxygen demand (BOD) and chemical oxygen demand (COD). The final step, tertiary stage

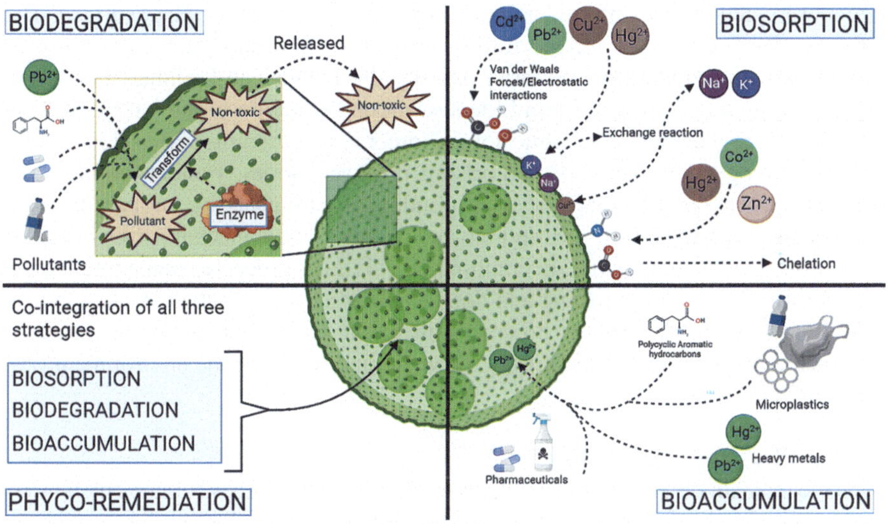

Fig. 1.3 Mechanistic overview of microalgae-mediated remediation strategies

treatment, involves a combination of advanced processes that may include filtration, nutrient removal, and disinfection to achieve the desired quality in the effluent. An overview of remediation strategies is illustrated in Fig. 1.3.

1.3.1 Biosorption

Biosorption is the capacity of biological materials to seize heavy metals from wastewater via metabolically driven mechanisms or physicochemical interactions. Microalgae biosorption is a passive physicochemical process involving the binding of pollutants to microalgal cell surfaces, which are composed of proteins, carbohydrates, and extracellular polymeric substances (EPS). Pollutants have included heavy metals, dyes, and organic compounds. The molecules in which the cells and EPS participate in the binding are mainly mediated through functional groups (carboxyl, amine, and phosphate) present on the EPS and cell wall (group interaction). Biosorption involves several simultaneous processes, including electrostatic attraction, chelation, and surface complexation. The post-mortem EPS-induced biochemical integrity and structural stability of the microalgal biomass is demonstrated by its ability to survive even when the biomass is non-living (Diankristanti & Ng, 2024). Pollutant removal by microalgae primarily occurs at the cell surface and within the EPS matrix, both of which contain numerous reactive functional groups, such as carboxyl, hydroxyl, amino, sulfhydryl, and phosphoryl moieties, that act as binding sites for diverse contaminants, particularly heavy metals. These groups engage in chelation, the development of stable coordination complexes with metal ions, through ion-exchange reactions in which toxic metals are incorporated in place of lighter cations naturally found on the algal surface. The pH-dependent net surface charge further promotes the electrostatic interaction of algal cells with pollutants of opposite polarity. Pollutants can be inner-sphere and complexed by direct chemical bond (dependent on the nature of the interaction), or entrapped with weaker electrostatic forces (outer-sphere complexes). Additionally, EPS, a heterogeneous network comprising polysaccharides, proteins, lipids, and nucleic acids, plays a crucial role in responding to pollutants by entrapping them through physical retention, adsorption, and complexation mechanisms within its three-dimensional architecture. In combination, all these processes make microalgae remarkably effective in purifying and decontaminating water bodies. A clear understanding of these biosorption processes is the basis for enhancing algal-based bioremediation strategies in treating wastewater and restoring the environment (Ali et al., 2024).

1.3.1.1 Physical Adsorption

It is a mechanism based on van der Waals and electrostatic forces between metal ions and the microbial cell surface. It is generally implicated with the first, passive phase of biosorption. Algae, fungal, and yeast biomass have been found to adsorb metals or ions of uranium, cadmium, copper, and cobalt through this process in a dead state (Parmar & Patel, 2025).

1.3.1.2 Ion Exchange

Cell walls of microorganisms, rich in polysaccharides and natural counter-ions (e.g., K^+, Na^+, Ca^{2+}), can exchange these ions with heavy metal ions (e.g., Cu^{2+}, Cd^{2+}, Zn^{2+}) in the surrounding solution. This ion exchange process is especially significant in marine algae that contain alginates (Parmar & Patel, 2025).

1.3.1.3 Complexation and Chelation

Heavy metals can form coordination complexes with active groups such as carboxyl and amino groups on the microbial cell wall. This binding mechanism is often stronger and more specific than simple adsorption. Complexation has been reported as the primary mechanism for the uptake of several metals, including copper, mercury, and zinc (Parmar & Patel, 2025).

1.3.1.4 Precipitation

Metal precipitation can occur via two mechanisms, one being a metabolism-dependent mechanism, where microbial cells respond to metal stress by producing compounds (e.g., organic acids) that facilitate precipitation, the other being independent of metabolism, where chemical interactions between metals and the cell surface result in metal salt formation and settling out of solution (Parmar & Patel, 2025).

1.3.2 Bioaccumulation

Bioaccumulation in microalgae is the mediated uptake and internal transport of contaminants across the cell membrane to the cytoplasm through mediated transport and energy-dependent mechanisms (active transport). This accumulation of contaminants within the cell causes physiological stress, alters metabolic pathways, and activates antioxidative systems (Diankristanti & Ng, 2024). In a comparative study of bioaccumulation capacity in microalgae, researchers examined the bioconcentration of two freshwater microalgae, *C. vulgaris* and *S. platensis,* using two sources of silver: silver nanoparticles (AgNPs) and silver nitrate ($AgNO_3$) (Nikokherad et al., 2022). Ultimately, *C. vulgaris* exhibited explicit bioconcentration capabilities, particularly with ionic silver, where its bioconcentration factor could exceed 14,000, indicating a strong capacity to uptake pollutants. *S. platensis*, on the other hand, had a greater capacity for the accumulation of AgNPs. Concentration-dependent toxicity was observed in *S. platensis* and *C. vulgaris*, as evidenced by reductions in growth, decreased cell viability, and a significant decline in pigment concentration, indicating a decline in photosynthetic flux. The results also suggested that silver nitrate is far more toxic than AgNPs.

1.3.2.1 Biosorption vs Bioaccumulation

Microalgae remove heavy metals from wastewater through two major processes—biosorption and bioaccumulation. Biosorption is a physicochemical process that enables microalgae to accumulate toxic metals on their cell surface without expending metabolic energy (ATP). As shown in the study, this mechanism may occur through either a physicochemical pathway, which does not require ATP, or through metal binding mediated by metabolic reactions that involve ATP. Biosorption typically takes place on the outer surface of algal cells, where functional groups such as carboxyl, hydroxyl, phosphate, and amino groups form complexes with metal ions (Marella et al., 2020). Because it does not depend on active metabolism, biosorption can also occur in dead or inactive cells, making it a cost-effective method for large-scale water purification.

1.3.2.2 Passive Uptake Mechanism

The passive uptake process is fundamentally equivalent to biosorption, wherein heavy metal ions adhere to the algal cell surface through various physicochemical interactions. This mechanism is governed by multiple environmental parameters, including pH, temperature, contact duration, ionic strength, and the concentration of biomass. Adsorption efficiency is determined by equilibrium dynamics and strongly influenced by the biochemical composition of the microalgal cell wall, which is enriched with polysaccharides, proteins, and polyalcohol constituents such as cellulose and pectin. These structural components possess reactive functional groups that facilitate metal ion binding via ion-exchange and complexation reactions. As this process operates independently of metabolic energy, passive uptake serves as a cost-effective, rapid, and efficient means for sequestering dissolved heavy metals from contaminated aqueous environments (Ding et al., 2017).

1.3.2.3 Active Uptake Mechanism

The process of bioaccumulation, on the other hand, is an active, energy-dependent process whereby living algal cells take up heavy metals into the cytoplasm via ATP-mediated transport systems. Metabolically active, this process enables the rapid absorption of metal ions, which are later converted into intracellular structures or bound to specific biomolecules, thereby facilitating their detoxification and ultimately sequestering them in the long term. At high levels of metal exposure, reactive oxygen species (ROS) are generated in microalgae, resulting in oxidative stress and potential cellular damage. To overcome this stress, the microalgae turn on enzymatic and non-enzymatic antioxidant defense mechanisms and produce metal-chelating peptides (metallothioneins (MTs) and phytochelatins (PCs)). Excess metal ions bind to them, neutralizing them, restoring redox balance, and preserving cellular homeostasis (Machado et al., 2024). Thus, while active uptake ensures the permanent sequestration of metals, it also requires metabolic activity and may cause physiological stress under high metal exposure.

1.3.3 Biodegradation

Algal biodegradation is the mechanism by which the algal group, primarily comprising microalgae and cyanobacteria (also known as blue-green algae), degrades environmental pollutants, including plastics, organic chemicals, dyes, hydrocarbons, pesticides, and phenol, into simpler and less toxic products through their enzymatic machinery and metabolic processes. This involves biofilm formation, the release of hydrolytic or oxidative enzymes, and sometimes photosynthetically mediated reactions, which aid in the natural detoxification of contaminated ecosystems. Mechanism of Algal Biodegradation: Algal biodegradation involves a chain of biochemical reactions in which pollutants are degraded or converted into less toxic substances.

1.3.3.1 Pollutant Uptake

The first stage in the biodegradation process is the adsorption of contaminants by algae. Algae take up organic contaminants across their cell membranes either by passive diffusion (an energy-independent, spontaneous process by which pollutants pass by the concentration gradient) or active transport (an energy-requiring process where algal cells employ ATP to transport pollutants against their concentration gradient) (Yang et al., 2025). Such an uptake is influenced by numerous key factors, such as the chemical nature of the contaminants, which may include their hydrophobicity, molecular size, and characteristics of the algal species. More lipophilic pollutants, for instance, are taken up more efficiently by algal cells. The efficiency of uptake is also influenced considerably by the algal species' capacity to metabolize and reduce pollutants. Within the algal cell, pollutants are either stored in vacuoles or enzymatically converted into non-toxic compounds, thereby reducing their potential toxicity. Under certain circumstances, pollutants can further break down or transform into intermediate compounds, allowing for their full mineralization or degradation into harmless substances (Yang et al., 2025).

1.3.3.2 Enzymatic Degradation

The most important process of biodegradation is the enzymatic degradation of contaminants. Algae secrete a range of enzymes that catalyze the degradation of complex organic chemicals. Some of the enzymes involved are peroxidases and laccases, which are responsible for the oxidative degradation of aromatic substances, such as phenols and dyes. They catalyze the oxidation of contaminants, cleaving chemical bonds and reducing their toxicity. Another class of enzymes is monooxygenases and dioxygenases, which facilitate hydrocarbon degradation, particularly the oxidation of hydrocarbons to more water-soluble substances that can be further degraded. They insert oxygen into the contaminant molecule, frequently increasing its biodegradability. Lastly, hydrolases are those that assist in degrading large, complex molecules (e.g., pesticides and plastics) into smaller, more manageable units. For instance, esterases and amylases hydrolyze ester and carbohydrate linkages (Touliabah et al., 2022).

1.3.3.3 Metabolism and Transformation

After the pollutant has been hydrolyzed or oxidized, the resulting intermediates are further metabolized by the algae. The metabolic processes are (a) oxidation (addition of oxygen results in phenols being converted to hydroxylated derivatives). (b) Reduction (gain of electrons or oxidation state decrement), e.g., as a case in point, nitrate or nitro-type pollutants are reduced by algae and are converted into nitrogenous substances that are more easily assimilated. (c) Conjugation and detoxification: Algae can detoxify toxic pollutants by conjugating them with amino acids, sugars, or other molecules. This makes the pollutants less toxic and more readily excreted or stored. Then, these pollutants are completely dissolved into inorganic compounds, such as water, carbon dioxide, and inorganic salts, through a process called mineralization. Sometimes, algae form symbiotic partnerships with bacteria to enhance the degradation process. Algae supply organic carbon and oxygen to bacteria, which in turn help algae degrade more complex pollutants. The synergy may enhance the efficiency of biodegradation, particularly in adverse environments where pollutant concentrations are high.

Efficiency of microalgae to biodegradation aromatic pollutants like BTEX (benzene, toluene, ethylbenzene, xylene), PAHs (pyrene, benzo[a]pyrene), and phenolic substances (phenol, bisphenol A, nonylphenol) is affected by environmental conditions (pH, light intensity, temperature, nutrient level, CO_2 concentration) and pollutant properties (chemical structure of pollutant, concentration, solubility). For increasing the efficiency, some technologies are used such as (a) bacteria-algae consortia—enhances biodegradation via mutual metabolic support; (b) immobilization techniques—increases cell stability and reuse potential; (c) photobioreactors—providing controlled light, temperature, and CO_2 levels for optimized degradation (Li & Meng, 2023), for example, *Chlorella vulgaris* [azo dye degradation with 90% efficiency] (Ishchi & Sibi, 2019). A bacterial consortium comprising *Pseudomonas* sp., *Agromyces* sp., *Chryseobacterium* sp., *Sphingobacterium* sp., and *Stenotrophomonas* sp. was utilized for the co-biodegradation of naphthalene and phenanthrene. This mixed culture (with a

Table 1.1 Comparative overview of different bioremediation strategies

Criteria	Biosorption	Bioaccumulation	Biodegradation
Definition	Passive binding of pollutants to biomass surface	Uptake and storage of pollutants inside living cells	Breakdown of complex pollutants into simpler, non-toxic forms
Mechanism	Adsorption to functional groups (e.g., carboxyl, hydroxyl)	Active transport and intracellular sequestration	Enzymatic degradation or transformation
Energy requirement	No energy required (non-metabolic process)	Requires cellular energy (metabolic)	Energy-dependent (requires metabolic activity)
Living biomass requirement	Can use dead or inactive biomass	Requires living, metabolically active cells	Requires living algae
Industrial scalability	High (simple setup, cheap biomass)	Moderate (needs live culture management)	Low to moderate (complex, requires optimization)
Integration potential	Can be used in columns, filters, biosorbent beds	Integrated into bioreactors	Suitable for in situ treatment, reactors
Examples of algal species	*Spirulina platensis*, *Chlorella vulgaris*	*Scenedesmus obliquus*, *Chlamydomonas reinhardtii*	*Anabaena*, *Oscillatoria*, *Chlorella*

concentration of 2000 mg/L) achieved very high degradation efficiencies (99.9% for naphthalene and 92.9% for phenanthrene) in just six days (Ahmad, 2021). A comparative view of different bioremediation methods is shown in Table 1.1.

1.3.4 Algal Species with High Bioremediation Potential

Various species of algae, microalgae (microscopic, unicellular photosynthetic organisms found in freshwater and marine environments), macroalgae (multicellular, eukaryotic algae commonly known as seaweeds), and cyanobacteria (also known as blue-green algae, are photosynthetic prokaryotes that belong to the domain Bacteria, unlike true algae, they lack a nucleus and membrane-bound organelles) have shown immense potential in the bioremediation of environmental pollutants. These microorganisms possess unique physiological and biochemical characteristics, including efficient nutrient uptake, metal binding, and the ability to grow in polluted environments, making them ideal organisms for remediation purposes. Among the microalgae, *Chlorella vulgaris* is the most widely studied species. It has been highly effective in removing nutrients such as nitrogen and phosphorus, as well as heavy metals like copper (Cu^{2+}), zinc (Zn^{2+}), and lead (Pb^{2+}) from industrial and municipal wastewater. *Scenedesmus obliquus* is another microalga that has demonstrated robust performance in conditions with abundant nutrients and pollution. The efficiency of *Scenedesmus* species in terms of wastewater treatment is excellent; that is, the organisms have proven efficient in removing ammonia, phosphate, and phenolic substances. *Scenedesmus* has been reported to attain an ammonium and phosphate removal efficiency of 98.17 and 96.87, respectively, with a reduction in the chemical oxygen demand (COD) of 87.93 in raceway pond systems (Iqbal et al., 2024). *Spirulina platensis*, a cyanobacterium often categorized among microalgae, also exhibits broad biosorptive potential for heavy metals such as copper and calcium. Additionally, its biomass serves as a valuable feedstock for biofuel and nutraceutical production. Among cyanobacteria, the cyanobacterium *Spirulina platensis*, commonly referred to as a microalgae, also exhibits a broad biosorptive capability towards heavy metals, including copper and calcium. Additionally, its biomass would make an excellent feedstock for the production of biofuels and nutraceuticals. *Oscillatoria* and *Anabaena* have demonstrated a high ability to remove pollutants. Nitrogen-fixing capabilities, phototrophic properties, and the ability to remove a wide range of other contaminants, such as nitrates, phosphates, and trace elements like cadmium and arsenic, among others, indicate that Anabaena has multifunctional bioremediating potential. *Oscillatoria*, which also shows resistance to industrial effluents, has been successfully employed to eliminate synthetic dyes and heavy metals in polluted water (Markou & Georgakakis, 2011). Algal species selection for bioremediation is done on various parameters, including pollutant type, environmental condition, and end-biomass utilization. Microalgae are widely used due to their high growth rate and large surface area-to-volume ratio, but macroalgae and cyanobacteria offer additional benefits in terms of structural stability and metabolic diversity. Various species have different growth conditions and pollutant affinities, and the proper algal strain selection plays a major role in optimizing bioremediation efficiency. Despite their promise, practical issues, such as sensitivity to high pollutant levels, competition within co-cultures, and harvesting challenges, must be addressed for large-scale use.

1.3.5 Microalgal Consortia

Algal-bacterial consortia (ABCs) are intricate, dynamic systems in which bacteria and microalgae interact through various ecological relationships, including mutualism, commensalism, parasitism, endosymbiosis, competition, and inhibition, which collectively control the efficacy of wastewater bioremediation. ABCs control nutrient exchange, turnover of metabolites, and signaling pathways that control pollutant degradation. Microalgae carry out photosynthesis to emit oxygen and organic carbon in mutualistic associations, promoting bacterial growth and respiration. In return, bacteria mineralize organic matter and provide CO_2, vitamins, or growth stimulators to the algae. Commensalistic relationships occur when bacteria exploit algal exudates without impeding algal growth, while parasitic or competitive relations may occur under nutrient stress or toxic conditions, usually repressing algal productivity. Endosymbiotic relationships, as observed in certain cyanobacteria and green algae, also enhance metabolic efficiency by facilitating the direct exchange of nutrients and electrons. Quorum-sensing and chemical communication also play significant roles in promoting biofilm development, consortium stability, and stress response management under dynamic wastewater conditions. Algal–bacterial consortia, from a biotechnological perspective, are more effective than single cultures in removing pollutants, recovering resources, and maintaining process stability. The dual systems utilize the contrasting metabolic processes of both members, incorporating phycoremediation, biodegradation, biosorption, and bio-oxidation processes. A *Chlorella vulgaris-Pseudomonas putida* consortium, for instance, removed more than 90% of ammonium and phosphate from simulated wastewater, where algae uptake nutrients and bacteria broke down organic matter (Wei et al., 2024).

A *Chlorella pyrenoidosa-Bacillus subtilis* consortium showed 82% elimination of hexavalent chromium (Cr (VI)) via combined biosorption bio-reduction, whereas a *Chlorella sorokiniana-Acinetobacter* sp. system showed 90% decolorization of methylene blue dye in 72 hours through bioadsorption and enzymatic degradation. Similarly, *the Microcystis aeruginosa-Aeromonas aeruginosa* consortium has shown remarkable degradation rates of phenolic substances in industrial effluents, which can be attributed to bacterial oxygenases and algal metabolic assimilation (S. Li et al., 2022). The high work of algal-bacterial consortia (ABCs) is, to a large extent, explained by the well-developed biofilm formation and the formation of a microscale nutrient gradient that facilitates the diffusion of substrates and transfer of mass of pollutants. Co-cultivation also reduces the energy requirements in terms of external aeration and added chemicals, thereby enhancing the system's overall efficiency and environmental sustainability. The recent breakthrough has shown the promise of genetically engineered (GE) strains and synthetically designed microbial consortia as a targeted approach to degrading challenging contaminants, including antibiotics, endocrine-disrupting compounds, and microplastics. In addition to the removal of pollutants, ABCs also play a major role in recycling nutrients and valorization of biomass. The resulting algal-bacterial biomass can be repurposed for the production of biofertilizers, biofuels, and bioplastics, aligning the process with the principles of a circular bioeconomy. Together, these consortia represent a synergistic and holistic approach to wastewater treatment that balances biological effectiveness with environmental sustainability.

1.3.6 Genetically Modified Algal Species

Genetically modified microalgae and cyanobacteria have gained increasing attention for enhancing wastewater treatment performance beyond the capabilities of wild-type microorganisms. Although genetically engineered (GE) microalgae have already been investigated for industrial applications such as carbon sequestration, lipids, and biohydrogen production, their use in wastewater bioremediation is still an advancing area with great promise. All recent research utilizes random mutagenesis strategies, such as chemical mutagens (e.g., ethyl methane sulfonate), UV or nuclear irradiation, and plasma exposure, followed by selective screening for favorable characteristics, including high pollutant tolerance or rapid growth in severe effluents.

These techniques have yielded strains that can survive in highly contaminated wastewaters, enhancing both biomass productivity and pollutant removal efficiency. For example, a mutant *Scenedesmus* sp. strain showed remarkable tolerance to undiluted cellulosic ethanol wastewater with biomass productivity of 40 mg L^{-1} day^{-1} and removal efficiency of 33.5% chemical oxygen demand (COD), 71.2% total ammoniacal nitrogen (TAN), and 46.4% total phosphorus (TP) (Zhang et al., 2017). A mutagenized strain of *Chlorella vulgaris* removed 54.8% COD, 97.6% TAN, and 84.2% TP from the same effluent type, whereas another *C. vulgaris* variant had more than 90% elimination of both total nitrogen (TN) and TP in anaerobically treated piggery wastewater (Wang et al., 2016). These developments collectively enhance the economic and operational viability of algal-based wastewater treatment (Calatrava et al., 2024). Aside from random mutagenesis, gene-targeted modifications are increasingly sought after to achieve precise functional improvements. The CRISPR/Cas9 technology and homologous recombination have already been utilized in organisms such as *Synechocystis* sp. PCC 6803, in which the deletion of phosphate regulator sphU resulted in overregulated phosphate transport and utilization for better phosphorus removal from shrimp wastewater (Krasaesueb et al., 2019). Likewise, heterologous gene expression in microalgae has added novel metabolic functionality; for example, *Chlamydomonas reinhardtii* genetically engineered to carry a sesquiterpene synthase gene from a plant grew well in anaerobic membrane bioreactor effluent, removing nitrogen and phosphorus in addition to producing the high-value compound patchoulol (De Freitas et al., 2022). In general, GE microalgae represent a revolutionary strategy for wastewater bioremediation, offering increased tolerance to pollutants, improved nutrient removal rates, and the potential for co-generation of high-value bioproducts. In addition, genetic tools can be leveraged for biocontainment techniques like synthetic auxotrophy and kill switches, limiting ecological hazards in open systems. With further advances in algal genomics and metabolic engineering, coupling GE microalgae with scalable bioremediation frameworks, particularly in combination with algal–bacterial consortia, could propel the circular bioeconomy model of wastewater management.

1.3.7 Management of Transformation Products in Microalgae

While bioremediation is efficient in lowering the concentration of parent contaminants, the production of intermediate or transformation products (metabolites) can cause further environmental harm. The metabolites can be more toxic, persistent, or mobile compared to the original substances, and the two-stage valorization technique can be used to mitigate the anomaly. Microalgae cultivated in wastewater to simultaneously achieve pollutant removal, metabolite recovery, and bioenergy generation, producing valuable cellular metabolites. Among these, natural pigments such as phycocyanin (up to 2.4 mg/g dry weight) and phycoerythrin (up to 1.3 mg/g dry weight) were extracted as high-value products from the algal biomass using mild aqueous extraction techniques. The residual biomass, still rich in organic compounds such as carbohydrates and proteins, was subjected to anaerobic digestion, yielding 159–199 mL CH_4/g volatile solids, indicating an efficient conversion of remaining metabolites into biogas (Arashiro et al., 2020). For the monitoring and management of metabolites, combining biological treatment (microalgae, microalgae-bacteria consortia) with advanced oxidation processes (AOPs), adsorption, or post-treatment units has been found to significantly improve the removal of recalcitrant micropollutants, decrease the toxicity of intermediates, and enhance the biodegradability of effluents. For instance, in a hybrid treatment for biodiesel industry wastewater, a moving-bed bioreactor (MBBR) followed by Fenton, photo-Fenton, or UV/H_2O_2 treatment resulted in more than 95% COD removal and efficiently decreased acute toxicity (de Oliveira Gonçalves et al., 2018).

Likewise, microalgae-native bacteria systems operating in continuous flow systems have been reported to provide consistent nutrient (N, P) removal, lipid and carbohydrate yield, CO_2 sequestration, as well as beneficial effluent water quality, if optimized for hydraulic retention time (HRT) (Li et al., 2023). Metabolite profiling methods (e.g., following drugs, transformation products) and toxicity bioassays are required to detect harmful byproducts or secondary metabolites. High-rate algae ponds were utilized in one study to eliminate pharmaceuticals and their metabolites; some compounds were effectively eliminated (>60%), but others (e.g., carbamazepine, metoprolol) were more resistant, indicating that bioadsorption/bioaccumulation is frequently a determinant in removal but not invariably sufficient (García-Galán et al., 2019). In addition, biological-oxidation treatment systems not only enhance the removal of pollutants but are also specifically tested for toxicity (i.e., a decrease in genotoxicity, bacterial toxicity, etc.) (Lu et al., 2022).

1.4 Process Optimization and Bioreactor Technologies

The large-scale applications of algal bioremediation rely crucially on the integration of optimized operational strategies that can be employed along with efficient bioreactor technologies. Microalgae are physiologically and metabolically adaptable with high physiological and metabolic capacity, which is the basis of their ability to absorb and convert various pollutants. This is despite the fact that these capabilities are inherently efficient but can only be maximized under well-regulated and optimized environmental conditions. Optimization is a process that involves adjusting operational parameters to approach ideal conditions, resulting in increased efficacy in removing pollutants, enhanced biomass productivity, and the recovery of value-added bioproducts (Asswad et al., 2024). It is also crucial to design and configure bioreactor systems that maintain optimal environments and facilitate efficient mass transfer of gases, nutrients, and light. Modern reactor technologies have enabled the transfer of pilot-scale experiments to full-scale industrial use, allowing for uniform algal cultivation across different wastewater streams with varying characteristics. Considering the increasing environmental sustainability requirements, the combination of new process optimization techniques and novel bioreactor design has proven indispensable for large-scale, cost-effective, and environmentally friendly algal bioremediation (Goh et al., 2022).

Recent developments in systems biology, process modeling, and automated reactor control have further transformed this area, introducing tools to monitor, predictively optimize, and simulate critical parameters such as growth kinetics, nutrient dynamics, and pollutant uptake. These are evidence-based solutions that significantly reduce uncertainty in experiments and accelerate the process of refining processes. Furthermore, the fact that circular principles of bioeconomy, i.e., the connection between wastewater treatment and the valorization of algal biomass, have become an integral part of the system has highlighted the importance of the simultaneous optimization of upstream and downstream processes (Shahid et al., 2020; Rout et al., 2022). This part thus reviews the various aspects of algal process optimization (Sect. 1.4.1), bioreactor design development (Sect. 1.4.2), operational issues and viability (Sect. 1.4.3), and integration aspects in wastewater treatment systems (Sect. 1.4.4).

1.4.1 Optimization Strategies

Algal bioremediation efficiency is dependent on the optimization of operational and physicochemical properties that regulate physiology and pollutant uptake, thereby enhancing the pollutant removal rate and maximizing biomass productivity, which is crucial for subsequent valorization processes. Macronutrients (nitrogen (N) and phosphorus (P)) are essential elements for most cellular metabolism and structure development in algae. According to their availability, growth rate, chlorophyll synthesis, and enzymatic activities involved in pollutant transformation. For instance, nitrate and ammonium, being the primary sources of nitrogen, can inhibit photosynthesis at higher concentrations. Meanwhile, phosphorus limitation can trigger lipid accumulation and also restrict nucleic acid synthesis, in turn reducing cell division. Microalgae exhibit species-specific responses to the concentrations of nutrients available; thus, optimization is tailored using N:P ratios, often closer to the ratio (12:1), depending on the targeted pollutant and the algal strain. Periodic/pulsed nutrient feeding has shown improvement in uptake mechanism and growth (Rout et al., 2018). Light being the primary source of energy for photosynthesis, its optimization, including intensity, duration, and quality, is critical. Typical photosynthetic photon flux densities (PPFD) for microalgae are 60 μmol m^{-2} s^{-1}. However, high intensity causes photoinhibition, while low intensity reduces productivity. LED arrays with tunable wavelengths have demonstrated improved chlorophyll absorption and biomass yield. Advanced strategies may include intermittent lighting, light dilutions, and internal light guides in closed bioreactors to maximize surface-to-volume ratios and minimize self-shading effects (Thongtha et al., 2025). The optimal range for microalgal strains has been found to be 20–30 °C. Temperature affects the fluidity of the membrane and plays a crucial role in regulating enzyme activity. Sub-optimal temperatures slow down metabolism, while high temperatures induce stress response and inhibit pollutant transformation. pH optimization is equally critical (Tian et al., 2024). The ideal pH for algae lies between 6.5 and 9.5. The fluctuation in them influences the metal ion speciation, phosphate availability, and

CO_2/bicarbonate equilibrium. For this purpose, buffer systems and automated pH controllers are integrated into bioreactor setups to ensure stability and reliability (Yu et al., 2022). For photoautotrophic growth, carbon supplementation is essential, and CO_2 availability enhances the photosynthetic rate, bioaccumulation, and synthesis of bioactive compounds involved in pollutant degradation. Industrial-grade CO_2 or flue gas is directly injected into the liquid culture media to support growth and act as a carbon sequestration mechanism. For high-density cultures, the mass transfer rates of gad and liquid are a limiting stage. Aeration rates, bubble size, and sparger design can be optimized for preventing the limiting stage and oxygen accumulation, which in many cases can become inhibitory (Yen et al., 2015). Efficient mixing ensures uniform nutrient and light distribution, preventing sedimentation while enhancing mass transfer in the chamber, reactor vessel, or photobioreactor. However, excessive mixing can be a factor in sheer stress and damage to algal cells. Therefore, an energy-efficient design, such as an air-lift system, paddle wheel, or impellers with low Reynolds numbers, is favored in large-scale operations (Massart et al., 2014). Response surface methodology (RSM), artificial neural networks (ANNs), and computational fluid dynamics (CFD) are increasingly being used to stimulate and optimize algal growth and pollutant kinetics under variable conditions, which provide precise control over process parameters and reduce the cost of experimental validation (García-Camacho et al., 2016).

1.4.2 Bioreactor Designs

Bioreactor technologies are crucial for cultivating algae under controlled conditions, thereby optimizing biomass productivity and pollutant removal. Bioreactor systems are designed to enhance the parameters crucial for the biodegradation and growth of algae, as mentioned in optimization strategies, while minimizing environmental contamination and resource inefficiencies. Algal bioreactors are typically classified into open systems and closed systems (photobioreactors (PBRs)), each with a specific configuration suited for different operational scales and effluent types.

1.4.2.1 Open Raceway Ponds

These are shallow, oval channels, typically 0.2–0.3 meters deep, where algal cultures are circulated by paddle wheels. These systems, owing to their low construction and operational costs, simple design, and inclusion of solar irradiance, make them ideal for large-scale, cost-effective bioremediation, particularly in rural and agricultural sectors. However, these systems have significant limitations, including vulnerability to environmental fluctuations, water loss due to evaporation, contamination, and inefficient carbon dioxide transfer (Skifa et al., 2024). To address these challenges, researchers have introduced innovations such as partial enclosures or floating covers, which can reduce evaporation and have less chances of contamination, while solar reflectors and concentration of light structures to help with photon capture, and CO_2 enrichment modules (connected to flue gas or anaerobic digestors) are used to improve carbon availability (Sun et al., 2025). Smart raceway ponds are now being introduced, which incorporate real-time sensors for monitoring key culture parameters such as pH, dissolved oxygen (DO), and nutrient levels (Igou et al., 2023). While open raceway ponds typically yield lower biomass than closed systems, their scalability and low operational cost considerations have made them suitable for decentralized wastewater treatment setups, especially in developing countries.

1.4.2.2 Closed Photobioreactors (PBRs)

Closed PBRs have been known for their better control over environmental conditions, safeguarding algal cultures from contamination and, in turn, enabling the production of high-value biomass, while also facilitating the treatment of not only industrial but also hazardous effluents. Recent advances in PBR design include tubular, flat-panel, and air-lift column configurations, which are geared towards optimizing spatial footprint, enhancing photon utilization, and managing metabolic by-products (Penloglou et al., 2024). Tubular PBRs typically contain long, transparent tubes (which can be made of glass, polycarbonate, or acrylic) that can be arranged in either horizontal, vertical, or helical configurations. Their high surface area-to-volume (S/V) ratio (exceeding 100 m^2/m^3) enables highly efficient light absorption and upregulates photosynthetic activity (Ortega et al., 2024). Helical or serpentine photobioreactor (PBR) arrangements enable the complex structural designs that are not attainable in traditional vertical or horizontal systems. The geometry increases fluid turbulence, minimizes algal sedimentation, and promotes even light distribution in the culture medium. However, such systems are usually characterized by the prevalence of oxygen oversaturation, which could trigger photoinhibition and oxidative stress in the algal cells. In response, the addition of degassing units serves to eliminate excess oxygen, and the peristaltic pumps are used to maintain constant circulation velocities (0.2–0.6 m s^{-1}) to ensure that the circulation occurs, and the units reduce the resistance to diffusion across the boundary layer (Kumar et al., 2011). Flat-panel PBRs consist of thin vertical or inclined chambers usually between 2 and 10 cm thick and are known to provide a high light-utilization efficiency in the least amount of spatial volume. Their small optical path length allows for better light penetration, making them especially suitable for dense algal cultures. The most recent advancements, such as the incorporation of optical fibers and reflective panels, have improved the redistribution of light internally and alleviated the shading effect in high-density systems. This planar geometry is also easier to clean, can be stacked on the module to scale up, and encourages natural convective mixing, which would reduce the amount of energy needed to circulate. These features make flat-panel PBR particularly beneficial for use in indoor settings and controlled conditions, which often utilize artificial lighting (Banerjee et al., 2023).

Bubble column PBRs, also known as air-lift column PBRs, utilize gas sparging to transfer the culture medium, thereby eliminating the need for mechanical agitation. Internal or external draft tubes are commonly used in these cylindrical reactors, forming loop-flow structures to facilitate effective mass transfer at low shear rates.

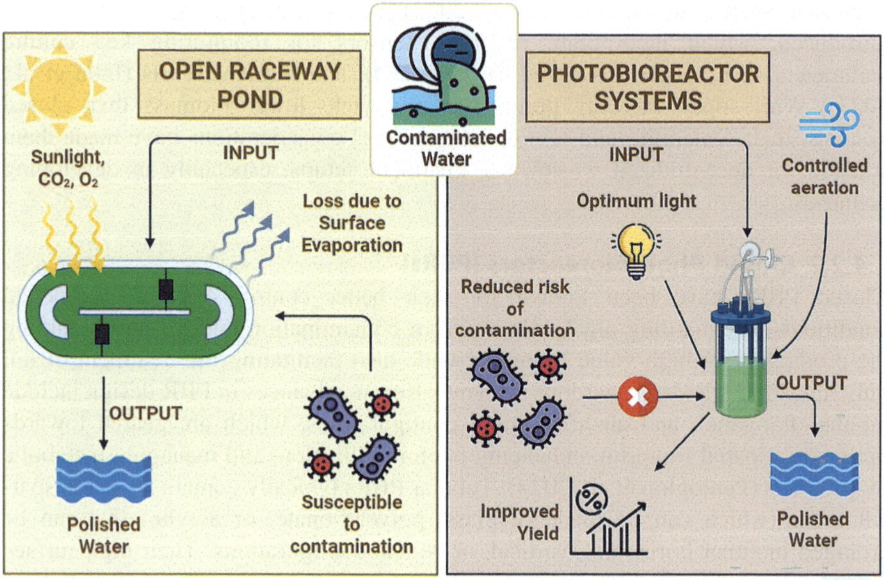

Fig. 1.4 Schematic comparison of open raceway ponds and photobioreactor systems used in algal pollutant removal. Photobioreactors offer improved yield and reduced contamination risk under controlled conditions compared to open ponds

These are especially favorable to shear-sensitive species like *Haematococcus pluvialis* and *Botryococcus braunii*. The integration of a dual-phase aeration system increases the volumetric mass transfer coefficient (kLa), improving carbon dioxide dissolution efficiency. Bubble size control and recirculation of gas strategies were also employed to enhance carbon utilization and oxygen stripping. The advantage of these designs is reduced biofouling and lower energy requirements compared to stirred designs (Uyar et al., 2024). A comparison between open raceway ponds and photobioreactor systems for algal-based wastewater treatment, highlighting differences in contamination risk, process control, and productivity, is depicted in Fig. 1.4.

Newly introduced hybrid systems aim to combine the advantages of each reactor type. For example, integrating vertical PBR modules with raceway ponds enables uninterrupted biomass production, as raceway ponds serve as the primary zone for nutrient absorption, and closed PBRs function as biomass intensification units. Additionally, an LED-based dynamic light integration strategy with programmable spectral composition enables PAR (photosynthetically active radiation) optimization, particularly targeting algal species with a unique pigmentation profile. Machine learning profiles are also being employed to dynamically adjust light, nutrient, and pH regimes based on real-time data (Tummawai et al., 2024).

1.4.3 Advantages and Limitations of Algal Bioremediation

1.4.3.1 Advantages

The speed of modern development has surpassed nature's ability to maintain equilibrium, pushing ecosystems toward imbalance and urging the search for sustainable alternatives. Amid this global search for greener solutions, microalgae have emerged as a potential resource. Microalgae are one of the most diverse classes of photosynthetic organisms, showing incredible promise as a resource for sustainable development.CO_2 is a greenhouse gas that widely contributes to global warming by trapping heat present in the atmosphere. Therefore, decarbonization is key to avoiding severe climate impacts. Decarbonization provides the benefit of reducing dependency on fossil fuels. CO_2 capture is one of the primary tools for decarbonizing emissions from industrial operations and transportation (Nagireddi et al., 2023). Microalgae, through the process of photosynthesis, convert carbon dioxide into glucose and oxygen with water and solar energy. Microalgae have the potential to form biomass and sequester carbon dioxide 5 to 10 times faster compared to fast-growing terrestrial plants (Kammerer et al., 2022). Moreover, microalgae can be readily grown in wastewater, saline water, and other sources besides freshwater (Jaiswal et al., 2021). Microalgae utilize CO_2 and transform it into useful metabolites through various pathways. Moreover, they exhibit remarkable carbon fixation capacity, with just 1 kg of microalgal biomass capable of assimilating about 1.83 kg of CO_2, contributing nearly 40% to the planet's total carbon sequestration. Green microalgae-based carbon sequestration is considered the most suitable method for carbon capture.

The twentieth century also faced the challenge of depleting fossil fuels. According to the 2016 International Energy Outlook report, approximately 10 kg of carbon dioxide (CO_2) is emitted per gallon of diesel fuel burned. A primary research challenge today lies in gradually transforming the traditional petroleum refining and reforming processes with biomass-based methods as we transition toward a new era of sustainable, bio-based economy. Biofuels are produced from food crops and non-food crops such as lignocellulosic biomass. The third-generation category considered for biofuel derivation is from microalgae (Hoang et al., 2022). Microalgal strains are often regarded as miniature biochemical factories capable of synthesizing a wide range of valuable compounds, including lipids, carotenoids, and proteins. Microalgae serve as a versatile source of biofuels because they produce all three key bioactive components, carbohydrates, lipids, and pigments, each of which can be converted into different forms of biofuels. Among these, their lipid content makes them particularly attractive for biofuel production, such as biodiesel (Dineshkumar & Sen, 2020).

The biofuels produced from microalgae have a higher potential than other biofuel alternatives. When the percentage of carbohydrates is high, the efficiency of bioethanol can be increased by a significant proportion, depending on the microalgal species. By absorbing nitrates, phosphates, and trace elements in wastewater, microalgae transform these substances into various bioactive compounds and value-added products through the use of solar energy (Hoang et al., 2022). The use of various algal species, including *Chlamydomonas, Chlorella,* and

Scenedesmus, has been proven to effectively assimilate essential nutrients (such as nitrogen and phosphorus) in wastewater and remove toxic pollutants, including heavy metals. Notably, *Chlorella vulgaris* cultivated in municipal wastewater achieved outstanding removals of 99.6% and 91.2% of nitrogen and phosphorus, respectively, and also produced biomethane. Similarly, *Chlorella variabilis* demonstrated effective purification of textile effluents, achieving 100% removal of nickel, aluminum, and iron, a biomass yield of 74 g m-2 d-1, and a lipid production rate of 20%. Moreover, the lipid-containing algae, named *Botryococcus* sp., showed excellent treatment in domestic wastewater, eliminating 59.9% nitrogen, 36.8% phosphate, 54.5% organic carbon, and biomass with 72.5% crude oil concentration (Shahid et al., 2019).

1.4.3.2 Limitations

Algae bioremediation is a desirable, low-cost, and viable method for numerous wastewaters and even polluted environments. Microalgae possess a unique capability to incorporate nutrients, trap heavy metals, and degrade organic pollutants, while simultaneously yielding biomass that can be further utilized to extract bioenergy and bio-products. However, the algal-based systems are facing many obstacles to mass adoption and sustainability. The major limitation is in the biomass recovery and harvesting. Microalgae are technically challenging and energy-consuming to separate from treated effluents due to their small cell size, colloidal stability, and low sedimentation rate. The traditional methods used in harvesting, such as centrifugation, flocculation, and membrane filtration, among others, substantially increase the operational cost, thereby limiting the cost-effectiveness of full-scale systems. Biomass accumulation may also be caused by incomplete or inefficient harvesting, which has an undesirable impact on water quality and stability of the processes (Abdelfattah et al., 2022). Another significant limitation is light penetration, especially with large-scale photobioreactors and open-pond systems. Algal productivity depends on the process of photosynthesis; hence, it is essential to have a uniform and adequate light distribution. Little light can be available due to high culture density, turbidity of wastewater, and self-shading in high population, resulting in low photosynthetic performance and low rates of pollutant removal. These restrictions can be overcome through optimized reactor design and light-management methods, ensuring that the entire culture volume is properly illuminated (Abdelfattah et al., 2022). Debilitation of the system is also caused by the toxicity of contaminants. High levels of poisonous heavy metals and organic toxicants alter pigment activity, enzyme functionality, and membrane integrity, which in turn affect algal metabolism and development. These toxicants can lead to cell lysis or a change in microbial community composition, which reduces the effectiveness of remediation in extreme cases. They have considered using metal-tolerant or genetically modified algal strains as a means of enhancing resistance and maintaining performance under stress conditions.

Bioremediation using algae is also operationally challenged by environmental dependency. Temperature, pH, dissolved oxygen, and nutrient balance are among the factors that significantly affect algal physiology and pollutant uptake. It is fundamental that in the case of outdoor or large-scale systems, maintaining optimal conditions is challenging due to climatic fluctuations, resulting in uncertain treatment outcomes (Yang et al., 2024; Srimongkol et al., 2022). Moreover, the non-target microorganisms, such as bacteria, fungi, and protozoa, can alter algal cultures in non-sterile wastewater. Such organisms can either be competitive or metabolize organic material differently, and this changes the system dynamics and decreases the overall effectiveness of pollutant removal. Although algal-bacterial consortia have the potential to enhance remediation through collaborative activity, non-selective microbial growth can disrupt the system (Abdelfattah et al., 2022). Lastly, process integration and scalability are the main challenges. Systems in the laboratory scale are indeed good controlled conditions, expanding them to industrial or municipal uses is technically and economically costly. Optimizing reactor design, effective harvesting methods, and integrating algal-based bioremediation with conventional wastewater treatment processes are necessary to make algal-based bioremediation economically feasible (Srimongkol et al., 2022).

1.4.4 Implementation Challenges and Feasibility

A significant hurdle is the high initial capital investment required for closed PBR systems, particularly during the scale-up process. The expenses of construction materials, monitoring sensors, automation systems, and sterilization equipment will lead to an increase in both capital and operational expenses. In fact, the cost per unit volume of treatment using PBRs can be up to 10 times higher than that of raceway systems. To offset these high costs, integrated biorefinery systems are being promoted, which co-produce high-value products such as polyunsaturated fatty acids (PUFAs), carotenoids, and biofertilizers, alongside water remediation, while improving the economic viability of the process (Figueroa-Torres & Theodoropoulos, 2023).

The transition from pilot or lab scale to full-scale introduces several challenges, contamination being the primary source of concern, especially in open systems where other microbes may invade and disrupt algal cultures. In most closed systems, biofouling is a persistent problem that interferes with light penetration, thereby reducing photosynthetic capability. Solutions that include the use of anti-fouling coatings, periodic back-flushing techniques, and pulsed lighting strategies, which disrupt biofilm formation (Soriano-Jerez et al., 2024). An effective carbon dioxide delivery system is necessary; imbalances in the system can lead to either carbon limitations or acidification, both of which can impair productivity. High-density cultures require additional aeration devices or membrane-based gas exchange units to manage delivery. Other major challenges lie in biomass harvesting, which is energy-intensive owing to the small size and low density of algal cells. While methods such as centrifugation and membrane filtration are commonly employed, new techniques like electro-flocculation and magnetic harvesting offer promising alternatives that require further validation (Hou et al., 2022).

The integration of algal bioreactors into existing wastewater infrastructures offers a unique opportunity to enhance process efficiency and sustainability. Algal-based tertiary treatment systems are effective, capable of removing 95% of residual nitrogen and phosphorus, while also sequestering heavy metals, disrupting chemicals, and microplastics from effluents. Furthermore, algae can assimilate carbon dioxide emitted from upstream aerobic digestion/combustion, thereby increasing carbon capture and climate mitigation efforts. Coupling anaerobic digestors with algal systems can create a closed-loop system where nutrients are recycled, and due to the co-digestion of algae and sewage sludge, energy generation is enhanced (Rajalakshmi et al., 2021). High-rate algal pond (HRAP) systems in California, for instance, have demonstrated improvements in effluent quality and a significant reduction in sludge (Magalhães et al., 2024). Similarly, photobioreactor retrofits implemented in Spain have yielded enhanced sustainability metrics and operational efficiencies (Blanco et al., 2023). These findings highlight the potential for integrating algal systems into conventional wastewater treatment plants to develop self-sustaining and resilient systems, as summarized in Table 1.2.

1.5 Case Studies

1.5.1 Microalgae for Freshwater Arsenic Bioremediation: Examining Cellular Toxicity, Bioconcentration Factor, and Eluding an Alternative Arsenic Detoxification Pathway

This study examined the arsenic-removal capacity of two microalgae strains, *Nostoc* (a cyanobacterium) and *Chlorella* (a green alga), under freshwater conditions (phosphate-rich and depleted) (Tang & Foo, 2024). Both strains removed arsenic (As), although *Nostoc* showed greater arsenic tolerance and uptake, especially in low-phosphate conditions. Whereas *Chlorella* relies on ATP-driven efflux, using pumps like ArsA–ArsB, Nostoc demonstrated phosphate- and energy-independent detoxification through the activation of the arsM gene. The arsM gene encodes for arsenic methylation, resulting in the relatively non-toxic methylated arsenic species MMA and DMA. As a result, *Nostoc* could persist in taking up As without relying on energy input. Furthermore, at the biomass level, while *Nostoc* experienced cell damage from As(III) exposure, it ultimately demonstrated a weight increase of 18.6%. In contrast, *Chlorella* achieved a lower weight increase of 7.5% and exhibited growth inhibition as a result of long-term exposure to soluble As(V). SEM pictures proved significant membrane damage in Nostoc, although it remained viable, whereas *Chlorella* was almost entirely degraded. Further molecular analysis revealed that Nostoc suppressed the expression of arsA and arsD genes but possessed strong arsM activity, indicating a methylation-based detoxification mechanism. In contrast, *Chlorella* lacked arsM expression and was unable to produce methylated arsenic species. All of these results indicate that *Nostoc* is a better candidate for bioremediation of As due to its energy-efficient uptake and biodegradation capabilities, particularly in nutrient-poor freshwater biomes (Tang & Foo, 2024).

Table 1.2 Implementation challenges and mitigation strategies

Challenges	Description	Mitigation strategies
High capital and operational costs	Closed PBRs need high-end construction materials, sensors, automation, and sterilization systems, which, for instance, can be up to 10 times costlier than open raceways	Integrated biorefineries; use of low-cost materials with modular PBR designs; co-production of bioproducts
Contamination risks	Open systems are vulnerable to invasion by native fungi, bacteria, or competitive algal species, disrupting culture stability	Semi-closed or hybrid systems with regular monitoring, selective media, and environmental control
Biofouling in closed PBRs	Reduction in light penetration, photosynthetic efficiency due to biofilm formation on reactor walls	Anti-fouling coatings; periodic back-flushing; pulsed lighting; mechanical cleaning
CO_2 delivery and pH balance	Poor carbon delivery leading to limitation or acidification, generally in dense cultures	Membrane-based gas exchange systems; dual-phase aeration; optimized CO_2 dosing schedules
Light distribution issues	Uneven lighting conditions lead to low photosynthetic capabilities	Internal light guides; reflectors; dynamic LED lighting; flat-panel and tubular geometries
Oxygen accumulation	Excess dissolved oxygen could inhibit growth and cause oxidative stress, common in tubular PBRs	Degassing systems; optimized circulation; bubble size control; loop flow systems
Mixing and hydrodynamic stress	Inadequate mixing could cause sedimentation; high shear stress damages algal species	Air-lift systems; external/internal draft tubes; low-shear design impellers for fragile species
Biomass harvesting	Algae, being small, low-density cells, make harvesting energy-intensive	Electro-flocculation; magnetic separation; bio-flocculant additives; low energy filtration
Scale-up complexity	Pilot-scale to industrial scale is inefficient due to system instability and logistical challenges	Pilot-scale validation; machine-learning control systems; real-time sensor integration; adaptive process design
Regulatory and environmental barriers	GMO risks, discharge compliance, and ecosystem safety concerns may delay development	Risk assessments; EIAs; alignments with national/environmental wastewater guidelines

1.5.2 Biomass Production and Phycoremediation of Microalgae Cultivated in Polluted River Water

As urbanization increases, the pollution of river water (in particular, river water in developing areas) has become a serious issue. Many river treatment options, especially in developed countries, are expensive. As a result, researchers are investigating the use of microalgae as an environmentally sustainable option for wastewater treatment. In a research project led by Ummalyma & Singh, 2022, five freshwater microalgae strains were assessed using the heavily polluted Nambul River (Manipur, India) and cultivated in a mixotrophic growth medium. Water quality analyses were conducted before and after the treatment, including pH, dissolved oxygen (DO), total dissolved solids (TDS), chemical oxygen demand (COD), and biological oxygen demand (BOD). The growth of the five microalgae strains showed significant improvements in pH (increase), DO (increase), compared with the final analyses for COD and BOD (reductions of 96% for COD and 85% for BOD). *Selenastrum* sp. SL7 produced the highest biomass level (660 mg/L) and lipid yields (194.5 mg/L), while the biomass had essential fatty acids: palmitic, oleic, linoleic, EPA, and DHA fatty acids. Their findings suggest that microalgae can be used for both water purification and biomass production, while providing a low-cost, sustainable alternative for remediation of environmental pollution on a bioremediation scale, while also providing a bioproduct for bioresource generation (Ummalyma & Singh, 2022). A comparative table of the two case studies is mentioned in Table 1.3.

1.6 Challenges, Regulatory Considerations, and Prospects

Algal bioremediation, despite its environmentally friendly advantages, faces challenges on different practical and technical fronts. Algal cultivation on a commercial scale necessitates rigorous control of environmental factors such as light intensity, pH, temperature, and nutrient availability, which are factors that increase cost. Open systems are vulnerable to contamination by bacteria, fungi, or protozoa that can dominate or destroy the algae. Harvesting and dewatering of algal biomass remain a major challenge due to their energy-demanding process. Additionally, not all algae capable of withstanding or degrading diverse pollutants exist, and the post-treatment biomass, which carries the pollutants, may require careful handling or destruction. Furthermore, the limited availability of genetic tools in many algal strains hinders efforts to enhance their bioremediation potential through genetic modification or synthetic biology. The implementation of algal bioremediation systems must comply with local and international environmental safety regulations. Guiding rules typically concern the biosafety of the algal organism, particularly in the case of GMOs, as there may be ecological risks involved. The effluents to be treated must satisfy stringent discharge standards, including limit levels of heavy metals, nutrients, and organic matter. Moreover, commercial-scale implementation of algal technology typically entails a careful risk assessment, validation research, and governmental clearances. There are also legal implications that arise from utilizing indigenous algal strains, which may be regulated by biodiversity conservation laws and international agreements, such as the Nagoya Protocol.

Continuous environmental monitoring, transparent data reporting, and adherence to biosafety protocols are vital components of any regulatory structure governing algal bioremediation. This technology holds significant promise as advancements in biotechnology and the growing demand for eco-friendly pollution control methods continue to expand. Progress in genetic engineering and synthetic biology is enabling the creation of algal strains with improved tolerance to contaminants and enhanced abilities to degrade pollutants. When integrated with circular economy principles, algal systems can simultaneously treat wastewater and utilize the

Table 1.3 Comparative analysis of key parameters in "microalgae for freshwater arsenic bioremediation: examining cellular toxicity, bioconcentration factor and eluding an alternative arsenic detoxification pathway" and "biomass production and phycoremediation of microalgae cultivated in polluted river water"

Title	Microalgae for freshwater arsenic bioremediation: examining cellular toxicity, bioconcentration factor and eluding an alternative arsenic detoxification pathway	Biomass production and phycoremediation of microalgae cultivated in polluted river water
Objective	To assess arsenic (As) removal efficiency, detoxification mechanism, and tolerance in two microalgae species under different phosphate conditions	To evaluate the ability of freshwater microalgae to treat polluted river water while generating useful biomass and lipids
Microalgae strains	*Nostoc* (cyanobacterium) and *Chlorella* (green alga)	Five freshwater strains; *Selenastrum* sp. *SL7* showed best performance
Type of pollutant/water source	Freshwater contaminated with *arsenic (As)*	Heavily polluted *Nambul River (Manipur, India)*
Experimental condition	Phosphate-rich and phosphate-depleted freshwater media; examined molecular and physiological responses	Mixotrophic cultivation in polluted river water with varying organic and inorganic contaminants
Mechanism of bioremediation	*Nostoc*: Energy-independent detoxification via *arsM gene* (arsenic methylation to MMA, DMA) *Chlorella*: ATP-driven efflux using *ArsA–ArsB pumps*	Nutrient uptake and *photosynthetic oxygenation*, reducing organic load (BOD, COD) and improving water quality
Key parameters	Arsenic uptake, bioconcentration factor, gene expression (arsA, arsD, arsM), biomass growth, and SEM imaging	pH, dissolved oxygen (DO), total dissolved solids (TDS), chemical oxygen demand (COD), biological oxygen demand (BOD), biomass, and lipid yield
Major findings	*Nostoc* showed higher As tolerance and uptake, especially under low phosphate. It demonstrated *18.6% biomass increase* under As(III) and *Chlorella* had lower growth (7.5%) with severe cell damage *Nostoc* detoxified as via methylation (arsM activation) producing less toxic MMA & DMA	Significant improvement in pH and DO reduction of *COD by 96%* and *BOD by 85%*. *Selenastrum* sp. *SL7* produced *660 mg/L biomass* and *194.5 mg/L lipids* Lipids contained essential fatty acids (palmitic, oleic, linoleic, EPA, DHA)
Observations	SEM showed membrane damage in *Nostoc* but overall viability; *Chlorella* cells degraded	No cellular imaging reported; biochemical analysis focused on water quality and biomass
Environmental significance	*Nostoc* is a promising candidate for *arsenic bioremediation*, especially in nutrient-poor waters, due to energy-efficient uptake and detoxification Demonstrated *molecular—level detoxification mechanisms* and *genetic adaptation* to heavy metal stress	Microalgae offer a *low-cost, sustainable alternative* for *river water purification* and *bioproduct generation* Demonstrated *dual benefit—*Pollution remediation and *bioresource (biomass/lipid) generation*

resulting biomass to produce valuable products, such as biofuels, bioplastics, or fertilizers. Modern innovations, such as automated photobioreactors and algae-bacteria co-culture systems, offer new avenues to enhance both operational efficiency and scalability (Behera et al., 2025).

Furthermore, algal cultivation contributes to climate change mitigation by capturing atmospheric CO_2 during growth. With supportive policies, increased investment, and stronger public engagement, algal bioremediation is poised to become a mainstream practice in environmental management. Although challenges remain, ongoing interdisciplinary research is gradually bridging existing knowledge gaps. The integration of omics technologies—encompassing genomics, transcriptomics, proteomics, and metabolomics—is deepening our understanding of algal biology, pollutant degradation pathways, and stress adaptation mechanisms. These findings are essential for the rational development of robust algal strains optimized for specific environmental applications. Combining algal systems with complementary treatment approaches, such as biochar adsorption, membrane filtration, or advanced oxidation, can further enhance pollutant removal efficiency while minimizing energy use and downtime. Collaboration among research institutions, industry, and regulatory authorities is accelerating the development of standardized methods and scalable models, facilitating the transition of algal bioremediation from experimental setups to field-scale deployment. With the growing global emphasis on sustainable technologies, algae-based remediation is likely to become a cornerstone of comprehensive, long-term ecological and economic sustainability strategies.

1.7 Conclusion

Algal systems in environmental remediation have become a significant advancement in sustainable pollution control technologies. Algal bioremediation, governed by mechanisms like biosorption, bioaccumulation, and enzymatic transformation, shows robustness to remove a wide array of environmental pollutants. Unlike traditional methods, which are energy-intensive and generate secondary by-products, algal bioremediation offers an ecologically compatible, cost-effective, and multifunctional approach. At the heart of algal bioremediation lies the remarkable adaptability of microalgae, which can thrive in a wide range of environmental conditions, even extreme ones, while simultaneously capturing pollutants and generating biomass of economic value. Their ability to fix carbon dioxide and assimilate nutrients such as nitrogen and phosphorus, along with their capacity to detoxify complex contaminants, makes them highly effective agents for both ecological restoration and the treatment of industrial effluents. This chapter highlights the crucial roles of cell surface functional groups, enzymes, and extracellular polymeric substances (EPS) in facilitating the removal of pollutants. It also explores how environmental factors including light intensity, temperature, pH, and nutrient availability, interact to influence algal physiology and remediation efficiency. Understanding these interactions supports the optimization of bioprocesses and the development of predictive models for improved reactor management and control.

From a technological standpoint, the scalability and performance of reactor systems are key to the commercial viability of algal remediation. Open raceway ponds are widely adopted in rural or decentralized settings due to their simplicity and low cost, yet they suffer from issues such as limited biomass productivity and vulnerability to contamination. In contrast, closed photobioreactors (PBRs) offer superior environmental control, higher yields, and reduced contamination risks; however, they require a greater capital investment and higher operational costs. Recent innovations—including internal light distribution systems, dual-phase aeration designs, and algorithm-based regulation—have led to the development of hybrid systems that combine the strengths of both open and closed configurations, thereby improving scalability, efficiency, and adaptability.

Looking ahead, advances in smart bioreactor design will be crucial in addressing current scalability constraints. Integrating intelligent monitoring systems for the real-time adjustment of light, nutrient, and gas parameters, coupled with next-generation biosensors, can enhance the resilience and responsiveness of algal cultures. Likewise, applying synthetic biology tools such as genome editing can yield algal strains with improved stress tolerance, nutrient uptake, and metabolic output. In parallel, innovations such as nanomaterial-assisted harvesting and biofilm-based reactors could reduce energy consumption and operational costs. Despite their numerous advantages, algal systems still face several challenges, including economic barriers, biofouling, inefficiencies in carbon dioxide delivery, uneven light distribution, and difficulties in biomass harvesting. Various solutions—such as electro-flocculation, magnetic harvesting, anti-fouling strategies, and hybrid reactor configurations—are being developed to mitigate these issues. Real-world applications, such as high-rate algal ponds in California and photobioreactor retrofits in Spain, demonstrate the feasibility of integrating algal systems into wastewater treatment. These systems not only improve effluent quality and minimize sludge production but also contribute to climate change mitigation through carbon capture and energy recovery. In conclusion, algal bioremediation represents a multifaceted approach to addressing modern pollution challenges. While further research and engineering refinement are necessary to overcome existing technical and economic barriers, ongoing innovations in reactor design, algal strain development, and value-added product recovery position these systems as pivotal components of future environmental remediation and sustainable resource recovery frameworks.

Key Takeaways

- Environmental pollution remains a major global concern, with contaminants from industrial, agricultural, and urban sources stressing ecosystems and human health.
- Algal bioremediation is highlighted as a sustainable and cost-effective alternative to traditional remediation methods, providing benefits such as biomass production, improved carbon footprint, and collective remediation potential.
- Algae remove pollutants through several complementary mechanisms—biosorption, bioaccumulation, and biodegradation.
- Biosorption is a quick, passive process where pollutants such as heavy metals and dyes attach to algal cell surfaces through specific functional groups.

- Bioaccumulation is an active, energy-dependent process where living algae absorb and store contaminants inside their cells.
- Biodegradation relies on enzymes to break down and detoxify organic pollutants, while phycoremediation combines these processes, allowing algae to absorb, transform, and remove multiple types of pollutants at once.
- The extracellular polymeric substances (EPS) released by algae help bind, immobilize, and detoxify pollutants. They also support cooperation with other microorganisms in biofilms, improving overall removal efficiency.
- Environmental conditions such as light intensity, temperature, pH, nutrient balance, and pollutant concentration have a major impact on how effectively algae can clean up contaminants.
- Certain species, including *Chlorella*, *Spirulina*, and cyanobacteria like *Nostoc* and *Anabaena*, are particularly effective at removing pollutants under a variety of environmental conditions.
- Bioreactor systems for algal remediation have evolved from simple open raceway ponds to more advanced closed photobioreactors. Open systems are easier and cheaper to operate, but they face contamination and yield issues. In contrast, closed systems offer better control and productivity, albeit at a higher cost in terms of setup and maintenance.
- Optimizing conditions such as nutrient ratios, light, temperature, CO_2 input, and mixing is key to improving both pollutant removal and biomass yield. Computational approaches, such as artificial neural networks (ANN) and computational fluid dynamics (CFD), are now being used to fine-tune these systems.
- Real-world applications have shown promising results; for example, *Nostoc* has been effective in removing arsenic, and microalgae have successfully treated river water contaminated with multiple pollutants, leading to better water quality.
- Despite these successes, some challenges still limit large-scale use, such as economic costs, biofouling, difficulties in harvesting, dependence on environmental conditions, and the need to meet regulatory standards.

Looking ahead, the future of algal bioremediation lies in integrating algae with wastewater treatment infrastructure, adopting circular bioeconomic models, and utilizing smart bioreactors supported by AI and biosensors. Advances in genetic engineering and stronger partnerships between researchers, industries, and policymakers will be crucial for standardization and large-scale implementation.

References

Abdelfattah, A., Ali, S. S., Ramadan, H., El-Aswar, E. I., Eltawab, R., Ho, S., Elsamahy, T., Li, S., El-Sheekh, M. M., Schagerl, M., Kornaros, M., & Sun, J. (2022). Microalgae-based wastewater treatment: Mechanisms, challenges, recent advances, and future prospects. *Environmental Science and Ecotechnology, 13*, 100205. https://doi.org/10.1016/j.ese.2022.100205

Ahmad, I. (2021). Microalgae–bacteria consortia: A review on the degradation of Polycyclic Aromatic Hydrocarbons (PAHs). *Arabian Journal for Science and Engineering, 47*(1), 19–43. https://doi.org/10.1007/s13369-021-06236-9

Ahmad, A., & Ashraf, S. S. (2024). Harnessing microalgae: Innovations for achieving UN Sustainable Development Goals and climate resilience. *Journal of Water Process Engineering, 68*, 106506. https://doi.org/10.1016/j.jwpe.2024.106506

Ali, S. S., Hassan, L. H., & El-Sheekh, M. (2024). Microalgae-mediated bioremediation: Current trends and opportunities-a review. *Archives of Microbiology, 206*(8). https://doi.org/10.1007/s00203-024-04052-x

Arashiro, L. T., Ferrer, I., Pániker, C. C., Gómez-Pinchetti, J. L., Rousseau, D. P. L., Van Hulle, S. W. H., & Garfí, M. (2020). Natural pigments and biogas recovery from microalgae grown in wastewater. *ACS Sustainable Chemistry & Engineering, 8*(29), 10691–10701. https://doi.org/10.1021/acssuschemeng.0c01106

Asswad, R., Djema, W., Bernard, O., Gouzé, J. L., & Cinquemani, E. (2024, December). Optimization of microalgae biosynthesis via controlled algal-bacterial symbiosis. In *IEEE 63rd Conference on Decision and Control (CDC)* (pp. 589–594). IEEE. https://doi.org/10.1109/CDC56724.2024.10886300

Ayilara, M. S., & Babalola, O. O. (2023). Bioremediation of environmental wastes: The role of microorganisms. *Frontiers in Agronomy, 5*. https://doi.org/10.3389/fagro.2023.1183691

Banerjee, S., Dasgupta, S., Atta, A., Das, D., Dayal, D., Malik, S., Kumar, H., Kishore, S., Rustagi, S., & Almutary, A. G. (2023). Flow rate optimization in a Flat-Panel photobioreactor for the cultivation of microalgae for mitigating waste gas. *Water (Basel), 15*(15), 2824. https://doi.org/10.3390/w15152824

Behera, B., Venkata, S. K., & Rout, P. R. (2025). Importance of biological knowledge in the downstream of microalgae-based processes and products. In *Algal Bioreactors* (pp. 17–35). Elsevier Science Ltd. https://doi.org/10.1016/B978-0-443-14059-4.00019-2

Blanco, E. C., Martín, M., & Vega, P. (2023). Achieving energy self-sufficiency in wastewater treatment plants by integrating municipal solid waste treatment: A process design study in Spain. *Journal of Environmental Chemical Engineering, 11*(5), 110673. https://doi.org/10.1016/j.jece.2023.110673

Calatrava, V., Gonzalez-Ballester, D., & Dubini, A. (2024). Microalgae for bioremediation: advances, challenges, and public perception on genetic engineering. *BMC Plant Biology, 24*(1), 1261. https://doi.org/10.1186/s12870-024-05995-5

Chakravorty, M., Nanda, M., Ahmed, W., Hussain, A., Vlaskin, M., Anna, K. I., & Kumar, V. (2024). In-vitro cr (III) alleviation and the concurrent biochemical responses by Chlorella minutissima to establish its phycoremediation potential and biofuel prospects. *Bioremediation Journal*, 1–11. https://doi.org/10.1080/10889868.2024.2352121

Chen, B., Li, F., Liu, N., Ge, F., Xiao, H., & Yang, Y. (2015). Role of extracellular polymeric substances from Chlorella vulgaris in the removal of ammonium and orthophosphate under the stress of cadmium. *Bioresource Technology, 190*, 299–306. https://doi.org/10.1016/j.biortech.2015.04.080

Ciobanu, A., Lucaci, A., & Bulgariu, L. (2024). Efficient metal ions biosorption on red and green algae biomass: Isotherm, kinetic and thermodynamic study. *Journal of Applied Phycology, 36*(6), 3809–3827. https://doi.org/10.1007/s10811-024-03332-9

De Freitas, B. B., Overmans, S., Medina, J. S., Hong, P., & Lauersen, K. J. (2022). Biomass generation and heterologous isoprenoid milking from engineered microalgae grown in anaerobic membrane bioreactor effluent. *Water Research, 229*, 119486. https://doi.org/10.1016/j.watres.2022.119486

De Oliveira Gonçalves, L., Starling, M. C. V. M., Leal, C. D., Oliveira, D. V. M., Araújo, J. C., Leão, M. M. D., & Amorim, C. C. (2018). Enhanced biodiesel industry wastewater treatment via a hybrid MBBR combined with advanced oxidation processes: Analysis of active microbiota and toxicity removal. *Environmental Science and Pollution Research, 26*(5), 4521–4536. https://doi.org/10.1007/s11356-018-2710-y

Diankristanti, P. A., & Ng, I. (2024). Marine microalgae for bioremediation and waste-to-worth valorization: Recent progress and future prospects. *Blue Biotechnology, 1*, 10. https://doi.org/10.1186/s44315-024-00010-w

Diengdoh, O. L., Ryntathiang, S., & Syiem, M. B. (2023). ZN tolerance in anabaena variabilis MEGCH1: An in-depth analysis of carbon and nitrogen assimilation; morphology and ultrastructure. *Journal of Applied Biological Sciences, 17*(3), 391–406. https://doi.org/10.71336/jabs.1138

Dineshkumar, R., & Sen, R. (2020). A sustainable perspective of microalgal biorefinery for co-production and recovery of high-value carotenoid and biofuel with CO2 valorization. *Biofuels, Bioproducts and Biorefining, 14*(4), 879–897. https://doi.org/10.1002/bbb.2107

Ding, T., Yang, M., Zhang, J., Yang, B., Lin, K., Li, J., & Gan, J. (2017). Toxicity, degradation and metabolic fate of ibuprofen on freshwater diatom Navicula sp. *Journal of Hazardous Materials, 330*, 127–134. https://doi.org/10.1016/j.jhazmat.2017.02.004

Dudeja, C., Masroor, S., Mishra, V., Kumar, K., Sansar, S., Yadav, P., Chaturvedi, N., Singh, R., & Kumar, A. (2025). Cyanobacteria-based bioremediation of environmental contaminants: Advances and computational insights. *Discover Agriculture, 3*(1). https://doi.org/10.1007/s44279-025-00193-9

Figueroa-Torres, G. M., & Theodoropoulos, C. (2023). Techno-economic analysis of a microalgae-based biorefinery network for biofuels and value-added products. *Bioresource Technology Reports, 23*, 101524. https://doi.org/10.1016/j.biteb.2023.101524

García-Camacho, F., López-Rosales, L., Sánchez-Mirón, A., Belarbi, E., Chisti, Y., & Molina-Grima, E. (2016). Artificial neural network modeling for predicting the growth of the microalga Karlodinium veneficum. *Algal Research, 14*, 58–64. https://doi.org/10.1016/j.algal.2016.01.002

García-Galán, M. J., Arashiro, L., Santos, L. H., Insa, S., Rodríguez-Mozaz, S., Barceló, D., Ferrer, I., & Garfí, M. (2019). Fate of priority pharmaceuticals and their main metabolites and transformation products in microalgae-based wastewater treatment systems. *Journal of Hazardous Materials, 390*, 121771. https://doi.org/10.1016/j.jhazmat.2019.121771

Goh, P. S., Ahmad, N. A., Lim, J. W., Liang, Y. Y., Kang, H. S., Ismail, A. F., & Arthanareeswaran, G. (2022). Microalgae-enabled wastewater remediation and nutrient recovery through membrane photobioreactors: Recent achievements and future perspective. *Membranes, 12*(11), 1094. https://doi.org/10.3390/membranes12111094

Hashmi, Z., Bilad, M. R., Fahrurrozi, N., Zaini, J., Lim, J. W., & Wibisono, Y. (2023). Recent progress in microalgae-based technologies for industrial wastewater treatment. *Fermentation, 9*(3), 311. https://doi.org/10.3390/fermentation9030311

Hoang, A. T., Sirohi, R., Pandey, A., Nižetić, S., Lam, S. S., Chen, W., Luque, R., Thomas, S., Arıcı, M., & Pham, V. V. (2022). Biofuel production from microalgae: Challenges and chances. *Phytochemistry Reviews, 22*(4), 1089–1126. https://doi.org/10.1007/s11101-022-09819-y

Hou, Y., Liu, C., Liu, Z., Han, T., Hao, N., Guo, Z., Wang, W., Chen, S., Zhao, L., Safavi, M., Ji, X., & Chen, F. (2022). A novel Salt-Bridge electroflocculation technology for harvesting microalgae. *Frontiers in Bioengineering and Biotechnology, 10*. https://doi.org/10.3389/fbioe.2022.902524

Igou, T., Zhong, S., Reid, E., & Chen, Y. (2023). Real-time sensor data profile-based deep learning method applied to open raceway pond Microalgal productivity prediction. *Environmental Science & Technology, 57*(46), 17981–17989. https://doi.org/10.1021/acs.est.2c07578

Ishchi, T., & Sibi, G. (2019). Azo dye degradation by Chlorella vulgaris: Optimization and kinetics. *International Journal of Biological Chemistry, 14*(1), 1–7. https://doi.org/10.3923/ijbc.2020.1.7

Iqbal, S., Nisa, K. U., Tarfeen, N., Wani, S., Nisa, Q., & Ali, S. (2024). Role of Algae in Bioremediation of Waste Disposal Sites. In Integrated Waste Management (pp. 50–65). https://doi.org/10.1201/9781003359326-3

Jaiswal, K. K., Dutta, S., Banerjee, I., Pohrmen, C. B., & Kumar, V. (2021). Photosynthetic microalgae–based carbon sequestration and generation of biomass in biorefinery approach for renewable biofuels for a cleaner environment. *Biomass Conversion and Biorefinery, 13*(9), 7403–7421. https://doi.org/10.1007/s13399-021-01504-y

Kammerer, S., Borho, I., Jung, J., & Schmidt, M. S. (2022). Review: CO2 capturing methods of the last two decades. *International Journal of Environmental Science and Technology, 20*(7), 8087–8104. https://doi.org/10.1007/s13762-022-04680-0

Krasaesueb, N., Incharoensakdi, A., & Khetkorn, W. (2019). Utilization of shrimp wastewater for poly-β-hydroxybutyrate production by Synechocystis sp. PCC 6803 strain ΔSphU cultivated in photobioreactor. *Biotechnology Reports, 23*, e00345. https://doi.org/10.1016/j.btre.2019.e00345

Kumar, K., Dasgupta, C. N., Nayak, B., Lindblad, P., & Das, D. (2011). Development of suitable photobioreactors for CO2 sequestration addressing global warming using green algae and cyanobacteria. *Bioresource Technology, 102*(8), 4945–4953. https://doi.org/10.1016/j.biortech.2011.01.054

Leong, Y. K., & Chang, J. (2020). Bioremediation of heavy metals using microalgae: Recent advances and mechanisms. *Bioresource Technology, 303*, 122886. https://doi.org/10.1016/j.biortech.2020.122886

Li, H., & Meng, F. (2023). Efficiency, mechanism, influencing factors, and integrated technology of biodegradation for aromatic compounds by microalgae: A review. *Environmental Pollution, 335*, 122248. https://doi.org/10.1016/j.envpol.2023.122248

Li, S., Zhang, C., Li, F., Ren, N., & Ho, S. (2022). Recent advances of algae-bacteria consortia in aquatic remediation. *Critical Reviews in Environmental Science and Technology, 53*(3), 315–339. https://doi.org/10.1080/10643389.2022.2052704

Li, X., Li, S., Xie, P., Chen, X., Chu, Y., Chang, H., Sun, J., Li, Q., Ren, N., & Ho, S. (2023). Advanced wastewater treatment with microalgae-indigenous bacterial interactions. *Environmental Science and Ecotechnology, 20*, 100374. https://doi.org/10.1016/j.ese.2023.100374

Li, W., Jin, W., Wu, D., Wang, C., Xu, H., & Song, N. (2024). The substantial generation of photochemically produced reactive intermediates (PPRIs) in algae-type zones from one large shallow lake promoted the removal of organic pollutants. *The Science of the Total Environment, 954*, 176821. https://doi.org/10.1016/j.scitotenv.2024.176821

Lu, J., Zhang, J., Xie, H., Wu, H., Jing, Y., Ji, M., & Hu, Z. (2022). Transformation and toxicity dynamics of polycyclic aromatic hydrocarbons in a novel biological-constructed wetland-microalgal wastewater treatment process. *Water Research, 223*, 119023. https://doi.org/10.1016/j.watres.2022.119023

Machado, A. A., Valiaparampil, J. G., & M, L. (2024). Unlocking the potential of algae for heavy metal remediation. *Water, Air, and Soil Pollution, 235*(10). https://doi.org/10.1007/s11270-024-07436-3

Magalhães, I. B., De Paula Pereira, A. S. A., Silva, T. A., Ferreira, J., Braga, M. Q., Couto, E. A., Assemany, P. P., & Calijuri, M. L. (2024). Advancements in high-rate algal pond technology for enhanced wastewater treatment and biomass production: A review. *Journal of Water Process Engineering, 66*, 105929. https://doi.org/10.1016/j.jwpe.2024.105929

Marella, T. K., Saxena, A., & Tiwari, A. (2020). Diatom mediated heavy metal remediation: A review. *Bioresource Technology, 305*, 123068. https://doi.org/10.1016/j.biortech.2020.123068

Markou, G., & Georgakakis, D. (2011). Cultivation of filamentous cyanobacteria (blue-green algae) in agro-industrial wastes and wastewaters: A review. *Applied Energy, 88*(10), 3389–3401. https://doi.org/10.1016/j.apenergy.2010.12.042

Massart, A., Mirisola, A., Lupant, D., Thomas, D., & Hantson, A. (2014). Experimental characterization and numerical simulation of the hydrodynamics in an airlift photobioreactor for microalgae cultures. *Algal Research, 6*, 210–217. https://doi.org/10.1016/j.algal.2014.07.003

Nagireddi, S., Agarwal, J. R., & Vedapuri, D. (2023). Carbon dioxide capture, utilization, and sequestration: Current status, challenges, and future prospects for global decarbonization. *ACS Engineering Au, 4*(1), 22–48. https://doi.org/10.1021/acsengineeringau.3c00049

Nasir, N. M., Jusoh, A., Harun, R., Ibrahim, N. N. L. N., Rasit, N., Ghani, W. a. W. a. K., & Kurniawan, S. B. (2023). Nutrient consumption of green microalgae, Chlorella sp. during the bioremediation of shrimp aquaculture wastewater. *Algal Research, 72*, 103110. https://doi.org/10.1016/j.algal.2023.103110

Nath, S., Astapati, A. D., Naha, A., Sharma, I., & Shah, M. P. (2024). Algal-based membrane bioreactors for effective removal of hazardous and toxic contaminants: A comprehensive review. *Current Research in Biotechnology, 7*, 100201. https://doi.org/10.1016/j.crbiot.2024.100201

Nikokherad, H., Esmaili-Sari, A., Moradi, A. M., Bahramifar, N., & Mostafavi, P. G. (2022). Bioaccumulation capacity of Chlorella vulgaris and Spirulina platensis exposed to silver nanoparticles and silver nitrate: Bio- and health risk assessment approach. *Algal Research, 64*, 102671. https://doi.org/10.1016/j.algal.2022.102671

Olguín, E. J. (2012). Dual purpose microalgae–bacteria-based systems that treat wastewater and produce biodiesel and chemical products within a Biorefinery. *Biotechnology Advances, 30*(5), 1031–1046. https://doi.org/10.1016/j.biotechadv.2012.05.001

Ortega, A. B., Bahena, P. D. F., Calderón, A. V., Del Río, J. A., & Arias, D. M. (2024). Impact of light spectrum on outdoors tubular photobioreactors used for microalgae-based wastewater treatment. *Journal of Environmental Chemical Engineering*, 114884. https://doi.org/10.1016/j.jece.2024.114884

Parmar, K. S., & Patel, K. M. (2025). Biosorption and bioremediation of heavy metal ions from wastewater using algae: A comprehensive review. *World Journal of Microbiology & Biotechnology, 41*(7). https://doi.org/10.1007/s11274-025-04424-5

Penloglou, G., Pavlou, A., & Kiparissides, C. (2024). Recent advancements in photo-bioreactors for microalgae cultivation: A brief overview. *Processes, 12*(6), 1104. https://doi.org/10.3390/pr12061104

Phiri, J. T., & Oh, S. (2024). Biosorption of Cd(II), Co(II), and Cu(II) onto microalgae under acidic and neutral conditions. *Sustainability, 16*(15), 6342. https://doi.org/10.3390/su16156342

Popa, M., Simionov, I., Petrea, S., Georgescu, P., Ifrim, G., & Iticescu, C. (2025). Efficiency of microalgae employment in nutrient removal (nitrogen and phosphorous) from municipal wastewater. *Water, 17*(2), 260. https://doi.org/10.3390/w17020260

Rajalakshmi, A. M., Silambarasan, T., & Dhandapani, R. (2021). Small scale photo bioreactor treatment of tannery wastewater, heavy metal biosorption and CO2 sequestration using microalga Chlorella sp.: A biodegradation approach. *Applied Water Science, 11*(7). https://doi.org/10.1007/s13201-021-01438-w

Rawat, I., Kumar, R. R., Mutanda, T., & Bux, F. (2010). Dual role of microalgae: Phycoremediation of domestic wastewater and biomass production for sustainable biofuels production. *Applied Energy, 88*(10), 3411–3424. https://doi.org/10.1016/j.apenergy.2010.11.025

Rout, P. R., Dash, R. R., Bhunia, P., & Rao, S. (2018). Role of Bacillus cereus GS-5 strain on simultaneous nitrogen and phosphorous removal from domestic wastewater in an inventive single unit multi-layer packed bed bioreactor. *Bioresource Technology, 262*, 251–260. https://doi.org/10.1016/j.biortech.2018.04.087

Rout, P. R., Zhang, T. C., Bhunia, P., & Surampalli, R. Y. (2021a). Treatment technologies for emerging contaminants in wastewater treatment plants: A review. *Science of the Total Environment, 753*, 141990. https://doi.org/10.1016/j.scitotenv.2020.141990

Rout, P. R., Shahid, M. K., Dash, R. R., Bhunia, P., Liu, D., Varjani, S., et al. (2021b). Nutrient removal from domestic wastewater: A comprehensive review on conventional and advanced technologies. *Journal of Environmental Management, 296*, 113246. https://doi.org/10.1016/j.jenvman.2021.113246

Rout, P. R., Goel, M., Mohanty, A., Pandey, D. S., Halder, N., Mukherjee, S., Bhatia, S. K., Sahoo, N. K., & Varjani, S. (2022). Recent advancements in microalgal mediated valorisation of wastewater from hydrothermal liquefaction of biomass. *BioEnergy Research, 16*(1), 45–60. https://doi.org/10.1007/s12155-022-10421-5

Santos, B., Freitas, F., Sobral, A. J., & Encarnação, T. (2025). Microalgae and circular economy: unlocking waste to resource pathways for sustainable development. *International Journal of Sustainable Engineering, 18*(1). https://doi.org/10.1080/19397038.2025.2501488

Sarma, U., Hoque, M. E., Thekkangil, A., Venkatarayappa, N., & Rajagopal, S. (2024). Microalgae in removing heavy metals from wastewater—An advanced green technology for urban wastewater treatment. *Journal of Hazardous Materials Advances, 15*, 100444. https://doi.org/10.1016/j.hazadv.2024.100444

Shahid, A., Malik, S., Zhu, H., Xu, J., Nawaz, M. Z., Nawaz, S., Alam, M. A., & Mehmood, M. A. (2019). Cultivating microalgae in wastewater for biomass production, pollutant removal, and atmospheric carbon mitigation; A review. *The Science of the Total Environment, 704*, 135303. https://doi.org/10.1016/j.scitotenv.2019.135303

Shahid, M. K., Kashif, A., Rout, P. R., Aslam, M., Fuwad, A., Choi, Y., J, R. B., Park, J. H., & Kumar, G. (2020). A brief review of anaerobic membrane bioreactors emphasizing recent advancements, fouling issues and future perspectives. *Journal of Environmental Management, 270*, 110909. https://doi.org/10.1016/j.jenvman.2020.110909

Sharma, B., Dangi, A. K., & Shukla, P. (2018). Contemporary enzyme based technologies for bioremediation: A review. *Journal of Environmental Management, 210*, 10–22. https://doi.org/10.1016/j.jenvman.2017.12.075

Skifa, I., Chauchat, N., Cocquet, P., & Guer, Y. L. (2024). Microalgae cultivation in raceway ponds: Advances, challenges, and hydrodynamic considerations. *EFB Bioeconomy Journal, 5*, 100073. https://doi.org/10.1016/j.bioeco.2024.100073

Soriano-Jerez, Y., Gallardo-Rodríguez, J., López-Rosales, L., García-Camacho, F., Bressy, C., Molina-Grima, E., & Cerón-García, M. (2024). Preventing biofouling in microalgal photobioreactors. *Bioresource Technology, 407*, 131125. https://doi.org/10.1016/j.biortech.2024.131125

Srimongkol, P., Sangtanoo, P., Songserm, P., Watsuntorn, W., & Karnchanatat, A. (2022). Microalgae-based wastewater treatment for developing economic and environmental sustainability: Current status and future prospects. *Frontiers in Bioengineering and Biotechnology, 10*. https://doi.org/10.3389/fbioe.2022.904046

Srivastava, A., Biswas, S., Yadav, S., Kumar, S., Srivastava, V., & Mishra, Y. (2020). Acute cadmium toxicity and post-stress recovery: Insights into coordinated and integrated response/recovery strategies of Anabaena sp. PCC 7120. *Journal of Hazardous Materials, 411*, 124822. https://doi.org/10.1016/j.jhazmat.2020.124822

Sun, Z., Bo, C., Cao, S., & Sun, L. (2025). Enhancing CO2 fixation in microalgal systems: Mechanistic insights and bioreactor strategies. *Marine Drugs, 23*(3), 113. https://doi.org/10.3390/md23030113

Tang, W. W., & Foo, S. C. (2024). Microalgae for freshwater arsenic bioremediation: Examining cellular toxicity, bioconcentration factor and eluding an alternative arsenic detoxification pathway. *3 Biotech, 14*(5). https://doi.org/10.1007/s13205-024-03977-w

Thongtha, S., Kittiwongwattana, C., Incharoensakdi, A., & Phunpruch, S. (2025). Light-emitting diode illumination enhances biomass, pigment, and lipid production in halotolerant cyanobacterium Aphanothece halophytica. *Phycology, 5*(2), 12. https://doi.org/10.3390/phycology5020012

Tian, X., Lin, X., Xie, Q., Liu, J., & Luo, L. (2024). Effects of temperature and light on microalgal growth and nutrient removal in turtle aquaculture wastewater. *Biology, 13*(11), 901. https://doi.org/10.3390/biology13110901

Touliabah, H. E., El-Sheekh, M. M., Ismail, M. M., & El-Kassas, H. (2022). A review of microalgae- and cyanobacteria-based biodegradation of organic pollutants. *Molecules, 27*(3), 1141. https://doi.org/10.3390/molecules27031141

Tummawai, T., Srinophakun, T. R., Padungthon, S., & Sukpancharoen, S. (2024). Application of artificial intelligence and image processing for the cultivation of Chlorella sp. using tubular photobioreactors. *ACS Omega, 9*(46), 46017–46029. https://doi.org/10.1021/acsomega.4c05971

Ummalyma, S. B., & Singh, A. (2022). Biomass production and phycoremediation of microalgae cultivated in polluted river water. *Bioresource Technology, 351*, 126948. https://doi.org/10.1016/j.biortech.2022.126948

Uyar, B., Ali, M. D., & Uyar, G. E. O. (2024). Design parameters comparison of bubble column, airlift and stirred tank photobioreactors for microalgae production. *Bioprocess and Biosystems Engineering, 47*(2), 195–209. https://doi.org/10.1007/s00449-023-02952-8

Wang, M., Yang, Y., Chen, Z., Chen, Y., Wen, Y., & Chen, B. (2016). Removal of nutrients from undiluted anaerobically treated piggery wastewater by improved microalgae. *Bioresource Technology, 222*, 130–138. https://doi.org/10.1016/j.biortech.2016.09.128

Wei, X., Yu, G., Cao, W., Feng, M., Xu, Y., Jin, M., Zhang, Y., Li, T., & Guo, L. (2024). Biomass producing and CO2 capturing simultaneously by Chlorella vulgaris: Effect of CO2 concentration and aeration rate. *Energy, 306*, 132321. https://doi.org/10.1016/j.energy.2024.132321

Xiao, R., & Zheng, Y. (2016). Overview of microalgal extracellular polymeric substances (EPS) and their applications. *Biotechnology Advances, 34*(7), 1225–1244. https://doi.org/10.1016/j.biotechadv.2016.08.004

Yadav, A. P. S., Dwivedi, V., Kumar, S., Kushwaha, A., Goswami, L., & Reddy, B. S. (2020). Cyanobacterial extracellular polymeric substances for heavy metal removal: A mini review. *Journal of Composites Science, 5*(1), 1. https://doi.org/10.3390/jcs5010001

Yang, K., Wang, J., Zheng, J., & Cai, W. (2024). Microalgae-based wastewater treatment: Advances and challenges in membrane harvesting technologies. *Separation and Purification Technology*, 130805. https://doi.org/10.1016/j.seppur.2024.130805

Yang, X., Wei, Y., Su, Y., Zhang, Z., Tang, X., Chen, Y., Yuan, M., & Yuan, S. (2025). The strategies Microalgae adopt to counteract the toxic effect of heavy metals. *Microorganisms, 13*(5), 989. https://doi.org/10.3390/microorganisms13050989

Yen, H., Ho, S., Chen, C., & Chang, J. (2015). CO2, NOx and SOx removal from flue gas via microalgae cultivation: A critical review. *Biotechnology Journal, 10*(6), 829–839. https://doi.org/10.1002/biot.201400707

Yu, H., Kim, J., Rhee, C., Shin, J., Shin, S. G., & Lee, C. (2022). Effects of different pH control strategies on microalgae cultivation and nutrient removal from anaerobic digestion effluent. *Microorganisms, 10*(2), 357. https://doi.org/10.3390/microorganisms10020357

Zhang, Q., Chang, C., Bai, J., Fang, S., Zhuang, X., & Yuan, Z. (2017). Mutants of Scenedesmus sp. for purifying highly concentrated cellulosic ethanol wastewater and producing biomass simultaneously. *Journal of Applied Phycology, 30*(2), 969–978. https://doi.org/10.1007/s10811-017-1311-3

Algal Bioremediation Strategies for the Removal of Heavy Metals, Dyes, and Hydrocarbons

2

Jogeswar Mahanta, Priyadarsani Patra, Balaram Sahoo, Arpita Patro, Puja Dokania, and Angana Sarkar

Abstract

Algal bioremediation leverages the metabolic and physicochemical properties of a diverse range of algae to remediate a broad spectrum of environmental pollutants, including heavy metals, synthetic dyes, and hydrocarbons. Algae remediate contaminants through a combination of complementary processes, including biosorption, bioaccumulation, enzymatic conversion, and synergistic systems with other related microorganisms. Functional groups are incorporated into the algal cell walls and extracellular polymeric substances (EPS), which generate large binding sites that promote the rapid accumulation of metals and dyes through ion exchange, complexation, electrostatic attraction, and hydrophobic interactions, particularly in the case of aromatic compounds. Since heavy metals are non-biodegradable, their removal is achieved by adsorption on the surface, immobilization, sequestration within the cell, and, in a few cases, a redox reaction, which decreases toxicity and allows for recovery. Synthetic dyes are mainly eliminated by adsorption and hydrogen bonding, whereas algal and microbial enzymes help to decolorate and partially transform complex dye molecules. Remediation of hydrocarbons by adsorption and emulsification through algal polymers and biosurfactants increases bioavailability and enzyme-mediated oxidation, which is usually catalyzed in algal-bacterial consortia to mineralize. This chapter describes the overall algal-based pollution reduction strategies and outlines the mechanisms of remediation for dyes, heavy metals, and hydrocarbons through microalgae, as well as identifies the major challenges and future opportunities for sustainable effluent treatment.

J. Mahanta · P. Patra · B. Sahoo · A. Patro · P. Dokania · A. Sarkar (✉)
Department of Biotechnology and Medical Engineering, National Institute of Technology, Rourkela, Odisha, India
e-mail: sarkara@nitrkl.ac.in

L. Kumar et al. (eds.), *Algal Bioremediation*,
https://doi.org/10.1007/978-981-95-8793-3_2

Keywords

Algal Bioremediation · Biosorption · Bioaccumulation · Heavy Metals · Dye Decolorization · Hydrocarbons

2.1 Introduction

Bioremediation utilizes living organisms, such as algae, bacteria, or plants, to clean up or detoxify environmental pollution. A less hazardous and less expensive alternative to conventional chemical and physical methods, this eco-friendly measure utilizes natural biological mechanisms to degrade, immobilize, or transform toxic materials into less harmful substances (Sharma, 2025; Qin et al., 2022). Environmental pollution, in the form of air, water, and land degradation, has increased in response to rapid industrialization, urbanization, and agricultural development. Heavy metals, hydrocarbons, dyes, and pesticides are just a few of the persistent pollutants that accumulate in ecosystems, presenting widespread risks to human health and the environment (Singh et al., 2025a). Wastewater treatment involves the elimination of heavy metals, fertilizers, and organic contaminants from municipal and industrial wastewater using microalgae and bacteria (Priya et al., 2022). Aquaculture waste and textile dye effluents can be effectively treated by algae-based systems (Nair et al., 2023). Petroleum hydrocarbons are transformed into safe molecules by adding fungus and bacteria that break down hydrocarbons, such as those found in marine oil spills (Gouthami et al., 2023). Bioremediation reduces pesticide and herbicide residues in agricultural soils, thereby increasing soil fertility and minimizing crop damage. Both macroalgae and microalgae have been used to eliminate heavy metals from polluted water bodies (Priya et al., 2022). These biosorbents are appealing due to their ease of production and natural abundance. In landfills, microorganisms decompose organic materials, lowering leachate toxicity and methane emissions (Bhardwaj et al., 2025).

The process of bioremediation is advantageous in removing heavy metals, hydrocarbons, and dyes from polluted environments (Verma & Kuila, 2019). It utilizes natural processes, such as biosorption, bioaccumulation, and bioaugmentation, which minimize the presence of harsh, toxic materials in the environment, making it eco-friendly (Visvanathan et al., 2024). Different microorganisms, such as *Chlorella*, *Scenedesmus*, and *Spirulina*, degrade hydrocarbons from oil spills, making the surrounding clean (Ahmad, 2022). These processes help in cleaning organic contaminants from air, water, and soil, making it versatile for a wide range of use (Liu et al., 2022). It restores the microbial diversity of the soil, which in turn helps increase agricultural productivity (Gupta et al., 2022). In comparison with the traditional methods (such as excavation and chemical treatment), bioremediation minimizes the cost, which makes it approachable for the consumers (Sharma, 2020). This process does not create secondary pollutants in the natural environment. Hence, no further clean-up is required to utilize natural resources (Bhaskar & Lakshminarayanachari, 2021). The effectiveness of the process depends on environmental conditions such as temperature, pH, nutrient availability, and oxygen levels (Mishra et al., 2021). Some pollutants are highly recalcitrant and cannot be easily degraded biologically (Kumari & Das, 2023). Additionally, large-scale applications may require continuous monitoring, and in some cases, the rate of degradation may be slower than that achieved by chemical or physical methods (Lan et al., 2024). Another challenge is ensuring that organisms used for bioremediation do not introduce invasive traits or ecological imbalances (Gaylarde & da Fonseca, 2025).

Microorganisms, such as bacteria, fungi, and algae, utilize processes like biosorption, bioaccumulation, and biotransformation to degrade or immobilize pollutants. Through the process of biosorption, metal ions are adsorbed onto functional groups on cell surfaces, including carboxyl, hydroxyl, and amino groups, resulting in passive elimination (Wang & Chen, 2009). Through bioaccumulation, pollutants are actively accumulated into cells and subsequently transformed or sequestered (Malik, 2004). The toxicity of industrial effluent can be reduced by microbes, such as *Pseudomonas*, which are capable of converting the highly toxic Cr^{6+} into the less toxic Cr^{3+} (Cheng et al., 2017). Due to their large surface area and potential for rapid growth under diverse environmental conditions, algae are highly effective (Wang et al., 2020). Hydrocarbons, pesticides, and solvents are biodegraded by bacteria such as *Pseudomonas, Bacillus,* and *Rhizobium* species (Das & Chandran, 2011). Organic pollutants and dyes are degraded by *Aspergillus* species-secreted and white-rot fungus-secreted enzymes (*Phanerochaete chrysosporium*) (Kumar et al., 2015). Macroalgae such as *Sargassum, Ulva,* and *Gracilaria* are used in wastewater treatment and biofilter systems (Mat et al., 2010; Davis et al., 2003), whereas microalgae such as *Chlorella, Scenedesmus,* and *Spirulina* are efficient in heavy metal adsorption such as Pb^{2+}, Cd^{2+}, Cu^{2+}, Ni^{2+}, and Zn^{2+} (Wang & Chen, 2009) (Table 2.1). Due to their rapid growth, high surface area, and metabolic flexibility, both microalgae and macroalgae are critical to bioremediation, also known as phycoremediation (Karnwal et al., 2024). The techniques, algae, and recent advances in algal-mediated pollution abatement are the focal areas of this chapter. It also identifies areas of research that are lacking and highlights how modern molecular tools, such as transcriptomics and proteomics, could enhance the efficiency of phycoremediation.

Bioremediation offers a sustainable and cost-effective approach to eliminate persistent environmental contaminants, including heavy metals, dyes, and hydrocarbons. Microorganisms and algae eliminate toxic heavy metals like Cr, Pb, Cd, Cu, Ni, and Zn through biosorption, bioaccumulation, and biotransformation (Wang & Chen, 2009). Degradation of industrial dyes and petroleum hydrocarbons is mediated through enzymatic and metabolic routes. The efficiency of these processes can be substantially influenced by the most crucial abiotic environmental parameters, which include pH, temperature, nutrient availability, oxygen levels, and pollutant concentration. Algal-based systems are considered most efficient for integrated wastewater treatment due to their quick growth rates, substantial surface area, and metabolic versatility (Karnwal et al., 2024). Although limited by issues of pollutant levels and scalability, this system can be further improved with

Table 2.1 Types of algae utilized for bioremediation

S. N.	Type	Scientific name	Pollutants removed	Mechanism	Applications	References
1	Microalgae	*Chlorella vulgaris*	Pb^{2+}, Cd^{2+}, Cu^{2+}, Zn^{2+}, dyes	Biosorption, bioaccumulation, and enzymatic degradation	Wastewater treatment, heavy metal removal	Wu (2024)
2	Microalgae	*Scenedesmus obliquus*	Cr^{6+}, Ni^{2+}, hydrocarbons	Cell wall adsorption, biofilm formation	Industrial effluent treatment	Mohebi et al. (2024)
3	Microalgae	*Spirulina platensis (Arthrospira)*	Pb^{2+}, dye molecules	Surface binding, intracellular uptake	Food industry wastewater	Chen (2025)
4	Microalgae	*Nostoc muscorum*	Hydrocarbons, heavy metals	EPS production, biodegradation	Oil spill bioremediation	Singh et al. (2025a, b)
5	Microalgae	*Oscillatoria tenuis*	Cu^{2+}, Zn^{2+}, hydrocarbons	Biosorption, biofilm growth	Aquatic ecosystem restoration	Sethi and Jonwal (2025)
6	Microalgae	*Navicula permitis*	Cr, Ni, Pb	Silica cell wall adsorption	Industrial effluent treatment	Elhamji et al. (2025)
7	Macroalgae	*Sargassum* sp.	Pb^{2+}, Cd^{2+}, dyes	Cell wall polysaccharides bind pollutants	Textile dye wastewater	Ahmad et al. (2025)
8	Macroalgae	*Gracilaria* sp.	Cu^{2+}, Zn^{2+}, hydrocarbons	Biosorption via agar, carrageenan matrix	Heavy metal and dye removal	Khattar et al. (2016)
9	Macroalgae	*Ulva lactuca*	Ni^{2+}, Cr^{6+}, Pb^{2+}	Biosorption, extracellular polymer secretion	Municipal wastewater	Younis (2025)
10	Macroalgae	*Ascophyllum nodosum*	Hg^{2+}, Pb^{2+}, dyes	Alginates in cell wall bind metals	Industrial effluent treatment	Foday Jr et al. (2021)

advancements in new molecular tools to increase remediation efficiency (Wang, 2025). Hence, algal bioremediation is a promising approach for managing heavy metal, dye, and hydrocarbon pollution in a sustainable manner.

2.2 Algal Remediation

Algal bioremediation occurs through various processes, including biosorption, bioaccumulation, and detoxification (Mishra et al., 2021). In biosorption, heavy metals are concentrated on a surface (Shabaan et al., 2025). Bioaccumulation processes accumulate toxic compounds in the body, whereas in the case of detoxification, algae convert these toxic substances into less toxic ones (Bai et al., 2025). Algal bioremediation functions through a combination of mechanisms, including fast cell-wall and extracellular polymeric substance (EPS) biosorption, emulsification and hydrophobic partitioning by biosurfactant and EPS, active uptake and intracellular sequestration, and enzymatic oxidation–reduction or co-metabolism for degradable organics (Murugesan et al., 2025). The algal cell wall and EPS contain high levels of functional groups, including carboxyl, hydroxyl, phosphate, sulphate, and amine that facilitate ion exchange, surface complexation, electrostatic attraction, π–π interaction, and micro-precipitation (Anand et al., 2023), which all together enable high-affinity capture of cationic metals and aromatic organics at low concentrations (Molebatsi et al., 2025). Depending on the intended application, both living cultures and immobilized/non-living algal biomasses are utilized. Living systems integrate pollutant removal with nutrient assimilation and oxygen production (Cavalletti, 2025), whereas dried or immobilized biomasses favor rapid, regenerable adsorption, which is beneficial in columns (Singh et al. 2024b).

2.2.1 Types of Algae

2.2.1.1 Microalgae

Microalgae are small and unicellular organisms (Thoré et al., 2023). They grow fast and have a high surface area (Shi et al., 2021). Their cell walls are rich in polysaccharides, proteins, lipids, and different pigments. Such pigments have different functional groups that bind the heavy metals (Ayele et al., 2021). Some of the functional groups are -OH, –COOH, $-SO_3H$, $-NH_2$ (Muñoz-Rivera et al., 2025). Numerous taxa, including *Chlorella vulgaris*, *Scenedesmus obliquus*, *Spirulina*, *Arthrospira*, *Nostoc* spp., and *Synechococcus* spp. are classified as microalgae (Hachicha et al., 2022). These creatures can be benthic, clinging to surfaces like rocks or sediments, or free-floating in aquatic habitats (phytoplankton) (Jackson et al., 2024). Microalgae can be found worldwide and thrive in a variety of habitats, including freshwater lakes, rivers, saltwater lagoons, deserts, and even the polar regions (Jana et al., 2024). One of the most remarkable features of microalgae is their ability to tolerate environmental extremes (Kumari et al., 2022). For instance, cyanobacteria (blue-green algae), such as *Nostoc* and *Oscillatoria*, can survive in hot springs with temperatures above 70 °C, while others can withstand high UV radiation in polar ice and deserts (Bataeva & Grigoryan, 2024). Their metabolic flexibility also allows them to utilize diverse nutrient sources, enabling growth in wastewater streams rich in organic matter, nitrates, phosphates, and even toxic heavy metals (Gärtner et al., 2021). This is due to their versatility; microalgae are excellent choices for biotechnological applications such as wastewater treatment, biofuel generation, medicine production, nutraceuticals, and feed additives for agriculture and aquaculture (Yaacob et al., 2022). As primary producers, they also serve as the foundation of aquatic food webs, providing nourishment for fish, zooplankton, and other higher trophic species (Wang, 2025).

2.2.1.2 Macroalgae

They are large, photosynthetic, multicellular algae that grow in freshwater and marine environments and are known as macroalgae, or seaweeds (Pereira, 2021). Macroalgae are visible to the human eye and frequently form extensive underwater forests or meadows (Flores-Moya et al., 2021), in contrast to microalgae, which are minuscule (Spalding et al., 2019). Based on their pigmentation, they can be generally divided into three groups: red algae (Rhodophyta), brown algae (Phaeophyceae), and green algae (Chlorophyta) (Taglioni et al., 2025) (Fig. 2.1). Each group has unique ecological responsibilities, pigments, and storage goods. They produce oxygen, store carbon dioxide, and provide food and habitat for a diverse range of marine creatures. Macroalgae are essential to aquatic ecosystems. They serve as the main

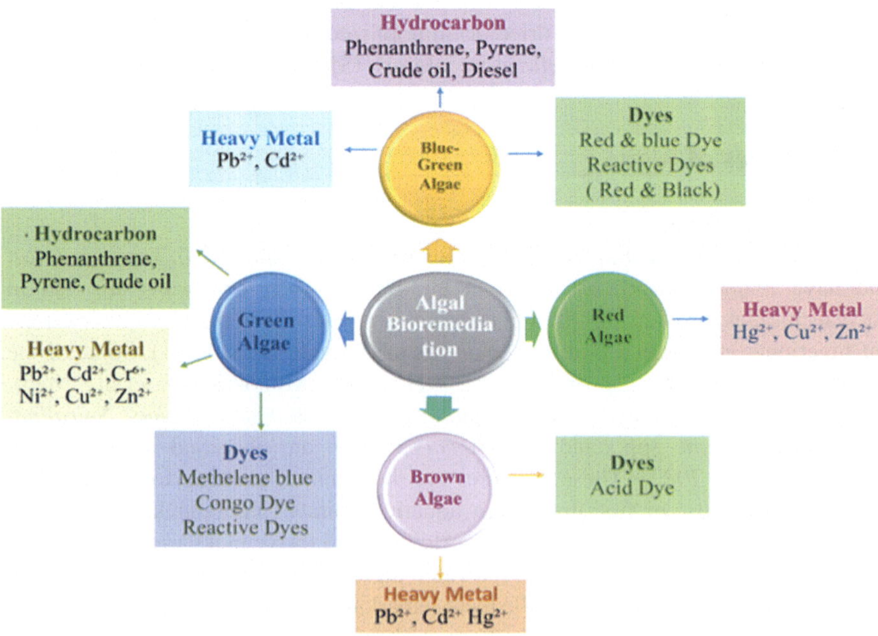

Fig. 2.1 Algal bioremediation schematic diagram for heavy metal, hydrocarbon, and dye removal

producers in the ecosystem and are the foundation of many marine food webs. They are harvested economically for their food (e.g., Porphyra, Laminaria), hydrocolloids (e.g., agar, carrageenan, and alginate), and bioactive chemicals that have medicinal uses. Furthermore, the function of macroalgae in bioremediation is becoming more widely acknowledged (Varabih & Nofirman, 2023). Through the polysaccharides in their cell walls, they can collect and accumulate harmful heavy metals like lead, cadmium, and arsenic, as well as excess nutrients like nitrogen and phosphorus from contaminated waterways (Iddrisu et al., 2024). They are therefore useful instruments for treating wastewater and restoring coastal ecosystems.

2.2.2 Removal of Contaminants by Algae

2.2.2.1 Heavy Metal Removal

Macroalgae and microalgae have both demonstrated significant promise in removing heavy metals through processes such as complexation, ion exchange, biosorption, and bioaccumulation. Through surface functional groups like carboxyl and hydroxyl, *Chlorella vulgaris* and *Chlorella pyrenoidosa* efficiently adsorb Pb^{2+}, Cd^{2+}, Cu^{2+}, Ni^{2+}, and Cr^{6+} (Wang, 2025). The removal of various metals via biosorption and extracellular polymeric substances (EPS) is another method used by *Scenedesmus obliquus* and *Desmodesmus* sp. The latter provides the advantages of both remediation and the generation of sustainable biofuel (Ganguly et al., 2024). *Spirulina platensis*'s excellent binding capacity and simple processing further enhance its large-scale application. *Synechococcus elongatus* combines rapid growth with genetic plasticity, making it a suitable fit for designed systems, while cyanobacteria like *Nostoc muscorum* and *Oscillatoria tenuis* utilize EPS and bioaccumulation for detoxification. For high-capacity metal adsorption, diatoms such as *Navicula permitis* and *Nitzschia palea* use their silica frustules and functional groups (Akbar et al., 2025). Additionally, macroalgae are important. *Sargassum wightii* and other *Sargassum* species are known to exhibit significant biosorption capabilities through their cell walls, which are rich in alginate (Salimi et al., 2025). While *Caulerpa racemosa* aids in wastewater treatment and aquaculture by lowering the accumulation of hazardous metals, *Ulva lactuca* is versatile in both its raw and processed forms (Imaduddin & Eilks, 2025) (Table 2.2). With its high surface area and filamentous structure, *Cladophora glomerata* provides effective, affordable, and sustainable cleanup. It also has the potential to be valuable in the manufacture of fertilizer and biofuel (Akbar et al., 2025).

The polysaccharide-rich cell walls of red and brown macroalgae have made them excellent biosorbents for heavy metal cleanup. *Sargassum muticum* exhibits remarkable elimination of Pb^{2+}, Cd^{2+}, Hg^{2+}, Cu^{2+}, Zn^{2+}, and Ni^{2+} among these. Its alginate, which is abundant and inexpensive for treating wastewater, is rich in negatively charged carboxyl groups that enable ion exchange and complexation with divalent cations (Selvakumar et al., 2023). The potential of modified seaweed-based sorbents is demonstrated by the improvement of *Ascophyllum nodosum* through chemical modification and nano-magnetite integration, which increased the absorption

Table 2.2 Types of microalgae utilized for heavy metal remediation

Sl No.	Scientific name	Heavy metals	Mechanism	Conditions	Reference
1	*Chlorella vulgaris*	Pb^{2+}, Cd^{2+}, Cu^{2+}, Zn^{2+}, Ni^{2+}, Cr^{6+}, As^{3+}	Biosorption via carboxyl/ hydroxyl groups; active intracellular bioaccumulation	Model organism for phycoremediation; fast growth	Cheng et al. (2017)
2	*Chlorella pyrenoidosa*	Pb^{2+}, Cd^{2+}, Cr^{6+}, Ni^{2+}	Surface binding via polysaccharides and proteins	Efficient Pb and Cd remover; used in lab-scale wastewater treatment	Lalhruaitluangi et al. (2025)
3	*Scenedesmus obliquus*	Pb^{2+}, Cu^{2+}, Cd^{2+}, Zn^{2+}, Ni^{2+}	EPS secretion + cell wall polymers bind metals	Often coupled with biofuel production	Naveed et al. (2019)
4	*Desmodesmus* sp.	Cr^{6+} Cd^{2+}, Pb^{2+}	Biosorption + bioaccumulation	High potential for Cr^{6+} detoxification	Ganguly et al. (2024)
5	*Spirulina platensis*	Pb^{2+}, Cd^{2+}, Cu^{2+}, Ni^{2+}, Zn^{2+}	Protein-rich cell wall → carboxyl and amino binding sites	Used as a powdered biosorbent	Malletzidou et al. (2025)
6	*Nostoc muscorum*	Cd^{2+}, Pb^{2+}, Cr^{6+}, Cu^{2+}	EPS-mediated sequestration; surface sorption	Strong capacity for Cd and Pb	Bandara (2025)
7	*Oscillatoria tenuis*	Pb^{2+}, Cu^{2+}, Cr^{6+}, Ni^{2+}	Surface biosorption + intracellular uptake	Studied in mixed metal wastewater	Sethi and Jonwal (2025)
8	*Synechococcus elongatus*	Cd^{2+}, Cu^{2+}, Zn^{2+}	Surface sorption, fast uptake kinetics	Model cyanobacterium for engineered remediation	Sha et al., (2025)
9	*Navicula permitis*	Pb^{2+}, Cd^{2+}, Cu^{2+}, Cr^{6+}	Silica frustule enhances adsorption sites	Two-step uptake: Surface then intracellular	Elhamji et al. (2025)
10	*Nitzschia palea*	Cr^{6+}, Cu^{2+}	Silica-based biosorption + metabolic uptake	Used in urban wastewater remediation studies	Nagar et al., (2025)

efficiencies of metals like Cu^{2+} to above 90% (Kumar et al., 2021). Due to their alginate concentration, other brown algae, such *Fucus vesiculosus*, also demonstrate a strong biosorption ability under a variety of circumstances, enhancing their status as environmentally benign substitutes. This potential is further expanded by red algae: Sulfated polysaccharides (agar, carrageenan) are used by *Gracilaria corticata* and *Gelidium* spp. to effectively sequester Pb^{2+}, Cd^{2+}, Cu^{2+}, and Zn^{2+} (Table 2.3). Widely grown as nori, *Porphyra* spp. exhibits adaptable Cd^{2+}, Cu^{2+}, and Zn^{2+} adsorption over a variety of pH ranges, and its edible nature attracts integrated biorefineries (Li et al., 2024).

Furthermore, laboratory investigations demonstrate that *Hypnea musciformis* exhibits high Pb^{2+}, Cu^{2+}, and Ni^{2+} absorption, as evidenced by cell wall thickening and color reductions following exposure. Its ability to concentrate trace elements without posing health hazards is confirmed by field evaluations, establishing it as a biosorbent and biomonitoring tool. When taken as a whole, these macroalgae provide economical, sustainable, and abundant methods for heavy metal bioremediation (Bai et al., 2025).

2.2.2.2 Hydrocarbon Removal

The hydrophobicity and phototoxicity of hydrocarbons, such as petroleum-derived alkanes and polycyclic aromatic hydrocarbons (PAHs), hinder algal photosynthesis, growth, and membranes (Fig. 2.1). For some PAHs, stress is often increased at higher irradiance. Nevertheless, algae combat hydrocarbons through hydrophobic adsorption to cell surfaces and EPS, biosurfactant/EPS-facilitated emulsification that increases bioavailability, and oxygenase/peroxidase-catalyzed conversions that detoxify lighter aromatics and n-alkanes. While bacterial consortia tend to increase mineralization above algal adsorption in isolation and improve treatment of mixed contaminants in wastewater and oil-contaminated waters, in practice, it is crucial to control light regime, pollutant load, and nutrients to balance productivity against hydrocarbon stress (Maglione et al., 2024). Hydrocarbons, particularly polycyclic aromatic hydrocarbons (PAHs), interfere with algal membranes, inhibit photosynthesis, and inhibit growth, with toxicity generally enhanced under elevated light due to photochemical stress. PAHs are capable of partitioning into lipid structures in algal cells, thereby modifying membrane integrity and reducing photosystem II efficiency, as indicated by reductions in chlorophyll fluorescence indices (e.g., Fv/Fm) under pyrene stress, particularly in sensitive species such as *Chlorella vulgaris* at elevated irradiance. Phototoxicity of PAHs has been reported at various trophic levels, starting from algae, highlighting the need for caution in managing irradiance and exposure when establishing algal remediation schemes. The extent of inhibition is species-specific, with a few algae (e.g., *Scenedesmus acutus*) exhibiting superior photosynthetic proficiency under PAH stress compared to others, suggesting species-specific tolerance and adaptive mechanisms (Patel et al., 2020). Table 2.4 illustrates the Removal of hydrocarbons by algae and associated aspects.

Table 2.3 Types of macroalgae utilized for heavy metal removal

S. N.	*Scientific name*	Heavy metals	Primary mechanism	Conditions	Reference
1	*Sargassum wightii*	Cr^{6+}, Cr^{3+}, Pb^{2+}, Cd^{2+}, Cu^{2+}, Zn^{2+}, Ni^{2+}	Biosorption via alginate carboxyl groups; ion exchange; surface complexation	High affinity for divalent cations; effective across pH ~4–6	Tamilselvan et al. (2012)
2	*Sargassum* spp.	Cd^{2+}, Pb^{2+}, Cu^{2+}, Ni^{2+}, Zn^{2+}	Carboxylic groups of alginate dominate binding; ion exchange	Classic high-capacity biosorbent among brown seaweeds	Davis et al. (2003)
3	*Ulva lactuca*	Pb^{2+}, Cd^{2+}, Cu^{2+}, Ni^{2+}, Zn^{2+}, Fe^{2+}	Biosorption via hydroxyl/carboxyl groups; ion exchange; sometimes with activated carbon	Effective across pH ~5–7; can be used raw or as activated carbon/ biochar	Ghoneim et al. (2014)
4	*Caulerpa racemosa*	Cr^{6+}, Pb^{2+}, Cu^{2+}	Biosorption; kinetic/thermo parameters studied; activated carbon comparison	Evaluates dosage, pH, contact time, initial concentration	Akbar et al. (2025)
5	*Cladophora glomerata*	Pb^{2+}, Zn^{2+}, Cu^{2+}, Cd^{2+}	Biosorption; batch experiments	Simultaneous removal of Pb2+ and Congo red	Zhang et al. (2025)
6	*Sargassum muticum*	Pb^{2+}, Cd^{2+}, Hg^{2+}, Cr^{6+}, Cu^{2+}, Zn^{2+}, Ni^{2+}	Biosorption; response surface methodology optimization	Statistical optimization for cadmium removal	Chaouay et al., (2025)
7	*Padina pavonica*	Pb^{2+}, Cd^{2+}, Ni^{2+}, Cu^{2+}	Biosorption via cell wall functional groups; ion exchange	Studied alongside *Sargassum wightii*	Tamilselvan et al. (2012)
8	*Laminaria digitata*	Pb^{2+}, Cd^{2+}, Zn^{2+}, Cu^{2+}	Alginate beads/ xerogels sorption; ion exchange with Ca/Na in alginate	Alginate-based beads widely tested for cations	Raab et al., (2025)
9	*Ascophyllum nodosum*	Pb^{2+}, Cd^{2+}, Hg^{2+}, Cu^{2+}	Immobilized biomass with alginate xerogels	Classical system for metal uptake studies	Ashok et al., (2025)

(continued)

Table 2.3 (continued)

S. N.	*Scientific name*	Heavy metals	Primary mechanism	Conditions	Reference
10	*Fucus vesiculosus*	Pb^{2+}, Cd^{2+}, Ni^{2+}, Zn^{2+}	Biochar/ bioadsorbent from seaweed biomass	High reported efficiencies in batch tests	Younis, (2025)
11	*Gracilaria corticata*	Pb^{2+}, Cd^{2+}, Cu^{2+}, Zn^{2+}, Ni^{2+}	Biosorption; simultaneous metal +dye removal; bioaccumulation/ depuration in cultivation	Demonstrated simultaneous Ni2+ and dye removal; cultivation reduces coastal metals	Agoun & Avci (2025)
12	*Gelidium* spp.	Cu^{2+}, Pb^{2+}, Zn^{2+}	Bioaccumulation in cultivation zones; risk and removal capacity assessment	Cultivation shown to decrease heavy metals in seawater	Carvalho et al. (2025)
13	*Porphyra* spp.	Cd^{2+}, Cu^{2+}, Zn^{2+}	Biosorption; comparison with activated carbon	Evaluated alongside *Ulva lactuca*	Park et al., (2025)
14	*Hypnea musciformis*	Pb^{2+}, Cu^{2+}, Ni^{2+}	Two-stage uptake: rapid adsorption then slower intracellular processes	Outdoor tank depuration study describes two-stage mechanism	Mishra et al. (2021)

2.2.2.3 Dyes Removal

Algae have shown promise as biosorbents, offering an affordable and environmentally responsible alternative to traditional methods for eliminating synthetic dyes. Regeneration cycles, dye specificity, and biosorption on cell-wall functional groups enabled species such as *Ulva fasciata* and *Oedogonium* sp. to remove reactive and methylene blue dyes 60–97% of the time (Sadiq et al., 2025). Using electrostatic attraction and enzymatic degradation, microalgae such as *Chlorella vulgaris* and *Scenedesmus obliquus* have been shown to remove up to 97% of methylene blue and other colors while simultaneously generating lipid-rich biomass for biofuel (Ali et al., 2023). Although performance deteriorates under changing pH and temperature conditions, filamentous green algae, such as *Spirogyra* and *Chara vulgaris*, were removed to a degree of over 90% (Hossain et al., 2023) (Table 2.5). According to Sani (2025), mixed algal consortia further improved removal effectiveness, reaching ~95–97% under ideal conditions for various dye types, demonstrating their potential for use in photobioreactors and large-scale wastewater ponds. All things considered, dye sequestration and biomass valorization into fertilizers, feed, and bioenergy are combined in algae-based systems (Das and Bhattarai, 2025). Algae offer a scalable and sustainable approach for treating industrial wastewater, despite their slower kinetics and environmental sensitivity compared to chemical methods (Ethiraj & Samuel, 2024). They also have the added benefit of remediation and resource

Table 2.4 Removal of hydrocarbons by algae

S. N.	Algal species	Target hydrocarbon	Removal efficiency	Removal mechanism	Advantages	Disadvantages	Large-scale production	References
1..	*Scenedesmus quadricauda*	Phenanthrene Benzo (a)anthracene	72.3% 61.8%	Biosorption; uptake and intracellular enzymatic breakdown; extracellular polymeric substance (EPS) binding	High growth rate, effective for PAHs, low-cost biomass production, synergistic removal by oxidation and biodegradation	Highly sensitive to environmental fluctuations, Fenton reagent handling and cost	Potential in wastewater treatment systems, but scaling requires stable environmental control	Rani et al. (2023)
2.	*Chlorella vulgaris*	Polycyclic aromatic hydrocarbons (PAHs)—phenanthrene, pyrene	Phenanthrene: ~60–70; Pyrene: ~55–65	Biosorption via cell wall functional groups; bioaccumulation; enzymatic degradation (lipases, oxygenases)	High biomass productivity, effective PAH degradation	Requires continuous light and nutrient supply	Suitable for photobioreactor and open pond systems for wastewater/oil spill treatment	Shourie & Vijayalakshmi (2022)
3.	*Scenedesmus obliquus*	Phenanthrene, pyrene, naphthalene	70–90%	Biosorption; uptake and intracellular enzymatic breakdown; extracellular polymeric substance (EPS) binding	High biodegradation rate of light PAHs Broad-spectrum hydrocarbon degradation	Limited efficiency for heavy PAHs Sensitive to sudden environmental changes	Feasible for industrial wastewater treatment in open ponds or bioreactors	Paniagua-Michel & Banat (2024)

4.	*Synechococcus* sp.	Light PAHs (phenanthrene, pyrene)	78–82%	Biosorption; uptake into cells; oxidative degradation by oxygenases	High tolerance to varying salinity and pH	Sensitive to extreme hydrocarbon levels; light limitation impacts performance	Potential in marine oil spill remediation	Hamouda et al. (2022)
5.	*Botryococcus braunii*	Crude oil fractions	~60%	Adsorption to extracellular matrix, bioaccumulation and enzymatic degradation	Hydrocarbon accumulation potential, possible biofuel production	Sensitive to environmental changes	Potential for integrated biofuel-remediation operations	Prasad et al. (2023)
6.	*Oscillatoria* sp.	Diesel, crude oil (n-alkanes C10–C20, PAHs)	Diesel: ~70–80; crude oil: ~65–75	Biosorption via extracellular sheath; biofilm-mediated trapping; enzymatic degradation of hydrocarbons	Can degrade complex hydrocarbon mixtures	Lower biomass productivity than green algae	Suitable for in situ oil spill bioremediation in tropical and subtropical waters	Saleh & Abdulhasan (2023)
7.	*Anabaena sp*	Crude oil, kerosene	Crude oil: ~55–65; kerosene: ~60–70	Biosorption on extracellular sheath; metabolic degradation via oxidative enzymes	Nitrogen fixation reduces fertilizer need	Slower degradation for heavy hydrocarbons	Applicable for large-scale pond-based remediation in warm climates	Akl et al. (2023)
8.	*Nostoc muscorum*	Diesel, lubricating oil	Diesel: ~50–60; lubricating oil: ~45–55	Biosorption on mucilaginous sheath; slow metabolic breakdown	Resilient to varied environments	Low efficiency for high-molecular-weight PAHs	Suitable for constructed wetlands or pond systems	Dell’Anno et al., (2021)

(continued)

Table 2.4 (continued)

S. N.	Algal species	Target hydrocarbon	Removal efficiency	Removal mechanism	Advantages	Disadvantages	Large-scale production	References
9.	*Nannochloropsis oculata*	Diesel, kerosene, gasoline (n-alkanes: C10–C18)	Diesel: ~65–75; kerosene: ~80–85; gasoline: ~70–75	Hydrophobic cell surfaces enhance adhesion; biosurfactant production; enzymatic oxidation of hydrocarbons	Tolerates wide hydrocarbon range; high removal rates; marine adaptability	Growth inhibition at high hydrocarbon concentrations; fuel-type dependent efficiency	Excellent for marine/coastal oil pollution treatment	Amran et al. (2022)
10.	*Chlamydomonas reinhardtii*	Phenanthrene, anthracene, pyrene	Phenanthrene: ~60; anthracene: ~55; Pyrene: ~50	Biosorption to cell wall; uptake into cells; enzymatic oxidation by oxygenases/ peroxidases; EPS secretion aiding emulsification and bioavailability	Genetic tractability for strain improvement; can be engineered for better degradation	Sensitive to high pollutant load; slow removal of heavy PAHs	Potential in specialized or genetically modified strains for targeted PAH cleanup	Perera et al., (2019)
11.	*Spirulina platensis*	Crude oil, diesel	Crude oil: ~70–80; diesel: ~60–70	Biosorption on cell surface; intracellular uptake; limited enzymatic degradation	High protein biomass; can be used as a co-product source	Lower tolerance to heavy PAHs; prefers moderate contamination	Possible in integrated biorefinery and remediation setups	Akl et al. (2023)

Table 2.5 Removal of dyes by algae

Sl. No.	Algal species	Targeted dye	Removal efficiency	Advantages	Disadvantages	Large-scale applications	Removal mechanism	References
1	*Ulva fasciata*	Reactive yellow 2 (RY2) Reactive red 195 (RR195) Reactive blue 19 (RB19) -reactive black 5 (RB5)	RY2: 82.75% RR195: 83.23% RB19: 60.06% RB5: 78.73%	High removal efficiency Low-cost biomass Environmentally friendly Versatility Simple operation Reusability	Slower process Sensitivity to environmental conditions Limited regeneration cycles Scaling challenges Disposal of spent biomass	Biomass sourcing and production Reactor design Integration into existing treatment plants	Biosorption to algal cell walls. Two-phase adsorption process. Enzymatic degradation (for living biomass).	El-Agawany et al., (2023)
2.	*Oedogonium* sp.	Methylene blue (MB)	97.43%	High removal efficiency Low-cost and readily available biomass Eco-friendly process Effective for cationic dyes	Limited dye specificity Sensitivity to environmental conditions Biomass preparation needed Regeneration limitations	Biomass sourcing and cultivation.	Adsorption onto cell wall functional groups.	Sadiq et al. (2025)
3	*Chlorella vulgaris*	Methylene blue (MB)	95.8%	High removal efficiency for cationic dyes Low-cost and eco-friendly biomass source No toxic byproducts	Lower efficiency for non-cationic dyes Sensitive to pH, temperature, and dye concentration	Feasible in both batch and continuous-flow systems	Primary mechanism: Biosorption via functional groups (–OH, –COOH, $–NH_2$, $–SO_3H$) on cell walls.	Ali et al. (2023)

(continued)

Table 2.5 (continued)

Sl. No.	Algal species	Targeted dye	Removal efficiency	Advantages	Disadvantages	Large-scale applications	Removal mechanism	References
4	*Spirogyra hyalina*	Methylene blue (MB)	99%	Very high removal efficiency Abundant and low-cost biomass source Eco-friendly process without toxic byproducts Works effectively for cationic dyes like MB	Lower efficiency for non-cationic dyes Sensitive to environmental factors like pH and temperature Biomass regeneration may cause capacity loss	Can be implemented in both batch and continuous systems Requires steady biomass supply through controlled cultivation or harvesting	Biosorption via functional groups (–OH, –COOH, $-NH_2$, –SO_3H) on algal cell walls.	Hossain et al., (2023)
5	*Spirogyra* sp. *Oscillatoria* sp.	Blue dye Red dye	*Spirogyra* sp.: 94.44% (blue dye), 58% (red dye) in 14 days at 3% biomass *Oscillatoria* sp.: 92.77% (blue dye), 40% (red dye) in same conditions	Effective for reactive dyes without chemical additives Blue dye removal very high (>92%) Non-toxic end products to beneficial soil bacteria (*Azotobacter* sp., *rhizobium* sp.)	Red dye removal efficiency much lower (40–58%) Long treatment time (14 days) Requires large biomass amounts for higher efficiency	Feasible for dye-contaminated industrial effluents where long retention times are acceptable. Potential use as a biological polishing step after primary/secondary treatment.	Biodegradation and biosorption: Functional groups on algal biomass bind dyes, followed by enzymatic or metabolic breakdown.	Brahmbhatt and Jasrai (2015)
6	*ADS-1.* *ADS-2.*	Direct blue dye (azo dye)	ADS-1: ~93.8%	Achieves high dye removal (>83% for low	Longer treatment time (15 days for	Can be integrated into existing wastewater	Biosorption of dye onto algal biomass.	Alseroury (2018)

			ADS-2: ~83.8%	concentrations) Produces algal biomass rich in fats (up to 75%), suitable for biofuel production	maximum decolorization). Lower efficiency at high initial dye concentrations.	treatment systems. Offers dual benefit of pollution removal and energy production.	Enzymatic degradation (azo-reductase breaking azo bonds; oxidative enzymes may also act).	
7	*Enteromorpha intestinalis*	Malachite green (MG)	94%	High removal efficiency at low biomass cost Simple process without harmful chemicals Biomass naturally abundant and renewable	Reduced efficiency at higher dye concentrations Sensitive to pH changes (optimal at pH 6)	Potential for integration into textile wastewater treatment plants Effective as a low-cost biosorbent for cationic dyes	Biosorption via negatively charged functional groups (–OH, –COOH, –SO_3H) on cell walls binding cationic MG molecules	Abo-Shady et al. (2021)
8	*Chara vulgaris*	Methylene blue (MB)	92.59%	High MB removal efficiency with low-cost biomass Eco-friendly and renewable adsorbent source Effective in natural pH conditions without chemical additives	Reduced efficiency at higher dye concentrations Sensitive to pH and temperature fluctuations Limited regeneration potential without efficiency loss	Feasible for integration into wastewater treatment for cationic dyes	Biosorption via functional groups (–OH, –COOH, –NH_2) on algal cell walls Electrostatic attraction between negatively charged biomass and cationic MB molecules	Gomaa et al. (2022)
9	*Scenedesmus obliquus*	Methylene blue (MB)	97.36%	Very high MB removal efficiency	Efficiency drops at higher dye concentrations	Can be implemented in both batch and	Biosorption through hydroxyl (–OH),	Shahi Khalaf Ansar et al. (2023)

(continued)

Table 2.5 (continued)

Sl. No.	Algal species	Targeted dye	Removal efficiency	Advantages	Disadvantages	Large-scale applications	Removal mechanism	References
				Abundant and easily cultivable microalga Environmentally friendly process without harmful byproducts	Biomass regeneration cycles may reduce adsorption capacity Requires careful pH control for optimal performance	column systems for textile wastewater treatment Suitable for integration into existing treatment plants as a polishing step	carboxyl (–COOH), and amino (–NH_2) groups on cell walls	
10	*Chlorella vulgaris, cyanobacteria & Nostoc linckia HA 46*	*Chlorella vulgaris*—Yellow 2G (azo dye) *Cyanobacteria & Nostoc linckia* HA 46—Reactive red 198	*Chlorella vulgaris*—63–69% *Cyanobacteria & Nostoc linckia* HA 46—94%	Cost-effective Environmentally friendly High biosorption capacity Versatile Dual benefit Potential for wastewater nutrient removal	Effective mainly at low dye concentrations and volumes Variable efficiency Slower process Sensitivity to pollutants Scalability challenges Bioavailability limitations	High rate treatment systems (HRTS) have been applied in developing countries to achieve near zero discharge from dye industries by cultivating specific plant/algal species	Biosorption via electrostatic attraction to cell wall functional groups Enzymatic breakdown Chromophore conversion into non-colored compounds	Gayathiri et al., (2022)
11	*Chlorella vulgaris Scenedesmus*	Methylene blue—Removed by	*Chlorella vulgaris*—90% MB	Low-cost and eco-friendly compared to	Efficiency drops at high dye concentrations	Potential in constructed wetlands, algal	Biosorption—Electrostatic attraction	Agarwal et al. (2016)

	obliquus *Spirogyra* sp. *Ulva lactuca*	*Chlorella vulgaris* and *Ulva lactuca* Congo red—Removed by *Scenedesmus obliquus* Reactive black 5—Removed by *spirogyra* sp.	*Scenedesmus obliquus*—80% CR *Spirogyra* sp.—Approximately 70% removal of RB-5. *Ulva lactuca*—85% MB	chemical treatments Can remove a wide variety of dyes, including toxic azo dyes	Sensitive to environmental changes (pH, temperature, light)	ponds, and integrated industrial effluent systems Often combined with bacteria or other plants for higher efficiency	between dye molecules and functional groups (–OH, –COOH, $-NH_2$) on algal cell walls Ion exchange—Replacement of ions on algal surfaces with dye ions, influenced by pH	
12	*Scenedesmus obliquus*	Disperse orange 2RL	98.14%	High dye removal efficiency Simultaneous lipid production for biodiesel Heterotrophic growth allows operation without light Lower cost and easier setup than mixotrophic cultivation	Requires external carbon source (e.g., glucose) Optimal removal only at specific pH and nutrient levels Lab-controlled conditions may differ from real wastewater	Suitable for wastewater treatment integrated with biofuel production; heterotrophic systems are cheaper, easier to maintain, and more scalable	Biosorption of dye molecules onto algal surface Biodegradation of dye via metabolic use as carbon source FT-IR evidence of structural change in dye after treatment	Hamouda et al. (2022)
13	*Chlorella vulgaris*, *Scenedesmus*	Methylene blue, Congo	~95%	Low cost, eco-friendly, simultaneous	Sensitive to environmental conditions,	Potential in algal ponds, integrated wastewater	Biosorption via cell wall functional	El-Sheekh et al. (2014)

(continued)

Table 2.5 (continued)

Sl. No.	Algal species	Targeted dye	Removal efficiency	Advantages	Disadvantages	Large-scale applications	Removal mechanism	References
	obliquus, *Spirulina platensis*	red, reactive black 5		nutrient removal, adaptable to different wastewater types	slower process than chemical methods, large-scale cultivation challenges	treatment with biomass valorization	groups, enzymatic degradation, ion exchange, physical entrapment	
14	*Chlorella vulgaris*, *Scenedesmus obliquus*, *Spirulina platensis*	Methylene blue, Congo red, reactive black 5	~95%	Low-cost, eco-friendly, capable of removing nutrients and dyes, adaptable to various wastewater types	Sensitive to environmental changes, slower removal rate than chemical methods, large-scale cultivation and harvesting challenges	Potential use in algal ponds, integrated wastewater treatment systems with biomass valorization (biofuels, feed)	Biosorption via surface functional groups (–OH, –COOH, $-NH_2$), enzymatic degradation, ion exchange, and physical entrapment of dye molecules	Sani (2025)
15	*Chlorella vulgaris*, *Scenedesmus obliquus*,	Methylene blue, Congo red, reactive	Up to ~97% under optimal pH, contact	Low cost, eco-friendly, can remove dyes and other pollutants,	Sensitive to environmental factors, slower than chemical	Potential in integrated wastewater treatment systems,	Biosorption (cell wall functional groups –OH, –COOH, $-NH_2$),	El-Sheekh et al. (2014)

	Oscillatoria sp., *Ulva lactuca*, *Sargassum* sp.	black 5, acid red 88	time, and biomass dosage	potential for biomass valorization	treatment, large-scale cultivation and harvesting challenges	high-rate algal ponds, combination with other biological treatments	enzymatic degradation, ion exchange, physical adsorption, and entrapment of dye molecules	
16	*Chlorella vulgaris* *Scenedesmus obliquus* *Spirogyra* sp.	Methylene blue (MB) Malachite green (MG) Congo red (CR)	*Chlorella vulgaris*: 92% MB *Scenedesmus obliquus*: 85% MG removal in 6 days *Spirogyra* sp.: 78% CR removal in 7 days	Cost-effective and eco-friendly dye removal method Can use wastewater as a nutrient source Biomass can be valorized for biofuels or fertilizers Simultaneous removal of nutrients and dyes	Longer treatment time compared to chemical methods Sensitivity to environmental conditions (light, pH, temperature) Risk of biomass contamination	Used in raceway ponds and photobioreactors for textile wastewater treatment Integrated in zero-liquid discharge (ZLD) textile effluent systems	Algae remove dyes mainly by bioadsorption (binding to cell wall functional groups), bioaccumulation (uptake into cells), biodegradation, and photosynthetic transformation, often aided by nutrient co-metabolism	Alaguprathana and Poonkothai (2017)

recovery. Algal/microbial cell toxicity: Many dyes, especially azo and anthraquinone dyes, are toxic or mutagenic (Fig. 2.1). They can damage algal cell membranes, inhibit enzymatic activity, limit photosynthesis, and decrease chlorophyll content (Kumar et al., 2021). For example, high concentrations of methylene blue destroy algal cells instead of breaking them down. Penetration of light: Vibrant dyes prevent sunlight from reaching the water. Since algae rely on light for photosynthesis, dye-rich wastewater prevents algal growth and lowers the efficacy of bioremediation (Keerthi et al., 2019).

2.2.3 Removal Mechanisms Using Algae

2.2.3.1 Metal Removal

These mechanisms operate synergistically, allowing algae to tolerate high metal concentrations while simultaneously reducing toxicity in the surrounding environment (Parmar and Patel, 2025). Biosorption is the passive attachment of metal ions to functional groups in cell walls without the need for metabolic metals actively enter algal cells through bioaccumulation, where they are coupled to proteins or stored in vacuoles (Fig. 2.2). EPS-mediated sequestration: metals are trapped in a protective matrix made of extracellular polymeric substances released by algae. Ion exchange: functional groups trade heavy metal ions in solution for cations (such as Na^+, K^+, and Ca^{2+}). Surface complexation: On the surfaces of algae, metals and ligands combine to generate coordination complexes.

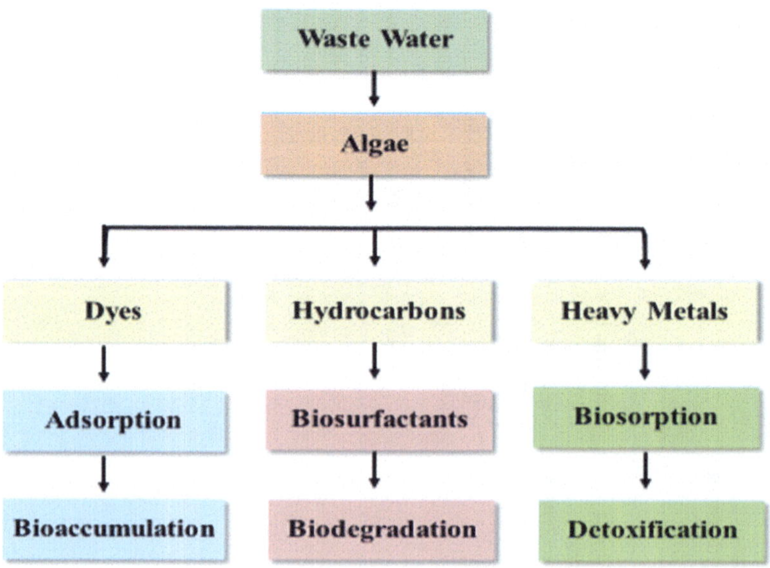

Fig. 2.2 Flowchart mechanism of algal bioremediation for the removal of heavy metals, hydrocarbons, and dyes

2.2.3.2 Hydrocarbon Removal

Hydrocarbons bind to hydrophobic regions on algal cell surfaces and extracellular polymeric substances (EPS), which concentrate PAHs and fuel-range compounds around cells and can allow subsequent transformation. Algal EPS and related biosurfactants emulsify hydrophobic hydrocarbons, enhancing their apparent solubility and bioavailability, and thereby increasing contact with degradative enzymes and co-microorganisms. It contains monooxygenases and dioxygenases that add hydroxyl groups to aromatic rings, forming hydroxylated or dihydroxylated intermediates on the way to subsequent cleavage and detoxification. These processes parallel microbial PAHs degradation pathways described above, though with capacities in each species. Certain hydrocarbons are accumulated and stored within cells, contributing to net removal, but may also subject cells to physiological stress if not metabolized (Patel et al., 2020). The remediation of hydrocarbons and PAHs by biosorption, bioaccumulation, and enzymatic degradation is a promising application for microalgae and cyanobacteria. *Scenedesmus quadricauda* needs steady conditions to break down benzo(a)anthracene (61.8%) and phenanthrene (72.3%) (Santos et al., 2025). While *Scenedesmus obliquus* removes 70–80% of light PAHs but is less effective with heavy hydrocarbons, *Chlorella vulgaris* uses enzymatic and surface processes to remove around 55–70% of pyrene and phenanthrene (Paniagua-Michel & Banat, 2024). 78–82% of light PAHs are removed by *Synechococcus* sp., making it suitable for cleaning up oil spills in marine environments. Approximately 60% of crude oil is broken down by *Botryococcus braunii*, which connects bioremediation to the potential for biofuel production (Prasad et al., 2023). Cyanobacteria such as *Oscillatoria* sp. and *Anabaena* sp. are suitable for tropical settings since they break down 65–80% of diesel and crude oil with the use of extracellular sheaths and enzymatic activity (Akl et al., 2023). Although it is limited in its ability to remove heavy PAHs, *Nostoc muscorum* can withstand a variety of environments and remove 45–60% of hydrocarbons. High efficiency (65–85%) across fuels makes *Nannochloropsis oculata* perfect for marine remediation (Amran et al., 2022). Approximately 50–60% of PAHs are eliminated by *Chlamydomonas reinhardtii*, which is pollutant-sensitive but genetically improvable. For integrated biorefineries, *Spirulina platensis* produces protein-rich biomass and removes 60–80% of oil and diesel (Akl et al., 2023).

2.2.3.3 Dyes Removal

Polysaccharides, proteins, and lipids with functional groups such as -OH, -COOH, $-NH_2$, and $-SO_4$ are abundant in the algal cell wall. These groups use van der Waals forces, ion exchange, hydrogen bonds, and electrostatic attraction to adsorb dye molecules. Even dead biomass undergoes this quick and passive process. Living algal cells actively transport dye molecules into their cytoplasm. Whether dyes are stored, altered, or mineralized within the cell depends on algal metabolism (Fig. 2.2). Although it proceeds more slowly than biosorption, long-term detoxification is achievable (Mata et al., 2010). Algae produce a variety of enzymes, including laccases, azoreductases, peroxidases, and oxidases, and these enzymes change

Table 2.6 Removal mechanism of dyes by algae

Mechanism	Process	Examples	References
Biosorption	Passive dye binding to cell wall functional groups	*Chlorella vulgaris*, *Scenedesmus* sp.	Gupta and Suhas (2009)
Bioaccumulation	Active uptake into cells	*Chlorella* sp.	Mata et al. (2010)
Biodegradation	Enzymatic breakdown (laccase, azoreductase, peroxidase)	*Chlorella vulgaris* degrading azo dyes	Kumar et al. (2021)
Algae–bacteria consortia	Symbiosis enhances degradation	Algal–bacterial wastewater treatment	Rawat et al. (2011)
Bioflocculation	Algae aggregate and settle dye particles	Green microalgae in textile effluent	Daneshvar et al., (2012)

complex dye molecules into simpler, less toxic forms, such as azo bonds (N=N) (Table 2.6).

2.2.4 Advantages of Algal Bioremediation

In comparison with the traditional procedures, algae-based cleanup techniques have several important advantages. Because algae can be grown on low-cost substrates, such as wastewater, they are incredibly cost-effective, as fewer expensive inputs are required (Wang et al., 2020). Since algae do not produce harmful byproducts, these techniques are more environmentally benign than chemical treatments (Verma & Kuila, 2019). The fact that the removal of metals is accompanied by the creation of useful biomass, which can be used to produce fertilizer, animal feed, or biofuels, is another significant advantage (Singh et al., 2024a). Furthermore, algae exhibit remarkable adaptability, as they can tolerate a wide range of metals under various environmental conditions (Wu, 2024). Lastly, these systems are practical and sustainable since they are easily scalable and allow for the large-scale cultivation of both macroalgae and microalgae in either controlled or natural environments.

2.2.5 Challenges and Limitations

Recovering biomass from harvested algae after cleanup can be costly and time-consuming. The toxicity of metals in algal development and metabolism may be inhibited by elevated metal concentrations (Sadiq et al., 2025). The changes in the environment that impact algal performance can be influenced by alterations in light, temperature, and pH (Rani et al., 2023). Secondary contamination of Biomass containing metals needs to be treated or disposed of properly to prevent recontamination. The financial feasibility of theoretically economical optimization is required for practical industrial application (Priya et al., 2022). If these problems are fixed through immobilization techniques, genetic engineering, and integration with existing wastewater treatment systems, algae bioremediation might become more practical and reliable (Mohebi et al., 2024).

2.3 Future Perspectives

The prospects for the future of algal bioremediation are promising, especially when combining the latest advances in biotechnology, nanotechnology, and systems engineering (Imaduddin & Eilks, 2025). Developments in metabolic engineering and genetic manipulation have the potential to produce algae strains with enhanced biosorption capacities and increased resistance to metals (Gouthami et al., 2023). Algal systems that utilize immobilized biomass, where the biomass is immobilized within matrices or beads, might reduce the cost of harvesting, increase the reusability, and provide increased stability (Ethiraj & Samuel, 2024.). The profitability of algal remediation systems may also be increased when combined with carbon sequestration, nutrient recovery, or biofuel production (Bhardwaj et al., 2025). Additionally, hybrid configurations that utilize a combination of algal processes and technologies, such as artificial wetlands, microbial consortia, or advanced oxidation processes, may improve the overall efficiency of the treatment processes (Anand et al., 2023). The use of algal bioremediation in treating wastewater produced by both industrial and municipal sources will further promote the utilization of natural technologies (Liu et al., 2022).

One of the most efficient, cost-effective, and environmentally friendly strategies for reducing pollution by heavy metals in aquatic environments is the use of algae. Such organisms possess distinct structural and biochemical attributes that enable them to take up and sequester a variety of poisonous metals (Patel et al., 2020). This process is highly resource-efficient, as their biomass has the potential for utilization in various industries (Shabaan et al., 2025). Despite the prevailing issues of toxicity management, biomass recovery, and scaling up, the area is evolving through sustained research activities and advances in technology (Wang, 2025). Given the increasing need for environmental sustainability and the necessity of constructing greener alternatives, algal bioremediation is a promising and feasible method for the remediation of polluted environments and the preservation of water for future generations (Zhang et al., 2025). The prospects of algal bioremediation will depend on the utilization of omics technologies, such as transcriptomics and proteomics (Sethi & Jonwal, 2025). Molecular technologies have the potential to describe protein-protein interaction patterns and gene patterns that govern degradation and pollution-resistant mechanisms (Rani et al., 2023). To enhance the efficiency of bioremediation, scientists may potentially modify the strains of algae genetically by identifying the key stress response genes and enzymes (Chen, 2025). The incorporation of these omics data, utilizing concepts from systems biology and bioengineering, will create algae cleanup systems that are scalable, affordable, and reliable (Cavalletti, 2025).

2.4 Conclusion

Algal bioremediation stands out as a practical, nature-based solution to stubborn pollutant classes. Its strength lies in a complementary toolkit: fast cell-surface biosorption and EPS-mediated binding/emulsification for immediate capture; active uptake and intracellular sequestration for stabilization; and enzyme-driven redox conversions that, especially in partnership with bacteria, facilitate the detoxification and even mineralization of degradable organics. For metals, where degradation is impossible, algae excel at immobilization and speciation control through ion exchange, complexation, electrostatic attraction, and micro-precipitation, with the added benefit of potential recovery. For dyes, electrostatic and hydrophobic interactions, π–π stacking, and oxidative enzymes enable robust decolorization, including in complex textile effluents. Translating this promise to full-scale demands careful engineering. High pollutant loads can inhibit growth; variable light, temperature, salinity, and competing ions challenge stability; and reliable hydrodynamics, harvesting, and biomass management are crucial for maintaining steady operation and facilitating downstream valorization. Even so, when systems are designed around species tolerance, EPS capacity, and controlled irradiance, and especially when integrated with bacterial partners or hybrid polishing steps, algal platforms deliver low-footprint, cost-conscious remediation with circular potential (e.g., metal recovery, biomass products). In short, algae offer a humane, eco-efficient pathway to clean water: adaptable enough for real-world effluents, powerful enough to address persistent pollutants, and scalable when biology and process engineering work in tandem. Thus, algal bioremediation is an effective and natural method of reducing environmental contaminants, especially hydrocarbons, heavy metals, and synthetic dyes.

References

Abo-Shady, A. M., El-Naggar, A. H., Motawea, M. M., El-Sheekh, M. M., Saleh, M. M., Mansour, A. T., & Abdel-Gawad, H. (2021). Removal efficiency of malachite green dye by green alga *Enteromorpha intestinalis*. *Egyptian Journal Of Aquatic Biology And Fisheries, 25*(5), 623–641. https://doi.org/10.21608/ejabf.2021.196250

Agarwal, S., Sadegh, H., Tyagi, I., Gupta, V. K., Ghasemi, M., & Maazinejad, B. (2016). Efficient removal of toxic dyes from aqueous solution using algal biomass: A review. *RSC Advances, 6*(63), 49452–49471. https://doi.org/10.1039/C6RA05414A

Agoun, N. A., & Avci, F. G. (2025). Phycoremediation: a path towards heavy metal bioremediation from wastewater. *Journal of Chemical Technology & Biotechnology, SCI where science meets business, 100*(1), 13–23. https://doi.org/10.1002/jctb.7745

Ahmad, I. (2022). Microalgae–Bacteria consortia: A review on the degradation of polycyclic aromatic hydrocarbons (PAHs). *Arabian Journal for Science and Engineering, 47*(1), 19–43.

Ahmad, I., Immanuel, J., & Evangelina, S. A. (2025). *Green technologies for wastewater treatment and bioenergy production treatment of wastewater using nanoparticles from seaweeds (Marine Algae)* (pp. 239–255). CRC Press, Boca Raton

Akbar, S. A., Lestari, A. N., Fazli, R. R., & Gunawan, G. (2025). Harnessing macroalgae for heavy metal phytoremediation: A sustainable approach to aquatic pollution control. In *BIO Web of Conferences* (Vol. 156, p. 02013). EDP Sciences.

Akl, F. M. A., Ahmed, S. I., El-Sheekh, M. M., & Makhlof, M. E. M. (2023). Bioremediation of n-alkanes, polycyclic aromatic hydrocarbons, and heavy metals from wastewater using seaweeds. *Environmental Science and Pollution Research, 30*, 104814–104832. https://doi.org/10.1007/s11356-023-29549-8

Alaguprathana, M., & Poonkothai, M. (2017). Bioremediation of textile dyeing effluent using algae–a review. *Journal of Advances in Microbiology, 7*(1), 1–12.

Ali, N., Nawaz, A., Ali, I., Batool, S., Rehman, K., Ullah, S., Zahra, A., Islam, N. U., Khan, M., & Khan, S. (2023). Efficient removal of methylene blue dye from aqueous solution using *Chlorella vulgaris*: A comparative analysis of live and dead biomass removal capability. *Frontiers in Marine Science, 10*, 1202362. https://doi.org/10.3389/fmars.2023.1202362

Alseroury, F. A. (2018). Simultaneous decolorization of dye contaminated wastewater and energy production using algae. *Journal of Biochemical Technology, 9*(4), 15–21.

Amran, R. H., Jamal, M. T., Pugazhendi, A., Al-Harbi, M., Ghandourah, M., Al-Otaibi, A., & Haque, M. F. (2022). Biodegradation and bioremediation of petroleum hydrocarbons in marine ecosystems by microorganisms: A review. *Nature Environment and Pollution Technology, 21*(3), 1149–1157. https://doi.org/10.46488/NEPT.2022.v21i03.019

Anand, U., Dey, S., Parial, D., Federici, S., Ducoli, S., Bolan, N. S., Dey, A., & Bontempi, E. (2023). Algae and bacteria consortia for wastewater decontamination and transformation into biodiesel, bioethanol, biohydrogen, biofertilizers and animal feed: A review. *Environmental Chemistry Letters, 21*(3), 1585–1609.

Ashok, A., Policegoudra, R., Nagaraj, R., Garlapati, P. K., Chauhan, O. P., & Semwal, A. D. (2025). Effects of different treatments on the volatile compounds heavy metals minerals amino acids and bioactive compounds of the edible brown alga Spatoglossum asperum. *Journal of Applied Phycology, 37*(4), 2715–2728. https://doi.org/10.1007/s10811-025-03519-8

Ayele, A., Suresh, A., & Benor, S. (2021). Phycoremediation of heavy metals, factors involved and mechanisms related to functional groups in the algae cell surface–A review. In *Strategies and tools for pollutant mitigation: avenues to a cleaner environment* (pp. 269–289).

Bai, R. G., Chandrasekharan Nair, S., Joller-Vahter, L., & Kikas, T. (2025). Microalgae in mitigating industrial pollution: Bioremediation strategies and biomagnification potential. *Biomass, 5*(4), 61.

Bandara, C., et al. (2025). Phycoremediation potential of Nostoc ellipsosporum and Spirulina subsalsa for pollutant removal from real textile wastewater (TWW) and synchronized biodiesel production from TWW-tolerant biomass. *Research Square*, 1. https://doi.org/10.21203/rs.3.rs-6947833/v1

Bataeva, Y. V., & Grigoryan, L. N. (2024). Ecological features and adaptive capabilities of cyanobacteria in desert ecosystems: A review. *Eurasian Soil Science, 57*(3), 430–445.

Bhardwaj, A., Bansal, M., Wilson, K., Gupta, S., & Dhanawat, M. (2025). Lignocellulose biosorbents: Unlocking the potential for sustainable environmental cleanup. *International Journal of Biological Macromolecules, 294*, 139497.

Bhaskar, C., & Lakshminarayanachari, K. (2021). Numerical model for primary and secondary air pollutants emitted from an area and point source in an urban area with chemical reaction and removal mechanisms. *Materials Today: Proceedings, 37*, 2961–2967.

Brahmbhatt, N. H., & Jasrai, R. T. (2015). Biodegradation of reactive dyes by two microalgal species. *International Journal of Science and Research (IJSR), 4*(5), 1697–1702.

Carvalho, M. F., Rodrigues, G., Pereira, D. T., Batista, D., Ouriques, L. C., & Simioni, C. (2025). Cultivation of Gelidium floridanum in different nitrate concentrations: Morphophysiological effects. *Journal of Applied Phycology*, 1–10.

Cavalletti, E. (2025). *Exposure of microalgae to heavy metals: Effects on growth, bioremediation strategies and identification of new methods to identify physiological damages* (Doctoral dissertation). The Open University.

Chaouay, J., Bentiss, F., Zbair, M., Belattmania, Z., Sabour, B., Lamonier, J.-F., Duquesne, S., & Jama, C. (2025). Study of mercury adsorption using biochars derived from the invasive brown seaweed "Sargassum muticum" as a low-cost and ecofriendly adsorbent in the aqueous phase. *International Journal of Environmental Science and Technology, 22*(5), 3451–3464. https://doi.org/10.1007/s13762-024-05765-8

Chen, H. (2025). *Cyanobacteria Anabaena sp. on human urine wastewater treatment and Phycobiliproteins production.* (Doctoral dissertation). Iowa State University.

Cheng, J., Yin, W., Chang, Z., Lundholm, N., & Jiang, Z. (2017). Biosorption capacity and kinetics of cadmium (II) on live and dead Chlorella vulgaris. *Journal of Applied Phycology, 29*(1), 211–221.

Daneshvar, E., Kousha, M., Sohrabi, M. S., Khataee, A., & Converti, A. (2012). Biosorption of three acid dyes by the brown macroalga Stoechospermum marginatum: Isotherm kinetic and thermodynamic studies. *Chemical Engineering Journal, 195–196*, 297–306. https://doi.org/10.1016/j.cej.2012.04.074

Das, B. D., & Bhattarai, A. (2025). The versatility of algae in addressing the global sustainability challenges. *Frontiers in Bioengineering and Biotechnology, 13*. https://doi.org/10.3389/fbioe.2025.1621817

Das, N., & Chandran, P. (2011). Microbial degradation of petroleum hydrocarbon contaminants: An overview. *Biotechnology Research International, 2011*, 1–13. https://doi.org/10.4061/2011/941810

Davis, T. A., Volesky, B., & Mucci, A. (2003). A review of the biochemistry of heavy metal biosorption by brown algae. *Water Research, 37*(18), 4311–4330.

Dell' Anno, F., Rastelli, E., Sansone, C., Brunet, C., Ianora, A., & Dell' Anno, A. (2021). Bacteria fungi and microalgae for the bioremediation of marine sediments contaminated by petroleum hydrocarbons in the omics era. *Microorganisms, 9*(8), 1695. https://doi.org/10.3390/microorganisms9081695

Elhamji, S., Sbihi, K., Lghoul, S., Aziz, K., El Maallem, A., Kurniawan, T. A., & Aziz, F. (2025). Addressing the challenge of heavy metal contamination in aquatic environment: Harnessing the bioremediation potential of Navicula permitis diatom for wastewater treatment. *Biomass and Bioenergy, 197*, 107776.

El-Agawany, N. I., Abdel-Razik, S. A. R., Abdel-Kareem, M. S., & Kaamoush, M. I. A. (2023). Environmental performance of two marine algae Ulva fasciata and Pterocladia capillacea in the biological treatment of four reactive dyes from aqueous solutions based on fresh and dried biomass. *Abstract Applied Water Science, 13*(3). https://doi.org/10.1007/s13201-023-01893-7

El-Sheekh, M. M., Hamouda, R. A., & El-Hafez, A. A. (2014). Biodegradation of dyes by some green algae and cyanobacteria. *Egyptian Journal of Aquatic Research, 40*(3), 301–308. https://doi.org/10.1016/j.ejar.2014.07.002

Ethiraj, S., & Samuel, M. S. (2024). A comprehensive review of the challenges and opportunities in microalgae-based wastewater treatment for eliminating organic, inorganic, and emerging pollutants. *Biocatalysis and Agricultural Biotechnology, 60*, 103316.

Flores-Moya, A., Moreno, D., De la Rosa, J., Altamirano, M., & Bañares-España, E. (2021). Seaweeds and seagrasses: The marine forests from the Alboran Sea. In *Alboran Sea-ecosystems and marine resources* (pp. 247–284). Springer International Publishing.

Foday, E. H., Jr., Bo, B., & Xu, X. (2021). Removal of toxic heavy metals from contaminated aqueous solutions using seaweeds: A review. *Sustainability, 13*(21), 12311.

Ganguly, A., Nag, S., Bhowmick, T. K., & Gayen, K. (2024). Phycoremediation of As (III) and Cr (VI) by Desmodesmus subspicatus: Impact on growth and biomolecules (carbohydrate, protein, chlorophyll and lipid)—A dual mode investigation. *Environmental Science and Pollution Research, 31*(35), 48545–48560.

Gayathiri, E., Prakash, P., Selvam, K., Awasthi, M. K., Gobinath, R., Karri, R. R., Ragunathan, M. G., Jayanthi. J., Mani, V., Poudineh, M. A., Chang, S. W., & Ravindran, B. (2022). Plant microbe based remediation approaches in dye removal: A review. *Bioengineered, 13*(3), 7798–7828. https://doi.org/10.1080/21655979.2022.2049100

Gaylarde, C. C., & da Fonseca, E. M. (2025). Biofertilization and bioremediation—How can microbiological technology assist the ecological crisis in developing countries? *Micro, 5*(2), 18. MDPI.

Ghoneim, M. M., El-Desoky, H. S., El-Moselhy, K. M., Amer, A., Abou El-Naga, E. H., Mohamedein, L. I., & Al-Prol, A. E. (2014). Removal of cadmium from aqueous solution using marine green algae, Ulva lactuca. *Egyptian Journal of Aquatic Research, 40*(3), 235–242.

Gomaa, M., El-Naeb, E. H., Hifney, A. F., Adam, M. S., & Fawzy, M. A. (2022). Coupling phenol bioremediation and biodiesel production by *Tetradesmus obliquus*: Optimization of phenol removal biomass productivity and lipid content. *South African Journal of Botany, 151*, 604–613. https://doi.org/10.1016/j.sajb.2022.10.044

Gouthami, K., Mallikarjunaswamy, A. M. M., Bhargava, R. N., Ferreira, L. F. R., Rahdar, A., Saratale, G. D., Bankole, P. O., & Mulla, S. I. (2023). Microbial biodegradation and biotransformation of petroleum hydrocarbons: Progress, prospects, and challenges. In *Genomics approach to bioremediation: Principles, tools, and emerging technologies* (pp. 229–247).

Gupta, V. K., & Suhas. (2009). Application of low-cost adsorbents for dye removal – A review. *Journal of Environmental Management 90*(8), 2313–2342. https://doi.org/10.1016/j.jenvman.2008.11.017

Gupta, A., Singh, U. B., Sahu, P. K., Paul, S., Kumar, A., Malviya, D., Singh, S., Kuppusamy, P., Singh, P., Paul, D., Rai, J. P., Singh, H. V., Manna, M. C., Crusberg, T. C., Kumar, A., & Saxena, A. K. (2022). Linking soil microbial diversity to modern agriculture practices: A review. *International Journal of Environmental Research and Public Health, 19*(5), 3141. https://doi.org/10.3390/ijerph19053141

Gärtner, G., Stoyneva-Gärtner, M., & Uzunov, B. (2021). Algal toxic compounds and their aeroterrestrial, airborne and other extremophilic producers with attention to soil and plant contamination: A review. *Toxins, 13*(5), 322.

Hachicha, R., Elleuch, F., Ben Hlima, H., Dubessay, P., de Baynast, H., Delattre, C., Pierre, G., Hachicha, R., Abdelkafi, S., Michaud, P., & Fendri, I. (2022). Biomolecules from microalgae and cyanobacteria: Applications and market survey. *Applied Sciences, 12*(4), 1924.

Hamouda, R. A., El-Ahmady El-Naggar, N., & Abou-El-Souod, G. W. (2022). Simultaneous bioremediation of disperse orange-2RL Azo dye and fatty acids production by *Scenedesmus obliquus* cultured under mixotrophic and heterotrophic conditions. *Scientific Reports, 12*, 20768. https://doi.org/10.1038/s41598-022-22825-6

Hossain, N., Nizamuddin, S., & Shah, K. (2023). Comparative study of solvothermal and catalytic solvothermal carbonization of rice husk for Fe(III), Zn(II), Cu(II), Pb(II) and Mn(II) adsorption, kinetics, surface chemistry and reaction mechanism. *Royal Society of Chemistry*. https://doi.org/10.1039/D3EW00068K

Iddrisu, L., Danso, F., Cheong, K. L., Fang, Z., & Zhong, S. (2024). Polysaccharides as protective agents against heavy metal toxicity. *Food, 13*(6), 853.

Imaduddin, M., & Eilks, I. (2025). Harnessing Indonesia's biodiversity for sustainable water treatment: A review of local plant-based solutions. *Abstract Environmental Science and Pollution Research, 32*(20), 12167–12190. https://doi.org/10.1007/s11356-025-36485-2

Jackson, T., Parker, J., & Hirst A. (2024). *Plankton: A worldwide guide*. Princeton University Press.

Jana, A., Banerjee, R., Ghosh, M., & Mukherjee, A. (2024). Potential phytoremediation of coal fly ash leachate using Lemna minor: A free floating macrophyte. *The Nucleus, 67*(3), 547–555. https://doi.org/10.1007/s13237-024-00507-0

Karnwal, A., Martolia, S., Dohroo, A., Al-Tawaha, A. R. M. S., & Malik, T. (2024). Exploring bioremediation strategies for heavy metals and POPs pollution: The role of microbes plants and nanotechnology. *Frontiers in Environmental Science 12*. https://doi.org/10.3389/fenvs.2024.1397850

Keerthi, A. T., Karthikeyan, S., & Salom Gnana Thanga, V. (2019). Occurrence and microbial degradation of fipronil residues in tropical highland rhizosphere soils of Kerala India. *Soil and Sediment Contamination: An International Journal, 28*(4), 360–379. https://doi.org/10.1080/15320383.2019.1578336

Khattar, J. S., Singh, Y., Parveen, S., & Singh, D. P. (2016). Microalgal biofuels. In *Biofuels: Productions and future perspectives* (p. 331).

Kumar, R., Singh, J., & Singh, D. P. (2015). White-rot fungi and their enzymes for the removal of industrial dyes from wastewater. *Environmental Chemistry Letters, 13*(4), 377–393.

Kumar, P., Singh, R., & Sharma, R. (2021). Microalgae-mediated removal of dyes from wastewater: Recent developments and challenges. *Bioresource Technology Reports, 15*, 100730.

Kumari, S., & Das, S. (2023). Bacterial enzymatic degradation of recalcitrant organic pollutants: Catabolic pathways and genetic regulations. *Environmental Science and Pollution Research, 30*(33), 79676–79705.

Kumari, S., Satapathy, S., Datta, M., & Kumar, S. (2022). Adaptation of microalgae to temperature and light stress. In *Plant stress: Challenges and management in the new decade* (pp. 123–134). Springer International Publishing.

Lalhruaitluangi, M., Ralte, L., Tiwari, D., & Jung, J. (2025). Highly efficient and toxicologically safe ZnO (NP)@ GO nanocomposite in the simultaneous detection of Cd^{2+}, Hg^{2+}, Pb^{2+}, and Zn^{2+} in aqueous medium. *Sensors and Actuators Reports*, 100373.

Lan, J., Liu, P., Hu, X., & Zhu, S. (2024). Harmful algal blooms in eutrophic marine environments: Causes monitoring and treatment. *Water, 16*(17), 2525. https://doi.org/10.3390/w16172525

Li, Y., Liang, H., Wang, L., Chen, G., Bai, Y., Tang, T., & Gao, D. (2024). Enhanced bioremediation of organically combined contaminated soil by white rot fungal agent: physiological characteristics and contaminants degradation. *Environmental Technology, 45*(28), 6039–6050. https://doi.org/10.1080/09593330.2024.2323025

Liu, J., Zhao, L., Liu, Q., Li, J., Qiao, Z., Sun, P., & Yang, Y. (2022). A critical review on soil washing during soil remediation for heavy metals and organic pollutants. *International journal of Environmental Science and Technology, 19*(1), 601–624.

Maglione, G., Zinno, P., Tropea, A., Mussagy, C. U., Dufossé, L., Giuffrida, D., & Mondello, A. (2024). Microbes' role in environmental pollution and remediation: A bioeconomy focus approach. *AIMS Microbiology, 10*(3), 723.

Malik, A. (2004). Metal bioremediation through growing cells. *Environment International 30*(2), 261–278. https://doi.org/10.1016/j.envint.2003.08.001

Malletzidou, L., Kyratzopoulou, E., Kyzaki, N., Nerantzis, E., & Kazakis, N. A. (2025). Towards the sustainable removal of heavy metals from wastewater using arthrospira platensis: A laboratory-scale approach in the context of a green circular economy. *Applied Sciences, 15*(2), 791. https://doi.org/10.3390/app15020791

Mata, T. M., Martins, A. A., & Caetano, N. S. (2010). Microalgae for biodiesel production and other applications: A review. *Renewable and Sustainable Energy Reviews, 14*(1), 217–232. https://doi.org/10.1016/j.rser.2009.07.020

Mishra, M., Singh, S. K., & Kumar, A. (2021). Environmental factors affecting the bioremediation potential of microbes. In *Microbe mediated remediation of environmental contaminants* (pp. 47–58). Woodhead Publishing.

Mohebi, M., Parashkoohi, M. G., & Mohammadi, A. (2024). A comparison of biofilm and suspension methods in removing heavy metals (chromium) from industrial wastewater with Scenedesmus obliquus and Chlorella vulgaris. *Results in Engineering, 24*, 103397.

Molebatsi, M., Nkoane, B., Keroletswe, N., Chigome, S., & Kabomo, M. T. (2025). The use of biosorbents in water treatment. *Environments 12*(9), 302. https://doi.org/10.3390/environments12090302

Muñoz-Rivera, M. P., Martínez-Morales, F., Morales-Guzmán, D., Rivera-Ramírez, A., Sánchez-Reyes, A., & Trejo-Hernández, M. R. (2025). Population dynamics of a bacterial consortium from a marine sediment of the Gulf of Mexico during biodegradation of the aromatic fraction of heavy crude oil. *International Microbiology, 28*(7), 1875–1885. https://doi.org/10.1007/s10123-025-00659-2

Murugesan, S., Sivamurugan, V., & Kathiresan, D. (2025). Potential use of extracellular substances from soil algae. In *Soil algae: Morphology, ecology and biotechnological applications* (pp. 261–292). Springer Nature Singapore.

Nagar, V., Aseri, V., Chopade, R., Pandit, P. P., Mavry, B., Singh, A., Awasthi, G., Awasthi, K. K., & Sankhla, M. S. (2025). Implications of diatoms for heavy metal bioremediation. In: Vinayak, V., & Gordon, R. (eds) *Diatom cultivation for biofuel food and high⍰value products* (pp. 323–340). Wiley.

Nair, V. K., Selvaraju, K., Samuchiwal, S., Naaz, F., Malik, A., & Ghosh, P. (2023). Phycoremediation of synthetic dyes laden textile wastewater and recovery of bio-based pigments from residual biomass: An approach towards sustainable wastewater management. *PRO, 11*(6), 1793.

Naveed, S., Li, C., Lu, X., Chen, S., Yin, B., Zhang, C., & Ge, Y. (2019). Microalgal extracellular polymeric substances and their interactions with metal(loid)s: A review. *Critical Reviews in Environmental Science and Technology, 49*(19), 1769–1802. https://doi.org/10.1080/10643389.2019.1583052

Paniagua-Michel, J., & Banat, I. M. (2024). Unravelling diatoms' potential for the bioremediation of oil hydrocarbons in marine environments. *Clean Technologies, 6*, 93–115. https://doi.org/10.3390/cleantechnol6010007

Park, S.-K., Han, S.-J., Jo, D.-M., Jo, J.-B., Lee, G., Park, K.-J., & Kim, Y.-M. (2025). Influence of environmental factors on the proximate components and heavy metal contents of raw laver (Pyropia spp.) from South Korea. *Marine Pollution Bulletin, 220*, 118372. https://doi.org/10.1016/j.marpolbul.2025.118372

Parmar, K. S., & Patel, K. M. (2025). Biosorption and bioremediation of heavy metal ions from wastewater using algae: A comprehensive review. *World Journal of Microbiology and Biotechnology, 41*(7). https://doi.org/10.1007/s11274-025-04424-5

Patel, A. B., Shaikh, S., Jain, K. R., Desai, C., & Madamwar, D. (2020). Polycyclic aromatic hydrocarbons: Sources, toxicity, and remediation approaches. *Frontiers in Microbiology, 11*, 562813.

Pereira, L. (2021). Macroalgae. *Encyclopedia, 1*(1), 177–188. https://doi.org/10.3390/encyclopedia1010017

Perera, I. A., Abinandan, S., Subashchandrabose, S. R., Venkateswarlu, K., Naidu, R., & Megharaj, M. (2019). Advances in the technologies for studying consortia of bacteria and cyanobacteria/microalgae in wastewaters. *Critical Reviews in Biotechnology, 39*(5), 709–731. https://doi.org/10.1080/07388551.2019.1597828

Prasad, R. K., Singh, R., & Choudhary, S. (2023). Bioremediation by using of microbes and their metabolic products. *Processes, 11*(8), 3036. https://doi.org/10.3390/pr11083036

Priya, A. K., Jalil, A. A., Vadivel, S., Dutta, K., Rajendran, S., Fujii, M., & Soto-Moscoso, M. (2022). Heavy metal remediation from wastewater using microalgae: Recent advances and future trends. *Chemosphere, 305*, 135375.

Qin, Z., Wei, C., Wei, T., Li, Z., Pang, Z., Luo, P., Feng, C., Qiu, G., Wei, C., Wu, H., & Peng, Y. (2022). Evolution of biochemical processes in coking wastewater treatment: A combined evaluation of material and energy efficiencies and secondary pollution. *Science of the Total Environment, 807*, 151072.

Raab, A., Stengel, D. B., & Feldmann, J. (2025). Differential prevalence of arsenic speciation in the kelps Laminaria digitata and L. hyperborea. *Marine Pollution Bulletin, 211*, 117473. https://doi.org/10.1016/j.marpolbul.2024.117473

Rani, R., Singh, P., Saini, N., Kumar, M., Kumar, A., Kumar, R., Kumar, V., & Saini, R. V. (2023). Recent advances in algae-based technologies for remediation of polycyclic aromatic hydrocarbons (PAHs) from the environment. *Environmental Advances, 12*, 100351. https://doi.org/10.1016/j.envadv.2023.100351

Rawat, I., Ranjith Kumar, R., Mutanda, T., & Bux, F. (2011). Dual role of microalgae: Phycoremediation of domestic wastewater and biomass production for sustainable biofuels production. *Applied Energy, 88*(10), 3411–3424.

Sadiq, I. S., Ibrahim, A. H., Abubakar, L., Yusuf, A. I., Suleiman, M. M., Usman, A., Mohammed, A. S., & Salihu, A. (2025). Assessment of biosorption potential of *Oedogonium sp.* biomass for removal of methylene blue from aqueous solution. *Beni-Suef University Journal of Basic and Applied Sciences, 14*(12). https://doi.org/10.1186/s44371-025-00111-4

Saleh, H. O. & Abdulhasan J. M. (2023). Evaluating the efficiency of chlorella vulgaris and spirulina microalgae in wastewater remediation under different light conditions. *International Information and Engineering Technology Association*. https://doi.org/10.18280/ijdne.180629

Salimi, A., Ghanbarizadeh, P., Mirvakili, A., & Moheimani, N. R. (2025). Optimizing heavy metal remediation of synthetic wastewater using Chlorella vulgaris and Sargassum angustifolium: A comparative analysis of biosorption and bioaccumulation techniques. *Science of the Total Environment, 992*, 179938. https://doi.org/10.1016/j.scitotenv.2025.179938

Sani, Z. M. (2025). Algal-based remediation of synthetic dyes: A mini review. *Asian Journal of Scientific Research, 18*(2), 72–81. https://doi.org/10.3923/asb.2025.72.81

Santos, A. D., Birolli, W. G., Souza, F. O., Giovanella, P., Cabral, L., Santana de Farias, G., Pilau, E. J., Sette, L. D., & Rodrigues-Filho, E. (2025). Leveraging Antarctic psychrotolerant fungi for PAH biodegradation unveiling key factors influencing the process. *Chemosphere, 373*, 144138. https://doi.org/10.1016/j.chemosphere.2025.144138

Selvakumar, R., Guhananthan, A., & Palanisami, T. (2023). Recent advances in micropollutant removal and mitigation from water using three dimensional adsorbent materials. *Current Opinion in Environmental Science & Health, 34*, 100475. https://doi.org/10.1016/j.coesh.2023.100475

Sethi, S., & Jonwal, H. (2025). Harnessing algae and nanotechnology for efficient remediation of environmental pollutants. In *Phyconanotechnology: Current research, challenges, and prospects* (pp. 129–144). Springer Nature Switzerland.

Sha, J.-Q., An, J., Wei, S.-H., & Song, H.-W. (2025). Low-carbon cadmium removal via cyanobacterial MICP: Metabolic mechanisms and species efficiency. *Bioresource Technology, 434*, 132775. https://doi.org/10.1016/j.biortech.2025.132775

Shabaan, A. M., Embaby, M. S., & Reyad, A. M. (2025). Potential application of Staphylococcus devriesei MS as a biosorbent agent for manganase, chromium, and cadmium heavy metals in contaminated water. *Scientific Reports, 15*(1), 9774.

Shahi Khalaf Ansar, B., Kavusi, E., Dehghanian, Z., Pandey, J., Asgari Lajayer, B., Price, G. W., Astatkie, T. (2023). Removal of organic and inorganic contaminants from the air soil and water by algae. *Environmental Science and Pollution Research, 30*(55), 116538-116566. https://doi.org/10.1007/s11356-022-21283-x

Sharma, I. (2020). Bioremediation techniques for polluted environment: Concept, advantages, limitations, and prospects. In *Trace metals in the environment-new approaches and recent advances*. IntechOpen.

Sharma, M. (2025). Advances in nature-based and nature-inspired solutions for ground improvement. *Indian Geotechnical Journal*, 1–20.

Shi, K., Liang, B., Guo, Q., Zhao, Y., Sharif, H. M. A., Li, Z., Chen, E., & Wang, A. (2021). Accelerated bioremediation of a complexly contaminated river sediment through ZVI-electrode combined stimulation. *Journal of Hazardous Materials, 413*, 125392. https://doi.org/10.1016/j.jhazmat.2021.125392

Shourie, A., & Vijayalakshmi, U. (2022). Fungal diversity and its role in mycoremediation. *Geomicrobiology Journal, 39*(3-5), 426–444. https://doi.org/10.1080/01490451.2022.2032883

Singh, V. P., Godara, P., & Srivastava, A. (2024a). Sustainable microalgal bioremediation of heavy metals and dyes from synthetic wastewater: Progressing towards United Nations sustainable development goals. *Waste Management Bulletin, 2*(4), 123–135.

Singh, V. P., Kumar, A., Srivastava, A., & Kumar, A. (2024b). Advancing environmental sustainability: A comprehensive review on alleviating carbon footprint and its application in microalgal fermentation and bioremediation. *Environment Development and Sustainability*. https://doi.org/10.1007/s10668-024-05796-8

Singh, C. K., Sodhi, K. K., V, N., Rajagopalan, V., Sharma, S., Kaur, J., & Kumar, Y. (2025a). Managing the complexity of emerging contaminants in aquatic environments: Exploring their ecotoxicological impacts, detection techniques, and the use of innovative technologies for their remediation. *Discover Catalysis, 2*(1), 9.

Singh, S. K., Yadav, N., Yadav, P., Shukla, L., Pradhan, T., Kumar, M., Singh, R., & Kumar, A. (2025b). Cyanobacterial based bioremediation of xenobiotics compounds. In *Advances in chemical pollution, environmental management and protection* (Vol. 12, pp. 507–524). Elsevier.

Spalding, H. L., Amado-Filho, G. M., Bahia, R. G., Ballantine, D. L., Fredericq, S., Leichter, J. J., Nelson, W. A., Slattery, M., & Tsuda, R. T. (2019). Macroalgae. In *Mesophotic coral ecosystems* (pp. 507–536). Springer International Publishing.

Taglioni, E., Cavaliere, C., Cerrato, A., Laganà, A., Montone, C. M., & Capriotti, A. L. (2025). Comprehensive profiling of sulfated phenolic compounds in edible and infesting seaweeds by a dedicated software-assisted platform. *Analytical and Bioanalytical Chemistry, 417*(23), 5199–5209.

Tamilselvan, N., Saurav, K., & Kannabiran, K. (2012). Biosorption of Cr (VI), Cr (III), Pb (II) and Cd (II) from aqueous solutions by Sargassum wightii and Caulerpa racemosa algal biomass. *Journal of Ocean University of China, 11*(1), 52–58.

Thoré, E. S. J., Muylaert, K., Bertram, M. G., & Brodin, T. (2023). Microalgae. *Current Biology 33*(3), R91-R95. https://doi.org/10.1016/j.cub.2022.12.032

Varabih, C. A., & Nofirman, N. (2023). The importance of seaweed as bioremediation natural agent: The importance of seaweed as bioremediation natural agent. *Journal of Oceanography and Aquatic Science, 1*(2), 48–53.

Verma, S., & Kuila, A. (2019). Bioremediation of heavy metals by microbial process. *Environmental Technology & Innovation, 14*, 100369.

Visvanathan, P., Kirubakaran, D., Selvam, K., Manimegalai, P., Rajkumar, M., & Vasantharaj, K. (2024). Recent strategies for natural bioremediation of emerging pollutants: Development of a green and sustainable environment. *Bioremediation of Emerging Contaminants in Water, 2*, 1–19.

Wang, L. (2025). From phytoplankton to fish: Exploring the trophic levels of aquatic ecosystems. *International Journal of Aquaculture, 15*.

Wang, J., & Chen, C. (2009). Biosorbents for heavy metals removal and their future. *Biotechnology Advances, 27*(2), 195–226. https://doi.org/10.1016/j.biotechadv.2008.11.002

Wang, S., Zhao, X., & Xing, M. (2020). Bioremediation of heavy metal-contaminated soils by microalgae: Mechanisms and future prospects. *Environmental Pollution, 265*, 114–125.

Wu, H. (2024). *Biosorption by green alga Chlorella vulgaris for decontamination of Pb (II) from wasters at near benign concentration* (Doctoral dissertation). Université d'Ottawa| University of Ottawa.

Yaacob, N. S., Abdullah, H., Ahmad, M. F., Maniyam, M. N., & Sjahrir, F. (2022). Microalgae biotechnology: Emerging biomedical applications. In *Algal biotechnology* (pp. 335–346). Elsevier.

Younis, A. (2025). Biosorption of heavy metals by algae: Recent advances, mechanisms, and applications in wastewater treatment–A review: Biosorption of heavy metals by algae: Recent advances, mechanisms, and applications in wastewater treatment–A review. *Journal of Qassim University for Science, 4*(1).

Zhang, L. S., Liu, Z. W., Qiu, C. F., Feng, X. Y., Ma, S. Y., Yin, Q., & Cao, D. J. (2025). 60Coγ activation of Cladophora rupestris biomass functional groups and its effect on Pb2+ adsorption. *Environmental Science and Pollution Research, 32*(3), 1293–1307.

Microalgae for Environmental Cleanup: A Holistic and Sustainable Approach for Pollution Management

3

Arun Kumar Mani, Suvetha Selvam, Sri Meenakshi Selvaraju, Poojasri Sowndarajan, Taehyeong Kim, Nazia Tabassum, and Fazlurrahman Khan

Abstract

Microalgae play a significant role in the bioremediation of various types of environmental pollutants, including heavy metals, organic compounds, pesticides, and pharmaceuticals. Algal bioremediation offers several advantages, including economic efficiency, resilience, and the production of valuable products. This chapter covers the principles of phycoremediation methods and explores the underlying mechanisms. It also demonstrates the involvement of algae in reducing the pollution from agricultural sources, industry, and urban areas. Nowadays, microalgae are considered one of the excellent tools in the bioremediation process due to their ease of cultivation, diverse metabolic activity, green, and environmental adaptability as a promising alternative technique when compared to the conventional methods. The excess nutrients present in the contaminated water bodies, such as nitrogen, phosphorus, heavy metals, and

A. K. Mani (✉) · S. Selvam · S. M. Selvaraju · P. Sowndarajan
Department of Chemistry and Biosciences, Srinivasa Ramanujan Centre, SASTRA Deemed University, Kumbakonam, Tamil Nadu, India
e-mail: arunkumar@src.sastra.edu

T. Kim
Department of Applied Biosciences, Kyungpook National University, Daegu, Republic of Korea

N. Tabassum
Marine Integrated Biomedical Technology Center, The National Key Research Institutes in Universities, Pukyong National University, Busan, Republic of Korea

F. Khan (✉)
Marine Integrated Biomedical Technology Center, The National Key Research Institutes in Universities, Pukyong National University, Busan, Republic of Korea

Ocean and Fisheries Development International Cooperation Institute, Pukyong National University, Busan, Republic of Korea
e-mail: fkhan055@pknu.ac.kr

L. Kumar et al. (eds.), *Algal Bioremediation*,
https://doi.org/10.1007/978-981-95-8793-3_3

organic compounds, can be effectively removed by photosynthetic microalgae. Bioadsorption, bio-uptake, biodegradation, and photodegradation are the major processes involved in this context. The effectiveness of algal bioremediation depends on numerous interrelated factors, such as pH, temperature, light intensity, and the nature of the pollutant and its concentration. Even though the algae play a major role in pollutant reduction, there are several hurdles, like slow growth rate, huge investment required for production, heavy contamination, stability loss, and complex recovery process, which are the major issues still facing in the development of industrial scaling processes, and hence, fine-tuning is much required for effective treatment. The integration of existing treatment methods and genetic engineering is the two pivotal methods that improve the pollution tolerance with greater potential. This chapter highlights the importance of algae to mitigate the wide range of environmental issues occurring in the current scenario, such as water and soil pollution, and other challenges in the environment. Also, phytoremediation and microbiological treatments are combined with algal bioremediation for better results. This field addresses the challenges and leverages genetic engineering, which helps in the development of industrial applications. Overall, this chapter encompasses the principles, practical use, and future prospects of phycoremediation.

Keywords

Algal cells · Environmental contaminants · Phycoremediation · Integrated approaches · Cellular pathway

3.1 Introduction

Large volumes of wastewater are generated every day due to overpopulation, urban development, and industrial growth (Kapoore et al., 2021). A significant portion of the pollution in freshwater and conventional water streams originates from industrial effluents, including those from municipalities, textile factories, pig farms, molasses facilities, and aquaculture operations (Ahmad et al., 2022). Many pollutants, including metals, oils and grease, herbicides, insecticides, volatile chemical compounds, and minerals, are generated in the wastewater. Furthermore, sewage or industrial effluent contains a significant amount of nutrients, such as nitrogen, phosphorus, and carbon, which are utilized for their growth and pollutant removal. The biomagnification of compounds such as nitrogen and phosphorus from low to high trophic levels in freshwater and saltwater ecosystems can have a significant ecological impact. Modern agriculture's excessive reliance on synthetic inputs has a negative impact on plants, soil, and even the quality of the water (Yong et al., 2021). The enhanced phosphate concentrations in aquatic ecosystems lead to the development of eutrophication. This results in the depletion of oxygen levels in the water. This low level of oxygen will result in a negative impact on aquatic creatures (Sperling & Chernicharo, 2005). The nitrate compound occurs naturally in groundwater and surface water bodies, one of the undesirable substances that makes the water unsuitable for drinking. It is necessary to remove this pollutant from the water sources. Conventional treatments like coagulation, sedimentation, and flocculation show high-energy costs, production of toxic compounds, and poor removal efficiency. To overcome this major issue, different biological approaches have been employed, including bacteria, algae, and fungi (He et al., 2013; Ratnasari et al., 2021). Bioremediation is one of the most powerful methods to clean environmental pollution, a method mostly suggested due to its low cost and effective performance. Nowadays, algae are considered as a promising candidate to remove environmental pollutants owing to their unique characteristics like generating oxygen by the photosynthetic process, diverse tolerant forms, ability to convert pollutants into biomass, and environmental niche. Algal species are widely known for their properties of biofuel production and wastewater cleanup. Heavy metals are accumulated by many algal species, and they are involved in degrading xenobiotic compounds (Suresh & Ravishankar, 2004). This process removes toxic or harmful compounds from the solid, liquid, or gaseous phase, and they are removed by mechanisms such as bioadsorption, bioaccumulation, and biotransformation (Upadhyay et al., 2024). This chapter deals with the kinetic mechanisms and effects of pH, temperature, and light intensity on the algal remediation process. It addresses the challenges in phycoremediation and implements physical, chemical, and biological remediation techniques to enhance removal efficiency through a synergistic bioremediation process. Furthermore, the final section explores the significant applications and future prospects of algal bioremediation for a greener environment.

3.2 Algal Species in Bioremediation

Algae are phytoplankton that appear in different shapes. They are categorized into microalgae and macroalgae. They are photosynthetic prokaryotic or eukaryotic organisms that grow very rapidly and adapt to extreme environmental conditions (Matamoros et al., 2016). Generally, the algae are classified based on their pollutant removal, habitat, cell wall composition and integrity, pigmentation, and storage materials. According to them, they are divided into three important groups such as green, red, and brown algae. The word "phycoremediation" is defined as the method to remove or mitigate pollutants from water, soil, and air by using algal species. The algae utilize the chemical and biological oxygen in water, thereby reducing the pollutants (Mohd Apandi et al., 2020). Algal species exhibited greater surface volume, binding affinity, and significant efficiency. These features are effectively involved in removing the textile dye, heavy metals, organic matter, and phase contaminants (Papazi et al., 2019). In addition to the removal of pollutants, algae can also use the nutrients present in the pollutants for their growth, such as nitrogen and phosphorus. Microalgae are considered to be the best alternative for removing different pollutants. They have high tolerance to the environment, overgrowth in wastewater, eco-friendly species, and greater ability to drug tolerance (Roostaei & Zhang, 2017). Algae demonstrate adaptability to the toxicity of organic and

Table 3.1 Algal species and their pollutant removal

S. No	Algae	Pollutant removal	References
1.	*Galdieria sulphuraria*	NH_3, Au, Pd, and Oc	Henkanatte-Gedera et al. (2017)
2.	*Gracilaria gracilis*	Y, Ce, Nd, Eu, and La	Jacinto et al. (2018)
3.	*Gracilaria lemaneiformis*	NH_4, No^{3-}, No^{2-}, and PO_4^{3-}	Wang et al. (2019)
4.	*Chlorella vulgaris*	Ni, Cu, P	He et al. (2013)
5.	*Parachlorella kessleri*	Ag	Sedlakova-Kadukova et al. (2019)
6.	*Chlamydomonas reinhardtii*	Cu	Flouty and Estephane (2012)
7.	*Amphora coffeaeformis*	Herbicide (mesotrione)	El-Eslamboly et al. (2019)

inorganic environmental pollutants through both intracellular and extracellular mechanisms. Table 3.1 represents the various forms of algae and their effectiveness in contaminant removal.

3.3 Kinetic Mechanisms of Pollutant Uptake by Phycoremediation

Phycoremediation utilizes microalgae to remove pollutants from contaminated water through several key mechanisms. Heavy metal uptake occurs via a two-phase process involving initial extracellular biosorption to cell wall functional groups, followed by slower intracellular bioaccumulation (Ibuot et al., 2019). Biosorption typically dominates, accounting for approximately 85.5% of uptake compared to 14.5% bioaccumulation in lead remediation studies (Danouche et al., 2021). Additional mechanisms include volatilization, bio-methylation, enzyme catalyzation, compartmentalization, and extracellular polymeric substance complexation. Pollutant removal efficiency depends on factors such as microalgae species, cell surface characteristics, nutrient availability, biosorbent size, and metal concentration (Nyika & Dinka, 2023). The process effectively removes dyes, heavy metals, and other toxic compounds from textile wastewater (Selvaraj et al., 2023). Enhancement strategies include chemical pretreatment, genetic engineering, and nanoparticle modification of cell surfaces (Kumar et al., 2023). This eco-friendly, cost-effective technology offers additional benefits, including bioenergy production and CO_2 mitigation (Selvaraj et al., 2023).

3.3.1 Adsorption

Adsorption is an extracellular process that uses solid materials to remove pollutants. Adsorbents are used to remove carbon nanomaterials and phenolic pollutants (Fu et al., 2018). The biosorption process requires functional groups, cellulose, and proteins found inside the algal cell wall. Adsorption and precipitation of heavy metals on the algal surface are mediated by the charged functional groups, including phosphate, carboxyl, amidogenic, sulfhydryl, and hydroxyl groups (Nagarajan et al., 2020). Through electrostatic attraction, the pollutants will bind to the algal cell surface, and it is a passive process that does not require energy. This method involves the formation of flocs and reduces the wastewater pollutants (Ahmed et al., 2021).

3.3.2 Bioaccumulation

Bioaccumulation is an intracellular bio-uptake process, where the pollutants are taken up within the cells. Pollutants that pass through the algal membrane accumulate inside the algal cells. Through the compartmentalization mechanism, pollutants and heavy metals accumulate in the cellular organelles, such as vacuoles, chloroplasts, and mitochondria (Danouche et al., 2021).

3.3.3 Biotransformation

Algal cells use chelators to convert toxic pollutants into non-toxic forms. The chelators are organic compounds that form complexes by linking themselves with metal ions, known as complexation. This can be a defense mechanism used by the algae to remove metal toxicity (Genchi et al., 2019). It has been removed by the phytoplankton using the carrier proteins. The chelation substances include acid residues, thiol molecules, enzymes, and peptides. Phytochelatins (PCs) are small cysteine-rich peptides that play a crucial role in heavy metal detoxification across diverse organisms, including algae, plants, and some animals. These non-genetically encoded peptides are enzymatically synthesized by phytochelatin synthase (PCS) from glutathione (Chia, 2021).

3.4 Algae-Based Bioremediation of Pollutants Across Diverse Environments

3.4.1 Heavy Metal Removal

Metal toxicity tends to be hazardous substances that lead to adverse environmental effects. Mostly, the heavy metals like lead, cadmium, mercury, silver, and arsenic originated from electric sources, automobiles, mines, and farm wastes such as herbicides. Algae remove heavy metals through two main processes. Initially, the algal cell adheres to the cell surface of contaminants, followed by attachment of ions on the cell wall due to the presence of various functional groups, including hydroxyl, amide, and sulfhydryl groups. Cationic molecules are attracted to the anionic charged molecules on the algal surface to mitigate the severity of heavy metal

Table 3.2 Algal species for heavy metal remediation

S. No	Heavy metals	Algae	Method of removal	References
1.	Arsenic	*Ulva lactuca*	Biosorption and bioaccumulation	Henriques et al. (2019)
2.	Boron	*Ulva reticulata (biochar)*	Biosorption	Senthilkumar et al. (2019)
3.	Cadmium	*Phormidium ambiguum*	Biosorption and bioaccumulation	Shanab et al. (2012)
4.	Chromium	*Durvillaea antarctica*	Biosorption	Guarín-Romero et al. (2019)
5.	Cobalt	*Chlorococcum humicola*	Biosorption	Borah et al. (2020)
6.	Mercury	*Ulva lactuca*	Biosorption and bioaccumulation	Henriques et al. (2019)
7.	Nickel	*Durvillaea antarctica*	Biosorption	Guarín-Romero et al. (2019)
8.	Zinc	*Fucus vesiculosus*	Biosorption	Brinza et al. (2019)

contaminants. Subsequently, the ions get embedded through the cell and slowly accumulate inside the cells (Jie et al., 2021; Usmani et al., 2020). Chromium is available in two different forms, which are trivalent and hexavalent chromium. The hexavalent cation is reduced to the trivalent form and can diffuse through the biological membrane. Complete reduction of heavy metals can be achieved using algae because they produce various intracellular and extracellular enzymes that facilitate the transformation of pollutants from complex structures (toxic) into simpler, non-toxic forms. This process requires energy; however, as photosynthetic organisms, algae are capable of producing their own energy to enhance the breakdown of pollutants. Due to their diverse metabolic activity and eco-friendly nature, algae have been widely employed as potent agents in the present bioremediation practice. Table 3.2 represents the diverse remediation mechanisms, including biosorption, bioaccumulation, and phytoremediation for heavy metals removal using microalgae that contribute to environmental detoxification and ecosystem restoration. Similarly, Fig. 3.1 highlights different biological pathways of microalgae employed to eradicate the pollutants.

3.4.2 Organic Pollutant Removal

Organic pollutants are considered to be stable and deposited, which leads to the buildup of toxicity in the water sources and the environment. They run off from agricultural and domestic waste, industrial effluents, and urban sources, which severely affect the health of aquatic life. Microalgae such as, *Aphanocapsa* spp., *Chlorella* spp., and *Scenedesmus* spp., which are effectively involved in dye bioremediation. It depends on parameters such as the type of algal species, the molecular

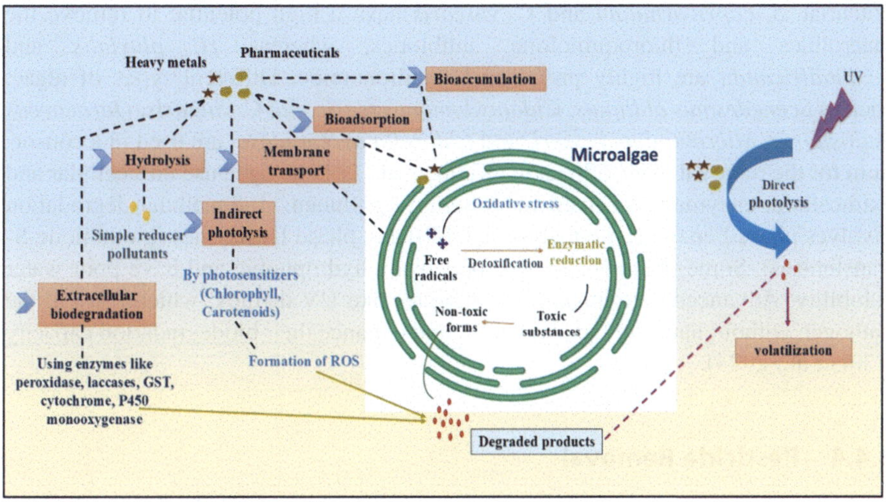

Fig. 3.1 Schematic representation of various pollutant removal mechanisms using phycoremediation

geometry of dyes, and azo-reductase metabolism (Premaratne et al., 2021). It is reported that 90% of the azo dyes were degraded by *Chlorella vulgaris* (Ishchi & Sibi, 2019). Remazol brilliant blue R dye and reactive 19 were degraded by *Scenedesmus quadricauda.*

3.4.3 Degradation of Pharmaceutical Products

A mixture of pharmaceutical products is present in wastewater, and these compounds can accumulate in the food web via biomagnification, affecting the environment, wildlife, and humans (Wang et al., 2019). Various microalgae have been reported to remove pharmaceuticals from wastewater. Pharmaceutical products are removed by mechanisms such as biodegradation, biomineralization, biosorption, stripping, and photodegradation. Bioaccumulation of pharmaceutical products by algal cells generates reactive oxygen species (ROS), which are molecules containing oxygen atoms with unpaired electrons, including superoxide radicals, hydroxyl radicals, hydroperoxyl radicals, and alkoxy radicals (Zou et al., 2017). Under normal conditions, ROS function as signaling molecules in cellular processes, but excessive production leads to oxidative stress and cellular damage (Rezayian et al., 2018). In algae, ROS can damage cell membranes, proteins, and lipids when antioxidant defense systems are overwhelmed (Ugya et al., 2019). Marine phytoplankton, particularly *Chattonella* species, generate high levels of extracellular ROS, including superoxide and hydroxyl radicals, which can cause tissue damage in surrounding organisms. *Haematococcus pluvialis*, *Selenastrum capricornutum*, *Scenedesmus quadricauda*, and *Chlorella vulgaris* were studied for the antibiotic removal potential. *S. capricornutum* and *C. vulgaris* have a high potential to remove the macrolides and fluoroquinolone antibiotics, whereas *H. pluvialis* and *S. quadiricauda* are highly preferred for sulfonamide. Different types of algae, such as *Scenedesmus obliquus*, *Chlamydomonas mexicana*, *C. vulgaris*, *Ourococcus multisporus*, *Micractinium resseri,* and *Chlorella pyrenoidosa*, are used in a consortium for the removal of enrofloxacin (Xiong et al., 2017). Algae use intracellular and extracellular enzymatic mechanisms to remove pollutants. Intracellular degradation involves phase I enzymes (cytochrome P450) and phase II enzymes (glutathione-S-transferases). Some pharmaceutical products are hydrophobic and have poor water solubility. Advanced detoxification techniques like UV therapy, which can kill the pathogen without harming the algal cells, and enhance their biodegradation capacity (Lim et al., 2024).

3.4.4 Pesticide Removal

Pesticides are natural or synthetic chemical compounds designed to control various pests across multiple sectors, including agriculture, forestry, aquaculture, and food production (Pathak et al., 2022). These substances can be classified according to multiple criteria such as toxicity, chemical composition, mode of action, target organisms, and source of origin (Ahamad et al., 2023). While pesticides are indispensable for agricultural production and crop protection, their extensive use poses significant threats to public health and ecosystems (Kaur et al., 2024). Synthetic organic pesticides include chlorinated hydrocarbons, organophosphates, carbamates, and pyrethroids (Ahamad et al., 2023). Environmental contamination occurs when pesticides spread beyond intended targets, with older compounds like DDT persisting in soil and water systems (Kaur et al., 2024). Herbicides are widely used in agricultural and wildland sectors to control undesirable weeds to increase economic profit (Alengebawy et al., 2021). Algal-mediated remediation for the removal of pesticides occurs through any of the four significant processes—adsorption, biodegradation, biouptake, and bioaccumulation. Algal cells provide a significant surface area ratio, rendering an ideal medium for the adsorption process and subsequent pesticide interaction. Bioaccumulation is a process that involves active transport mechanisms in which the pesticide products are attached to the algal surface and then are transported inside and bind with the proteins and organelles present intracellularly. This accumulation will induce the production of reactive oxygen species and lead to the oxidation of DNA and membrane lipids. In turn, antioxidative enzymes produced by the microalgae can eliminate the excess ROS production (Nicodemus et al., 2020). Biodegradation is one of the effective mechanisms for the removal of contaminants. It converts the complex pesticide compounds into simpler molecules by catalytic metabolic conversion. Activation of pesticides by oxidation, reduction, and hydroxylation for increased solubility, degradability, and hydrophilicity is the major step in pesticide biodegradation. The enzyme transfers to the pesticide to form conjugates, which are then transported to the vacuoles. Algal cells also have the capability to accumulate and degrade pesticides simultaneously.

3.5 External Factors Shaping the Effectiveness of Algal Bioremediation

3.5.1 Effect of pH

pH is the crucial factor that determines the growth of microorganisms, including microalgae. Different microbes prefer different levels of pH for their growth, while changes in pH can affect the function of enzymes and proteins. Microalgae exhibit remarkable pH tolerance, with most species thriving under neutral conditions, while some extremophiles can survive in highly acidic or alkaline environments. Several studies demonstrate the cultivation of organisms at extreme pH levels. *Chlorella sorokiniana* can grow at pH >10 for enhanced atmospheric CO_2 capture (Vadlamani et al., 2017), while acid-tolerant strains like *Stichococcus bacillaris* and *Chlamydomonas acidophila* successfully grow at pH below 3, achieving biomass productivities only 10–39% lower than neutral-pH species (Abiusi et al., 2022). Non-acidophilic species can be acclimated to extreme acidic conditions for sustainable biomass production (Abinandan et al., 2018). However, the growth of microalgae can change the pH of the medium, which affects the growth of algal cells (Li et al., 2020). pH is the factor that influences algal growth and the utilization of ammonia nitrogen. Changes in the pH can reduce the ability of algal cells to reduce nitrogen and nutrient removal. Because pH level affects the activity of the enzyme, nutrient disintegration, and the imbalance between absorption and dissociation. Elevated pH levels restrict the growth of algae and enzymatic reactions, whereas at high pH, it promotes volatilization of ammonium into ammonia gas. This leads to nitrogen loss, which affects the biological efficiency of algae. Conversely, at a low pH level, the algal nutrient absorption and growth are disrupted (Delgadillo-Mirquez et al., 2016). The study showed that Pb was removed by the algal cell over different pH levels, and 64% of contaminants were removed at pH 5.5. 42% of the pollutants are removed at neutral pH.

3.5.2 Effect of Temperature

Temperature is one of the essential environmental factors that maintains the algal growth. Improper temperature can affect the algal growth and their metabolism. The optimum temperature for algal growth is 20°C to 35°C. An increase in temperature can lead to protein denaturation, enzyme inactivation, and metabolic disorders, which result in algal death. Different temperature profiles are studied for nutrient removal efficiency, which shows that metabolic activities in algae have increased in elevated temperature, and are helpful in nutrient removal (Xu et al., 2019).

3.5.3 Effect of Light

Algae are photosynthetic organism that requires light as an important source for photosynthesis, and produce ATP, NADPH, and other products of photosynthesis. The usage of light varies among different algal species. Under high light concentration, the increase in light intensity can increase the algal biomass, but photooxidation leads to photoinhibition (Ma & Jian, 2022). Overexposure to light is considered a stress condition that leads to the generation of reactive oxygen species due to electron accumulation in the photosynthetic electron transport chain. This leads to inhibition of photosynthesis, which affects the removal of pollutants. Algae like *Chlorella,* placed under high light levels, can lower its absorption and accumulation of heavy metals like cadmium and lead. High-light stress destroys the machinery of photosynthesis and regulates the ROS production, which affects the removal of heavy metals (Bajguz, 2010). For instance, elevated light levels limit the growth of freshwater algae, thereby hindering their ability to absorb dissolved compounds from polluted water (Rochaix, 2011).

3.6 Current Challenges in Phycoremediation

Algae are considered excellent bioremediators due to their exceptional properties, such as superior metal tolerance, rapid growth, excellent efficacy in metal-binding, large surface area, reusable and natural characteristics like photosynthetic efficiency, metabolic activity, and eco-friendliness. Interestingly, the inactive algal cells are also employed in the bioremediation process, where their effectiveness in heavy metal removal occurs through a passive mechanism (biosorption) that is not significantly constrained by nutrients or other external factors. However, the phycoremediation technique faces certain challenges due to some drawbacks. Algae exhibit resistance to heavy metal toxicity, and prolonged exposure negatively impacts their growth. This leads to decreased biomass yield. This decline affects the production of valuable compounds like lipids, nanoparticles, and pigments (Chugh et al., 2022). Although heavy metal bioremediation has been widely studied, the underlying mechanisms are not completely known. Researchers have introduced the concept of genetic engineering by modifying genes in microalgae. This leads to the overexpression of protein for bioremediation and also enhances the efficiency. Some studies have reported that the genetically modified *Chlamydomonas reinhardtii* removed the diclofenac from water even at high concentrations, showing exceptional metabolic activity. It exhibits strong bioremediation potential while enhancing the pharmaceutical pollutant removal (Liakh et al., 2023). *Anabaena* sp. PCC 7120 metabolizes the lindane, a toxic pesticide, by stimulating the *lin* genes associated with the degradation process (Guio et al., 2023). These reports highlight the potential of genetically modified algae in bioremediation. Despite these advantages, the genetic alterations in algae cause significant effects on their growth, metabolism, and interactions with their surrounding microorganisms. It reduced their effectiveness in removing environmental pollutants and created new environmental issues like ecological disruption, altered nutrient cycles, challenges in monitoring, gene dissemination, and risk of toxic algal blooms. In real-world applications, the genetically modified strain should be tested to ensure its safety and effectiveness for humans. Additionally, legal and ethical considerations are appropriate in their implementation. Public concerns and government support are needed to permit the use of genetic algal strains in bioremediation (Calatrava et al., 2024). Environmental factors like temperature, pH, and light intensity affect the algal metabolism, growth, and pollution removal processes. Temperature fluctuations stimulate the growth of algae, which results in algal death. Conversely, shifts in pH limit the uptake of nutrients and mitigate the removal of pollutants. The quantity of pollutants potentially affects the algal population. To combat this problem, experts proposed a hybrid approach, which facilitates a synergistic effect for pollutant removal as well as enhancement of algal bioremediation.

3.7 Hybrid Technique: Synergistic Effect of Phycoremediation with Other Methodologies

Algal remediation possesses significant potential for diminishing the contaminants in the environment. Its efficacy can be greatly improved by combining it with advanced remediation techniques. Integrating algal bioremediation with other approaches, such as physical, chemical, and biological, enhances pollutant removal, improves tolerance in diverse environmental conditions, and optimizes sustainability. These hybrid methods not only increase the efficiency of pollutant degradation but also could be a novel, eco-friendly approach.

3.7.1 Physical Remediation Techniques

3.7.1.1 Integration of Phycoremediation with Thermal Desorption

Microalgae possess an exceptional ability through absorption and accumulation mechanisms and reduce various kinds of pollutants, such as heavy metals, nutrients, and organic pollutants. Generally, the pollutants adhere to the algal surfaces by the biosorption process, and the organic pollutants are taken up by algal cells through a bioaccumulation mechanism. Thermal desorption is a technique to remove pollutants from the soil by the method of heating. It is used to eliminate contaminants via extreme temperatures or other thermal processes. The process of thermal desorption technique heats the contaminated soil at a specified temperature. The impurities present in the soil get liberated and transmitted into the gas stream (Nie et al., 2024). The combination of these two techniques allows a long-term solution. Harmful compounds are neutralized by algal utilization. The condensation of chemicals and pollutants is carried out in a thermal technique. This technique helps extract the pollutants from the environment.

3.7.1.2 Phycomediated Membrane Bioreactor

Microalgae-based membrane bioreactors (MBRs) are one of the best solutions for removing environmental pollutants in municipal wastewater. The nutrients and contaminants are absorbed by the algal cells, whereas the algal biomass is separated by physical separation facilitated by a membrane unit. The MBR is an integrated bioprocess with a membrane filter, and it is an advanced system. The algal cells and high molecular weight pollutants are removed by membrane filtration. Phosphate-accumulating bacteria and nitrifying bacteria are inhibited by high aeration within the reactor. Although it can enhance the growth of microbes by allowing the uptake of dissolved oxygen and organic carbon. The suspended solids, microorganisms, are filtered by the membrane and are involved in effluent purification (Zahmatkesh et al., 2023). The synergy of algal action and membrane technology is a powerful effect for removing heavy metals, organic compounds, and pathogens. It not only reduces the sludge generation but is also involved in the production of biofuel from algae. It is one of the eco-friendly methods and has positive effects on the environment. It mitigates the fouling of the membrane and increases the membrane durability, and lowers the cost.

3.7.1.3 Electrokinetic-Based Phycoremediation Technique

The combined method of electrokinetic and algal bioremediation presents an effective hybrid approach to get rid of pollutants in low-permeability soils. The electrokinetic remediation technique is environment-friendly, which facilitates in situ remediation. This system uses two electrodes (cathode and anode) that are directly inserted into the polluted soil. The separation of contaminants from the soil is done through three processes: electrophoresis, electroosmosis, and electromigration. The effect of this method is based on the concentration and type of pollutants, ionic movement, solubility, chemical and physical properties of the soil. It shows some advantages, such as pollutants being separated only between the electrodes, resulting in lower costs, and no harmful substances being used (Sun et al., 2023). The synergistic combination of electrokinetic (EK) and phycoremediation/bioremediation technologies significantly enhances soil remediation efficiency while reducing energy demands. EK processes apply low-intensity electric fields to mobilize contaminants through electro-osmotic flow, electromigration, and electrophoresis, particularly effective in low hydraulic conductivity soils (Gnanasundar & Akshai Raj, 2020). When coupled with phytoremediation, this electrokinetic-assisted approach increases contaminant bioavailability and reduces treatment time compared to standalone phytoremediation (Rodríguez et al., 2021; Cameselle et al., 2021). EK-bioremediation combinations enhance biodegradation rates and microbial enzyme secretion while improving contaminant mobilization (Ramadan et al., 2018). The low operating energy requirements of EK systems, combined with the sustainable nature of biological processes, make these hybrid approaches cost-effective alternatives to conventional remediation methods (Moghadam et al., 2016). The applied electric field in an environment can significantly improve the bioavailability of organic pollutants by exploiting them through electrokinetic effects. In an underground polluted area, organic pollutants can be degraded using electrode reactions and electrical thermal effects, with biological effects. This creates a synergistic interaction for the remediation of soil contaminants and heavy metals. It could be a promising approach in the future.

3.7.2 Chemical Remediation Techniques

3.7.2.1 Algal-Based Solidification Technique

This approach mitigates the pollutant mobility for long-term environmental sustainability. Solidification and stabilization treatment consists of two steps. The process of solidification traps pollutants and restricts their movement, while the stabilization process lowers bioavailability and leaching. Typically, a binding agent consists of a stabilizer and curing substances. The most commonly used curing agents are concrete, ashes, and blast furnaces, which weaken the pollutants in soil. The stabilizing agents are introduced to minimize the leaching toxicity during the period of the solidification process (Han et al., 2020). Algal bioremediation decreases the harshness of chemical substances and energy processes. Meanwhile, this solidification process developed a stabilized matrix. Algae-derived biomass might be separated and retrieved by a solidification process and used in various applications, like biofertilizers with high nutrient content, biofuels, bioenergy, high-value bioproducts for pharmaceuticals, nutraceuticals, and food additives (Sarwer et al., 2022; Sun et al., 2022; Bhalamurugan et al., 2018). This interaction approach increases the long-term stability of bioremediation.

3.7.2.2 Algal-Driven Soil Decontamination Technique

The algae-assisted soil washing method integrates surfactants and chelating agents, merging traditional chemical soil washing with the beneficial biological actions of algae. This technique has evolved to effectively eliminate contaminants from the soil. Soil contaminant scan be removed using washing agents like surfactants, chelating agents, and inorganic compounds through the process of dissolution, chelation, and desorption (Trellu et al., 2021). Apart from the type of agents, the time of washing, the concentration used, the ratio of solid-liquid, and the physico-chemical properties of the soil influence the removal performance. The chemicals used might reduce the combined ability of soil and organic pollutants, thus increasing their movement in the soil. However, it had some problems with removal efficiency and was expensive. This could be further improved (Zhu et al., 2021). So, combining both soil washing and phycoremediation will improve the degradation efficiency of pollutants. This coupled technique achieves greater efficiency. Soil washing extract the heavy metals and organic pollutants through chemical action, while phycoremediation uses the algae to absorb and modify the residual toxins in treated effluents. Research demonstrates that soil washing effectively mobilizes hydrocarbons from crude oil-contaminated soils, with removal efficiencies reaching up to 100% for polycyclic aromatic hydrocarbons and 95.7% for total petroleum hydrocarbons (Offiong et al., 2021). Following soil washing, cyanobacteria like *Anabaena* sp. show significant potential for treating contaminated effluents and degrading residual organic compounds (Bhattacharya et al., 2024). This combined approach of soil washing followed by biological treatment represents an effective strategy for hydrocarbon remediation, as bioremediation technologies are environmentally friendly, cost-effective, and capable of converting organic pollutants to innocuous products (Okoh et al., 2020; Abdullah et al., 2020). This approach overall improves efficiency, minimizes the level of harsh substances, and supports the sustainable reuse of algal biomass.

3.7.2.3 Oxidative Phycoremediation

The combined action of phycoremediation and chemical oxidants represents an effective technique for the improved breakdown of pollutants and absorption in a contaminated environment. Chemical oxidation is a process of using oxidizing agents that break down the organic pollutants into non-toxic or less harmful substances. It mostly detoxifies the organic pollutants, including pesticides, petroleum, and PAHs. The most common oxidizing agents that are used for the treatment process are $KMnO_4$, persulfate, and Fenton's reagents. During this process, oxidation, hydrolysis, and adsorption occur. Oxidizing agents will be added to the sewage water, which will react with pollutants. This chemical reaction reduces and stabilizes the particles, rendering them easier to treat and remove. A new chemical oxidation technique, like the advanced oxidation process, effectively removes contaminants. This process emits reactive oxygen species such as OH^-, H^+, and free radicals to oxidize the contaminants and treat effluents. They convert harmful chemicals into non-toxic compounds. It is a quick and simple method to treat pollutants, particularly in wastewater (Aparicio et al., 2022). This dual technique could enhance the remediation of urban and industrial wastewater and offer advantages over conventional treatments. The chemical oxidation process will break down pollutants, while microalgae absorb the by-products and convert these into less harmful compounds. The integration of advanced oxidation processes with biological treatment enhances pollutant degradation and improves biodegradability (Nidheesh et al., 2021). Industrial applications demonstrate significant potential, with microalgae successfully treating various wastewater streams, including textile and tannery effluents (Amin et al., 2022). This integrated approach supports circular bioeconomy principles by transforming waste into resources while addressing environmental pollution challenges (Ali et al., 2024). This combination can also mitigate the production of recalcitrant pollutants. This approach can be suitable for sustainable wastewater treatment systems, and the yielded algal biomass can be processed into biofuels and organic fertilizers.

3.7.3 Biological Remediation Techniques

3.7.3.1 Synergistic Phycoremediation with Phytoremediation

The combined application of phyto-phycoremediation provides a sustainable and eco-friendly technique to remove pollutants from the contaminated environment. Plant remediation technique eliminates toxic metals, volatile compounds, and contaminants. The plant compounds have the ability to metabolize, detoxify, stabilize, and dissolve chemicals that reside in soil, including hydrocarbons, heavy metals, and pesticides. This process induces a wide range of detoxifying techniques such as phytovolatilization, rhizofiltration, plant decomposition, phytoaccumulation, and phytostabilization. This phenomenacreates an eco-friendly strategy through the combination of algae and plants. It possesses the greatest advantages over the traditional methods, namely, cost-effectiveness, non-toxicity, and reusability. Phytoremediation absorbs and detoxify the contaminants in the environment, while phycoremediation increases the efficiency of the phytoremediation process through the enzymatic reaction of the microorganisms. The enzymes produced accelerate the degradation of pollutants and improve the bioavailability. This mechanism is called rhizodegradation. Meanwhile, the algal cells produce extracellular polymeric substances that enhance pollutant absorption on the soil surfaces (Paul et al., 2024). This dual process generates a renewable environment for bioenergy production and bioremediation.

3.7.3.2 Tri-Bioremediation

This approach leverages the unique abilities of bacteria, fungi, and algae to create a synergistic system that effectively removes pollutants and heavy metals from contaminated soil. Microbial bioremediation involves introducing specific strains or communities of microorganisms into the soil to break down harmful substances. It has gained significant interest due to its cost-effectiveness, high efficiency, and minimal environmental impact during use. Microbes eliminate contaminants through their metabolic processes, employing mechanisms such as bioaccumulation, biosorption, and biodegradation. The microbial groups involved—bacteria, fungi, and algae—work together to reduce pollutant toxicity and concentration. This combined strategy shows promise for reclaiming petroleum hydrocarbons in marine environments. This could be a tri approach in marine environments for the reclamation of petroleum hydrocarbons. Bacteria and fungi generate oxidoreductase enzymes for degrading organic matter and immobilize the inorganic pollutants. The hazardous substances are neutralized by the microalgae and produce exopolysaccharides like algal biofilm, which facilitates the absorption of pollutants from the environmental surface and converts them to less soluble forms. Various organisms use different cellular processes for petroleum hydrocarbon degradation with improved efficiency (Dell' Anno et al., 2021). This is a promising solution for addressing various environmental challenges in the future. Figure 3.2 explains the synergistic bioremediation strategies that include physical, chemical, and biological remediation techniques with phycoremediation for pollutant removal.

3.8 Algal Bioremediation in Various Application Conditions

Algal bioremediation has drawn interest as a sustainable technique for cleansing contaminated surroundings and different kinds of wastewater. Microalgae can effectively eliminate viruses, organic pollutants, heavy metals, and nutrients from

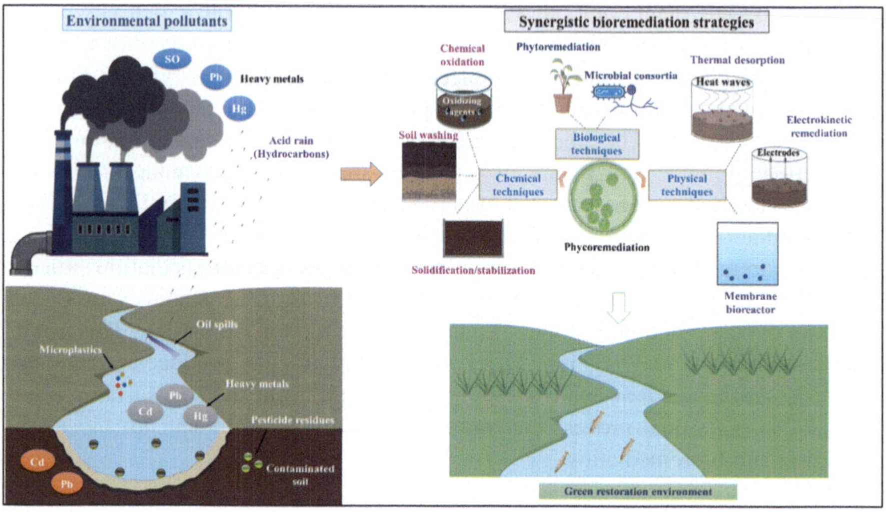

Fig. 3.2 Hybrid bioremediation strategies with phycoremediation for pollutant degradation

wastewater. This process has a number of benefits, including being economical, requiring low energy, and producing valuable biomass that can be used to produce biofuel and other products. Algal bioremediation is remarkable for its cost, sustainability, and possibility to yield valuable byproducts when compared to conventional methods (Gondi et al., 2021). Algal bioremediation is a technology capable of being used in various settings, including wastewater treatment facilities, polluted rivers, and contaminated soils (Dubey et al., 2023). Figure 3.3 shows how algal-based bioremediation is implemented across various ecological systems.

3.8.1 Wastewater Treatment

Microalgae have emerged as a potential tool for wastewater treatment method that additionally produces useful byproducts. Algae-based treatment technologies, such as photobioreactors and waste stabilization ponds, offer economical and sustainable substitutes for conventional techniques. Biofuels, charcoal, pigments, and other beneficial products can be derived from the algal biomass generated during treatment (Arun et al., 2020). Microalgae play a crucial role in ecosystem wellness through oxygen production and carbon dioxide sequestration. Globally, algae are estimated to produce nearly half of the atmospheric oxygen, despite comprising less than 1% of the total photosynthetic biomass (Sengupta et al., 2017). Their efficient carbon concentrating mechanisms enable high photosynthetic rates, making them effective for biosequestration with approximately 1.83 kg of CO_2 converted per kg of dry algal biomass (Viswanaathan & Sudhakar, 2018). Beyond their atmospheric benefits, microalgae enhance ecosystem health by serving as natural biofilters, absorbing

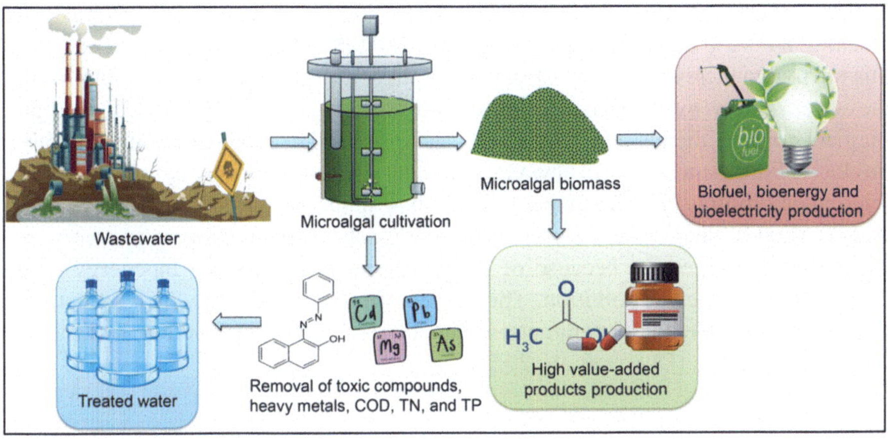

Fig. 3.3 Microalgae-based remediation of pollutants from different environments. (Reprinted from (El-Sheekh et al., 2025). Copyright © 2025 by Author(s) and distributed under the terms of the Creative Commons CC BY license (http://creativecommons.org/licenses/by/4.0/))

excess nutrients and contaminants while improving water quality. They support aquatic food webs, contribute to habitat creation, and maintain biodiversity (Kiranmayee et al., 2025). In aquatic systems, microalgae create biological pumps that transport carbon from surface waters to depths (Sengupta et al., 2017). Additionally, they produce oxygen while providing essential nutrients through bacterial interactions, supporting sustainable ecosystem functioning (Solomon et al., 2023; Ende et al., 2024). However, challenges such as biomass harvesting and the need for large areas of land remain obstacles to broader adoption.

3.8.2 Algal Bioremediation in Polluted River Systems

Microalgae have demonstrated strong potential for cleaning polluted river water through phycoremediation, while simultaneously generating valuable biomass. *Chlorella vulgaris* demonstrates exceptional efficiency in removing nitrogen and phosphorus from various wastewater sources while producing lipid-rich biomass suitable for biofuel production. Multiple studies confirm high nutrient removal rates, with nitrogen removal ranging from 72.1% to 99% and phosphorus removal from 87% to over 99% (Venckus et al., 2017; Yousif et al., 2022). For lead removal, *Scenedesmus obliquus* achieved over 50% efficiency after 18 days, with biosorption being the predominant mechanism (Danouche et al., 2021). Additionally, *S. obliquus* biomass grown in wastewater contains high sugar content (up to 44.5%), making it suitable for bioethanol production, while also achieving high removal rates of nutrients like ammonium and phosphate (>97%) (Hamouda et al., 2016; Oliveira et al., 2018). *Spirulina platensis* demonstrates significant potential for heavy metal biosorption, particularly for lead and cadmium removal from contaminated water.

Multiple studies confirm its high adsorption efficiency, with lead removal rates reaching 84–92% under optimal conditions (Al-Homaidan et al., 2015). The use of this microalga increased the effectiveness of phycoremediation while also improving the water quality by lowering hazardous substances. Because of its high lipid and pigment content, the generated biomass can be utilized to produce biofuel and other products. Furthermore, in wastewater treatment, mixed microbial communities and microalgal biofilms performed much better than single-species cultures (Ugya et al., 2021). Algal biomass offers a sustainable approach for both resource recovery and wastewater management because of its dual capacity to produce bioenergy while clearing environmental pollution. The degree of effectiveness to which a treatment works depends on external parameters, namely pH, biomass production, and starting contaminant levels (Dubey et al., 2023).

3.8.3 Algal Bioremediation in Contaminated Soils

An effective and environmentally conscious technique of addressing contamination in both soil and water is algal bioremediation. *Chlorella vulgaris* shows particularly high efficiency, achieving 65–99% removal rates for various heavy metals in single-metal systems and 49–99% in multi-metal conditions within 3–7 days (Kyratzopoulou et al., 2025). Heavy metal removal occurs through both intracellular and extracellular mechanisms, with functional groups like amino, carboxyl, and hydroxyl groups on cell surfaces binding metal ions (Leong & Chang, 2020). Comparative studies reveal species-specific performance differences, with *Coelastrella* sp. demonstrating superior lead and cadmium uptake compared to other microalgal strains (Qader & Shekha, 2023). This microalgae-based approach offers advantages including cost-effectiveness, eco-friendliness, and high removal efficiency, making it a promising alternative to conventional chemical and physical treatment methods (Ankit et al., 2020; Yeheyo et al., 2024). Using a variety of mechanisms, including bioaccumulation, biosorption, biodegradation, and pH modulation, microalgae and cyanobacteria can eliminate heavy metal pollutants. These microorganisms are notable for their great remediation efficiency, affordability, and easy accessibility (Sarker et al., 2023). Phycoremediation depends on a number of complex biological processes, such as the function of metal transport systems inside cells, the activity of extracellular polymeric substances, and the role of functional groups in cell walls (Danouche et al., 2021).

3.9 Limitations and Future Prospects

Despite the great potential of algal bioremediation, issues persist, particularly in developing the technology and optimizing the conditions required for algal growth. Future research should focus on creating resilient algal strains, establishing successful microbial consortia, and enhancing biofilm production to make this strategy both profitable and sustainable (Alazaiza et al., 2022). To expand the use of algal bioremediation at larger scales, further studies are needed to improve the selection of algae species, investigate genetic modification for enhanced efficiency, and integrate algal-based strategies with traditional treatment technologies (Touliabah & Ismail, 2021). Selecting suitable strains of algae is vital for preventing risks, including overgrowth or the production of toxic secondary metabolites. It has been demonstrated that genetic and metabolic engineering tools enable microalgae to serve as robust cell factories, tolerating a wide range of environmental conditions while maintaining productivity for biofuels and valuable compounds (Guihéneuf et al., 2016). Hence, engineered algal strains demonstrates their ability to resist harsh environmental conditions, with significant potential for pollutant bioremediation. The financial sustainability of bioremediation procedures can be significantly enhanced by converting algal biomass into useful products, such as bioplastics, biofertilizers, and biofuels. The risk of algal overgrowth or toxin production must be mitigated through careful selection of species.

3.10 Conclusion

Microalgae offer a promising tool for treating diverse environmental contaminants due to their rapid growth, adaptation to various environmental settings, and the ability to produce various intracellular and extracellular enzymes that transform toxic forms into non-toxic ones. This eco-friendly approach is largely determined by several interrelated factors, including the nature and condition of the algae used in this process, pollutant concentration, and external factors. Selecting an appropriate algal strain for effective pollution removal is a major challenge in the industrial scaling process. To overcome this issue, a synergistic approach, such as a combination of physical, chemical, and biological methods with phycoremediation, demonstrates a novel and promising technology in the bioremediation process. Phyco-remediation is an effective method for degrading pollutants present in wastewater, including heavy metals. When optimally executed, it can effectively remove pollutants, improve scalability, and mitigate the toxic effects of chemical treatment. It also explores the diverse applications in environmental conditions and could be a sustainable strategy for green environmental restoration.

Acknowledgments The authors gratefully thank the management of SASTRA Deemed University and the Department of Chemistry and Biosciences, Srinivasa Ramanujan Centre, for their invaluable support and provision of the necessary resources that facilitated the preparation of this article. This research was also a part of the project titled 'Global Bluefood leadership project (RS-2025-02373103)', funded by the Ministry of Oceans and Fisheries, Republic of Korea.

References

Abdullah, S. R. S., Al-Baldawi, I. A., Almansoory, A. F., Purwanti, I. F., Al-Sbani, N. H., & Sharuddin, S. S. N. (2020). Plant-assisted remediation of hydrocarbons in water and soil: Application, mechanisms, challenges and opportunities. *Chemosphere, 247*, 125932. https://doi.org/10.1016/j.chemosphere.2020.125932

Abinandan, S., Subashchandrabose, S. R., Cole, N., Dharmarajan, R., Venkateswarlu, K., & Megharaj, M. (2018). Sustainable production of biomass and biodiesel by acclimation of non-acidophilic microalgae to acidic conditions. *Bioresource Technology, 271*, 316–324. https://doi.org/10.1016/j.biortech.2018.09.140

Abiusi, F., Trompetter, E., Pollio, A., Wijffels, R. H., & Janssen, M. (2022). Acid tolerant and acidophilic microalgae: An underexplored world of biotechnological opportunities. *Frontiers in Microbiology, 13*, 820907. https://doi.org/10.3389/fmicb.2022.820907

Ahamad, A., Ahamad, J., & Naim, M. J. (2023). Current perspective on pesticides: Their classification, behaviour, potential use and toxic effects. *Journal of Angiotherapy, 7*. https://doi.org/10.25163/angiotherapy.719360

Ahmad, A., Banat, F., Alsafar, H., & Hasan, S. W. (2022). Algae biotechnology for industrial wastewater treatment, bioenergy production, and high-value bioproducts. *Science of the Total Environment, 806*, 150585. https://doi.org/10.1016/j.scitotenv.2021.150585

Ahmed, D. A. E. A., Gheda, S. F., & Ismail, G. A. (2021). Efficacy of two seaweeds dry mass in bioremediation of heavy metal polluted soil and growth of radish (*Raphanus sativus* L.) plant. *Environmental Science Pollution Research, 28*, 12831–12846. https://doi.org/10.1007/s11356-020-11289-8

Alazaiza, M. Y., Albahnasawi, A., Ahmad, Z., Bashir, M. J., Al-Wahaibi, T., Abujazar, M. S. S., Abu Amr, S. S., & Nassani, D. E. (2022). Potential use of algae for the bioremediation of different types of wastewater and contaminants: Production of bioproducts and biofuel for green circular economy. *Journal of Environmental Management, 324*, 116415. https://doi.org/10.1016/j.jenvman.2022.116415

Alengebawy, A., Abdelkhalek, S. T., Qureshi, S. R., & Wang, Q. (2021). Heavy metals and pesticides toxicity in agricultural soil and plants: Ecological risks and human health implications. *Toxics, 9*(3), 42. https://doi.org/10.3390/toxics9030042

Al-Homaidan, A. A., Al-Abbad, A. F., Al-Hazzani, A. A., Al-Ghanayem, A. A., & Alabdullatif, J. A. (2015). Lead removal by *Spirulina platensis* biomass. *International Journal of Phytoremediation, 18*(2), 184–189. https://doi.org/10.1080/15226514.2015.1073673

Ali, S. S., Hassan, L. H., & El-Sheekh, M. (2024). Microalgae-mediated bioremediation: Current trends and opportunities-a review. *Archives of Microbiology, 206*, 343. https://doi.org/10.1007/s00203-024-04052-x

Amin, M., Tahir, F., Ashfaq, H., Akbar, I., Razzaque, N., Haider, M. N., Xu, J., Zhu, H., Wang, N., & Shahid, A. (2022). Decontamination of industrial wastewater using microalgae integrated with biotransformation of the biomass to green products. *Energy Nexus, 6*, 100089. https://doi.org/10.1016/j.nexus.2022.100089

Ankit, Bordoloi, N., Tiwari, J., Kumar, S., Korstad, J., & Bauddh, K. (2020). Efficiency of algae for heavy metal removal, bioenergy production, and carbon sequestration. In *Emerging eco-friendly green technologies for wastewater treatment. Microorganisms for sustainability* (Vol. 18). https://doi.org/10.1007/978-981-15-1390-9_4

Aparicio, J. D., Raimondo, E. E., Saez, J. M., Costa-Gutierrez, S. B., Álvarez, A., Benimeli, C. S., & Polti, M. A. (2022). The current approach to soil remediation: A review of physicochemical and biological technologies, and the potential of their strategic combination. *Journal of Environmental Chemical Engineering, 10*(2), 107141. https://doi.org/10.1016/j.jece.2022.107141

Arun, S., Sinharoy, A., Pakshirajan, K., & Lens, P. N. (2020). Algae based microbial fuel cells for wastewater treatment and recovery of value-added products. *Renewable and Sustainable Energy Reviews, 132*, 110041. https://doi.org/10.1016/j.rser.2020.110041

Bajguz, A. (2010). Suppression of Chlorella vulgaris growth by cadmium, Lead, and copper stress and its restoration by endogenous Brassinolide. *Archives of Environmental Contamination and Toxicology, 60*(3), 406. https://doi.org/10.1007/s00244-010-9551-0

Bhalamurugan, G. L., Valerie, O., & Mark, L. (2018). Valuable bioproducts obtained from microalgal biomass and their commercial applications: A review. *Environmental Engineering Research, 23*, 229–241. https://doi.org/10.4491/eer.2017.220

Bhattacharya, P., Jana, S., & Banerjee, S. (2024). Phytoremediation capability of *Anabaena* sp. for high organic and chromium-loaded wastewater in membrane bioreactors. *Water Science & Technology, 89*, 1142–1154. https://doi.org/10.2166/wst.2024.061

Borah, D., Kennedy, B., Gopalakrishnan, S., et al. (2020). Bioremediation and biomass production with the green microalga Chlorococcum humicola and textile mill effluent (TE). *Proceedings of the National Academy of Sciences, India Section B: Biological Sciences., 90*, 415–423. https://doi.org/10.1007/s40011-019-01112-x

Brinza, L., Geraki, K., Cojocaru, C., Holdt, S. L., & Neamtu, M. (2019). Baltic Fucus vesiculosus as potential bio-sorbent for Zn removal: Mechanism insight. *Chemosphere, 238*, 124652. https://doi.org/10.1016/j.chemosphere.2019.124652

Calatrava, V., Gonzalez-Ballester, D., & Dubini, A. (2024). Microalgae for bioremediation: Advances, challenges, and public perception on genetic engineering. *BMC Plant Biology, 24*, 1261. https://doi.org/10.1186/s12870-024-05995-5

Cameselle, C., Gouveia, S., Cabo, A., & Reddy, K. R. (2021). Electrokinetic-assisted phytoremediation of heavy metal contaminated soil: Present status, challenges, and opportunities. In *Phytoremediation technology for the removal of heavy metals and other contaminants from soil and water* (pp. 537–555). https://doi.org/10.1016/B978-0-323-85763-5.00031-3

Chia, J. C. (2021). Phytochelatin synthase in heavy metal detoxification and xenobiotic metabolism. *Biodegradation Technology of Organic and Inorganic Pollutants*. https://doi.org/10.5772/intechopen.99077

Chugh, M., Kumar, L., Shah, M. P., & Bharadvaja, N. (2022). Algal bioremediation of heavy metals: An insight into removal mechanisms, recovery of by-products, challenges, and future opportunities. *Energy Nexus, 7*, 100129. https://doi.org/10.1016/j.nexus.2022.100129

Danouche, M., El Ghachtouli, N., & El Arroussi, H. (2021). Phycoremediation mechanisms of heavy metals using living green microalgae: Physicochemical and molecular approaches for enhancing selectivity and removal capacity. *Heliyon, 7*(7), e07609. https://doi.org/10.1016/j.heliyon.2021.e07609

Delgadillo-Mirquez, L., Lopes, F., Taidi, B., & Pareau, D. (2016). Nitrogen and phosphate removal from wastewater with a mixed microalgae and bacteria culture. *Biotechnology Reports, 11*, 18–26. https://doi.org/10.1016/j.btre.2016.04.003

Dell' Anno, F., Rastelli, E., Sansone, C., Brunet, C., & Ianora, A. (2021). Bacteria, fungi and microalgae for the bioremediation of marine sediments contaminated by petroleum hydrocarbons in the omics era. *Microorganisms, 9*(8), 1695. https://doi.org/10.3390/microorganisms9081695

Dubey, S., Chen, C., Haldar, D., Tambat, V. S., Kumar, P., Tiwari, A., Singhania, R. R., Dong, C., & Patel, A. K. (2023). Advancement in algal bioremediation for organic, inorganic, and emerging pollutants. *Environmental Pollution, 317*, 120840. https://doi.org/10.1016/j.envpol.2022.120840

El-Eslamboly, A. A. S. A., Abd. El. Wanis, M. M., & Amin, A. W. (2019). Algal application as a biological control method of root-knot nematode Meloidogyne incognita on cucumber under protected culture conditions and its impact on yield and fruit quality. *Egyptian Journal of Biological Pest Control, 29*(1), 1–9. https://doi.org/10.1186/s41938-019-0122z

El-Sheekh, M. M., El-Kassas, H. Y., & Ali, S. S. (2025). Microalgae-based bioremediation of refractory pollutants: An approach towards environmental sustainability. *Microbial Cell Factories, 24*, 19. https://doi.org/10.1186/s12934-024-02638-0

Ende, S., Henjes, J., Spiller, M., Elshobary, M., Hanelt, D., & Abomohra, A. (2024). Recent advances in recirculating aquaculture systems and role of microalgae to close system loop. *Bioresource Technology, 407*, 131107. https://doi.org/10.1016/j.biortech.2024.131107

Flouty, R., & Estephane, G. (2012). Bioaccumulation and biosorption of copper and lead by a unicellular algae Chlamydomonas reinhardtii in single and binary metal systems: A comparative study. *Journal of Environmental Management, 111*, 106–114. https://doi.org/10.1016/j.jenvman.2012.06.042

Fu, Y., Shen, Y., Zhang, Z., Ge, X., & Chen, M. (2018). Activated bio-chars derived from rice husk via one- and two-step KOH-catalyzed pyrolysis for phenol adsorption. *Science of the Total Environment, 646*, 1567–1577. https://doi.org/10.1016/j.scitotenv.2018.07.423

Genchi, G., Sinicropi, M. S., Lauria, G., Carocci, A., & Catalano, A. (2019). The effects of cadmium toxicity. *International Journal of Environmental Research and Public Health, 17*(11), 3782. https://doi.org/10.3390/ijerph17113782

Gnanasundar, V., & Akshai Raj, R. (2020). Remediation of inorganic contaminants in soil using electrokinetics, phytoremediation techniques. *Materials Today: Proceedings, 45*, 950–956. https://doi.org/10.1016/j.matpr.2020.03.038

Gondi, R., Kavitha, S., Yukesh Kannah, R., Parthiba Karthikeyan, O., Kumar, G., Kumar Tyagi, V., & Rajesh Banu, J. (2021). Algal-based system for removal of emerging pollutants from wastewater: A review. *Bioresource Technology, 344*, 126245. https://doi.org/10.1016/j.biortech.2021.126245

Guarín-Romero, J. R., Rodríguez-Estupiñán, P., Giraldo, L., & Moreno-Piraján, J. C. (2019). Simple and competitive adsorption study of nickel (II) and chromium (III) on the surface of the Brown algae Durvillaea Antarctica biomass. *ACS Omega, 4*(19), 18147. https://doi.org/10.1021/acsomega.9b02061

Guihéneuf, F., Khan, A., & Tran, L. (2016). Genetic engineering: A promising tool to engender physiological, biochemical, and molecular stress resilience in green microalgae. *Frontiers in Plant Science, 7*, 190468. https://doi.org/10.3389/fpls.2016.00400

Guio, J., Fillat, M. F., Peleato, M. L., & Sevilla, E. (2023). Responses of Anabaena sp. PCC7120 to lindane: Physiological effects and differential expression of potential lin genes. *MicrobiologyOpen, 12*(3), e1355. https://doi.org/10.1002/mbo3.1355

Hamouda, R., Yeheia, D. S., Hamzah, H. A., & Hussein, M. H. (2016). Removal of heavy metals and production of bioethanol by green alga *Scenedesmus obliquus* grown in different concentrations of wastewater. *Sains Malaysiana, 45*(3), 467–476.

Han, L., Li, J., Xue, Q., Chen, Z., Zhou, Y., & Poon, C. S. (2020). Bacterial-induced mineralization (BIM) for soil solidification and heavy metal stabilization: A critical review. *Science of the Total Environment, 746*, 140967. https://doi.org/10.1016/j.scitotenv.2020.140967

He, P., Mao, B., Lu, F., Shao, L., Lee, D., & Chang, J. (2013). The combined effect of bacteria and Chlorella vulgaris on the treatment of municipal wastewaters. *Bioresource Technology, 146*, 562–568. https://doi.org/10.1016/j.biortech.2013.07.111

Henkanatte-Gedera, S., Selvaratnam, T., Karbakhshravari, M., Myint, M., Nirmalakhandan, N., Van Voorhies, W., & Lammers, P. J. (2017). Removal of dissolved organic carbon and nutrients from urban wastewaters by Galdieria sulphuraria: Laboratory to field scale demonstration. *Algal Research, 24*, 450–456. https://doi.org/10.1016/j.algal.2016.08.001

Henriques, B., Teixeira, A., Figueira, P., Reis, A. T., Almeida, J., Vale, C., & Pereira, E. (2019). Simultaneous removal of trace elements from contaminated waters by living Ulva lactuca. *Science of the Total Environment, 652*, 880–888. https://doi.org/10.1016/j.scitotenv.2018.10.282

Ibuot, A. A., Gupta, S. K., Ansolia, P., & Amit, K. B. (2019). Heavy metal bioremediation by microalgae, mechanisms and applications. *Microbial Degradation of Xenobiotic Compounds, 19*.

Ishchi, T., & Sibi, G. (2019). Azo dye degradation by *Chlorella vulgaris*: Optimization and kinetics. *International Journal of Biological Chemistry, 14*, 1–7.

Jacinto, J., Henriques, B., Duarte, A., Vale, C., & Pereira, E. (2018). Removal and recovery of critical rare elements from contaminated waters by living *Gracilaria gracilis*. *Journal of Hazardous Materials, 344*, 531–538. https://doi.org/10.1016/j.jhazmat.2017.10.054

Jie, W., Zhenyu, L., Xin, H., et al. (2021). Porous materials prepared by magnesium phosphate cement for the effective immobilization of lead ions. *International Journal of Environmental Research, 15*, 681–694. https://doi.org/10.1007/s41742-021-00344-y

Kapoore, R. V., Wood, E. E., & Llewellyn, C. A. (2021). Algae biostimulants: A critical look at microalgal biostimulants for sustainable agricultural practices. *Biotechnology Advances, 49*, 107754. https://doi.org/10.1016/j.biotechadv.2021.107754

Kaur, R., Choudhary, D., Bali, S., Bandral, S. S., Singh, V., Ahmad, M. A., Rani, N., Singh, T. G., & Chandrasekaran, B. (2024). Pesticides: An alarming detrimental to health and environment. *Science of the Total Environment, 915*, 170113. https://doi.org/10.1016/j.scitotenv.2024.170113

Kiranmayee, J., Gujjarlapudi, S. L., Kelam, N., Rao, V. M. M., & Kokkanti, M. (2025). Microalgae as environmental helpers: A comprehensive review on their role in climate mitigation, ocean health, and ecosystem restoration. *International Journal of Science and Research Archive, 14*(03), 1467–1478. https://doi.org/10.30574/ijsra.2025.14.3.0820

Kumar, A., Ponmani, S., Sharma, G., Sangavi, P., Chaturvedi, A., Singh, A., Malyan, S., Kumar, A., Khan, S., Shabnam, A. A., Jigyasu, D., & Gull, A. (2023). Plummeting toxic contaminates from water through phycoremediation: Mechanism, influencing factors and future outlook to enhance the capacity of living and non-living algae. *Environmental Research, 239*, 117381. https://doi.org/10.1016/j.envres.2023.117381

Kyratzopoulou, E., Kyzaki, N., Malletzidou, L., Nerantzis, E., & Kazakis, N. (2025). The efficiency of Chlorella vulgaris in heavy metal removal: A comparative study of mono- and multi-component metal systems. *Clean Technologies., 7*, 35. https://doi.org/10.3390/cleantechnol7020035

Leong, Y. K., & Chang, J. (2020). Bioremediation of heavy metals using microalgae: Recent advances and mechanisms. *Bioresource Technology, 303*, 122886. https://doi.org/10.1016/j.biortech.2020.122886

Li, K., Li, M., He, Y., Gu, X., Pang, K., Ma, Y., & Lu, D. (2020). Effects of pH and nitrogen form on Nitzschia closterium growth by linking dynamic with enzyme activity. *Chemosphere, 249*, 126154. https://doi.org/10.1016/j.chemosphere.2020.126154

Liakh, I., Harshkova, D., Hrouzek, P., Bišová, K., Aksmann, A., & Wielgomas, B. (2023). Green alga Chlamydomonas reinhardtii can effectively remove diclofenac from the water environment—A new perspective on biotransformation. *Journal of Hazardous Materials, 455*, 131570. https://doi.org/10.1016/j.jhazmat.2023.131570

Lim, H. R., Khoo, K. S., Chew, K. W., Tao, Y., Xia, A., Ma, Z., Munawaroh, H. S. H., Huy, N. D., & Show, P. L. (2024). Upstream bioprocessing of Spirulina platensis microalgae using rainwater and recycle medium from post-cultivation for C-phycocyanin production. *Journal of the Taiwan Institute of Chemical Engineers, 166*, 104986. https://doi.org/10.1016/j.jtice.2023.104986

Ma, X., & Jian, W. (2022). Growth conditions and growth kinetics of chlorella vulgaris cultured in domestic sewage. *Sustainability, 15*(3), 2162. https://doi.org/10.3390/su15032162

Matamoros, V., Uggetti, E., García, J., & Bayona, J. M. (2016). Assessment of the mechanisms involved in the removal of emerging contaminants by microalgae from wastewater: A laboratory scale study. *Journal of Hazardous Materials, 301*, 197–205.

Moghadam, M. J., Moayedi, H., Sadeghi, M. M., et al. (2016). A review of combinations of electrokinetic applications. *Environmental Geochemistry and Health, 38*, 1217–1227. https://doi.org/10.1007/s10653-016-9795-3

Mohd Apandi, N., Muhamad, M. S., Radin Mohamed, R. M., Mohamed Sunar, N., & Gani, P. (2020). Optimizing of microalgae Scenedesmus sp. Biomass production in wet market wastewater using response surface methodology. *Sustainability, 13*(4), 2216. https://doi.org/10.3390/su13042216

Nagarajan, D., Lee, D., Chen, C., & Chang, J. (2020). Resource recovery from wastewaters. *Technology, 302*, 122817. https://doi.org/10.1016/j.biortech.2020.122817

Nicodemus, T. J., DiRusso, C. C., Wilson, M., & Black, P. N. (2020). Reactive Oxygen Species (ROS) mediated degradation of organophosphate pesticides by the green microalgae Coccomyxa subellipsoidea. *Bioresource Technology Reports, 11*, 100461. https://doi.org/10.1016/j.biteb.2020.100461

Nidheesh, P. V., Couras, C., Karim, A. V., & Nadais, H. (2021). A review of integrated advanced oxidation processes and biological processes for organic pollutant removal. *Chemical Engineering Communications, 209*(3), 390–432. https://doi.org/10.1080/00986445.2020.1864626

Nie, J., Wang, Q., Han, L., & Li, J. (2024). Synergistic remediation strategies for soil contaminated with compound heavy metals and organic pollutants. *Journal of Environmental Chemical Engineering, 12*(4), 113145. https://doi.org/10.1016/j.jece.2024.113145

Nyika, J., & Dinka, M. O. (2023). Factors and mechanisms regulating heavy metal phycoremediation in polluted water. *Discover Water, 3*, 14. (2023). https://doi.org/10.1007/s43832-023-00041-1

Offiong, N. A. O., Fatunla, O. K., Essien, J. P., Yang, C., & Dong, J. (2021). Soil washing of total petroleum and polycyclic aromatic hydrocarbons from crude oil-contaminated ultisol using aqueous extracts of waterleaf. *Environmental Technology, 44*(1), 35–44. https://doi.org/10.1080/09593330.2021.1961875

Okoh, E., Yelebe, Z. R., Oruabena, B., et al. (2020). Clean-up of crude oil-contaminated soils: Bioremediation option. *International journal of Environmental Science and Technology, 17*, 1185–1198. https://doi.org/10.1007/s13762-019-02605-y

Oliveira, A. C., Barata, A., Batista, A. P., & Gouveia, L. (2018). Scenedesmus obliquus in poultry wastewater bioremediation. *Environmental Technology, 40*(28), 3735–3744. https://doi.org/10.1080/09593330.2018.1488003

Papazi, A., Karamanli, M., & Kotzabasis, K. (2019). Comparative biodegradation of all chlorinated phenols by the microalga Scenedesmus obliquus — The biodegradation strategy of microalgae. *Journal of Biotechnology, 296*, 61–68. https://doi.org/10.1016/j.jbiotec.2019.03.010

Pathak, V. M., Verma, V. K., Rawat, B. S., Kaur, B., Babu, N., Sharma, A., Dewali, S., Yadav, M., Kumari, R., Singh, S., Mohapatra, A., Pandey, V., Rana, N., & Cunill, J. M. (2022). Current status of pesticide effects on environment, human health and it's eco-friendly management as bioremediation: A comprehensive review. *Frontiers in Microbiology, 13*, 962619. https://doi.org/10.3389/fmicb.2022.962619

Paul, I., Biswas, R., & Halder, G. (2024). Traversing the potential of phytoremediation and phycoremediation as pioneering technologies in microplastic mitigation—A critical review. *Science of the Total Environment, 956*, 177200. https://doi.org/10.1016/j.scitotenv.2024.177200

Premaratne, M., Nishshanka, G., Liyanaarachchi, V., Nimarshana, P., & Ariyadasa, T. U. (2021). Bioremediation of textile dye wastewater using microalgae: Current trends and future perspectives. *Journal of Chemical Technology & Biotechnology, 96*(12), 3249–3258. https://doi.org/10.1002/jctb.6845

Qader, M., & Shekha, Y. (2023). Role of microalgae in environmental biotechnology to remove heavy metals. *Journal of Applied Sciences and Nanotechnology, 3*, 174–184. https://doi.org/10.53293/jasn.2022.5346.1183

Ramadan, B. S., Sari, G. L., Rosmalina, R. T., & Effendi, A. J. (2018). An overview of electrokinetic soil flushing and its effect on bioremediation of hydrocarbon contaminated soil. *Journal of Environmental Management, 218*, 309–321. https://doi.org/10.1016/j.jenvman.2018.04.065

Ratnasari, A., Syafiuddin, A., Kueh, A. B. H., et al. (2021). Opportunities and challenges for sustainable bioremediation of natural and synthetic estrogens as emerging water contaminants using bacteria, fungi, and algae. *Water, Air, and Soil Pollution, 232*, 242. https://doi.org/10.1007/s11270-021-05183-3

Rezayian, M., Niknam, V., & Ebrahimzadeh, H. (2018). Oxidative damage and antioxidative system in algae. *Toxicology Reports, 6*, 1309–1313. https://doi.org/10.1016/j.toxrep.2019.10.001

Rochaix, J. (2011). Regulation of photosynthetic electron transport. *Biochimica et Biophysica Acta – Bioenergetics, 1807*(3), 375–383. https://doi.org/10.1016/j.bbabio.2010.11.010

Rodríguez, L., Sánchez, V., & López-Bellido, F. J. (2021). Electrokinetic-assisted phytoremediation. *Assisted Phytoremediation*, 371–398. https://doi.org/10.1016/B978-0-12-822893-7.00005-7

Roostaei, J., & Zhang, Y. (2017). Spatially explicit life cycle assessment: Opportunities and challenges of wastewater-based algal biofuels in the United States. *Algal Research, 24*, 395–402. https://doi.org/10.1016/j.algal.2016.08.008

Sarker, A., Masud, M. A. A., Deepo, D. M., Das, K., Nandi, R., Ansary, M. W. R., Islam, A. R. M. T., & Islam, T. (2023). Biological and green remediation of heavy metal contaminated water and soils: A state-of-the-art review. *Chemosphere, 332*, 138861. https://doi.org/10.1016/j.chemosphere.2023.138861

Sarwer, A., Hamed, S. M., Osman, A. I., et al. (2022). Algal biomass valorization for biofuel production and carbon sequestration: A review. *Environmental Chemistry Letters, 20*, 2797–2851. https://doi.org/10.1007/s10311-022-01458-1

Sedlakova-Kadukova, J., Kopcakova, A., Gresakova, L., Godany, A., & Pristas, P. (2019). Bioaccumulation and biosorption of zinc by a novel Streptomyces K11 strain isolated from highly alkaline aluminium brown mud disposal site. *Ecotoxicology and Environmental Safety, 167*, 204–211. https://doi.org/10.1016/j.ecoenv.2018.09.123

Selvaraj, D., Dhayabaran, N. K., & Mahizhnan, A. (2023). An insight on pollutant removal mechanisms in phycoremediation of textile wastewater. *Environmental Science and Pollution Research, 30*, 124714–124734. https://doi.org/10.1007/s11356-022-21307-6

Sengupta, S., Gorain, P. C., & Pal, R. (2017). Aspects and prospects of algal carbon capture and sequestration in ecosystems: A review. *Chemistry and Ecology, 33*(8), 695–707. https://doi.org/10.1080/02757540.2017.1359262

Senthilkumar, R., Reddy Prasad, D. M., Govindarajan, L., Saravanakumar, K., & Naveen Prasad, B. S. (2019). Synthesis of green marine algal-based biochar for remediation of arsenic(V) from contaminated waters in batch and column mode of operation. *International Journal of Phytoremediation, 22*(3), 279–286. https://doi.org/10.1080/15226514.2019.1658710

Shanab, S., Essa, A., & Shalaby, E. (2012). Bioremoval capacity of three heavy metals by some microalgae species (Egyptian isolates). *Plant Signaling & Behavior, 7*(3), 392–399. https://doi.org/10.4161/psb.19173

Solomon, W., Mutum, L., Janda, T., et al. (2023). Potential benefit of microalgae and their interaction with bacteria to sustainable crop production. *Plant Growth Regulation, 101*, 53–65. https://doi.org/10.1007/s10725-023-01019-8

Sperling, M. V., & Chernicharo, C. A. D. L. (2005). *Biological wastewater treatment in warm climate regions*. IWA Publishing.

Sun, J., Norouzi, O., & Mašek, O. (2022). A state-of-the-art review on algae pyrolysis for bioenergy and biochar production. *Bioresource Technology, 346*, 126258. https://doi.org/10.1016/j.biortech.2021.126258

Sun, Z., Zhao, M., Chen, L., Gong, Z., Hu, J., & Ma, D. (2023). Electrokinetic remediation for the removal of heavy metals in soil: Limitations, solutions and prospection. *Science of the Total Environment, 903*, 165970. https://doi.org/10.1016/j.scitotenv.2023.165970

Suresh, B., & Ravishankar, G. A. (2004). Phytoremediation—A novel and promising approach for environmental clean-up. *Critical Reviews in Biotechnology, 24*(2–3), 97–124. https://doi.org/10.1080/07388550490493627

Touliabah, H. E., El-Sheekh, M. M., & Ismail, M. M. (2021). A review of microalgae- and cyanobacteria-based biodegradation of organic pollutants. *Molecules, 27*(3), 1141. https://doi.org/10.3390/molecules27031141

Trellu, C., Pechaud, Y., Oturan, N., Mousset, E., Van Hullebusch, E. D., Huguenot, D., & Oturan, M. A. (2021). Remediation of soils contaminated by hydrophobic organic compounds: How to recover extracting agents from soil washing solutions? *Journal of Hazardous Materials, 404*, 124137. https://doi.org/10.1016/j.jhazmat.2020.124137

Ugya, A. Y., Imam, T. S., Li, A., Ma, J., & Hua, X. (2019). Antioxidant response mechanism of freshwater microalgae species to reactive oxygen species production: A mini review. *Chemistry and Ecology, 36*(2), 174–193. https://doi.org/10.1080/02757540.2019.1688308

Ugya, A. Y., Ajibade, F. O., & Hua, X. (2021). The efficiency of microalgae biofilm in the phycoremediation of water from River Kaduna. *Journal of Environmental Management, 295*, 113109. https://doi.org/10.1016/j.jenvman.2021.113109

Upadhyay, M., Hansa, A., Devi, A., Asgari Lajayer, B., Price, G., & Sharma, R. (2024). Status and future scope of algal biomass-based remediation for various environmental contaminants. *Journal of Water Process Engineering, 65*, 105809. https://doi.org/10.1016/j.jwpe.2024.105809

Usmani, Z., Sharma, M., Lukk, T., Karpichev, Y., Thakur, V. K., Kumar, V., et al. (2020). Developments in enzyme and microalgae based biotechniques to remediate micropollutants from aqueous systems—A review. *Critical Reviews in Environmental Science and Technology, 52*(10), 1684–1729. https://doi.org/10.1080/10643389.2020.1862551

Vadlamani, A., Viamajala, S., Pendyala, B., & Varanasi, S. (2017). Cultivation of microalgae at extreme alkaline pH conditions: A novel approach for biofuel production. *ACS Sustainable Chem. Eng., 5*(8), 7284–7294. https://doi.org/10.1021/acssuschemeng.7b01534

Venckus, P., Kostkevičienė, J., & Bendikienė, V. (2017). Green algae chlorella vulgaris cultivation in municipal wastewater and biomass composition. *Journal of Environmental Engineering and Landscapes Management, 25*, 56–63. https://doi.org/10.3846/16486897.2016.1245661

Viswanaathan, S., & Sudhakar, M. (2018). Microalgae: Potential agents for CO_2 mitigation and bioremediation of wastewaters. In *New and future developments in microbial biotechnology and bioengineering* (pp. 129–148). https://doi.org/10.1016/B978-0-12-818258-1.00008-X

Wang, L., Xiao, H., He, N., Sun, D., & Duan, S. (2019). Biosorption and biodegradation of the environmental hormone Nonylphenol by four marine microalgae. *Scientific Reports, 9*(1), 1–11. https://doi.org/10.1038/s41598-019-41808-8

Xiong, J., Kurade, M. B., Patil, D. V., Jang, M., Paeng, K., & Jeon, B. (2017). Biodegradation and metabolic fate of levofloxacin via a freshwater green alga, Scenedesmus obliquus in synthetic saline wastewater. *Algal Research, 25*, 54–61. https://doi.org/10.1016/j.algal.2017.04.012

Xu, K., Zou, X., Wen, H., et al. (2019). Effects of multi-temperature regimes on cultivation of microalgae in municipal wastewater to simultaneously remove nutrients and produce biomass. *Applied Microbiology and Biotechnology, 103*, 8255–8265. https://doi.org/10.1007/s00253-019-10051-6

Yeheyo, H. A., Ealias, A. M., George, G., & Jagannathan, U. (2024). Bioremediation potential of microalgae for sustainable soil treatment in India: A comprehensive review on heavy metal and pesticide contaminant removal. *Journal of Environmental Management, 363*, 121409. https://doi.org/10.1016/j.jenvman.2024.121409

Yong, J. J. J. Y., Chew, K. W., Khoo, K. S., Show, P. L., & Chang, J. (2021). Prospects and development of algal-bacterial biotechnology in environmental management and protection. *Biotechnology Advances, 47*, 107684. https://doi.org/10.1016/j.biotechadv.2020.107684

Yousif, Y. I. D., Mohamed, E. S., & El-Gendy, A. S. (2022). Using chlorella vulgaris for nutrient removal from hydroponic wastewater: Experimental investigation and economic assessment. *Water Science & Technology, 85*, 3240–3258. https://doi.org/10.2166/wst.2022.157

Zahmatkesh, S., Karimian, M., Pourhanasa, R., Ghodrati, I., Hajiaghaei-Keshteli, M., & Ismail, M. A. (2023). Wastewater treatment with algal based membrane bioreactor for the future: Removing emerging contaminants. *Chemosphere, 335*, 139134. https://doi.org/10.1016/j.chemosphere.2023.139134

Zhu, Z., Wang, J., Liu, X., Yuan, L., Liu, X., & Deng, H. (2021). Comparative study on washing effects of different washing agents and conditions on heavy metal contaminated soil. *Surfaces and Interfaces, 27*, 101563. https://doi.org/10.1016/j.surfin.2021.101563

Zou, Z., Chang, H., Li, H., et al. (2017). Induction of reactive oxygen species: An emerging approach for cancer therapy. *Apoptosis, 22*, 1321–1335. https://doi.org/10.1007/s10495-017-1424-9

Algal Bioremediation: A Sustainable Approach for Emerging Contaminant Removal

4

Eliana Marcela Jiménez-Bambague, Carlos Arturo Madera-Parra, Fiderman Machuca-Martínez, Jefferson E. Contreras-Ropero, Janet B. García-Martínez, Andres Fernando Barajas-Solano, and Antonio Zuorro

Abstract

Traditional treatment systems employed in wastewater treatment plants continue to face significant limitations regarding a broad range of emerging contaminants, mainly due to increased domestic, agricultural, and industrial use. Given the long-term environmental persistence of these compounds, they pose a potential hazard to human health and aquatic ecosystems; therefore, alternative treatment methods are urgently needed. In this context, algal bioremediation has been considered an effective alternative for this purpose, as microalgae naturally possess the potential to adsorb, accumulate, and convert numerous environmentally significant chemicals. This chapter presents a critical comparison of the published performance of different algal configurations (HRAPs, closed PBRs, and alga–bacterium consortia) in removing complex mixtures of emerging contaminants. It also examines the primary operating parameters that influence the performance of these technologies in practice, including relevant environmental and process

E. M. Jiménez-Bambague · C. A. Madera-Parra · F. Machuca-Martínez
School of School of Natural Resources and the Environment, Universidad del Valle, Ciudad Universitaria Meléndez, Cali, Colombia

J. E. Contreras-Ropero
Research Center for Sustainable Development in Industry and Energy, Program of Chemical Engineering, Universidad Industrial de Santander, Bucaramanga, Colombia

J. B. García-Martínez · A. F. Barajas-Solano (✉)
Department of Environmental Sciences, Universidad Francisco de Paula Santander, Cúcuta, Colombia
e-mail: andresfernandobs@ufps.edu.co

A. Zuorro (✉)
Department of Chemical Engineering, Materials, and Environment, Sapienza University, Rome, Italy
e-mail: antonio.zuorro@uniroma1.it

L. Kumar et al. (eds.), *Algal Bioremediation*,
https://doi.org/10.1007/978-981-95-8793-3_4

parameters. Finally, this chapter explores the potential of integrating algal systems with other advanced and complementary technologies to increase the removal of highly persistent contaminants. In doing so, this chapter provides technical insight into the capability and technical requirements for the effective integration of algal bioremediation into advanced treatment technologies addressing contemporary contaminants of emerging concern.

Keywords

Microalgae · Emerging contaminants · Bioremediation · Wastewater Treatment · Additional technologies

4.1 Introduction

The sustained increase in the use of chemical substances across urban, agricultural, and industrial sectors has given rise to a new class of compounds whose environmental detection—or recognition as hazardous—has occurred only recently, owing to advances in analytical techniques and growing environmental exposure to novel chemical formulations (Sutherland & Ralph, 2019). These substances, known as emerging contaminants (ECs), encompass a wide array of synthetic or natural chemicals and biological agents that, unlike "legacy" pollutants such as heavy metals or organochlorine pesticides, have historically neither been regulated nor routinely monitored (Gondi et al., 2022). The categories include pharmaceuticals (e.g., antibiotics, analgesics, and hormonal contraceptives), personal care products (synthetic fragrances, UV filters, and antibacterial soaps), modern pesticides (neonicotinoids and newer herbicides), flame retardants, and industrial compounds such as plasticizers (phthalates) and per- and polyfluoroalkyl substances (PFAS), as well as antibiotic resistance genes and emerging pathogens. All of these compounds exhibit environmental persistence, low biodegradability, and chronic toxicity even at trace concentrations (Dubey et al., 2023).

ECs enter the environment through various routes, mirroring their multiple origins. In urban environments, unutilized pharmaceuticals and cosmetic products are disposed of via domestic wastewater discharges, whereas in agriculture, excessive chemicals such as pesticides and fertilizers are applied, contributing to leachates and runoff that pollute water bodies devoid of pretreatment (Yong et al., 2021). In agricultural animal habitats, the application of manure to soils causes the release of veterinary drugs along with their metabolites into the environment, and untreated or partially treated effluents from the pharmaceutical, textile, and plastic industries also notably contribute to the introduction of such long-lasting compounds (Satpati et al., 2024). Therefore, ECs are present in aquatic systems (rivers, lakes, and groundwaters), where they exist as complex mixtures of chemical and biological pollutants and may even travel to remote areas via atmospheric transport or riverine flows (Gondi et al., 2022).

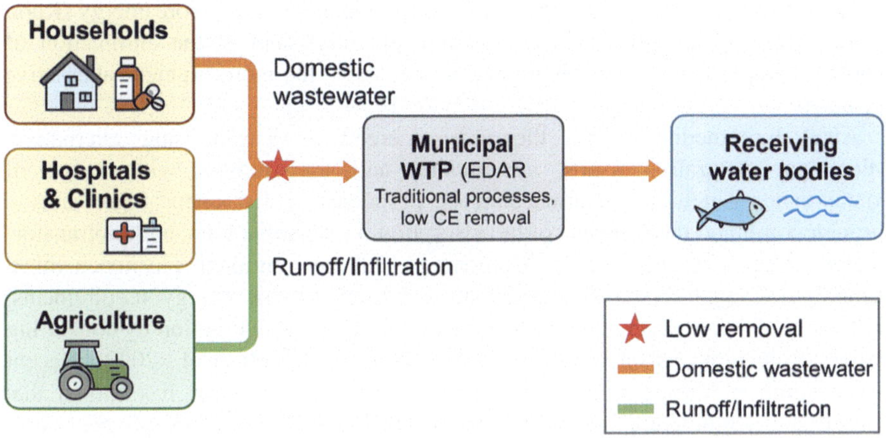

Fig. 4.1 Transfer dynamics of emerging contaminants from multiple anthropogenic sources to environmental compartments

This impairment flow is not just the aggregation of single independent sources. Nevertheless, it illustrates the numerous clues that stream (concurring from urban areas, hospitals, and agricultural areas) and reach receiving waters, such as rivers, coastal waters, and aquifers. The importance of this design is not only for the motion of transport from one point to another but also for the intricate behaviors of different pollutants with a variety of physicochemical characteristics (Sutherland & Ralph, 2019). Effluents from hospitals bring antibiotics and pharmaceutical metabolites along with trace metals and multidrug-resistant bacteria, causing selection of the microbial population (Ajala et al., 2022). Additionally, while industrial wastewater is being discharged, agricultural runoff adds yet other persistent pesticides, synthetic hormones, and nitrogenous fertilizers, which, when combined with urban pharmaceuticals, may have synergistic or antagonistic effects on aquatic biota that are not predicted from single-compound assessments (Singh et al., 2024). These processes are further complicated by industrial pollutants, such as flame retardants and plasticizers, and are extremely common in crowded large cities (Fig. 4.1).

As traditional treatment lines are not very efficient against ECs, several WWTPs have started implementing advanced tertiary treatments—activated carbon adsorption, ozonation, advanced oxidation processes (e.g., UV/H_2O_2 or photoFenton), and membrane filtration—to improve the removal of these recalcitrant compounds (Gondi et al., 2022). However, each has its downside: Chlorination can result in more persistent and often more toxic chlorinated byproducts when it reacts with certain pharmaceuticals (Dubey et al., 2023); advanced oxidation processes can achieve >90% degradation of some ECs, but often produce intermediate metabolites that remain biologically active or toxic, and are energy-intensive and specialized reagents (Satpati et al., 2024); activated carbon adsorption works well, but the bed may fill up and have to be reactivated, and it is expensive to regenerate; and nanofiltration or reverse osmosis concentrates ECs in saltwater streams in need of further treatment, and they are susceptible to fouling and require more energy (Khoo et al., 2021). Coagulation and flocculation are inefficient in the elimination of dissolved impurities, which highlights the necessity for more efficient alternative techniques.

Algal bioremediation has therefore emerged as a promising alternative. Microalgae naturally adsorb, accumulate, and transform a wide range of contaminants—including pharmaceuticals, pesticides, and cosmetic ingredients—through combined mechanisms of bioadsorption, bioaccumulation, and biotransformation (Dubey et al., 2023). Compared with conventional physicochemical technologies, algal systems offer advantages such as low energy requirements, utilization of solar resources, and the potential for circular integration by converting the resulting biomass into biofuels or biofertilizers (Gondi et al., 2022). Recent optimization of drying regimes for *Potamosiphon* sp. biomass has shown that appropriate temperature–moisture control significantly increases phycoerythrin extraction yields, strengthening the circular-economy argument for value-added pigment recovery (Vergel-Suarez et al., 2023).

Pharmaceuticals—spanning analgesics/anti-inflammatories, antibiotics, psychiatric drugs, and antihypertensives—enter receiving waters via household and hospital discharges and incomplete removal in wastewater treatment, with typical levels in the ng–μg L^{-1} range associated with chronic ecological effects (Yong et al., 2021; Gondi et al., 2022; Dubey et al., 2023). Conventional tertiary steps can underperform for recalcitrant molecules such as diclofenac or carbamazepine and may yield persistent intermediates. By contrast, algal processes combine rapid biosorption with intracellular accumulation and enzymatic biotransformation; for instance, *Chlorella sorokiniana* hydroxylates sulfamethoxazole, and controlled photobioreactors (PBRs) have reported high removals for antibiotics and psychiatric pharmaceuticals at pilot scale (Chu et al., 2022; Pereira et al., 2023; López-Serna et al., 2024).

Personal care products—including synthetic fragrances, UV filters, and antimicrobials such as triclosan—are widely detected at low concentrations and can display endocrine-disrupting or antibacterial activity (Gondi et al., 2022; Dubey et al., 2023). In engineered algal systems, removal typically proceeds via fast sorption to cell surfaces followed by enzyme-mediated transformations; for triclosan, oxidation–reduction and subsequent conjugation generate less toxic metabolites. Performance gains are consistently observed under closed or hybrid operation that stabilizes light, pH, and nutrient supply (Wang et al., 2018b; Pereira et al., 2023).

Modern pesticides, notably organophosphates and neonicotinoids, reach aquatic environments through runoff and leaching, present persistence and neuro/endocrine activity, and contribute to mixture toxicity (Yong et al., 2021; Gondi et al., 2022). Several are amenable to algal biodegradation—chlorpyrifos being a representative case with metabolic pathways implicated in its breakdown—while algal–bacterial consortia can enhance cometabolism when redox conditions and irradiance are tightly controlled (Chen et al., 2016; Kundu et al., 2024; López-Serna et al., 2024).

Among flame retardants, hydrophobic brominated compounds such as TBBPA are persistent and bioaccumulative; microalgae effect sequential debromination, sulfation, and glycosylation that facilitate detoxification and downstream removal, with stable closed reactors supporting these Phase II routes (Gondi et al., 2022; Peng et al., 2014; García-Galán et al., 2021). A broader group of emerging contaminants—plasticizers (phthalates), bisphenol A and parabens, PFAS, and biological agents including antibiotic-resistance genes and pathogens—shows heterogeneous treatability: many organics respond to algal biotransformation or to integrated trains (e.g., photocatalysis or ozonation followed by algal polishing), whereas highly persistent species such as PFAS generally require membrane or advanced-oxidation pretreatment to reduce toxicity and improve subsequent assimilation (Sousa et al., 2022; Zhang et al., 2023; Wang et al., 2023; Pereira et al., 2023; López-Serna et al., 2024).

This chapter evaluates the performance of various algal bioremediation configurations—including high-rate algal ponds (HRAPs), closed photobioreactors (PBRs), and alga–bacterium consortia—in removing complex mixtures of emerging contaminants. It also examines the main operational and environmental parameters that govern their effectiveness under real-world conditions and explores possibilities for coupling algal systems with advanced, complementary technologies. Finally, this study provides a technical overview of the capabilities, limitations, and implementation requirements to integrate algal processes into broader treatment schemes aimed at controlling contemporary contaminants.

4.2 Fundamentals of Algal Bioremediation

Microalgae as potential biotechnological tools for the alleviation of emerging contaminants. Notably, microalgae have attracted attention as potential biotechnological tools for the attenuation of ECs through three main mechanisms: biosorption, bioaccumulation, and biotransformation (Dubey et al., 2023; Satpati et al., 2024). Biosorption is the phenomenon of bonding and sequestering pollutants to the surface of a cell through ionic links, hydrogen bridges, or van der Waals forces. Since biosorption is based on surface interactions, it is possible with either living or inactivated biomass, and it does not destroy the contaminant but reduces its free concentration in water by adsorbing it temporarily on the cell wall, resulting in the theft of the binding sites of intracellular proteins (Gondi et al., 2022). Concurrently, bioaccumulation is facilitated as toxicants are actively imported into the cell, where they can be sequestered into vacuoles or assimilated as nutrients by algal metabolism over extended periods and, consequently, can be retained within the cell for longer periods (Dubey et al., 2023).

In contrast, biotransformation (or metabolic biodegradation) is pivotal for the effective removal of organic ECs because microalgae can chemically modify pollutants, reduce their toxicity, or convert them into simpler, less persistent metabolites. A highly specialized enzymatic arsenal drives biotransformation. During phase I, enzymes such as mono-oxygenases (most notably cytochrome P450) catalyze oxidation, hydroxylation, or dealkylation reactions, increasing contaminant polarity (Satpati et al., 2024; Satpati et al., 2024). For example, *Chlorella sorokiniana* can hydroxylate the antibiotic sulfamethoxazole, initiating its breakdown (Chu et al., 2022). Phase II reactions then neutralize the phase I intermediates via conjugation with endogenous compounds: enzymes such as glutathione S-transferases (GSTs), sulfotransferases, or glycosyltransferases attach glutathione, sulfate, or glucose, thereby increasing water solubility and facilitating excretion (Dubey et al., 2023). *Scenedesmus quadricauda*, for example, transforms the flame retardant TBBPA through sequential debromination, sulfation, and glycosylation, producing less toxic derivatives that are easier to remove (Gondi et al., 2022).

Complementary processes also operate in algal bioremediation systems. Solar-induced photodegradation, often enhanced by photosynthetic pigments, and cometabolic degradation mediated by heterotrophic bacteria in combination with algae create versatile, more efficient symbiotic systems (Khoo et al., 2021). The algal treatment of wastewater is not new: it has long been applied to remove nutrients such as nitrogen and phosphorus as well as certain heavy metals, mainly through assimilation and biosorption (Dubey et al., 2023). Treating organic ECs, however, poses an additional challenge because they require chemical breakdown rather than simple physical removal. Unlike heavy metals—which can be re-released if environmental conditions change—organics degraded enzymatically lose their toxic structure irreversibly. A further advantage of algal bioremediation is its sustainability: microalgae harness solar energy and atmospheric CO_2 for growth, lowering the carbon footprint of treatment and enabling low-cost implementations such as open ponds or algal wetlands while demanding less energy than advanced physicochemical processes do (Dubey et al., 2023).

In challenging matrices, such as hospital or agricultural effluents, microalgae are highly resistant to large loads and highly effective in eliminating recalcitrant compounds that are not entirely removed by conventional treatments (particularly pharmaceuticals, pesticides, and personal-care products) (Kundu et al., 2024). The potential of these bacteria to modulate the pH of the medium and compete for nutrients constrains pathogen expansion, and cooperation with heterotrophic bacteria increases the complementary metabolic pathways that fortify the degradation of recalcitrant pollutants (Satpati et al., 2024). This promiscuity is also corroborated by the multiple examples of interactions reported in the literature between EC classes and specific algae (Table 4.1), which we summarize here. The table shows how contaminant chemistry and algal metabolism are the predominant elimination mechanisms. For example, *Chlorella sorokiniana* has a remarkable bioconversion ability for the degradation of antibiotics and pesticides, which is effective for decomposing compounds of different polarities and structural complexities (Chen et al., 2016; Chu et al., 2022). In contrast, *S. quadricauda* can perform diverse complex phase II reactions of brominated compounds, such as TBBPA, that lead to decreased toxic potential (Peng et al., 2014). This range of metabolic responses across microalgal strains suggests that the choice of microalgal strain for the removal of contaminants depends not only on the nature of the contaminant but also on environmental factors and cofactors, including light, nutrients, and adjacent bacteria.

Table 4.1 Microalgal removal mechanisms for emerging contaminants

Emerging contaminant	Microalga	Predominant removal mechanism	Reference
Pharmaceutical (antibiotic sulfamethoxazole)	*Chlorella sorokiniana*	Biotransformation via phase I CYP450 mono-oxygenase hydroxylation	Chu et al. (2022)
Pharmaceutical (anti-inflammatory diclofenac)	Immobilized *Chlamydomonas reinhardtii*	Metabolic biodegradation (≈80% intracellular degradation; remainder by accumulation)	Kariyawasam et al. (2024)
Personal-care product (triclosan)	*Scenedesmus obliquus*	Biotransformation: oxidation–reduction followed by conjugation (hydroxylated, dechlorinated, and glucose/methyl conjugates)	Wang et al. (2018b)
Pesticide (organophosphate insecticide chlorpyrifos)	*Chlorella sorokiniana*	Biodegradation (>97% removal via algal metabolic pathways, likely including phosphatase-mediated hydrolysis)	Chen et al. (2016)
Flame retardant (brominated TBBPA)	*Scenedesmus quadricauda*	Near-complete biotransformation; key phase II reactions include sulfation, glycosylation, O-desmethylation, and debromination	Peng et al. (2014)
Antibiotics (mixture: ciprofloxacin, clarithromycin, erythromycin, metronidazole, ofloxacin, sulfamethoxazole, trimethoprim)	*Tetradesmus obliquus*	Rapid biosorption (dominant), followed by slower metabolic transformation	Frascaroli et al. (2024)
Antibiotic (ciprofloxacin)	*Chlorella pyrenoidosa*	Bioaccumulation + biodegradation as main pathways	Li et al. (2024)
Antibiotics (same 7-compound mixture as above)	*Auxenochlorella protothecoides*	Biosorption-dominated uptake with ancillary biodegradation	Frascaroli et al. (2024)
Antibiotic (sulfamethoxazole)	*Chlorella pyrenoidosa*	Bioaccumulation/ biodegradation (supported by recent physiological response + mechanism review)	Huang et al. (2023)

(continued)

Table 4.1 (continued)

Emerging contaminant	Microalga	Predominant removal mechanism	Reference
Personal-care preservatives (propylparaben; triclosan)	*Mixed microalgae (Chlorella/ Scenedesmus) in anoxic–aerobic photobioreactor*	Sorption + biodegradation under sequential redox conditions	Ruas et al. (2021)
Pharmaceuticals (e.g., azithromycin, sertraline; tertiary WWTP)	*Mixed microalgal consortium (flat-panel PBR)*	Sorption + biodegradation under controlled PBR operation	Pereira et al. (2023)

4.3 Algal Configurations for Emerging-Contaminant Removal

The main configurations employed in algal systems to eliminate emerging contaminants (ECs) are high-rate algal ponds (HRAPs), various types of closed photobioreactors (PBRs), and algal–bacterial symbiotic consortia (Leong et al., 2021; Torres-Franco et al., 2021). These technologies differ structurally and operationally, and those differences translate directly into removal efficiency, technical applicability, and scalability in real-world wastewater-treatment contexts (García-Galán et al., 2021; Pereira et al., 2023). Common strategies for incorporating algae into advanced treatments include HRAPs and tubular, flat-panel, membrane, bubble-column, and internal-loop air-lift PBRs (Leong et al., 2021; Torres-Franco et al., 2021). Hybrid variants have also been developed that integrate aerobic and anoxic zones within the same unit to optimize both nutrient assimilation and denitrification (Wang et al., 2018a). Such approaches can achieve tertiary-level treatment—removing ECs while simultaneously generating biomass of energetic value.

Although many technological options exist, three stand out in industrial and field applications because of their performance and operational feasibility: HRAPs, closed PBRs, and hybrid algal–bacterial systems. The following sections present a comparative analysis of these technologies, focusing on removal efficiencies, operational constraints, and representative case studies (Pereira et al., 2023; Mantovani et al., 2024).

HRAPs are shallow open systems that are generally operated as raceways with paddlewheels to facilitate mixing and maintain uniform exposure to sunlight. Under these conditions, the rapid growth of microalgae and their symbiosis with heterotrophic bacteria in wastewater culture are encouraged. Microalgae can be photosynthetic producers, whereas bacteria consume organic matter and release CO_2, which is then assimilated by microalgae, and an efficient treatment cycle is performed (Leong et al., 2021; Torres-Franco et al., 2021). The main merits are the lower capital and operational costs of HRAPs compared to closed-PBRs, the reasonable energy requirement per treated wastewater volume for large systems, and the physical scalability to sizable dimensions suitable for municipal applications. The cultivation of microalgal–bacterial consortia enhances system stability and promotes the elimination of nutrients and emerging contaminants. Nonetheless, HRAPs are open systems with inherent vulnerability to climatic variability (seasons, solar irradiance, and ambient temperature), which have appreciable effects on removal efficiency and algal growth, particularly in non-tropical climates (Farias et al., 2023). Environmental exposure also poses risks of microbial contamination, evaporation, and pH swings; thus, the process must be tightly controlled, and the composition of microorganisms in the soil can be destabilized. Field-scale evidence under tropical Colombian conditions shows that nutrient-rich farm wastewaters can sustain productive algal growth while removing nutrients, reinforcing the suitability of open HRAP configurations in warm climates (Urbina-Suarez, Barajas-Solano, et al., 2022b).

Applied research demonstrates the opportunities as well as the limitations of HRAPs. Torres-Franco et al. (2021) reported that HRAPs (operating under tropical conditions) removed more than 70% of frequently detected pharmaceuticals, including ibuprofen and paracetamol, at a hydraulic retention time (HRT) of 3 days (Leong et al., 2021), similar to diclofenac, which is a more resistant compound but achieves removal yields ranging from 40% to 60%. Farias et al. (2023) reported that the intermittent-feeding regime affected the removal of carbamazepine, reaching values of more than 50% at the best irradiance and mixing conditions. Cumulatively, these results demonstrate that HRAPs can be competitive with other technology types where operating parameters are tightly optimized, albeit with some constraints on operation.

PBRs are used as closed systems that provide excellent control of the algal culture environment. They also completely isolate biomass from the external environment and significantly minimize the risk of cross-contamination and operation under aseptic conditions, which is not the case in HRAPs. Various styles, including tubular, flat-panel, and column styles, may be custom-designed for each process. With parameters such as pH, temperature, CO_2, and light availability under controlled ranges, PBRs offer ideal conditions for long-term algal growth and contaminant selectivity degradation (Liao et al., 2024; López-Serna et al., 2024). One of the main advantages of PBRs is their ability to grow specialized or genetically modified algal strains that cannot survive outdoors. The optimized environment facilitates high biomass production and high levels of enzyme expression in biotransformation pathways. PBRs also optimize photosynthetic efficiency with optimized LED lighting, which increases the metabolic rate and thus contaminant removal. Together with these technical advantages, however, there are several challenges: the implementation costs are low because of special material requirements and the need for sustained mixing, aeration, and light exposure. Fouling, that is, the deposition of biomass on internal surfaces, also requires periodic cleaning and can be a source of long-term operational issues (Torres-Franco et al., 2021).

With respect to pollutant removal, many studies have documented the effectiveness of PBRs. For example, López-Serna et al. (2024) operated a flat-panel PBR with a *Chlorella* strain and achieved 85% removal of antibiotics such as sulfamethoxazole and azithromycin with a 24-hour hydraulic retention time (HRT). Similarly, Liao et al. (2024) reported >90% elimination of ibuprofen and naproxen in a column PBR with controlled internal lighting. In a complementary study, Razaviarani et al. (2023) used a tubular PBR and obtained removals ranging from 45% to 100% for a mixture of 20 pharmaceuticals, underscoring the process's sensitivity to specific operating conditions. Collectively, these results show that (despite their greater complexity and cost) PBRs can achieve outstanding efficiencies in short treatment times, especially when custom-designed for the contaminant profile and operated under well-controlled parameters.

Microalgae and bacteria generally coexist as symbiotic consortia in biological wastewater treatment systems. Such interactions can be intentionally emphasized via hybrid system configurations that optimize the metabolic synergies of these categories (Wang et al., 2022). Most frequently, such systems are based on anaerobic and aerobic high-rate algal pond (APHRP, HPARP) or open pond biomass systems with oxygenated and non-oxygenated zones, an indirect photobioreactor (IPBR), and photosynthetically activated sludge systems. In such arrangements, microalgae produce oxygen from photosynthesis during the daytime, which supports bacterial respiration, and bacteria produce CO_2 and metabolites that increase algal growth, resulting in a highly efficient positive feedback loop (Bej et al., 2024). The added value of these hybrid systems is the possibility of driving out organic and new emerging pollutants. Complex aromatic links can be cleaved by bacteria via enzymes (e.g., monooxygenases), leading to the production of intermediate metabolites that are further cometabolized or utilized by algae (Bej et al., 2024).

Furthermore, the mixed biofilm structure improved the adsorption concentration of contaminants that are easy to biodegrade. Moreover, algal–bacterial systems can reduce the COD, Cr, and N and P from municipal wastewater by 89%, 80%, and 90%, respectively (Moondra et al., 2020). In more complex methods, such as elimination of triclosan and propylparaben, complete removal of persistent compounds has also been demonstrated (Ji et al., 2019).

The efficient performance of these systems, however, depends critically on controlling multiple parameters with precision, and sufficient light penetration into the biomass is required for photosynthesis (Leong et al., 2021; Torres-Franco et al., 2021; García-Galán et al., 2021). In addition, diel pH may oscillate strongly as algal–bacterial metabolism alternates between photosynthesis and respiration, which can destabilize consortia and alter removal activity (Wang et al., 2022; Ji et al., 2019; Kang & Kim, 2021). These variations could impact the stability of consortia and the removal activity of contaminants. In addition, direct competition for essential nutrients (e.g., phosphorus and ammonium) might exist, which may favor the growth of one group of strains over the other, given that the culture conditions are not appropriately balanced (Wang et al., 2022). The potential for heavy or dense floc development can limit the penetration of light and access to nutrients, directly affecting the rate of contaminant removal. It must also be considered in the design.

However, in practice, there is strong empirical evidence in favor of these methods. With a pilot scale constructed using a *Chlorella vulgaris* and *Bacillus licheniformis* consortium, removal effectiveness of 88.8, 84.9, and 82.3% (w/w) for total nitrogen, ammonium, and COD, respectively, could be achieved after only 6 d of operation (Ji et al., 2019). A similar study exhibited the application of a consortium in an aerated HRAP reactor for the removal of 87% COD and 80% total nitrogen from complex industrial effluents (Wang et al. (2022). In support of these findings, Bej et al. (2024) reported (across more than ten studies) that hybrid systems achieved >85% removal of antibiotics such as SMX, CPX, and AMP under multiple configurations. In another study, a mobile system associated with photobioreactors had NH_4-N removal over 95% and total nitrogen removal of 87.7%, with a retention time of less than 3 days (Kang & Kim, 2021). These results demonstrate that algal-bacterial consortia contribute new removal mechanisms, in addition to diversifying operational conditions, thereby enhancing treatment reliability and efficiency for a wide range of emerging contaminants.

The available experimental data on different algal configurations, presented in Table 4.2, allow for the identification of operational patterns for contaminant removal across current research schemes. First, removal efficiency is closely linked to the level of environmental control in the system. Closed photobioreactors (tubular or flat panels) consistently outperform open systems in removing complex pharmaceutical contaminants (López-Serna et al., 2024; Razaviarani et al., 2023). For example, a semi closed tubular photobioreactor operated with mixed microalgae achieved 94% removal efficiency for diazepam, 83% for lorazepam, and 70% for ibuprofen (García-Galán et al., 2021). Conversely, open systems such as HRAPs, even under favorable climatic conditions, generally exhibit lower efficiency. A study involving two HRAPs with varying hydraulic retention times (HRTs) reported removals above 90% for certain compounds but lower efficiencies for others, depending on the season and specific contaminant (Matamoros et al., 2015). This contrast suggests that maintaining key parameters, such as pH, light intensity, and the nutrient-to-carbon ratio, is critical for activating specific algal biotransformation mechanisms. These parameters are more effectively controlled in closed systems, enhancing removal performance (Kishi et al., 2023).

Another notable pattern is the influence of structural complexity on system functionality. Hybrid configurations that integrate anoxic and aerobic zones enable the sequential removal of recalcitrant contaminants. For example, a combined system with anaerobic digestion coupled with an anoxic-aerobic photobioreactor achieved removals exceeding 80% for several pharmaceutical contaminants, including ibuprofen, acetaminophen, triclosan, and propylparaben (Ruas et al., 2021). Furthermore, selecting specific microalgal strains is critical. The use of *Chlorella* and *Scenedesmus* in PBRs has resulted in removal efficiencies ranging from 62% to 100% for emerging contaminants such as triclosan, ibuprofen, and propylparaben through bioaccumulation and sorption mechanisms under controlled conditions (López-Serna et al., 2024).

Table 4.2 Summary of microalgae-based wastewater treatment configurations for emerging contaminant removal

Configuration	Emerging contaminant treated	Microalgae	Removal efficiency	Operational conditions	Reference
High-rate algal pond (HRAP)—open, 3-day HRT (tropical climate)	Pharmaceutical mixture in urban wastewater (analgesics: Ibuprofen, acetaminophen; anti-inflammatories, etc.)	Natural consortium of native Chlorophyta (green microalgae) cocultured with influent bacteria	>70% for ibuprofen and acetaminophen; 30–70% for diclofenac, naproxen; <30% for carbamazepine (overall average ~60%)	3-day HRT; continuous flow 0.2 m^3/d; raceway pond (0.3 m depth); outdoor operation (≈25–30 °C); no artificial aeration (photosynthetic oxygenation)	Jiménez-Bambague et al. (2020)
Closed tubular photobioreactor—1200 L pilot-scale (outdoor)	Pharmaceuticals in graywater (bathroom effluent): mixture of anti-inflammatories (ibuprofen, diclofenac, ketoprofen), antiepileptics, etc.	Autochthonous wastewater microalgae (consortium dominated by *chlorella* sp. and *Scenedesmus* sp.)	30–80% removal depending on compound (e.g., ~80% ibuprofen; ~50% diclofenac)	HRT ~4.6 days; outdoor tubular reactor (1200 L) with recirculation; initial inoculation with lake microalgae; solar illumination; supplementary CO_2; ambient temperature (~20 °C)	Hom-Diaz et al. (2017)
Closed flat-panel photobioreactor—GreenDune© system (tertiary WWTP)	Pharmaceuticals in municipal postsecondary effluent (antibiotics, psychiatric drugs, antihypertensives, etc.; 20 compounds total)	Mixed microalgal consortium adapted to effluent (mainly green Chlorococcales)	~82.5% global average (up to 100% for azithromycin, sertraline; minimum ~65% for ofloxacin)	1-day HRT; two flat-panel photobioreactors (750 L each) operated in parallel; solar illumination + aeration with CO_2; optimized nutrient control (N:P); day/night cycle, T ≈ 18–25 °C	Pereira et al. (2023)
Hybrid algal-bacterial HRAP—sequential anoxic/aerobic stages	Preservatives and biocides: triclosan (antimicrobial),	Green microalgae + heterotrophic bacteria (floc consortium; algal genera:	~100% (complete removal detected for both compounds)	Modified HRAP reactor with anoxic zone (coupled settler) followed	Pereira et al. (2023)

	propylparaben (cosmetic paraben) in synthetic wastewater	*Chlorella*/*Scenedesmus*; bacterial: varied)		by aerobic-photosynthetic zone; total HRT ~6 days; intermittent aeration; algal sludge recirculation; controlled carbon source addition for anoxia	
High-rate algae-bacteria pond (HRAP)—pilot, municipal centrate	Mixture of pharmaceuticals (e.g., sulfamethoxazole, lamotrigine, metoprolol, fluoxetine, diclofenac, carbamazepine, clarithromycin, etc.)	Native algal–bacterial consortium dominated by *Chlorella*/*Scenedesmus*	>85% (SMX, lamotrigine); ~65–70% (metoprolol, fluoxetine, diclofenac); ~30–40% (amisulpride, ofloxacin, carbamazepine, clarithromycin)	Outdoor HRAP; continuous operation (May–Nov); HRT ≈ 6 d	Mantovani et al. (2024)
Thin-layer cascade photobioreactor (TLC-PBR)—pilot	Veterinary CECs and co-occurring pollutants in swine-farm effluent	Mixed consortium (≈70–90% *Chlorella*, 10–25% *Scenedesmus*)	62–86% overall CEC removal	Semi-continuous TLC-PBR; controlled day/night; outdoor	López-Serna et al. (2024)
Pilot PBR (swine manure)	Veterinary antibiotics: tetracycline (TET), ciprofloxacin (CIP), sulfadiazine (SDZ)	Algal–bacterial consortium (dominant *chlorella*/*Scenedesmus*)	TET 77 ± 5%, CIP 90 ± 14%, SDZ 60 ± 27%	Pilot photobioreactor, quasi-continuous; 35-day campaign	Zambrano et al. (2023)
Tubular PBR—outdoor pilot	Pesticides (acetamiprid, propanil; mixture)	Adapted microalgal community	Propanil 99%, Acetamiprid 71% (steady state)	Outdoor tubular PBR; HRT ≈ 8 d; transformation-product tracking	Avila et al. (2022)
Passive maturation pond (alga–alga consortium)	Antibiotics (SMX, AMX, TMP, OFX, CLR)	*Chlorella protothecoides* + *C. vulgaris*	SMX 77.3% (10 ppb); OFX 55.1% (100 ppb) (10 d)	Maturation-pond simulated tests; HRT 7–10 d	Ndlela et al. (2023)
Closed lab PBR (batch)	EDCs: parabens (MeP, PrP, BuP), BPA, benzophenone, estrone	*Scenedesmus* sp.; *Chlorella vulgaris*	Parabens ≈100% (7 d); BPA 82–90% (7 d)	Closed PBRs; photoautotrophic; controlled lab conditions	García et al. (2024)

4.4 Technological Integration of Algal Systems with Advanced Technologies

The combination of microalgae and selected physicochemical methods enables the treatment of recalcitrant pollutants through complementary approaches. The role of microalgae in capture and degradation mechanisms is enhanced, and several technologies, such as photocatalysis, advanced oxidation, or membrane separation, improve treatment efficiency. Such synergistic effects have been well documented in the literature, with a positive impact on both removal efficiency and operational stability (Kundu et al., 2024; Sousa et al., 2022). For example, optimization of a UV/H_2O_2 pretreatment in real tannery effluent (adjusting pH, temperature, oxidant dose, and lamp power) enhanced COD removal and nitrification, illustrating how advanced oxidation can condition complex matrices for subsequent algal polishing (Urbina-Suarez et al., 2023). Some of the popular integrated techniques are.

4.4.1 Photocatalysis and Microalgae

In this system, microalgae (e.g., *Chlorella* sp.) sequester contaminants on the cell surface or through intracellular bioadsorption and bioaccumulation. On the one hand, photocatalytic processes, whose active materials include materials such as TiO_2 or metallic nanoparticles that are activated by UV light, produce very reactive hydroxyl radicals that can oxidize these pollutants to less noxious or even mineralized compounds (Zhang et al., 2023). The synergism between them makes microalgae a concentration platform, and photocatalysts can enhance the localized degradation of adsorbed pollutants such that the toxicity of effluent is reduced and algal viability is promoted (Zhang et al., 2023). This analogy has been demonstrated experimentally: a combination system of a *Chlorella* sp. and a doped TiO_2 photocatalyst for bisphenol A and an antibiotic (oxytetracycline) in synthetic effluents under UV (Sousa et al., 2022).

4.4.2 Ozonation and Microalgae

In these two-phase systems, ozonation serves as the key oxidizing agent, breaking down hard-to-degrade compounds such as pharmaceuticals and pesticides (etc.) into more biodegradable intermediates. This pretreatment also lowers effluent toxicity and thereby aids in subsequent assimilation by microalgae, which metabolize these intermediates via enzymatic pathways such as lipid peroxidation and monooxygenase activity (Wang et al., 2023). The results for *Chlorella pyrenoidosa* indicated that ozone (1 mg/L) pretreatment resulted in an increase in the removal of carbamazepine from 45% to 77% compared with that of non-ozonated reactors. Furthermore, they prompt algal lipid production under controlled conditions (Kundu et al., 2024).

4.4.3 Biochar and Microalgae

Biochar is a porous framework with a large surface area, which allows the effective adsorption of organic pollutants and could act as a physical support for immobilizing algal biomass. This structure plays a role in the long-term exposure of microalgae that adhere to biochar to contaminants, and they are involved in the biotransformation of adsorbed contaminants through internal metabolism and the release of oxidative enzymes (Liu et al., 2023). In pilot studies, iron-activated biochar-supported algae, *Scenedesmus obliquus*, have been associated with greater total removal rates of 91% for TCS and 84% for BPA, that is, an increase of 30% compared with that of Chlorella sp. (Ahmad et al., 2021).

4.4.4 Constructed Wetlands and Microalgae

In such a combination, microalgae provide mainly dissolved oxygen via photosynthesis, which increases aerobic microbial activities in the wetland bed (Zhou et al., 2022; Chang et al., 2012). Moreover, algae absorb nutrients and accumulate new pollutants through biological adsorption and transformation. Wetlands behave like filter media by attenuating pollutants through sedimentation, retention at sorption sites, and biofilms (Abouhend et al., 2018; Kundu et al., 2024). This synergy enhances the removal process by establishing a favorable redox environment in the porous medium (García-Galán et al., 2021). Wang et al. reported that *Chlorella* sp. can remove up to 93% of ammonium, 76% of ciprofloxacin, and 65% of triclosan after 10 days of operation (Wang et al., 2018b).

4.4.5 Membrane Bioreactor and Microalgae

Membrane bioreactors (ABR) are membrane-facilitated algae systems that integrate the physical properties of membranes with the biotransformation capability of microalgal cells. Microalgae, including *Chlorella vulgaris*, filter and detoxify emerging pollutants through unique metabolic pathways and enzymatic and intracellular oxidation (López-Serna et al., 2024; Leong et al., 2021). The membrane acts as a physical obstruction to the passage of biomass and undegraded pollutants, therefore preventing them from being carried away into the produced mate and maintaining high cell densities in the reactor, supporting system growth (Farias et al., 2023). More than 96% of steroid hormones and more than 88% of antibiotics, such as erythromycin, from complex organic matrices, including those in AMBR configurations, have been removed from *C. vulgaris* (Yang et al., 2025).

4.4.6 Electrochemical Processes and Microalgae

In bioelectrochemical cells, microalgae at the cathode supply oxygen through photosynthesis, facilitating cathodic reduction reactions. Meanwhile, electroactive bacteria at the anode degrade organic matter, generating electrons that flow to the cathode and produce electrical energy (Santoro et al., 2017; Logan et al., 2015; Strik et al., 2011). This cooperation removes organic contaminants and simultaneously recovers energy. Algal photosynthesis replaces traditional mechanical aeration, improving system energy efficiency (Sun et al., 2020). A photobioelectrochemical cell with *Chlorella* sp. achieved 78% removal of sulfamethoxazole and generated up to 0.95 V electrical potential, validating its dual potential for treatment and energy generation (Kumar & Shukla, 2023).

4.5 Operational and Regulatory Challenges of Integrated Algal Systems

Technical, regulatory, and economic limitations that preclude the full-scale implementation of IAS, along with the state-of-the-art technologies for eliminating (emerging) contaminants, hinder their use on a global scale (Leong et al., 2021). These obstacles include the fact that microalgae are sensitive to environmental conditions, effluents are complex, biomass collection is difficult, specific regulations do not exist, and related costs are high (Farias et al., 2023; Gondi et al., 2022; Kundu et al., 2024).

4.5.1 Scale-Up and Environments

Moving from the laboratory to the actual operational environment introduces its own set of considerations. In terms of changing solar radiation, variable temperature, and biological competition, environmental conditions have a direct effect on the growth and metabolic activity of microalgae and lead to suboptimal contaminant removal. An unstable trend of biomass growth undermines the effectiveness of biosorption and biodegradation processes (Do & Du, 2024). It has been reported that species of the strain, such as the *Scenedesmus* sp., can reduce pharmaceutical removal efficiency by up to 50% under such nonoptimal environmental conditions (Mendonça et al., 2023). The presence of biological competitors in open systems and seasonal effects further enhances these instabilities. To circumvent these challenges, methods using wild strains or closed photobioreactors have been suggested (Yusoff et al., 2019).

4.5.2 Chemical Compatibility and System Stability

The chemical composition of the treated effluent affects the viability of the microalgae and the treatment efficiency. Photosynthesis and algal growth are frustrated by heavy metals, antibiotics, and other poisonous substances, which cause physiological stress and low pollutant removal efficiency (Bhatt et al., 2022). For example, the addition of fluoxetine in the presence of QACs caused a collapse in *Chlorella pyrenoidosa* populations by directly damaging the photosynthetic system and inducing oxidative stress (Xie et al., 2022). A lack of proper conditioning of the influent, i.e., improper pH setting or poor removal of inhibitory agents, may cause osmotic stress or blooms of unwanted organisms (e.g., cyanobacteria) (Gondi et al., 2022). Compatibility with upstream and/or downstream processes (e.g., ozonation, membrane filtration) also needs to be addressed to prevent problematic conversion products (e.g., residual oxidants, fouling metabolites) (Wang et al., 2023; Torres-Franco et al., 2021; López-Serna et al., 2024). To address this, states require real-time water quality monitoring and advanced pretreatments, which has therefore led to greater operational complexity (Mehanni et al., 2023; Li et al., 2024). Empirical optimization of the photoperiod and influent dilution in real tannery wastewater has demonstrated that the photoperiod and wastewater concentration markedly influence microalgal metabolite production and stress tolerance, identifying operational levers to mitigate chemical inhibition (Urbina-Suarez, Ayala-González, et al., 2022a).

4.5.3 Harvesting and Disposal of Biomass

Efficient removal of the algal biomass from the treated effluent is needed to prevent the loss of dissolved algal biomass, maintain water quality, and enable potential biomass valorization. Because of their low density and fine cell size, microalgae require methods such as centrifugation or flocculation to be effectively harvested (Xu et al., 2024). Incomplete biomass recovery leads to increased COD in effluents and higher clean water requirements (Wang et al., 2024). Although alternative strategies such as immobilization on solid supports and magnetic bioadsorbents have been investigated, they face technical and economic barriers. Additionally, biomass containing toxicants is subject to regulatory restrictions and may require treatment before reuse, or it may be classified as hazardous waste, which undermines the sustainability of the system.

4.5.4 Regulations Constraint

A lack of guidelines regarding emerging pollutants creates limitations for implementing integrated algal systems (IAS). Existing regulations are oriented mainly toward typical pollutants, with no direct instructions for the removal of pharmaceuticals or persistent organic pollutants (Sutherland & Ralph, 2019). Owing to this discrepancy, technical and legal uncertainty is raised, hindering the validation of new treatment technologies and discouraging technology development (Kumar & Shukla, 2023). Although the EU has PMI-based guidelines and both the WHO and the EPA have developed recommendations, there is no united, compulsory system of regulations encouraging the broad implementation of novel therapies. Therefore, the institutional pressure for replacing the old treatment plant infrastructure is insufficient, making strategic planning for sound solutions more challenging. Technoeconomic simulation of an integrated microalgal plant treating inland-fisheries wastewater has quantified the achievable biomass output and unit production costs, revealing the value of process modeling in identifying cost drivers and risk scale-up decisions(García-Martínez et al., 2022).

4.5.5 Operational Costs and Sustainability

The coupling of algal systems with leading-edge technologies requires enormous initial investment and high operational costs. Equipment costs, such as those of closed photobioreactors, ozone generators, and monitoring sensors, are challenging for any economy. The operational requirements for continued CO_2 delivery, agitation, illumination, and harvesting techniques, such as centrifugation, result in increased expenses (Mehanni et al., 2023; Li et al., 2024). Although some reports claim that these systems can have lower energy requirements than conventional systems do and can form interesting coproducts such as lipids and bioplastics, the commercialization of these systems is still challenging (Mehariya et al., 2024). The economic value chain and economy of IAS thus rely on financial incentives, enabling policy environments and existing markets to support bioproducts (Maryjoseph & Ketheesan, 2020). A lack of a clear regulatory safety net and durable financial incentives has made economic justification for scaling these technologies difficult.

4.6 Future Perspectives and Innovation Opportunities

Although microalgal bioprocesses have shown potential for combating ECs (emerging contaminants), their integration as a tertiary treatment option is still limited by metabolic inefficiency, susceptibility to the environment, and limited integration with advanced operational systems. Multiple opportunities arise for innovation to optimize performance and anchor algal bioremediation as a functional element in the circular economy infrastructure and transformation toward more resilient water management. One of the most innovative strategies is the exploitation of omics instruments for understanding and optimizing the intracellular microalgae degradation process. The integration of genomic, transcriptomic, proteomic, and metabolomic technologies enables the reconstruction of metabolic pathways associated with biotransformations of pharmaceuticals, pesticides, and personal care products. For example, transcriptome research revealed differentially activated genes linked to oxidative enzymatic activity in response to *Chlorella vulgaris* challenge with compounds such as diclofenac and triclosan, indicating a potential path for genetic exploration (Mishra et al., 2019).

These results suggest that bioengineering approaches can be used to develop algal strains with enhanced metabolic functions. In particular, the integration of human drug-metabolizing cytochrome P450 genes into microalgae offers an innovative approach for incorporating liver detoxification functions into aquatic systems. This model has been recently proposed as a potential alternative for removing emerging recalcitrant compounds at WWTPs. However, technical conundrums associated with gene expression, the availability of cofactors, and host cell physiological integrity remain (Kumar et al., 2020).

Similarly, the integration of comparative multiomics analyses has proven valuable for identifying secondary metabolites and degradation byproducts that may present residual toxicity. The simultaneous characterization of microbial communities in algal–bacterial consortia is proposed to optimize functional complementarity. Recent research has shown that specific bacterial species can complete metabolic pathways initiated by microalgae, suggesting that the rational design of synthetic consortia could significantly increase EC removal efficiency (Shah et al., 2024). Additionally, machine learning (ML) and artificial intelligence (AI) are revolutionizing algal bioremediation optimization. ML tools have successfully modeled extensive experimental datasets to predict optimal operational parameter combinations, such as light intensity, CO_2 concentration, N:P ratio, or hydraulic retention time. In a recent study, decision tree models predicted algal growth under 18 different configurations with less than 10% error, demonstrating practical applicability in real-world optimization scenarios (Yusof et al., 2025).

In summary, the future of algal bioremediation depends not only on biological fundamentals but also on its capacity to integrate into broader technological, economic, and social ecosystems. The convergence of omics tools, intelligent automation, and circular economy principles outlines a clear roadmap for consolidating this technology as an advanced treatment option in urban and industrial scenarios.

4.7 Conclusion

In this context, the use of microalgae is an efficient method for eliminating a broad spectrum of emerging contaminants through mechanisms that include bioadsorption, bioaccumulation, and biotransformation, with applications including carbon capture, oxygen production, and the production of valuable biomass. This multifunctionality allows them to be applied in the treatment of complex effluents and incorporated into circular economy and resource recovery strategies. Nevertheless, particular metabolic limitations, physiological sensitivity to environmental fluctuations, and uneven efficiency against highly recalcitrant chemicals, such as PFASs or some recalcitrant pharmaceuticals, limit their effectiveness. In such a case, the performance can be unstable or insufficient for them to be used alone.

Considering its shortcomings, the cultivation of microalgae in hybrid treatment systems that combine biological and physicochemical processes such as biochar adsorption, advanced oxidation, or UV disinfection seems to be more efficient. This approach provides optimal overall efficiency and makes it possible to sequence technologies that match the effluent mix and the final quality desired in the discharge. This would be possible through careful technical planning, which includes influent pretreatment—pH adjustment, inhibitor removal, nutrient balance, and selection of resilient algal strains or consortia that are complementary to the different types of contaminants. The decision between open and closed systems should be a function of climatic, spatial, and financial conditions. It should include inline instrumentation for measuring key parameters, such as biomass density, dissolved oxygen, or remaining organic load, which are essential for adjusting the process to maintain dynamic performance levels.

On the one hand, the integrated management of lignocellulosic biomass—from harvesting to valorization or final disposal—must be accounted for in system-level design, with conditioning to processes such as anaerobic digestion, pelletization, and safe incineration, according to the level of toxicity achieved. The holistic approach promotes the evolution of traditional plants into modern, multifunctional infrastructures for resource recovery, decarbonization, and pollutant removal. Driven by both regulatory and societal pressures for industrial water quality, robust, flexible, microalgae-based solutions can provide significant augmentation in addition to conventional system removal capabilities while still being operationally and ecologically sustainable when integrated innovatively.

References

Abouhend, A. S., McNair, A., Kuo-Dahab, W. C., Watt, C., Butler, C. S., Milferstedt, K., Hamelin, J., Seo, J., Gikonyo, G. J., El-Moselhy, K. M., & Park, C. (2018). The oxygenic photogranule process for aeration-free wastewater treatment. *Environmental Science & Technology, 52*(6), 3503–3511. https://doi.org/10.1021/acs.est.8b00403

Ahmad, I., Abdullah, N., Koji, I., Yuzir, A., & Mohamad, S. E. (2021). Potential of microalgae in bioremediation of wastewater. *Bulletin of Chemical Reaction Engineering & Catalysis, 16*(2), 413–429. https://doi.org/10.9767/bcrec.16.2.10616.413-429

Ajala, O. J., Tijani, J. O., Salau, R. B., Abdulkareem, A. S., & Aremu, O. S. (2022). A review of emerging micro-pollutants in hospital wastewater: Environmental fate and remediation options. *Results in Engineering, 16*, 100671. https://doi.org/10.1016/j.rineng.2022.100671

Avila, R., García-Vara, M., López-García, E., Postigo, C., López de Alda, M., Vicent, T., & Blánquez, P. (2022). Evaluation of an outdoor pilot-scale tubular photobioreactor for removal of selected pesticides from water. *Science of The Total Environment, 804*, 150040. https://doi.org/10.1016/j.scitotenv.2021.150040

Bej, S., Swain, S., Bishoyi, A. K., Mandhata, C. P., Sahoo, C. R., & Padhy, R. N. (2024). Recent advancements on antibiotic bioremediation in wastewaters with a focus on algae: An overview. *Environmental Technology, 45*(21), 4214–4229. https://doi.org/10.1080/09593330.2023.2245166

Bhatt, P., Bhandari, G., Bhatt, K., & Simsek, H. (2022). Microalgae-based removal of pollutants from wastewaters: Occurrence, toxicity and circular economy. *Chemosphere, 306*, 135576. https://doi.org/10.1016/j.chemosphere.2022.135576

Chang, J.-J., Wu. S.-Q., Dai, Y.-R., Liang, W., & Wu, Z.-B. (2012). Treatment performance of integrated vertical-flow constructed wetland plots for domestic wastewater. *Ecological Engineering, 44*, 152-159. https://doi.org/10.1016/j.ecoleng.2012.03.019

Chen, S., Chen, M., Wang, Z., Qiu, W., Wang, J., Shen, Y., Wang, Y., & Ge, S. (2016). Toxicological effects of chlorpyrifos on growth, enzyme activity and chlorophyll a synthesis of freshwater microalgae. *Environmental Toxicology and Pharmacology, 45*, 179–186. https://doi.org/10.1016/j.etap.2016.05.032

Chu, Y., Zhang, C., Wang, R., Chen, X., Ren, N., & Ho, S.-H. (2022). Biotransformation of sulfamethoxazole by microalgae: Removal efficiency, pathways, and mechanisms. *Water Research, 221*, 118834. https://doi.org/10.1016/j.watres.2022.118834

Do, S., & Du, Z.-Y. (2024). Exploring the impact of environmental conditions and bioreactors on microalgae growth and applications. *Energies, 17*(20), 5218. https://doi.org/10.3390/en17205218

Dubey, S., Chen, C.-W., Haldar, D., Tambat, V. S., Kumar, P., Tiwari, A., Singhania, R. R., Dong, C.-D., & Patel, A. K. (2023). Advancement in algal bioremediation for organic, inorganic, and emerging pollutants. *Environmental Pollution, 317*, 120840. https://doi.org/10.1016/j.envpol.2022.120840

Farias, S. L., Ruas, G., Serejo, M. L., & Boncz, M. Á. (2023). Evaluation of the effect of the feeding regime on the removal of metals and pathogens in microalgae–bacterial systems. *Water Science & Technology, 88*(1), 11–22. https://doi.org/10.2166/wst.2023.194

Frascaroli, G., Hunter, C., Roberts, J., & Escudero, A. (2024). Antibiotic removal by three promising microalgae strains: Biotic, abiotic routes, and response mechanisms. *Water, Air, & Soil Pollution, 235*(9), 600. https://doi.org/10.1007/s11270-024-07385-x

García-Galán, M. J., Matamoros, V., Uggetti, E., Díez-Montero, R., & García, J. (2021). Removal and environmental risk assessment of contaminants of emerging concern from irrigation waters in a semi-closed microalgae photobioreactor. *Environmental Research, 194*, 110278. https://doi.org/10.1016/j.envres.2020.110278

García-Martínez, J. B., Contreras-Ropero, J. E., Urbina-Suarez, N. A., López-Barrera, G. L., Barajas-Solano, A. F., Kafarov, V., Barajas-Ferreira, C., Ibarra-Mojica, D. M., & Zuorro, A. (2022). A simulation analysis of a microalgal-production plant for the transformation of inland-fisheries wastewater in sustainable feed. *Water, 14*(2), 250. https://doi.org/10.3390/w14020250

García, N., Rodríguez, R., Vicente, G., Espada, J. J., & Bautista, L. F. (2024). Comprehensive study on endocrine disruptor removal from wastewater using different microalgae species. *Applied Sciences, 15*(1), 132. https://doi.org/10.3390/app15010132

Gondi, R., Kavitha, S., Yukesh Kannah, R., Parthiba Karthikeyan, O., Kumar, G., Kumar Tyagi, V., & Rajesh Banu, J. (2022). Algal-based system for removal of emerging pollutants from wastewater: A review. *Bioresource Technology, 344*, 126245. https://doi.org/10.1016/j.biortech.2021.126245

Hom-Diaz, A., Jaén-Gil, A., Bello-Laserna, I., Rodríguez-Mozaz, S., Vicent, T., Barceló, D., & Blánquez, P. (2017). Performance of a microalgal photobioreactor treating toilet wastewater: Pharmaceutically active compound removal and biomass harvesting. *Science of the Total Environment, 592*, 1–11. https://doi.org/10.1016/j.scitotenv.2017.02.224

Huang, R., Liu, W., Su, J., Li, S., Wang, L., Jeppesen, E., & Zhang, W. (2023). Keystone microalgae species determine the removal efficiency of sulfamethoxazole: A case study of Chlorella pyrenoidosa and microalgae consortia. *Frontiers in Plant Science, 14*. https://doi.org/10.3389/fpls.2023.1193668

Ji, X., Li, H., Zhang, J., Saiyin, H., & Zheng, Z. (2019). The collaborative effect of Chlorella vulgaris-Bacillus licheniformis consortia on the treatment of municipal water. *Journal of Hazardous Materials, 365*, 483–493. https://doi.org/10.1016/j.jhazmat.2018.11.039

Jiménez-Bambague, E. M., Madera-Parra, C. A., Ortiz-Escobar, A. C., Morales-Acosta, P. A., Peña-Salamanca, E. J., & Machuca-Martínez, F. (2020). High-rate algal pond for removal of pharmaceutical compounds from urban domestic wastewater under tropical conditions. Case study: Santiago de Cali, Colombia. *Water Science and Technology, 82*(6), 1031–1043. https://doi.org/10.2166/wst.2020.362

Kang, D., & Kim, K. (2021). Real wastewater treatment using a moving bed and wastewater-borne algal–bacterial consortia with a short hydraulic retention time. *Processes, 9*(1), 116. https://doi.org/10.3390/pr9010116

Kariyawasam, T., Petkovich, M., & Vriens, B. (2024). Diclofenac degradation by immobilized *Chlamydomonas reinhardtii* and *Scenedesmus obliquus*. *MicrobiologyOpen, 13*(6). https://doi.org/10.1002/mbo3.70013

Khoo, K. S., Chia, W. Y., Chew, K. W., & Show, P. L. (2021). Microalgal-bacterial consortia as future prospect in wastewater bioremediation, environmental management and bioenergy production. *Indian Journal of Microbiology, 61*(3), 262–269. https://doi.org/10.1007/s12088-021-00924-8

Kishi, M., Tanaka, K., Tagawa, M., Akizuki, S., & Toda, T. (2023). Energy-efficient algal culture through aeration-less oxygen removal in a gas-permeable bag photobioreactor. *Algal Research, 69*, 102959. https://doi.org/10.1016/j.algal.2022.102959

Kumar, G., Shekh, A., Jakhu, S., Sharma, Y., Kapoor, R., & Sharma, T. R. (2020). Bioengineering of microalgae: Recent advances, perspectives, and regulatory challenges for industrial application. *Frontiers in Bioengineering and Biotechnology, 8*. https://doi.org/10.3389/fbioe.2020.00914

Kumar, N., & Shukla, P. (2023). Microalgal-based bioremediation of emerging contaminants: Mechanisms and challenges. *Environmental Pollution, 337*, 122591. https://doi.org/10.1016/j.envpol.2023.122591

Kundu, P., Dutta, N., & Bhattacharya, S. (2024). Application of microalgae in wastewater treatment with special reference to emerging contaminants: A step towards sustainability. *Frontiers in Analytical Science, 4*. https://doi.org/10.3389/frans.2024.1513153

Leong, Y. K., Huang, C.-Y., & Chang, J.-S. (2021). Pollution prevention and waste phycoremediation by algal-based wastewater treatment technologies: The applications of high-rate algal ponds (HRAPs) and algal turf scrubber (ATS). *Journal of Environmental Management, 296*, 113193. https://doi.org/10.1016/j.jenvman.2021.113193

Li, Z., Li, S., Wu, Q., Gao, X., & Zhu, L. (2024). Physiological responses and removal mechanisms of ciprofloxacin in freshwater microalgae. *Journal of Hazardous Materials, 466*, 133519. https://doi.org/10.1016/j.jhazmat.2024.133519

Liao, Y., Fatehi, P., & Liao, B. (2024). A study of theoretical analysis and modelling of microalgal membrane Photobioreactors for microalgal biomass production and nutrient removal. *Membranes, 14*(12), 245. https://doi.org/10.3390/membranes14120245

Liu, T., Cui, K., Li, C.-X., Chen, Y., Wang, Q., Yuan, X., Chen, Y., Liu, J., & Zhang, Q. (2023). Efficient peroxymonosulfate activation by biochar-based nanohybrids for the degradation of pharmaceutical and personal care products in aquatic environments. *Chemosphere, 311*, 137084. https://doi.org/10.1016/j.chemosphere.2022.137084

Logan, B. E., Wallack, M. J., Kim, K.-Y., He, W., Feng, Y., & Saikaly, P. E. (2015). Assessment of microbial fuel cell configurations and power densities. *Environmental Science & Technology Letters, 2*(8), 206–214. https://doi.org/10.1021/acs.estlett.5b00180

López-Serna, R., Franco, B., Bolado, S., & Jiménez, J. J. (2024). Removal of contaminants of emerging concern from pig manure in different operation stages of a thin-layer cascade photobioreactor. Relationship with concentrations in microalgae and manure. *Journal of Environmental Management, 354*, 120340. https://doi.org/10.1016/j.jenvman.2024.120340

Mantovani, M., Rossi, S., Ficara, E., Collina, E., Marazzi, F., Lasagni, M., &Mezzanotte, V. (2024). Removal of pharmaceutical compounds from the liquid phase of anaerobic sludge in a pilot-scale high-rate algae-bacteria pond. *Science of The Total Environment, 908*, 167881. https://doi.org/10.1016/j.scitotenv.2023.167881

Maryjoseph, S., & Ketheesan, B. (2020). Microalgae based wastewater treatment for the removal of emerging contaminants: A review of challenges and opportunities. *Case Studies in Chemical and Environmental Engineering, 2*, 100046. https://doi.org/10.1016/j.cscee.2020.100046

Matamoros, V., Gutiérrez, R., Ferrer, I., García, J., & Bayona, J. M. (2015). Capability of microalgae-based wastewater treatment systems to remove emerging organic contaminants: A pilot-scale study. *Journal of Hazardous Materials, 288*, 34–42. https://doi.org/10.1016/j.jhazmat.2015.02.002

Mehanni, M. M., Gadow, S. I., Alshammari, F. A., Modafer, Y., Ghanem, K. Z., El-Tahtawi, N. F., El-Homosy, R. F., & Hesham, A. E.-L. (2023). Antibiotic-resistant bacteria in hospital wastewater treatment plant effluent and the possible consequences of its reuse in agricultural irrigation. *Frontiers in Microbiology, 14*, 1141383. https://doi.org/10.3389/fmicb.2023.1141383

Mehariya, S., Das, P., Thaher, M. I., Abdul Quadir, M., Khan, S., Sayadi, S., Hawari, A. H., Verma, P., Bhatia, S. K., Karthikeyan, O. P., Zuorro, A., & Al-Jabri, H. (2024). Microalgae: A potential bioagent for treatment of emerging contaminants from domestic wastewater. *Chemosphere, 351*, 141245. https://doi.org/10.1016/j.chemosphere.2024.141245

Mendonça, I., Cunha, C., Kaufmann, M., Faria, M., & Cordeiro, N. (2023). Microplastics reduce microalgal biomass by decreasing single-cell weight: The barrier towards implementation at scale. *Science of the Total Environment, 877*, 162950. https://doi.org/10.1016/j.scitotenv.2023.162950

Mishra, A., Medhi, K., Malaviya, P., & Thakur, I. S. (2019). Omics approaches for microalgal applications: Prospects and challenges. *Bioresource Technology, 291*, 121890. https://doi.org/10.1016/j.biortech.2019.121890

Moondra, N., Jariwala, N. D., & Christian, R. A. (2020). Microalgal-bacterial consortia: An alluring and novel approach for domestic wastewater treatment. *Water Conservation and Management, 4*(1), 51–56. https://doi.org/10.26480/wcm.01.2020.51.56

Ndlela, L. L., Schroeder, P., Genthe, B., & Cruzeiro, C. (2023). Removal of Antibiotics Using an Algae-Algae Consortium (Chlorella protothecoides and Chlorella vulgaris). *Toxics, 11*(7), 588. https://doi.org/10.3390/toxics11070588

Peng, F.-Q., Ying, G.-G., Yang, B., Liu, Y.-S., Lai, H.-J., Zhou, G.-J., Chen, J., & Zhao, J.-L. (2014). Biotransformation of the flame retardant tetrabromobisphenol-A (TBBPA) by freshwater microalgae. *Environmental Toxicology and Chemistry, 33*(8), 1705–1711. https://doi.org/10.1002/etc.2589

Pereira, A., de Morais, E. G., Silva, L., Pena, A., Freitas, A., Teixeira, M. R., Varela, J., & Barreira, L. (2023). Pharmaceuticals removal from wastewater with microalgae: A pilot study. *Applied Sciences, 13*(11), 6414. https://doi.org/10.3390/app13116414

Razaviarani, V., Arab, G., Lerdwanawattana, N., & Gadia, Y. (2023). Algal biomass dual roles in phycoremediation of wastewater and production of bioenergy and value-added products. *International journal of Environmental Science and Technology, 20*(7), 8199–8216. https://doi.org/10.1007/s13762-022-04696-6

Ruas, G., López-Serna, R., Scarcelli, P. G., Serejo, M. L., Boncz, M. Á., & Munoz, R. (2021). Influence of the hydraulic retention time on the removal of emerging contaminants in an anoxic-aerobic algal-bacterial Photobioreactor coupled with anaerobic digestion. *SSRN Electronic Journal.* https://doi.org/10.2139/ssrn.3978608

Santoro, C., Arbizzani, C., Erable, B., & Ieropoulos, I. (2017). Microbial fuel cells: From fundamentals to applications. A review. *Journal of Power Sources, 356*, 225-244 https://doi.org/10.1016/j.jpowsour.2017.03.109

Satpati, G. G., Kundu, D., Rajak, R. C., Gupta, S., Kim, J.-W., & Davoodbasha, M. (2024). Algal-based membrane reactor for the remediation of emerging contaminants from wastewater: Mechanism, synthesis and technological advancement. *Algal Research, 79*, 103465. https://doi.org/10.1016/j.algal.2024.103465

Shah, B. A., Malhotra, H., Papade, S. E., Dhamale, T., Ingale, O. P., Kasarlawar, S. T., & Phale, P. S. (2024). Microbial degradation of contaminants of emerging concern: Metabolic, genetic and omics insights for enhanced bioremediation. *Frontiers in Bioengineering and Biotechnology, 12*. https://doi.org/10.3389/fbioe.2024.1470522

Singh, G., Singh, A., & Kumar Mishra, V. (2024). A critical review of occurrence, sources, fate, ecological risk, and health effect of emerging contaminants in water and wastewater. *Environmental Nanotechnology, Monitoring & Management, 22*, 100994. https://doi.org/10.1016/j.enmm.2024.100994

Sousa, H., Sousa, C. A., Simões, L. C., & Simões, M. (2022). Microalgal-based removal of contaminants of emerging concern. *Journal of Hazardous Materials, 423*, 127153. https://doi.org/10.1016/j.jhazmat.2021.127153

Strik, D. P. B. T. B., Timmers, R. A., Helder, M., Steinbusch, K. J. J., Hamelers, H. V. M., & Buisman, C. J. N. (2011). Microbial solar cells: applying photosynthetic and electrochemically active organisms. *Trends in Biotechnology, 29*(1), 41–49. https://doi.org/10.1016/j.tibtech.2010.10.001

Sun, J., Li, N., Yang, P., Zhang, Y., Yuan, Y., Lu, X., & Zhang, H. (2020). Simultaneous antibiotic degradation, nitrogen removal and power generation in a microalgae-bacteria powered biofuel cell designed for aquaculture wastewater treatment and energy recovery. *International Journal of Hydrogen Energy, 45*(18), 10871–10881. https://doi.org/10.1016/j.ijhydene.2020.02.029

Sutherland, D. L., & Ralph, P. J. (2019). Microalgal bioremediation of emerging contaminants – Opportunities and challenges. *Water Research, 164*, 114921. https://doi.org/10.1016/j.watres.2019.114921

Torres-Franco, A., Passos, F., Figueredo, C., Mota, C., & Muñoz, R. (2021). Current advances in microalgae-based treatment of high-strength wastewaters: Challenges and opportunities to enhance wastewater treatment performance. *Reviews in Environmental Science and Bio/Technology, 20*(1), 209–235. https://doi.org/10.1007/s11157-020-09556-8

Urbina-Suarez, N. A., Ayala-González, D. D., Rivera-Amaya, J. D., Barajas-Solano, A. F., & Machuca-Martínez, F. (2022a). Evaluation of the light/dark cycle and concentration of tannery wastewater in the production of biomass and metabolites of industrial interest from microalgae and cyanobacteria. *Water, 14*(3), 346. https://doi.org/10.3390/w14030346

Urbina-Suarez, N. A., Barajas-Solano, A. F., Garcia-Martinez, J. B., Lopez-Barrera, G. L., & González-Delgado, A. D. (2022b). Prospects for using wastewater from a farm for algae cultivation: The case of Eastern Colombia. *Journal Of Water And Land Development*, 172–179. https://doi.org/10.24425/jwld.2022.140387

Urbina-Suarez, N. A., López-Barrera, G. L., García-Martínez, J. B., Barajas-Solano, A. F., Machuca-Martínez, F., & Zuorro, A. (2023). Enhanced UV/H2O2 system for the oxidation of organic contaminants and ammonia transformation from tannery effluents. *PRO, 11*(11), 3091. https://doi.org/10.3390/pr11113091

Vergel-Suarez, A. H., García-Martínez, J. B., López-Barrera, G. L., Barajas-Solano, A. F., & Zuorro, A. (2023). Impact of biomass drying process on the extraction efficiency of C-Phycoerythrin. *BioTech, 12*(2), 30. https://doi.org/10.3390/biotech12020030

Wang, J., Wang, X., Yu, Z., Huang, S., Yao, D., Xiao, J., Chen, W., Wang, Z., & Zan, F. (2022). Using algae bacteria consortia to effectively treat coking wastewater: Performance, microbial community, and mechanism. *Journal of Cleaner Production, 334*, 130269. https://doi.org/10.1016/j.jclepro.2021.130269

Wang, M., Keeley, R., Zalivina, N., Halfhide, T., Scott, K., Zhang, Q., van der Steen, P., & Ergas, S. J. (2018a). Advances in algal-prokaryotic wastewater treatment: A review of nitrogen transformations, reactor configurations and molecular tools. *Journal of Environmental Management, 217*, 845–857. https://doi.org/10.1016/j.jenvman.2018.04.021

Wang, S., Poon, K., & Cai, Z. (2018b). Removal and metabolism of triclosan by three different microalgal species in aquatic environment. *Journal of Hazardous Materials, 342*, 643–650. https://doi.org/10.1016/j.jhazmat.2017.09.004

Wang, T., Hosseinzadeh, M., Cuccagna, A., Alakenova, R., Casademunt, P., Reyes Rovatti, A., López-Rubio, A., & Porte, C. (2023). Comparative toxicity of conventional versus compostable plastic consumer products: An in-vitro assessment. *Journal of Hazardous Materials, 459*, 132123. https://doi.org/10.1016/j.jhazmat.2023.132123

Wang, Y., Ma, J., Chu, H., Zhou, X., & Zhang, Y. (2024). Advances in microalgae-based livestock wastewater treatment: Mechanisms of pollutants removal, effects of inhibitory components and enhancement strategies. *Chemical Engineering Journal, 483*, 149222. https://doi.org/10.1016/j.cej.2024.149222

Xie, Z., Wang, X., Gan, Y., Cheng, H., Fan, S., Li, X., & Tang, J. (2022). Ecotoxicological effects of the antidepressant fluoxetine and its removal by the typical freshwater microalgae Chlorella pyrenoidosa. *Ecotoxicology and Environmental Safety, 244*, 114045. https://doi.org/10.1016/j.ecoenv.2022.114045

Xu, S., Li, Z., Yu, S., Chen, Z., Xu, J., Qiu, S., & Ge, S. (2024). Microalgal–bacteria biofilm in wastewater treatment: Advantages, principles, and establishment. *Water (Basel), 16*(18), 2561. https://doi.org/10.3390/w16182561

Yang, K., Wang, J., Zheng, J., & Cai, W. (2025). Microalgae-based wastewater treatment: Advances and challenges in membrane harvesting technologies. *Separation and Purification Technology, 360*, 130805. https://doi.org/10.1016/j.seppur.2024.130805

Yong, J. J. J. Y., Chew, K. W., Khoo, K. S., Show, P. L., & Chang, J.-S. (2021). Prospects and development of algal-bacterial biotechnology in environmental management and protection. *Biotechnology Advances, 47*, 107684. https://doi.org/10.1016/j.biotechadv.2020.107684

Yusof, Z., Tong, Y. W., Selvarajoo, K., Parakh, S. K., & Foo, S. C. (2025). Overcoming challenges in microalgal bioprocessing through data-driven and computational approaches. *Current Opinion in Food Science, 61*, 101253. https://doi.org/10.1016/j.cofs.2024.101253

Yusoff, F. M., Nagao, N., Imaizumi, Y., & Toda, T. (2019). *Bioreactor for microalgal cultivation systems: strategy and development* (pp. 117–159). https://doi.org/10.1007/978-3-030-14463-0_4

Zambrano, J., García-Encina, P. A., Jiménez, J. J., Ciardi, M., Bolado-Rodríguez, S., & Irusta-Mata, R. (2023). Removal of veterinary antibiotics in swine manure wastewater using microalgae–bacteria consortia in a pilot scale photobioreactor. *Environmental Technology & Innovation, 31*, 103190. https://doi.org/10.1016/j.eti.2023.103190

Zhang, M., Ning, R., Zheng. Q., & Gao, K. (2023). Microalgae-based biotechnology as a promising strategy for removing antibiotics from wastewater: Opportunities, challenges and future directions. *Frontiers in Bioengineering and Biotechnology, 11*. https://doi.org/10.3389/fbioe.2023.1248765

Zhou, J.-L., Yang, L., Huang, K.-X., Chen. D.-Z., & Gao, F. (2022). Mechanisms and application of microalgae on removing emerging contaminants from wastewater: A review. *Bioresource Technology, 364*, 128049. https://doi.org/10.1016/j.biortech.2022.128049

5 Microalgal Bioremediation of Environmental Pollutants: Mechanisms, Applications, and Challenges

Adriane Terezinha Schneider, Richard Luan Silva Machado, Darissa Alves Dutra, Eduarda Funari Machado, Ana Julia de Lima Grutzmacher, Rosangela Rodrigues Dias, Mariany Costa Deprá, Leila Queiroz Zepka, and Eduardo Jacob-Lopes

Abstract

Environmental pollution has a profound impact on environmental quality and poses substantial risks to human health. Industrial and agricultural activity generate large amounts of pollutants, which have direct and irreversible impacts on Earth's ecosystems. In this scenario, microalgae-based bioremediation emerges. It is an environmentally friendly and effective alternative for mitigating the toxicity of various chemical pollutants and physical materials that are harmful to the environment. Through the mechanisms of biosorption, bioaccumulation, and biodegradation, microalgae are capable of removing these contaminants from wastewater while simultaneously generating value-added biomass. Its applications include the bioremediation of heavy metals, hydrocarbons, pesticides, pharmaceuticals, radionuclides, and even microplastics, reinforcing its versatility. However, much progress has already been made at laboratory and pilot scales; large-scale implementation faces bottlenecks that are difficult to overcome. In light of all this, microalgae offer a unique contribution compared to conventional approaches. Therefore, the primary objective of this chapter is to present an integrative perspective on the principles of the circular bioeconomy and the role of microalgae-based bioremediation. Its principles, foundations, mechanisms, and applications in the use of microalgae for pollutant removal

A. T. Schneider · R. L. S. Machado · D. A. Dutra · E. F. Machado · A. J. de Lima Grutzmacher · R. R. Dias · M. C. Deprá · L. Q. Zepka · E. Jacob-Lopes (✉)
Bioprocess Intensification Group, Federal University of Santa Maria, UFSM, Santa Maria, Rio Grande do Sul, Brazil

L. Kumar et al. (eds.), *Algal Bioremediation*,
https://doi.org/10.1007/978-981-95-8793-3_5

will be discussed. Furthermore, case studies on industrial applications will be covered, along with the main factors influencing efficiency, technical and economic limitations, and future prospects.

Keywords

Emerging contaminants · Environmental pollutants · Microalgae · Sustainability · Bioremediation · Heavy metals

5.1 Introduction

Currently, global environmental pollution impacts are the greatest contemporary challenge we face. Many of these impacts arise silently, yet they have reached alarming levels. The intensification of anthropogenic activities and rapid industrialization in recent decades have led to the release of industrial effluents, combustion gases, automobile emissions, solid waste, and agricultural runoff. These emissions are a significant contributor to ecological imbalances, harming air, water, and soil quality (Yuvraj, 2022). To minimize this problem, a scenario involving the adoption of efficient, accessible, and environmentally sustainable technologies has attracted attention.

Microalgae emerge as a fundamental driver in bioremediation due to their ability to adsorb, accumulate, and degrade pollutants. In addition to their use for pollutant removal, they offer several benefits, including CO_2 consumption and the complete removal of nutrients (N and P), resulting in the generation of value-added biomass. Through a circular bioeconomy approach, biomass can be utilized and redirected to produce byproducts such as biochar, biogas, bioethanol, and biodiesel (Mandal et al., 2024).

Therefore, the main mechanisms involved in pollutant removal processes include biosorption, bioaccumulation, and biodegradation. These processes are discussed in detail in Sect. 5.3 (Microalgae-based Bioremediation Mechanisms). Here, it is only necessary to note that these mechanisms enable the transformation, sequestration, and detoxification of various pollutants (Kumar & Shukla, 2023).

In light of these mechanisms, and as far as the scientific literature allows us to affirm, a diverse group of substances is susceptible to removal by microalgae-based bioremediation. The inorganic compounds include heavy metals, greenhouse gases (CO_2, SO_2, NO_2), nitrates, nitrites, and fluorides, as well as radioactive substances. These compounds originate from agro-industrial processes, semiconductor manufacturing, food processing, chemical and metallurgical industries, as well as domestic, agricultural, and industrial waste. Organic compounds include petroleum hydrocarbons and tributyltin (TBT), originating from industrial, municipal, and agricultural effluents. Pesticides are generally classified as organic pollutants; however, they are sometimes categorized as emerging contaminants due to their persistence and regulatory gaps. Technically, emerging contaminants are newly detected substances that are not yet regulated by existing standards. This is the case with

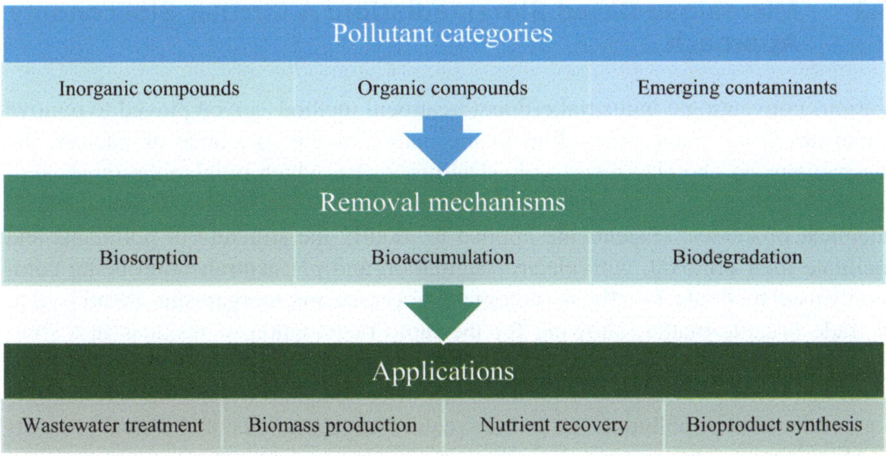

Fig. 5.1 Microalgae-based bioremediation

personal hygiene products, medications, and flame retardants. However, these contaminants have significant environmental persistence, impact the reproductive systems of aquatic organisms, and bioaccumulate throughout the food chain (Rempel et al., 2021; Dubey et al., 2023). The following schematic diagram (Fig. 5.1) presents the categories of pollutants addressed, the mechanisms of microalgae removal, and their potential applications.

Although significant advances have been made, both at laboratory and pilot scales, large-scale implementation still faces critical barriers. The main issues are related to technological readiness and cost. This translational gap between experimental results and commercial application remains one of the sector's biggest obstacles (Dey et al., 2024; Dias et al., 2025; Rossi et al., 2024). In contrast, databases demonstrate growing scientific interest, focusing on the importance of factors such as strain selection, cultivation strategy, and production system design to increase efficiency. Despite this, current microalgae-based remediation processes remain a highly ambitious goal in the biotechnology sector. Yet, it is essential to consider some important factors that contribute to efficiency throughout the bioremediation process, such as strain selection, cultivation strategy, system, and method to obtain the best results (Pacheco et al., 2020).

Taking into account the issues addressed above, although these technologies are already widely used, these processes and mechanisms have not yet truly bridged the translational gap between successful research and commercial application. Therefore, the objective of this chapter is to discuss the state of the art in microalgae-based bioremediation, with an emphasis on circularity, including the progress of treatment processes and the mechanisms of action. Furthermore, the chapter also discusses the gaps that need to be addressed to increase process efficiency levels.

5.2 Microalgae-Based Bioremediation: A Circular Bioeconomy Approach

Various conventional industrial effluent treatment methods are employed to remove impurities from water. According to the nature of the substance of interest, the mechanisms can be classified as physical processes, which involve the removal of solid objects using techniques such as sieving, flotation, and sedimentation. In chemical processes, reagents are applied to modify the structure of pollutants and facilitate their removal, with electrocoagulation and pH neutralization being commonly used methods. Finally, in biological processes, microorganisms are utilized to degrade organic matter, allowing for the rapid degradation of residues in a short period, such as a few days, rather than years (Liu & Wang, 2023).

In this sense, while these methodologies offer adequate water treatment and the correct disposal of polluting waste, they require large amounts of chemical products and high energy consumption. Besides that, microalgae demonstrate strong potential to improve both sustainability and economics in wastewater treatment (Abuhasheesh et al., 2025). Through photosynthesis, they absorb greenhouse gases (GHGs), such as CO_2, release oxygen, and generate microalgal biomass. This high-value biomass can be utilized to produce food supplements, dyes, biofuels, and biofertilizers, thereby promoting the use and consumption of more sustainable raw materials. For example, pilot-scale studies have reported CO_2 removal efficiencies exceeding 80% and nitrogen/phosphorus recovery rates above 70%, with biomass yields ranging from 0.5 to 1.2 g/L, depending on cultivation conditions (Dias et al., 2025). These results reinforce the viability of microalgae as a sustainable option.

In this way, microalgae function both as a means of generating rich bioproducts and as a method of treating industrial effluents, making them an attractive alternative that combines environmental protection with economic benefits (Jacob-Lopes et al., 2018). Table 5.1 compares conventional treatment methods versus microalgae-based approaches in terms of energy demand, burdens, co-products, and sustainability.

Considering the above, microalgae play a significant role in the circular bioeconomy by transforming waste into value-added products. Due to the contribution of microalgae to sustainability, their importance is even more highlighted in achieving the Sustainable Development Goals (SDGs). The SDGs are a global initiative proposed by the United Nations General Assembly, comprising 17 goals that aim to ensure global well-being through social, economic, and environmental changes. For example, some proposed goals aim to improve quality of life, health, and education, while also conserving the environment (Weiland et al., 2021). Thus, microalgae can play a strategic role in combating hunger and promoting food security (SDG 2). Since they do not require fertile soil or traditional agricultural areas for cultivation, their production is possible in regions where agriculture is limited (Abdelfattah et al., 2023). Furthermore, microalgae are a source of biomass that contains essential nutrients used in supplements, and they can be incorporated into the diet. If included in regions where there is an insufficient intake of essential nutrients, it can help combat malnutrition and serve as a pathway to achieving SDG 3 (good health and well-being). Furthermore, microalgae production is related to

Table 5.1 Conventional treatment methods and microalgae-based treatment methods

Aspect	Conventional methods	Approaches with microalgae
Energy demand	High	Moderate/low
Operating cost	High (pumping and aeration)	Potentially reduced when implemented in integrated systems
Co-products	Reusing byproducts as raw material for a new cycle	Valuable bio-based products; supplements, pigments, enzymes, feed, biofuels, biofertilizers
Environmental sustainability	High resource consumption, production of toxic byproducts	Capture of 1.83 $kgCO_2/kg$ of biomass
Scalability	Well-established globally	Still under development. Promising results from pilot-scale studies
Treatment time	From hours to days	Days to weeks
Risks/ limitations	Generation of toxic secondary waste, high energy demand	Intensive water and land use, crop contamination, high downstream processing costs

Adapted from Thapa (2020), Dębowski et al. (2021), Kuok et al. (2022), Srimongkol et al. (2022), Hamawand (2023), Gupta et al. (2024), Kundu et al. (2024), Velásquez-Orta et al. (2024), Dias et al. (2025), and Pant et al. (2025)

action against global climate change (SDG 13). In turn, throughout their cultivation and the photosynthesis process, microalgae absorb carbon dioxide and thus help to reduce the concentration of the gas in the atmosphere, which intensifies the greenhouse effect. Studies demonstrate a CO_2 capture potential of approximately 1.83 $kgCO_2/kg$ of biomass, placing microalgae as a powerful tool in mitigating global warming (Razzak et al., 2024).

On the other hand, beyond these advantages, it's essential to acknowledge that there are certain limitations and trade-offs. Large-scale cultivation may require significantly more land and water, thereby raising concerns about sustainability. Furthermore, there are risks of crop contamination, high costs associated with subsequent biomass processing steps, and limitations on achieving productivity that is independent of environmental conditions.

Finally, microalgae cultivation has proven to be an effective alternative for bioproduct generation and sustainable wastewater treatment, and it is possible to conclude that they can be considered an important factor in economic wastewater treatment strategies and an alternative in progress towards achieving the SDGs. However, research and investment in microalgal biotechnology, as well as renewable technologies and energy sources, are still necessary to provide a more sustainable world, and what proves efficient in theory ultimately becomes viable in practice.

5.3 Microalgae-Based Bioremediation Mechanisms

During the wastewater treatment (WWT) process, three main steps are generally applied. The first involves the preliminary removal of larger particles and debris through screening and sedimentation. Then comes the secondary step, in which aerobic bacteria oxidize organic compounds and ammonia, converting them into carbon dioxide (CO_2) and water (H_2O) (Qin et al., 2022). This step is widely known in the academic context as the biological oxidation process or activated sludge system, where nutrients such as phosphorus and nitrogen are assimilated by microalgae, contributing to the reduction of both biochemical and chemical oxygen demand (BOD and COD, respectively) (Maltsev et al., 2023). Finally, the third step consists of the combination of processes such as filtration, disinfection, and nutrient removal, depending on the required quality of the final effluent.

In this context, the use of microalgae for bioremediation appears as a viable and innovative alternative to the conventional biological oxidation step, altering the dynamics of aerobic bacterial activity by leveraging the photosynthetic capabilities of these organisms. This process not only removes key nutrients like nitrogen and phosphorus but also generates biomass that can be applied in various sectors, including the production of renewable biofuels (Deepika et al., 2025).

Additionally, microalgae play a central role in bioremediation through strategies such as adsorption, intracellular accumulation, and pollutant breakdown, aiming to eliminate contaminants present in aquatic systems (Machado et al., 2025). These strategies are integral to the broader concept of bioremediation, which involves using biological organisms to eliminate, neutralize, or convert environmental pollutants. In the case of microalgae, these processes manifest as biosorption (when binding to the surface occurs), bioaccumulation (when intracellular absorption occurs), and biodegradation (when enzymatic transformation occurs). The predominance of these processes depends exclusively on environmental conditions—contaminant concentration, pH, and light availability (Kumar & Shukla, 2023; Altaf et al., 2023).

For instance, adsorption is a non-metabolic and passive mechanism by which living or non-living algal biomass binds pollutants via interactions with specific functional groups on the cell surface, such as hydroxyl (OH), carboxyl (COOH), amine (NH2), and phosphate (PO_4^{3-}). The algal cell wall, composed of a flexible and porous fibrous network, provides sites that enhance the binding of heavy metals and trace elements like manganese (Mn), cobalt (Co), copper (Cu), zinc (Zn), molybdenum (Mo), boron (B), and iron (Fe) (Rempel et al., 2021). These interactions can also occur with new and emerging contaminants, such as nanomaterials, agrochemicals, and pharmaceuticals, which tend to adhere to the surface of the cells before potentially being absorbed. Thus, the biosorption process predominates under conditions of acidic pH and high metal concentrations, while bioaccumulation and biodegradation prevail under conditions with high nutrient levels and optimized by light (Leng et al., 2020; Quan et al., 2023).

As illustrated in Fig. 5.2, this includes the stages of adsorption (attachment to the algal surface), bioaccumulation (transport and retention within the cell), and biodegradation (biochemical transformation of toxic agents into safer compounds).

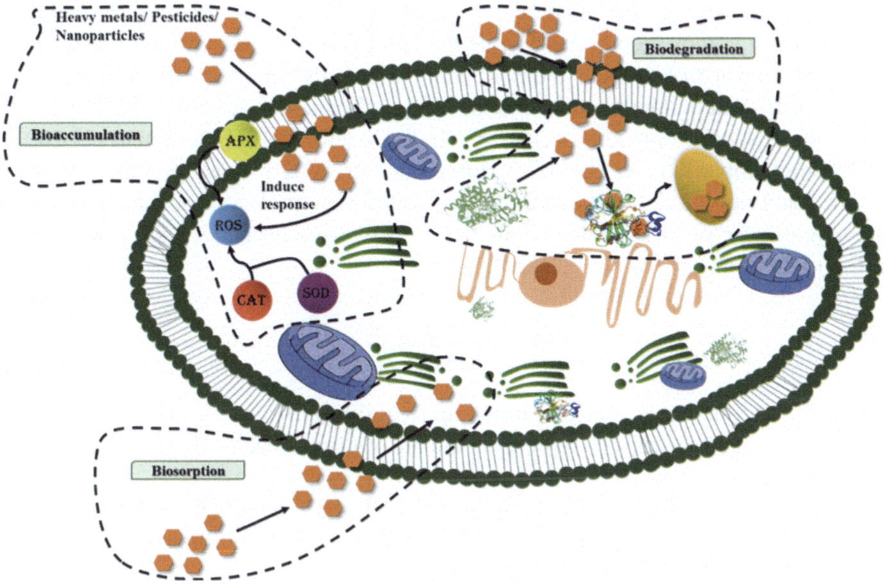

Fig. 5.2 Schematic representation of microalgal bioremediation mechanisms

Biosorption involves the attachment of contaminants to the cell surface via electrostatic and chemical interactions. Bioaccumulation is the process by which pollutants are actively transported into cells, where intracellular accumulation can trigger the activation of antioxidant defenses. Biodegradation, initiated by enzymes such as cytochrome P450, transforms complex pollutants into less toxic, more soluble compounds. ROS (reactive oxygen species) are generated as part of the oxidative stress response, with enzymes such as SOD (superoxide dismutase), CAT (catalase), and APX (ascorbate peroxidase) mitigating their effects.

Although these elements are essential in low concentrations, they can become toxic when accumulated in excess, such as chromium (Cr), cadmium (Cd), mercury (Hg), lead (Pb), and arsenic (As). On the other hand, some micronutrients promote cell growth through hormesis, in which low concentrations of potentially toxic substances induce beneficial and adaptive biological responses (Machado et al., 2025). Still, biosorption can occur through physisorption (weak interactions, such as hydrogen bonds, van der Waals forces, and electrostatic interactions) or chemisorption (ionic or covalent bonds) (Kumar & Shukla, 2023).

Going a step further, recent studies have included kinetic and mathematical models to represent biosorption dynamics. The microalgae biosorption process can be described mathematically by models that express the relationship between the pollutant concentration in solution and the amount adsorbed on the cell wall (Tattibayeva et al., 2022). These models, known as *adsorption isotherms*, are fundamental tools for understanding the capacity and binding layer of biosorption systems used in the removal of organic toxins. The Langmuir and Freundlich isotherms are among the most widely applied: the former assumes monolayer adsorption on homogeneous sites, while the latter describes adsorption on heterogeneous surfaces in an empirical and nonlinear manner. Pseudo-first-order and pseudo-second-order kinetic models describe the temporal dynamics and the mechanism by which the adsorption process occurs (Ayele & Godeto, 2021; Foroutan et al., 2021, 2022; Peighambardoust et al., 2021; Hosseini et al., 2022; Mansour et al., 2022).

The Langmuir model suggests that the adsorption of metal ions occurs on shallow and single-layer surfaces, without interaction between adjacent cell sites, as shown in Eq. (5.1) (Tattibayeva et al., 2022).

$$\frac{C_e}{q_e} = \frac{1}{K_L Q_m} + \frac{C_e}{Q_m} \tag{5.1}$$

where C_e are the initial concentrations and equilibrium of ions (mg/L); q_e is the adsorption value (mg/g); Q_m represents the adsorption capacity (mg/g); and K_L the adsorption energy (L/g).

Considering constants in the Langmuir model, the Freundlich model is used to illustrate the adsorption process on inhomogeneous and multilayer surfaces, as shown in Eq. (5.2) (Tattibayeva et al., 2022).

$$\ln\ q_e = \ln K_f + \frac{1}{n}\ \ln\ C_e \tag{5.2}$$

where K_f and n are considered constants of the Freundlich model, representing the relationship between adsorption capacity and intensity, respectively.

To estimate the parameters $1/n$ and K_f, $\ln q_e$ is usually described as a function of $\ln C_e$. In the literature, the value of n is generally reported to vary between 1 and 10. This parameter indicates the physicochemical nature of adsorption: when $n = 1$, the process follows a linear relationship; for $n > 1$, adsorption is predominantly physical and considered favorable; when $n < 1$, the mechanism is suggested to be associated with chemical interactions.

The pseudo-first-order and pseudo-second-order models serve to delineate the kinetic behavior of the absorption process and are described in Eqs. (5.3 and 5.4) respectively (Mansour et al., 2022; Tattibayeva et al., 2022).

$$\ln\ (q_e - q_t) = \ln\ q_e - tk_1 \tag{5.3}$$

$$\frac{t}{q_t} = \left(\frac{1}{K_2 q_e^2}\right) + \frac{t}{q_e} \tag{5.4}$$

where q_t and q_e are the adsorption capacity per gram of adsorbent (mg/g); k_1 (1/min), the adsorption rate constant; k_2 (g/mg min), the quasi-square velocity constant of the kinetic model.

Bioadsorption, one of the mechanisms within biosorption, is considered non-selective and reversible, allowing the concomitant removal of several contaminant bodies such as heavy metals and emerging organic compounds (ECs), including pharmaceuticals. Its efficiency depends on the polarity of the compounds: lipophilic contaminants (usually cationic) are more easily adsorbed than hydrophilic ones (usually anionic) (Prosenc et al., 2021). In addition, extracellular structures such as extracellular polymeric substances (EPS) favor the adhesion of contaminants, acting as active sites for retention and facilitating subsequent removal or degradation. Studies report significant removals, such as 91% of the drug Tradmol by *Scenedesmus obliquus* and 100% of metronidazole by *Chlorella vulgaris*.

It is important to highlight that these mechanisms can manifest themselves in both live and inactive microalgae. The use of inactive biomass has several advantages, including greater tolerance to toxic compounds, lower costs by eliminating the need for culture media, and the possibility of reuse after contaminant desorption. Studies indicate that extracted biomass (lipids removed) has a greater adsorption capacity due to the increase in surface area (Suárez-Martínez et al., 2022).

At the same time, microalgae can absorb pollutants through bioaccumulation, an active and energy-dependent process that involves the internalization of compounds by living cells. This mechanism, although slower than biosorption, enables the intracellular storage or transformation of toxic substances, making it effective in removing heavy metals, pesticides, and nitrates (Prosenc et al., 2021). During this process, contaminants cross the cell membrane and can cause damage to the cell structure, inducing defense responses mediated by antioxidant enzymes such as catalase (CAT), peroxidase (POD), ascorbate peroxidase (APX), and superoxide dismutase (SOD), which neutralize reactive toxic species (ROS) generated in response to cellular stress. The bioaccumulation process tends to prevail in conditions where pollutant concentrations are low and exposure times are prolonged (Rempel et al., 2021).

Both processes, biosorption and bioaccumulation, occur simultaneously and dynamically, making it difficult to isolate them experimentally. However, microalgae have a high capacity for adaptation, even in environments with low concentrations of pollutants, thanks to the resistance of their cell wall (Rempel et al., 2021).

This resilience extends its applications in different contexts, from household waste to industrial effluents. However, factors such as pH, temperature, exposure time, and contaminant concentration need to be optimized to maximize bioaccumulation (Kumar & Shukla, 2023). Selecting strains that are tolerant to contaminated environments is also an effective strategy. After internalization, the compounds are capable of metabolization, which leads to the next and most efficient treatment mechanism: biodegradation.

Biodegradation is considered the most effective method for removing emerging contaminants (ECs) because it promotes their chemical conversion into less toxic or harmless substances, such as CO_2 and H_2O. This conversion occurs through enzymatic reactions and can follow the pathway of biotransformation (generation of intermediate metabolites) or complete biomineralization (Mokrani & Nabti, 2024). Initially, the activation of the molecules occurs through oxidation catalyzed by cytochrome P450 enzymes, facilitating hydroxylation, reduction, or conjugation reactions. These substances are then transported to organelles such as vacuoles for storage or elimination. In environments with satisfactory light and nutrient availability, biodegradation processes predominate. This process is mostly enhanced by phytoremediation strategies (Quan et al., 2023; Altaf et al., 2023).

This process can occur intracellularly, through the direct action of enzymes, or extracellularly, with the aid of EPS that act as biosurfactants, increasing the availability of pollutants (Leng et al., 2020). Species such as *Chlorella* and *Scenedesmus* have already demonstrated a reduction of more than 80% of antibiotics and pesticides, mainly through biodegradation (Quan et al., 2023). Enzymes such as γ-glutamylcysteine synthetase and phytochelatin synthetase facilitate the detoxification of heavy metals by forming complexes with glutathione and phytochelatins. Additionally, proteins such as metallothioneins and antioxidant enzymes (SOD and CAT) protect cells from oxidative stress induced by these compounds (Altaf et al., 2023). Biodegradation can also be enhanced by the presence of light (photoremediation), which activates reactions with reactive oxygen species (ROS), contributing to the breakdown of persistent compounds.

5.4 Microalgae-Mediated Bioremediation of Organic and Inorganic Pollutants

Among the most pressing environmental challenges today, the growing contamination of water resources stands out. To lessen these impacts, microalgae offer a promising bioremediation solution for contaminated environments. In this context, researchers have investigated various microalgae species for their ability to remove organic and inorganic substances using the mechanisms outlined in Sect. 5.3 (Faruque et al., 2024). Persistent organic pollutants—such as hydrocarbons, pesticides, and industrial solvents—have high toxicity and low degradation, becoming a significant environmental risk (Kuppan et al., 2024). As a result, the use of microalgae to treat such contaminants has been explored in scientific studies.

Marine ecosystems worldwide face a severe environmental challenge from contamination by petroleum-derived hydrocarbons. These pollutants are highly resistant to natural degradation and have toxic effects on aquatic life (Ahmed & Fakhruddin, 2018). Conventional technologies are commonly applied for their removal — mechanical or chemical. However, these technologies have limitations in both effectiveness and cost. To find other effective bioremediation methods, studies have focused on using microalgae. Hamouda et al. (2023) demonstrated that a consortium of the green microalgae *Chlorella vulgaris* and the cyanobacterium *Synechococcus* sp. efficiently degraded kerosene, leading to hydrocarbon removal. At the same time, the process generated biomass with a high lipid content—a characteristic that favors its application in the production of biofuels. Several authors, including Li et al. (2018), Das and Deka (2019), and Al-Hussieny et al. (2020), highlight the microalgae *Chlorella vulgaris* as particularly effective in hydrocarbon degradation.

Liu et al. (2019) investigated the tolerance of five marine microalgae species to oil contamination, including *Dunaliella salina*, *Chlorella* sp., *Cryptococcus weissflogii*,

Phaeodactylum tricornutum, and *Prorocentrum donghaiense*. The results demonstrated that *D. salina* and *Chlorella* sp. presented high resistance to water-soluble fractions of diesel oil and were also effective in the biodegradation of these hydrocarbons. Beyond conventional hydrocarbons, polycyclic aromatic hydrocarbons (PAHs) constitute a highly toxic class of pollutants, primarily arising from the incomplete combustion of organic matter. They are notable for their carcinogenicity, persistence, and genotoxic effects (Satpati et al., 2023). Studies show that species such as *Chlorella vulgaris* and *Selenastrum capricornutum* have demonstrated high efficiency in removing fluoranthene, pyrene, and benzo[a]pyrene, compounds common in environments contaminated by fossil fuels. Such microalgae can perform this removal through these mechanisms, which were described in Sect. 5.3, mostly involving enzymes such as glutathione-S-transferase and dioxygenases (Tomar & Jajoo, 2021). Other species, such as *Scenedesmus acutus*, *Oscillatoria* sp., and *Nostoc calcicola*, also showed removal rates above 95% for pyrene (Ghanbarzadeh et al., 2022).

Furthermore, intensive agricultural practices have caused significant impacts on surface and groundwater bodies. Excessive use of nutrients such as nitrogen (N) and phosphorus (P), along with the application of pesticides and the release of heavy metals, contributes to eutrophication and aquatic contamination (Lisetskii & Buryak, 2023). Ali et al. (2023) in their study showed that the use of microalgae such as *Chlorella vulgaris*, *Chlorella salina*, *Scenedesmus dimorphus*, and *Arthrospira platensis* is efficient in eliminating nutrients such as N and P, in addition to bioremediating heavy metals, with rates ranging from 72% to 100%. Additionally, microalgae have shown a high capacity to absorb toxic and persistent metals such as zinc (Zn), nickel (Ni), arsenic (As), mercury (Hg), copper (Cu), cadmium (Cd), lead (Pb), chromium (Cr), and manganese (Mn). Removal efficiency can reach up to 100%, depending on environmental conditions (Ali et al., 2023; Sarma et al., 2024). According to Chandrashekharaiah et al. (2021), while *Chlorella pyrenoidosa* showed variable performance, *Scenedesmus acutus* achieved a cadmium adsorption rate of 57.14%, with 98.5% of the metal retained on the cell surface.

Additionally, inorganic pollutants include, in addition to heavy metals and halides, radioactive substances. Recently, there has been growing concern regarding water contamination by radionuclides; these radioactive substances are equally difficult to remove from water (Dinis et al., 2025). Radionuclides such as uranium (U), cesium (Cs), and radium (Ra) have been the subject of studies that point to *Chlorella sorokiniana* and *Arthrospira platensis* as organisms effective in the bioaccumulation of these elements (Zinicovscaia et al., 2020). The microalgae *Chlorella sorokiniana* also demonstrated high performance in uranium biosorption in a study conducted by Embaby et al. (2022), where it reached a maximum adsorption rate of 188.7 mg/g. This same species was identified by León-Vaz et al. (2021) as capable of accumulating cadmium to an exceptional level, removing 65% of the initial concentrations.

Another relevant aspect of the use of microalgae for bioremediation of water bodies concerns the ability of these microorganisms to remove pesticides commonly used in agriculture. These substances infiltrate groundwater and surface water through various processes, primarily leaching and surface runoff (Singhal et al., 2021). Castellanos-Estupiñan et al. (2022) demonstrated that *Chlorella* sp. achieved 100% removal efficiency for the pesticide chlorpyrifos, while *Scenedesmus* sp. removed 75%. Through laboratory tests and applications in photobioreactors, it was possible to demonstrate removals of over 80% for herbicides such as atrazine, 2,4-D, and 2-methyl-4-chlorophenoxyacetic acid (MCPA) by microalgae. In some cases, such as atrazine, this bioremediation occurred in a few days, with limited impacts on microalgal growth depending on the concentration and by-products present (García-Galán et al., 2020). Furthermore, studies on wastewater from agricultural greenhouses have shown that these same microalgae not only absorb pesticides such as metalaxyl and triclopyr, but also promote their active degradation (La bella et al., 2022).

Regarding drugs and antibiotics, their presence in aquatic environments represents a growing concern due to their bioactivity even at low concentrations. Substances such as diclofenac, carbamazepine, sulfamethoxazole, and ciprofloxacin are frequently detected in effluents from wastewater treatment plants (Onchoke et al., 2023). Microalgae such as *Chlorella vulgaris*, *Scenedesmus obliquus*, and *Arthrospira platensis* have been widely studied for their ability to remove such compounds through the mechanisms described in Sect. 5.3. Laboratory tests have demonstrated removals greater than 80% for ibuprofen and paracetamol (Bhatt et al., 2022). Furthermore, *Chlamydomonas reinhardtii* has demonstrated efficacy in degrading antibiotics, including reducing microbial resistance genes (Gasana et al., 2025).

Concerning water bodies polluted by emerging substances, the bottleneck of removing microplastics and metallic nanoparticles stands out. Even though traditional methods show slow efficiency, microalgae, including *Scenedesmus* sp. and *Chlorella pyrenoidosa,* have proven capable of adsorbing polystyrene particles and silver nanoparticles, respectively, which assists in their environmental removal (Tarbajova et al., 2023). However, the application of microalgae for large-scale removal of emerging contaminants remains challenging. Some of these challenges stem from recovery difficulties, limited biodegradability, and the risk of byproduct toxicity (Velásquez-Orta et al., 2024).

Finally, among the broad range of compounds that microalgae are capable of bioremediating are phenolic compounds such as bisphenol A (BPA) and textile dyes such as methylene blue and reactive red 198. These substances have also been efficiently degraded through microalgal bioremediation. *Arthrospira platensis* and *Dunaliella salina* do not just adsorb these molecules; they also facilitate their enzymatic breakdown, leading to over 90% removal (Tarbajova et al., 2023). It is important to highlight that, although microalgae can perform complex pollutant degradation processes, in some cases, the formation of toxic intermediate metabolites has been observed. Therefore, further investigations must be carried out into their fate and the potential related ecological risks (Quan et al., 2023). Through efficient mechanisms such as biosorption, bioaccumulation, and enzymatic biodegradation, these microorganisms demonstrate a broad capacity to remove several pollutants mentioned in this chapter. In addition to their effectiveness in remediation, microalgae are capable of offering additional benefits, such as the generation of biomass with energy potential and adaptation to different environments. Therefore, their application in wastewater treatment systems, industrial effluents, and areas impacted by agricultural and urban activities consolidates it as a sustainable, versatile approach aligned with the principles of bioeconomy and environmental conservation.

5.5 The State-of-the-Art of Microalgae-Mediated Bioremediation

Microalgae-based bioremediation, also called phycoremediation, has proven to be a promising alternative for treating organic and inorganic pollutants, with the potential to transform residual resources into a strategic input within the logic of the circular bioeconomy (Kaloudas et al., 2021; Dias et al., 2021). Bibliometric analyses in databases like ScienceDirect reveal increasing academic interest in this area. The search for the term "bioremediation" generated more than 21,800 research articles and 5100 review articles from 2014 to 2024, with about 66% of these publications published in the last 5 years. When combining the keywords "bioremediation" and "microalgae," over 3800 indexed publications were found during the same period, showing noticeable annual growth (Fig. 5.3). The data provided by bibliometric analyses highlight the prominence of bioremediation and microalgae-based bioremediation as emerging and disruptive technologies in effluent treatment.

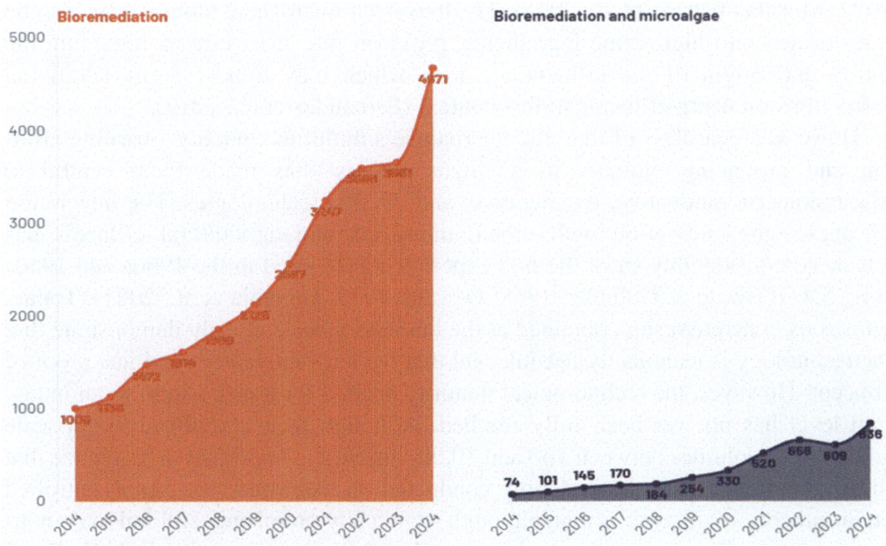

Fig. 5.3 Number of articles published in the last 10 years

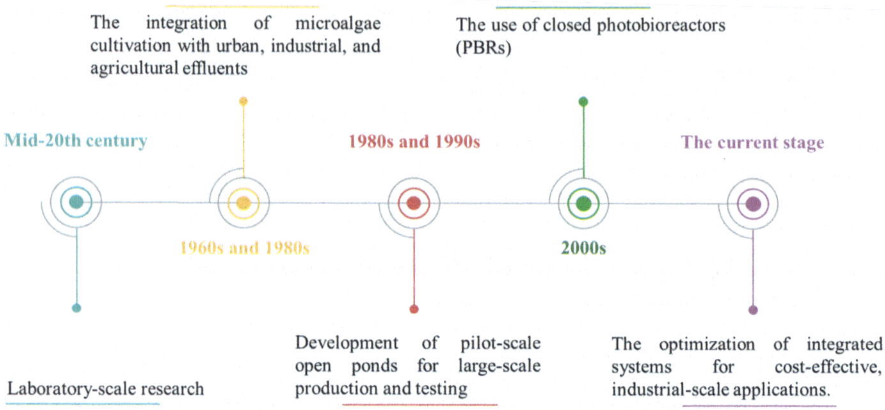

Fig. 5.4 Schematic timeline of the inclusion of the use of microalgae

Microalgae such as *Chlorella* and *Arthrospira*, for example, are widely studied for their ability to efficiently remove nutrients like nitrogen and phosphorus, as well as other pollutants such as heavy metals and pharmaceuticals (Ansari et al., 2025). After some experimental studies, it was verified that the influence of environmental parameters—pH, temperature, and light intensity—is related to removal efficiencies, showing the importance of process optimization (Magalhães et al., 2022; Yang et al., 2025). Additionally, it is important to note that bioremediation technology based on these microorganisms offers significant advantages over traditional effluent treatment methods, as it enables both environmental debugging and the production of biomass with potential uses in bioenergy, biofertilizers, and feed (Kumar et al., 2022; Morillas-España et al., 2025). The harvested microalgae biomass can also be transformed into high-value ingredients, provided that strict criteria regarding the purity and origin of the effluent are met, which may impose some additional restrictions on using effluents in this context (Fernández et al., 2019).

However, regardless of that, the microalgae's multifunctionality—treating effluent and producing biomass in a single process—has made them central to discussions on innovative, regenerative, and circular technologies. The integration of microalgae cultivation with urban, industrial, and agricultural effluents has advanced considerably since the first experiments recorded in the 1960s and 1980s (Fig. 5.4) (Oswald & Golueke, 1968; Oswald, 1973; Geremia et al., 2021). Today, numerous concrete results obtained at the laboratory scale already demonstrate that the technology is technically feasible and that we have moved beyond just proof of concept. However, the technological maturity needed for transposition to an industrial level has not yet been fully reached. Although there are already pilot-scale studies with volumes between 100 and 10,000 liters, it is important to recognize that these experiences are limited and conducted in controlled or semi-controlled environments—with results that, although technically promising, still fail to demonstrate sustainability, scalability, and replicability (Morillas-España et al., 2021; Rossi et al., 2024). For example, innovative pilot systems operated in municipal wastewater treatment lagoons have achieved nutrient removal rates above 70%. However, they still face challenges regarding biomass collection and cost-effectiveness (Velásquez-Orta et al., 2024).

Fernández et al. (2019) demonstrated that, even in demonstration facilities of up to 5 hectares using raceway and thin-layer cascade reactors, biomass production costs are around 3.6 and 1.4 €/kg—considering the use of effluents as a cultivation medium. In a complementary way, Dias et al. (2025) reported values ranging from 1.98 to 9.69 €/kg in raceway pond systems fed with wastewater. Such costs, still far from the critical threshold of 1.0 €/kg required for competitive insertion in the bioenergy, biofertilizer, and, ultimately, animal feed markets, highlight an obstacle to the technological readiness of phycoremediation.

More than a technical issue, the viability of integrating microalgae cultivation with effluents rests, above all, on the composition of the effluent and its influence on biomass productivity—factors that have already been shown to dictate the results of technical, economic, and environmental analyses (Depra et al., 2020). In other words, if the strategy of using industrial, urban, and agricultural pollutants substantially compromises productivity, there is a risk of subverting the environmentally virtuous logic of this approach (Togarcheti et al., 2017). Thus, instead of transforming an environmental liability into an input, the system may result in systemic inefficiencies that entomb the benefits generated and the promise of mitigating environmental impacts. In this scenario, evidently, microalgae-based bioremediation may cease to be a solution and become part of the very problem that it proposed to resolve. This has currently called into check the optimistic narrative with which microalgae-based bioremediation technology is often presented, reinforcing the need for integrated, transparent, and critical analyses regarding its application viability. In sum, technological enthusiasm is not enough—it must be confronted with consistent metrics of technical-economic and technical-environmental feasibility on real and more relevant operational scales. Finally, the state of the art offers solid promise, but the evidence is still partial and restricted to initiatives on a demonstration and pilot scale (Dias et al., 2025).

5.6 Factors Affecting the Efficiency of Microalgal Bioremediation

Although there is a diversity of technologies aimed at effluent treatment, a significant number of technologies prove to be ineffective. It is clear that ineffective chemical treatments generate waste with high levels of unstable by-products, and ineffective biological treatments generate a lot of ecotoxicity. However, to address these challenges, efforts have been focused on research involving microalgae-based bioremediation. For example, in industrial effluents, the biodegradation of recalcitrant pollutants occurs concomitantly at low cost, also adding environmental advantages. This is because microalgae use sunlight as energy, reducing the amount of energy applied compared to conventional treatments, capturing CO_2, and providing value-added biomass. In turn, for microalgae-based bioremediation to be adequately efficient, requirements such as the composition and characteristics of the effluent and the selection of strains are fundamental (Sousa et al., 2021).

The composition of the effluent demonstrates, above all, which polluting compounds are present in the environment. Effluents containing pollutants, such as heavy metals and pharmaceutical residues, pose an imminent risk to the environment. However, microalgae are capable of removing these pollutants. Furthermore, the efficiency of the removal process is directly linked to environmental conditions such as light intensity, temperature, and pH. These factors primarily modulate growth and biosorption/bioaccumulation capacity (Yang et al., 2025).

Light intensity is one of the key factors determining the growth of microalgae, as well as their ability to remove nutrients such as nitrogen and phosphorus from the environment. Research by Palikrousis et al. (2024) showed an approximately 100% reduction in $N\text{-}NH_4$ (ammonium nitrogen) and phosphorus when *C. sorokiniana* was subjected to photosynthetic photon flux density (PPFD) of 162 μmol m^{-2} s^{-1}. When subjected to a PPFD of 20 μmol m^{-2} s^{-1}, the removal rate dropped to around 55%. The temperature factor has a strong relationship with the metabolic rates of microalgae, resulting in increased nutrient removal efficiency at high temperatures. At a temperature of 30 °C, removal efficiencies of 82.62%, 97.94%, and 99.37% were observed for $N\text{-}NH_4$, $NO_3\text{-}N$, and $NO_2\text{-}N$, respectively, by the microalgae *Desmodesmus* sp. CHX1. When exposed to a temperature of 25 °C, the removal efficiencies were lower, at 77.27% ($N\text{-}NH_4$), 83.59% (NO3-N), and 97.02% (NO_2-N) (Tian et al., 2024). Similarly, pH substantially affects the removal of nutrients, including $N\text{-}NH_4$, total nitrogen (TN), and total phosphorus (TP). *Desmodesmus* sp. SNN1 was subjected to secondary effluent treatment at pH 9.0 and resulting in removal rates of 99.95, 88.90, and 97.92% for $N\text{-}NH_4$, TN, and TP, respectively. At pH 5.0, these removal rates were significantly reduced (Wang et al., 2023).

However, in general, high concentrations, such as heavy metals like chromium (Cr), cadmium (Cd), arsenic (As), copper (Cu), zinc (Zn), nickel (Ni), mercury (Hg), and lead (Pb), end up resulting in significant inhibition of microalgae growth (Yang et al., 2025). Table 5.2 presents the removal efficiency of heavy metals by a variety of microalgae species. Species such as *Chlamydomonas reinhardtii*, *Chlorella vulgaris*, *Coelastrum proboscideum*, *Scenedesmus acuminatus*, *Scenedesmus quadricauda*, *Scenedesmus* sp., and *Spirulina platensis* showed great efficiency in the removal of heavy metals, such as Tl, Cu, Pb, N, S, P, and Fe. Furthermore, compounds such as Cu and Cd achieved a removal efficiency below 30% when using the microalgae *Chlorella vulgaris*, non-flocculating *Chlorella vulgaris* CNW11, and *Scenedesmus incrassatulus*. However, the initial pollution load is a crucial factor, and research focused on specific strains may enhance their bioremediation efficiency.

Other significant elements that need to be highlighted are nitrogen oxides (NO_x). These compounds, when discarded in large quantities in unsuitable environments, contribute to the formation of acid rain, photochemical SMOG, and fog, resulting in environmental and human health problems. Although species such as *Chlorella*, *Chlamydomonas*, *Scenedesmus*, *Synechococcus*, and *Spirulina* are tolerant to NO_x, the removal of this pollutant by microalgae requires the pollutant to be dissolved in

Table 5.2 Bioremediation of heavy metals from industrial wastewater using microalgae

Microalgae	Pollutants	Efficiency (%)
Aphanothess sp.	Pb (II)	93.00%
C. reinhardtii (wild-type)	Cd (II)	90.20%
Chlamydomonas reinhardtii	Tl	100% (150 mg/L); 94% (250 mg/L); 95.00% (500 mg/L)
Chlorella sorokiniana TU5	Mo (VI)	57.80% at 115.65 mg/L
Chlorella sp.	Cu	69.90%
Chlorella vulgaris	Co (II)	94.00%
Chlorella vulgaris	Ni	32.00% at 5.7 mg/L
Chlorella vulgaris	Tl	100.00% (150 mg/L); 89.00% (250 mg/L); 96% (500 mg/L)
Chlorella vulgaris	Mn	99.40% at 3 mg/L
Chlorella vulgaris	Zn	88.80% at 3 mg/L
Chlorella vulgaris	Cu	100.00%, 74.00%, 38.00%, and 26.00% for 0.1, 0.3, 0.6, and 0.9 mg/L
Chlorella vulgaris	Mo (VI)	80.30% at 0.5 mg/L
Desmodesmus sp.	Cu	43.00% at 11.9 mg/L
Desmodesmus sp.	Ni	39.00% at 5.7 mg/L
Scenedesmus obliquus	Ni	62.00%
Scenedesmus obliquus	Zn	90.00%
Scenedesmus quadricauda	N	100.00%
Scenedesmus quadricauda	S	100.00%
Scenedesmus sp.	P	100.00%
Scenedesmus sp.	Hg (II)	64.00%
Spirulina platenses	Cu	79.20%
Spirulina platenses	Fe	100.00%

Adapted from Dubey et al. (2023) and Yang et al. (2025)

water before treatment. However, the dissolution of NO_x in water still needs to be improved, and strategies such as increasing the surface area and reducing the bubble diameter can increase the efficiency of pollutant removal by microalgae (Chen & Wang, 2020).

Another strategy that contributes to increased bioremediation efficiency is cell immobilization. Cell immobilization is based on the confinement of biocatalysts, as in the case of microalgae cells, and is carried out within or on support materials. In this case, the difference between immobilized cells and free cells is the ease with which they can be separated and reused. Furthermore, this new formation provides greater tolerance in more aggressive environments, where variations in pH, temperature, and contaminant toxicity occur. On the other hand, consortia between microalgae and bacteria also result in better performance in the bioremediation of pollutants. Consortia of this type are particularly favorable for the bioremediation of heavy metals, pesticides, naphthenic acids, dyes, and phenolic compounds. From this perspective, the consortium helps mainly with variations in the environment that can become very sensitive to microorganisms. In general, microalgae secrete the organic carbon present, transforming it into dissolved form, and thus acting as a direct carbon source for the growth and development of bacteria. In response, bacteria promote the growth of microalgae by mineralizing elements such as N, P, and S (Liu et al., 2023).

Regarding microalgae cultivation systems, when focused on pollutant removal, it is important to address points such as biomass productivity. Low biomass productivity corresponds to lower system efficiency, resulting in lower nutrient removal from the environment. In closed systems, cultivation conditions can be controlled throughout the entire process, resulting in greater biomass production. On the contrary, open systems do not have this control over factors, resulting in an unfavorable biomass value. For example, when comparing the removal rate in a horizontal air-lift tubular photobioreactor and a high-rate open pond, the nutrient removal capacity was significantly better for the closed system (Magalhães et al., 2022).

Finally, the efficiency of microalgae-based bioremediation is fostered by details, mainly about the strains and the environment. Perspectives on improvements in removal parameters provide currently tangible and viable ways. However, it is clear that more enlightening research tends to demonstrate other, even more enlightening methods and foundations for microalgae-based pollutant bioremediation.

5.7 Conclusion

Microalgae-based bioremediation is emerging as a versatile, sustainable, and promising technology for mitigating environmental pollution caused by contaminants. Its mechanisms of action contribute to the transformation and sequestration of pollutants, generating biomass. When integrated into wastewater treatment systems, it also contributes to the principles of circularity and the SDGs. Although a body of scientific evidence exists at laboratory and pilot scales, many obstacles still impede its expansion to industrial levels. Effluent composition, strain selection, cultivation systems, and process optimization are key factors that significantly impact the efficiency of large-scale processes. However, the application of metabolic engineering to improve pollutant degradation remains a development gap. On the other hand, the inclusion of AI, digital monitoring, and hybrid treatment systems can expedite the implementation of microalgae-based bioremediation. Ultimately, joint efforts are essential to make microalgae-based bioremediation a favorable and sustainable process.

References

Abdelfattah, A., Ali, S. S., Ramadan, H., El-Aswar, E. I., Eltawab, R., Ho, S. H., et al. (2023). Microalgae-based wastewater treatment: Mechanisms, challenges, recent advances, and future prospects. *Environmental Science and Ecotechnology, 13*, 100205.

Abuhasheesh, Y., Ghazal, A., Tang, D. Y. Y., Banat, F., Hasan, S. W., & Show, P. L. (2025). Advances in chlorella microalgae for sustainable wastewater treatment and bioproduction. *Chemical Engineering Journal Advances, 22*, 100715.

Ahmed, F., & Fakhruddin, A. N. M. (2018). A review on environmental contamination of petroleum hydrocarbons and its biodegradation. *International Journal of Environmental Sciences & Natural Resources, 11*(3), 1–7.

Al-Hussieny, A. A., Imran, S. G., & Jabur, Z. A. (2020). The use of local blue-green algae in the bioremediation of hydrocarbon pollutants in wastewater from oil refineries. *Plant Archives, 20*, 797–802.

Ali, A., Khalid, Z., & Ajarem, J. S. (2023). Wastewater treatment by using microalgae: Insights into fate, transport, and associated challenges. *Chemosphere, 338*, 139501.

Ansari, F. A., Hassan, H., Gani, K. M., Rawat, I., Gupta, S. K., & Bux, F. (2025). Influence of nitrogen sources on growth and biochemical composition of Chlorella sorokiniana. *Biomass and Bioenergy, 197*, 107832.

Ayele, A., & Godeto, Y. G. (2021). Bioremediation of chromium by microorganisms and its mechanisms related to functional groups. *Journal of Chemistry, 2021*(1), 7694157.

Bhatt, P., Bhandari, G., Bhatt, K., & Simsek, H. (2022). Microalgae-based removal of pollutants from wastewaters: Occurrence, toxicity and circular economy. *Chemosphere, 306*, 135576.

Castellanos-Estupiñan, M. A., Carrillo-Botello, A. M., Rozo-Granados, L. S., Becerra-Moreno, D., García-Martínez, J. B., Urbina-Suarez, N. A., et al. (2022). Removal of nutrients and pesticides from agricultural runoff using microalgae and cyanobacteria. *Water (Basel), 14*(4), 558.

Chandrashekharaiah, P. S., Sanyal, D., Dasgupta, S., & Banik, A. (2021). Cadmium biosorption and biomass production by two freshwater microalgae Scenedesmus acutus and Chlorella pyrenoidosa: An integrated approach. *Chemosphere, 269*, 128755.

Chen, H., & Wang, Q. (2020). Microalgae-based nitrogen bioremediation. *Algal Research, 46*, 101775.

Das, B., Deka, S. (2019). A cost-effective and environmentally sustainable process for phycoremediation of oil field formation water for its safe disposal and reuse. *Abstract Scientific Reports 9*(1). https://doi.org/10.1038/s41598-019-51806-5

Dębowski, M., Krzemieniewski, M., Zieliński, M., & Kazimierowicz, J. (2021). Immobilized microalgae-based photobioreactor for CO2 capture (IMC-CO2PBR): Efficiency estimation, technological parameters, and prototype concept. *Atmosphere, 12*(8), 1031.

Deepika, C., Frascaroli, G., Gowri, A., & Silkina, A. (2025). Microalgae-based bioremediation: A sustainable approach for the removal of emergent pollutants. In *Biotechnological interventions in the removal of emerging pollutants* (pp. 101–139). Springer Nature Singapore.

Depra, M. C., Severo, I. A., dos Santos, A. M., Zepka, L. Q., & Jacob-Lopes, E. (2020). Environmental impacts on commercial microalgae-based products: Sustainability metrics and indicators. *Algal Research, 51*, 102056.

Dey, S., Samanta, P., Ghosh, A. R., Banerjee, S., & Sen, K. (2024). State-of-the-art microalgae-based bioreactor wastewater treatment for the elimination of emerging contaminants: A mechanistic review. *Cleaner Water, 2*, 100027.

Dias, R. R., Deprá, M. C., Zepka, L. Q., & Jacob-Lopes, E. (2021). Microalgae-based bioremediation. *Applied Water Science: Remediation Technologies, 2*, 357–380.

Dias, R. R., Deprá, M. C., de Menezes, C. R., Zepka, L. Q., & Jacob-Lopes, E. (2025). Microalgae cultivation in wastewater: How realistic is this approach for value-added product production? *Processes, 13*(7), 2052.

Dinis, M. D. L., Al-Shomali, Z., Pereira, A., & Marques, A. C. (2025). State-of-the-art review on the removal of naturally occurring radioactive materials in water. *International Journal of Environmental Research and Public Health, 22*(5), 727.

Dubey, S., Chen, C. W., Haldar, D., Tambat, V. S., Kumar, P., Tiwari, A., et al. (2023). Advancement in algal bioremediation for organic, inorganic, and emerging pollutants. *Environmental Pollution, 317*, 120840.

Embaby, M. A., Haggag, E. S. A., El-Sheikh, A. S., & Marrez, D. A. (2022). Biosorption of uranium from aqueous solution by green microalga Chlorella sorokiniana. *Environmental Science and Pollution Research, 29*(38), 58388–58404.

Faruque, M. O., Uddin, S., Hossain, M. M., Hossain, S. Z., Shafiquzzaman, M., & Razzak, S. A. (2024). A comprehensive review on microalgae-driven heavy metals. *Journal of Hazardous Materials Advances, 16*, 100492.

Fernández, F. A., Sevilla, J. M. F., & Grima, E. M. (2019). Costs analysis of microalgae production. In *Biofuels from algae* (pp. 551–566). Elsevier.

Foroutan, R., Peighambardoust, S. J., Hemmati, S., Khatooni, H., & Ramavandi, B. (2021). Preparation of clinoptilolite/starch/CoFe2O4 magnetic nanocomposite powder and its elimination properties for cationic dyes from water and wastewater. *International Journal of Biological Macromolecules, 189*, 432–442.

Foroutan, R., Peighambardoust, S. J., Mohammadi, R., Peighambardoust, S. H., & Ramavandi, B. (2022). Development of new magnetic adsorbent of walnut shell ash/starch/Fe3O4 for effective copper ions removal: Treatment of groundwater samples. *Chemosphere, 296*, 133978.

García-Galán, M. J., Monllor-Alcaraz, L. S., Postigo, C., Uggetti, E., de Alda, M. L., Díez-Montero, R., & García, J. (2020). Microalgae-based bioremediation of water contaminated by pesticides in peri-urban agricultural areas. *Environmental Pollution, 265*, 114579.

Gasana, Z., Kayiranga, A., Nizeyimana, J. C., Tian, S., Rugema, J., You, L., Huang, X., & Su, J.-Q. (2025). Removal of antibiotics and antibiotic resistance genes using microalgae-based wastewater treatment system: A bibliometric review and mechanism analysis. *Journal of Water Process Engineering, 72*, 107496.

Geremia, E., Ripa, M., Catone, C. M., & Ulgiati, S. (2021). A review about microalgae wastewater treatment for bioremediation and biomass production—A new challenge for Europe. *Environments, 8*(12), 136.

Ghanbarzadeh, M., Niknam, V., Soltani, N., Ebrahimzadeh, H., & Shahavi, M. H. (2022). Removal of Phenanthrene by some microalga species and study of antioxidative compounds in Nostoc calcicola ISC 89. *Journal of Soils and Sediments, 22*, 109–119.

Gupta, R., Mishra, N., Singh, G., Mishra, S., & Lodhiyal, N. (2024). Microalgae cultivation and value-based products from wastewater: Insights and applications. *Blue Biotechnology, 1*(1), 20.

Hamawand, I. (2023). Energy consumption in water/wastewater treatment industry—Optimisation potentials. *Energies, 16*(5), 2433.

Hamouda, R. A., Alhumairi, A. M., & Saddiq, A. A. (2023). Simultaneous bioremediation of petroleum hydrocarbons and production of biofuels by the micro-green alga, cyanobacteria, and its consortium. *Heliyon, 9*(6), e16656.

Hosseini, S. S., Hamadi, A., Foroutan, R., Peighambardoust, S. J., & Ramavandi, B. (2022). Decontamination of Cd2+ and Pb2+ from aqueous solution using a magnetic nanocomposite of eggshell/starch/Fe3O4. *Journal of Water Process Engineering, 48*, 102911.

Jacob-Lopes, E., Zepka, L. Q., & Queiroz, M. I. (Eds.). (2018). *Energy from microalgae*. Springer.

Kaloudas, D., Pavlova, N., & Penchovsky, R. (2021). Phycoremediation of wastewater by microalgae: A review. *Environmental Chemistry Letters, 19*, 2905–2920.

Kumar, N., & Shukla, P. (2023). Microalgal-based bioremediation of emerging contaminants: Mechanisms and challenges. *Environmental Pollution, 337*, 122591.

Kumar, N., Banerjee, C., Chang, J. S., & Shukla, P. (2022). Valorization of wastewater through microalgae as a prospect for generation of biofuel and high-value products. *Journal of Cleaner Production, 362*, 132114.

Kundu, P., Dutta, N., Bhattacharya, S. (2024). Application of microalgae in wastewater treatment with special reference to emerging contaminants: a step towards sustainability. *Frontiers in Analytical Science, 4*. https://doi.org/10.3389/frans.2024.1513153

Kuok, K. K., Chiu, P. C., Rahman, M. R., Bakri, M. K. B., & Chin, M. Y. (2022). Effectiveness of centralized wastewater treatment plant in removing emerging contaminants: A case study at Kuching, Malaysia. *Journal of Water Resource and Protection, 14*(9), 650–663.

Kuppan, N., Padman, M., Mahadeva, M., Srinivasan, S., & Devarajan, R. (2024). A comprehensive review of sustainable bioremediation techniques: Eco friendly solutions for waste and pollution management. *Waste Management Bulletin, 2*, 154.

La Bella, E., Baglieri, A., Fragalà, F., & Puglisi, I. (2022). Multipurpose agricultural reuse of microalgae biomasses employed for the treatment of urban wastewater. *Agronomy, 12*(2), 234.

Leng, L., Wei, L., Xiong, Q., Xu, S., Li, W., Lv, S., et al. (2020). Use of microalgae based technology for the removal of antibiotics from wastewater: A review. *Chemosphere, 238*, 124680.

León-Vaz, A., León, R., Giráldez, I., Vega, J. M., & Vigara, J. (2021). Impact of heavy metals in the microalga Chlorella sorokiniana and assessment of its potential use in cadmium bioremediation. *Aquatic Toxicology, 239*, 105941.

Li, J., Chen, Q., Bao, B., Liu, M., Bao, M., Liu, J., & Mu, J. (2018). RNA-seq analysis reveals the significant effects of different light conditions on oil degradation by marine Chlorella vulgaris. *Marine Pollution Bulletin, 137*, 267–276.

Lisetskii, F. N., & Buryak, Z. A. (2023). Runoff of water and its quality under the combined impact of agricultural activities and urban development in a small river basin. *Water, 15*(13), 2443.

Liu, H., & Wang, Z. (2023). Treatment and resource utilization for a non-biodegradable organophosphorus wastewater using micro-channel reactor. *Engenharia Sanitaria e Ambiental, 28*, e20220235.

Liu, F., Tu, T., Li, S., Cai, M., Huang, X., & Zheng, F. (2019). Relationship between plankton-based β-carotene and biodegradable adaptablity to petroleum-derived hydrocarbon. *Chemosphere, 237*, 124430.

Liu, C. J., Deng, S. G., Hu, C. Y., Gao, P., Khan, E., Yu, C. P., & Ma, L. Q. (2023). Applications of bioremediation and phytoremediation in contaminated soils and waters: CREST publications during 2018–2022. *Critical Reviews in Environmental Science and Technology, 53*(6), 723–732.

Machado, R. L. S., Dutra, D. A., Schneider, A. T., Dias, R. R., Deprá, M. C., Zepka, L. Q., & Jacob-Lopes, E. (2025). Future prospect of development of integrated wastewater and algal biorefineries and its impact on biodiversity and environment. In *Algal biorefinery* (pp. 371–383). Elsevier.

Magalhães, I. B., Ferreira, J., de Siqueira Castro, J., de Assis, L. R., & Calijuri, M. L. (2022). Agro-industrial wastewater-grown microalgae: A techno-environmental assessment of open and closed systems. *Science of the Total Environment, 834*, 155282.

Maltsev, Y., Kulikovskiy, M., & Maltseva, S. (2023). Nitrogen and phosphorus stress as a tool to induce lipid production in microalgae. *Microbial Cell Factories, 22*(1), 239.

Mandal, R. R., Bashir, Z., Mandal, J. R., & Raj, D. (2024). Potential strategies for phytoremediation of heavy metals from wastewater with circular bioeconomy approach. *Environmental Monitoring and Assessment, 196*(6), 502.

Mansour, A. T., Alprol, A. E., Abualnaja, K. M., El-Beltagi, H. S., Ramadan, K. M., & Ashour, M. (2022). The using of nanoparticles of microalgae in remediation of toxic dye from industrial wastewater: Kinetic and isotherm studies. *Materials, 15*(11), 3922.

Mokrani, S., & Nabti, E. H. (2024). Recent status in production, biotechnological applications, commercial aspects, and future prospects of microbial enzymes: A comprehensive review. *International Journal of Agriculture and Food Science Technology, 10*, 006–020.

Morillas-España, A., Lafarga, T., Sánchez-Zurano, A., Acién-Fernández, F. G., Rodríguez-Miranda, E., Gómez-Serrano, C., & González-López, C. V. (2021). Year-long evaluation of microalgae production in wastewater using pilot-scale raceway photobioreactors: Assessment of biomass productivity and nutrient recovery capacity. *Algal Research, 60*, 102500.

Morillas-España, A., López-Serna, R., Chikri, L. Y. R., Jiménez, J. J., Lafarga, T., Uggetti, E., et al. (2025). Microalgae wastewater treatment: Pharmaceutical removal and biomass valorization. *Journal of Environmental Management, 380*, 124942.

Muhammad Ahsan, Altaf Nitin, Sharma Dipali, Srivastava Sayanti, Mandal Sandeep, Adavi Rupak, Jena Rakesh Kumar, Bairwa Abilash Valsala, Gopalakrishnan Awadhesh, Kumar Abhijit, Dey Milan Kumar, Lal Rahul Kumar, Tiwari Ravinder, Kumar Parvaiz, Ahmed (2023) Deciphering the melatonin-mediated response and signalling in the regulation of heavy metal stress in plants Planta 257(6). https://doi.org/10.1007/s00425-023-04146-8

Onchoke, K. K., Lopez, G., & Broom, A. M. (2023). Detection of carbamazepine, diclofenac, and ketoprofen via a SPE-HPLC-PDA method in a municipal wastewater treatment plant in East Texas, USA. *Analytical Chemistry Letters, 13*(2), 127–140.

Oswald, W. J. (1973). Productivity of algae in sewage disposal. *Solar Energy, 15*(1), 107–117.

Oswald, W. J., & Golueke, C. G. (1968). Harvesting and processing of waste-grown microalgae. *Algae, Man and the Environment, 1*, 371–389.

Pacheco, D., Rocha, A. C., Pereira, L., Verdelhos, T. (2020). Microalgae Water Bioremediation: Trends and Hot Topics. *Appl. Sci. 10*(5), 1886. https://doi.org/10.3390/app10051886

Palikrousis, T. L., Manolis, C., Kalamaras, S. D., & Samaras, P. (2024). Effect of light intensity on the growth and nutrient uptake of the microalga Chlorella sorokiniana cultivated in biogas plant digestate. *Water, 16*(19), 2782.

Pant, S., Goel, M., Sahoo, N. K., Yuan, Q., & Rout, P. R. (2025). Microalgae-based treatment for wastewater management and valorisation. *Current Opinion in Environmental Science & Health, 48*, 100662.

Peighambardoust, S. J., Foroutan, R., Peighambardoust, S. H., Khatooni, H., & Ramavandi, B. (2021). Decoration of Citrus Limon wood carbon with Fe3O4 to enhanced Cd2+ removal: A reclaimable and magnetic nanocomposite. *Chemosphere, 282*, 131088.

Prosenc, F., Piechocka, J., Škufca, D., Heath, E., Bulc, T. G., Istenič, D., & Buttiglieri, G. (2021). Microalgae-based removal of contaminants of emerging concern: Mechanisms in Chlorella vulgaris and mixed algal-bacterial cultures. *Journal of Hazardous Materials, 418*, 126284.

Qin, Z., Wei, C., Wei, T., Li, Z., Pang, Z., Luo, P., et al. (2022). Evolution of biochemical processes in coking wastewater treatment: A combined evaluation of material and energy efficiencies and secondary pollution. *Science of the Total Environment, 807*, 151072.

Quan, L., Cheng, Y., Wang, J., Chen, Y., Li, D., Wang, S., et al. (2023). Efficient removal of thiamethoxam by freshwater microalgae Scenedesmus sp. TXH: Removal mechanism, metabolic degradation and application. *Journal of Environmental Management, 332*, 117388.

Razzak, S. A., Bahar, K., Islam, K. O., Haniffa, A. K., Faruque, M. O., Hossain, S. Z., & Hossain, M. M. (2024). Microalgae cultivation in photobioreactors: Sustainable solutions for a greener future. *Green Chemical Engineering, 5*(4), 418–439.

Rempel, A., Gutkoski, J. P., Nazari, M. T., Biolchi, G. N., Cavanhi, V. A. F., Treichel, H., & Colla, L. M. (2021). Current advances in microalgae-based bioremediation and other technologies for emerging contaminants treatment. *Science of the Total Environment, 772*, 144918.

Rossi, S., Pizzera, A., Bellucci, M., Marazzi, F., Mezzanotte, V., Parati, K., & Ficara, E. (2024). Piggery wastewater treatment with algae-bacteria consortia: Pilot-scale validation and techno-economic evaluation at farm level. *Bioresource Technology, 351*, 127051. Authorea Preprints.

Sarma, U., Hoque, M. E., Thekkangil, A., Venkatarayappa, N., & Rajagopal, S. (2024). Microalgae in removing heavy metals from wastewater–an advanced green technology for urban wastewater treatment. *Journal of Hazardous Materials Advances, 15*, 100444.

Satpati, G. G., Gupta, S., Biswas, R. K., Choudhury, A. K., Kim, J. W., & Davoodbasha, M. (2023). Microalgae mediated bioremediation of polycyclic aromatic hydrocarbons: Strategies, advancement and regulations. *Chemosphere, 344*, 140337.

Singhal, M., Jadhav, S., Sonone, S. S., Sankhla, M. S., & Kumar, R. (2021). Microalgae based sustainable bioremediation of water contaminated by pesticides. *Biointerface Research in Applied Chemistry, 12*, 149–169.

Sousa, C. A., Sousa, H., Vale, F., & Simoes, M. (2021). Microalgae-based bioremediation of wastewaters-influencing parameters and mathematical growth modelling. *Chemical Engineering Journal, 425*, 131412.

Srimongkol, P., Sangtanoo, P., Songserm, P., Watsuntorn, W., & Karnchanatat, A. (2022). Corrigendum: Microalgae-based wastewater treatment for developing economic and environmental sustainability: Current status and future prospects. *Frontiers in Bioengineering and Biotechnology, 10*, 1048819.

Suárez-Martínez, D., Angulo-Mercado, E., Mercado-Martínez, I., Vacca-Jimeno, V., Tapia-Larios, C., & Cubillán, N. (2022). Enhanced tetracycline removal from highly concentrated aqueous media by lipid-free Chlorella sp. biomass. *ACS Omega, 7*(16), 14128–14137.

Tarbajova, V., Kolackova, M., Chaloupsky, P., Dobesova, M., Capal, P., Pilat, Z., et al. (2023). Physiological and transcriptome profiling of *Chlorella sorokiniana*: A study on azo dye wastewater decolorization. *Journal of Hazardous Materials, 460*, 132450.

Tattibayeva, Z., Tazhibayeva, S., Kujawski, W., Zayadan, B., & Musabekov, K. (2022). Peculiarities of adsorption of Cr (VI) ions on the surface of Chlorella vulgaris ZBS1 algae cells. *Heliyon, 8*(9), e10468.

Thapa, B. (2020). Study of performance of completely mixed activated sludge process with varying hydraulic retention time (HRT) and solid retention time (SRT) using lab-scale plant. *Journal of Development Innovations, 4*(1), 80–88.

Tian, X., Lin, X., Xie, Q., Liu, J., & Luo, L. (2024). Effects of temperature and light on microalgal growth and nutrient removal in turtle aquaculture wastewater. *Biology, 13*(11), 901.

Togarcheti, S. C., kumar Mediboyina, M., Chauhan, V. S., Mukherji, S., Ravi, S., & Mudliar, S. N. (2017). Life cycle assessment of microalgae based biodiesel production to evaluate the impact of biomass productivity and energy source. *Resources, Conservation and Recycling, 122*, 286–294.

Tomar, R. S., & Jajoo, A. (2021). Enzymatic pathway involved in the degradation of fluoranthene by microalgae Chlorella vulgaris. *Ecotoxicology, 30*(2), 268–276.

Velásquez-Orta, S. B., Yáñez-Noguez, I., Ramírez, I. M., & Ledesma, M. T. O. (2024). Pilot-scale microalgae cultivation and wastewater treatment using high-rate ponds: A meta-analysis. *Environmental Science and Pollution Research, 31*(34), 46994–47021.

Wang, P., Shao, Y., Geng, Y., Mushtaq, R., Yang, W., Li, M., et al. (2023). Advanced treatment of secondary effluent from wastewater treatment plant by a newly isolated microalga Desmodesmus sp. SNN1. *Frontiers in Microbiology, 14*, 1111468.

Weiland, S., Hickmann, T., Lederer, M., & Schwindenhammer, S. (2021). The 2030 agenda for sustainable development: Transformative change through the sustainable development goals? *Politics and Governance, 9*(1), 90–95.

Yang, X. Y., Wei, Y. X., Su, Y. Q., Zhang, Z. W., Tang, X. Y., Chen, Y. E., et al. (2025). The strategies microalgae adopt to counteract the toxic effect of heavy metals. *Microorganisms, 13*(5), 989.

Yuvraj. (2022). Microalgal bioremediation: A clean and sustainable approach for controlling environmental pollution. In *Innovations in environmental biotechnology* (pp. 305–318). Springer.

Zinicovscaia, I., Safonov, A., Zelenina, D., Ershova, Y., & Boldyrev, K. (2020). Evaluation of biosorption and bioaccumulation capacity of cyanobacteria Arthrospira (spirulina) platensis for radionuclides. *Algal Research, 51*, 102075.

Fate of Environmental Pollutants in Algal Cells

6

Jefferson E. Contreras-Ropero, Janet B. García-Martínez, Andres Fernando Barajas-Solano, Crisóstomo Barajas-Ferreira, and Viatcheslav Kafarov

Abstract

Conventional wastewater treatment methods based on physicochemical processes and activated sludge exhibit limited efficiency in removing trace metals, dissolved nutrients, and light hydrocarbon fractions, allowing these contaminants to persist in receiving ecosystems. In this context, the photoautotrophic physiology of microalgae has emerged as a promising tool for capturing and transforming such pollutant loads. However, their precise role as "living filters" depends on a rigorous understanding of the pathways each contaminant follows through the algal cell wall. Accordingly, this chapter explores how microalgae integrate negatively charged surface biosorption with intracellular ion transport mediated by P-type ATPases and ZIP (Zrt/Irt-like protein) channels, forming a continuous uptake pathway that mitigates effluent toxicity. Drawing on recent transcriptomic and metabolomic evidence, this chapter details how parameters such as pH, ionic strength, the nitrogen-to-phosphorus ratio (N:P), and light intensity influence contaminant capture and transformation dynamics across various taxa cultivated in urban, industrial, and agricultural wastewater matrices. In addition, it examines posttreatment biomass valorization pathways, including microbial carbonates for low-carbon biocement production, phosphate-based fertilizers derived from intracellular polyphosphate reserves, and lipid-rich oils targeted for biofuel generation. In doing so, this chapter presents the cellular

J. E. Contreras-Ropero · C. Barajas-Ferreira · V. Kafarov (✉)
Research Center for Sustainable Development in Industry and Energy, Program of Chemical Engineering, Universidad Industrial de Santander, Bucaramanga, Colombia
e-mail: kafarov@uis.edu.co

J. B. García-Martínez · A. F. Barajas-Solano (✉)
Department of Environmental Sciences, Universidad Francisco de Paula Santander, Cúcuta, Colombia
e-mail: andresfernandobs@ufps.edu.co

L. Kumar et al. (eds.), *Algal Bioremediation*,
https://doi.org/10.1007/978-981-95-8793-3_6

mechanisms, operational frameworks, and valorization strategies essential for integrating algal bioremediation into advanced wastewater treatment schemes.

Keywords

Microalgae · Algal cellular fate · Bioremediation · Biomineralization · Coproducts

6.1 Introduction

The increasing pressure on water resources has made wastewater a key environmental indicator of the complexity of human operations. In addition to common pollutants, effluents are enriched with elements as well as dissolved nutrients and volatile organic compounds (VOCs), including cadmium, zinc, ammonium, orthophosphate, benzene, and toluene, whose persistence at trace levels (<100 μg/L) poses hazards in several aspects, including ecosystem quality and public health (Ng et al., 2019). It is believed that 10–40% of trace heavy metals, such as cadmium (Cd), lead (Pb), and chromium (Cr), and up to 30% of dissolved nitrogen and phosphorus can persist in effluents after advanced treatment processes. This deficit in removal contributed to the exceedance of regulatory levels at receptors, particularly for compounds such as BTEX hydrocarbons, which cannot be effectively removed with less efficient technologies.

Traditional techniques such as activated sludge and coagulation–flocculation achieve acceptable removal efficiencies for solids and organic materials, but their performance for structurally complex and recalcitrant pollutants remains limited (Whitton et al., 2015). In addition, these plants have high energy requirements (~0.3–0.6 kWh/m^3) and produce significant amounts of waste sludge, which increases costs and limits long-term sustainability. Industrial effluents typically contain three priority groups that shape environmental and health risk. First, trace metals (Cd, Pb, Cr) persist after advanced treatment. They can impair aquatic communities by disrupting growth and reproduction under prolonged exposure. In contrast, chronic human exposure is linked to renal, cardiovascular, and developmental effects, making trace-level control essential when reuse or biomass valorization is envisioned (Jomova et al., 2025; Saravanan et al., 2024). Second, reactive nutrients (NH_4^+, NO_3^-, PO_4^{3-}) degrade receiving waters because excess nitrogen and phosphorus intensify eutrophication, lower dissolved oxygen, and promote harmful algal blooms, so polishing must target the bioavailable fraction to protect ecological function and any subsequent uses of water (Heisler et al., 2008; Yang et al., 2008). Finally, aromatic BTEX (benzene, toluene, ethylbenzene, xylenes) often remain in complex industrial matrices at microgram-per-liter ranges, which compromises safety when effluents are reused or when process derivatives enter value chains, and benzene is particularly critical because it is carcinogenic and drinking-water standards set very low limits, therefore advanced polishing needs selective abatement at trace levels before reuse or biomass valorization (Mrowiec & Suschka, 2009; Fayemiwo et al., 2017).

Given that risk profile and the regulatory emphasis on trace-level control and reuse, current practice deploys algal configurations with proven reliability in tertiary treatment. High-rate algal ponds (HRAPs) are operated at full scale with low energy demand and consistent nitrogen and phosphorus removal under real effluents, supported by recent scale-up reports and state-of-the-art reviews that define design and operational windows in practice (Magalhães et al., 2024). Rotating algal biofilms increases areal productivity and simplifies harvesting while maintaining nitrogen and phosphorus abatement during continuous operation in complex matrices, with recent studies documenting their performance and transfer mechanisms that support deployment in municipal and industrial contexts (Vo et al., 2025; Li et al., 2026). Closed photobioreactor trains have shown robust phosphorus removal and recovery from real secondary effluents, with documented operation at around 568 m^3 day^{-1} and biomass capture compatible with downstream valorization, confirming stability and controllability at plant conditions (Molitor et al., 2024). In channels and flowways dedicated to nutrient control, algal turf systems (ATS) intercept dissolved loads and stabilize water quality under controlled harvesting regimes, with recent evidence on operating levers that enable field performance tuning (Hariz et al., 2025; Gan et al., 2022).

Building on these priority contaminants and their impacts, this lack of functionality continues to drive the quest for improved, selective, and sustainablc platforms that can effectively detoxify these compounds while integrating into circular economy schemes. In this context, microalgae have been suggested as alternative biotechnology tools. Their photoautotrophic physiology allows them to fix inorganic carbon, assimilate nutrients, and immobilize metal ions and organic pollutants from complex liquid matrices (Wang et al., 2019; Vo et al., 2024). The high surface-area-to-volume ratio and anionic functional groups (e.g., carboxylates and sulfonates) on the cell wall make biosorption processes efficient. In contrast to conventional mechanisms, the microalgal mechanism generates oxygen through photosynthesis; therefore, there is less need for mechanical aeration, and less sludge is produced. Furthermore, an open reactor is low-cost and energy-efficient for cultivation. Pilot-scale studies have reported 70–90% removal of nitrogen and phosphorus, along with significantly lower energy demand. The biochemical complexity of the algal cell wall itself permits an efficient surface-based biosorption process, and its metabolic flexibility allows dynamic adaptation to changes in the aquatic milieu (Bagasariya et al., 2021). However, measuring their effectiveness solely on overall removal oversimplifies. Greater insight into the intracellular fate of contaminants is necessary to confirm that algal systems remain fully functional and to establish operational and regulatory standards. Indeed, a large proportion of pollutants can still adsorb to the cell surface. Still, they can also be internalized by the cell through metal carriers such as ZIPs (Zrt/Irt-like proteins) or P-type ATPases, metabolized via specific metabolic pathways, or sequestered within subcellular organelles (Fujie et al., 2022). This variety of routes clearly affects both removal efficiency and the final destination and valorization potential of algal biomass (Slocombe et al., 2020). One unresolved "black box" is the distribution and transformation of metals, nutrients, and organic ligands within algal cells, which is a barrier to regulatory acceptance. It is thus vital to quantitatively clarify the cellular processes involved in surface adsorption, active transport, and intracellular sequestration. Recent advances in transcriptomics, proteomics, and metabolomics have enabled the identification of molecular pathways associated with intracellular detoxification. Studies have reported differential induction of genes encoding metal transporters, phytochelatin (PC) biosynthesis, and polyphosphate accumulation as adaptive responses to the presence of contaminants in the medium (Vo et al., 2024). Environmental factors such as pH, ionic strength, the nitrogen-to-phosphorus ratio (N:P), and light intensity further modulate these metabolic pathways, affecting contaminant uptake and transformation both directly and indirectly (Wei, 2024). Differentiating intracellular fate by contaminant type—such as heavy metals, nutrients, or BTEX compounds—requires specific methodologies for traceability, as each class follows distinct internalization, metabolism, or subcellular storage patterns.

In parallel, the strategic potential of valorizing the resulting algal biomass has been increasingly recognized. Depending on its composition, biomass can be directed toward biocement production through biologically induced carbonate precipitation (Solovchenko et al., 1834), the development of slow-release fertilizers enriched in polyphosphates (Slocombe et al., 2020), or the synthesis of biofuels from intracellular lipids (Li et al., 2022). These valorization routes position microalgae as biofactories capable of closing material loops, enabling the integration of remediation and production of strategic inputs within a circular economy framework. However, the scalability of such systems remains a significant challenge. Factors such as influent variability, microbial competition, and the absence of specific regulations for the use of microalgae in tertiary treatment hinder their widespread adoption (Janpum et al., 2022). Moreover, the lack of standardized methods for assessing the intracellular fate of pollutants limits interstudy comparability and impedes the validation of predictive models. Considering this context, the present chapter provides a detailed review of the cellular fate of contaminants in algal systems. It outlines the mechanisms of biosorption, transmembrane transport, and intracellular transformation, considering the operational and environmental variables that influence their efficiency. Additionally, it explores biomass valorization routes and discusses emerging perspectives, including genetic engineering, life cycle assessment (LCA), and regulatory alignment. This approach aims to establish a robust scientific foundation to support the sustainable implementation of algal bioremediation within advanced wastewater treatment schemes.

6.2 Mechanisms of Capture, Transport, and Sequestration

Microalgae remove contaminants through a continuous sequence of processes: initially, they trap ions or molecules on their cell surface, then actively internalize them via membrane transporters, and finally sequester or transform them within cellular compartments. Each stage of this purification pathway is detailed below at the mechanistic level.

6.2.1 Surface Biosorption

Microalgae exhibit a remarkable capacity for passive biosorption of heavy metals via functional groups on their cell surfaces. The algal cell wall—typically composed of polysaccharides such as cellulose, alginates, and peptidoglycans—and extracellular polymeric substances (EPSs) provide numerous negatively charged binding sites, including carboxyl, hydroxyl, phosphate, sulfate, and amine groups, among others (Yang et al., 2025; Ranjbar & Malcata, 2022). These ionizable functional groups confer an electronegative surface that attracts metal cations through electrostatic interactions (Li et al., 2020). Dissolved heavy metals (e.g., Cd^{2+}, Pb^{2+}, Zn^{2+}, and Cr^{6+} as chromates) may be rapidly adsorbed onto the cell wall through various chemical mechanisms: chelation/complexation, ion exchange (e.g., replacing Ca^{2+} or K^{+} bound to the wall), van der Waals forces, hydrogen bonding with EPS components, and even surface precipitation (Balzano et al., 2020). For example, precipitates such as lead phosphate or cadmium sulfide have been observed to form at the cell periphery following initial adsorption, immobilizing part of the metal within the wall or periplasmic space (Yang et al., 2025).

The effectiveness of surface biosorption varies significantly among species, depending on the abundance and accessibility of active groups in the cell wall. Algae with walls rich in alginates and sulfates generally exhibit a high affinity for metal cations (Alharbi et al., 2025). A representative adsorption model is the Langmuir isotherm, which assumes a monolayer of homogeneous binding sites. Remarkable maximum biosorption capacities (q_max) have been reported in various studies: *Chlamydomonas* sp. (dry biomass) reached ~40 mg Cd^{2+}/g (Mahlangu et al., 2024) (similar to the previously cited range of ~37–91 mg/g for *Chlorella marina*), whereas *Parachlorella* sp. achieved up to ~96 mg/g for Cd^{2+} at 35 °C (Mahlangu et al., 2024). Similarly, *Spirulina platensis* (free biomass) presented q_max ≈ 304 mg/g for Pb^{2+} in batch systems (Villen-Guzman et al., 2021), and diatoms such as *Craticula subminuscula* adsorbed ~296 mg/g Cr(VI) under optimized conditions (Sbihi et al., 2024). These high capacities underscore the potential of surface biosorption in microalgae, independent of their cellular metabolism.

6.2.2 Active Transmembrane Transport

A fraction of the adsorbed metals may be internalized into the cell via membrane-dependent mechanisms. Like plants and other eukaryotes, microalgae possess families of metal transporters located in the plasma and organelle membranes, some of which are activated by trace elements or toxic metals. Among these, ZIP channels/permeases ("Zrt/IRT-like proteins") are prominent; they mediate the uptake of divalent cations such as Zn^{2+} or Fe^{2+} and can inadvertently facilitate the entry of Cd^{2+} and other metals by analogy (Ranjbar & Malcata, 2022). Additionally, natural resistance-associated macrophage protein (NRAMP) transporters exploit proton gradients to transport divalent metals into the cytosol (Puente-Sánchez et al., 2018). P-type ATPases of the P1B subfamily mediate metal efflux or compartmentalization—referred to as heavy metal ATPases (HMAs)—which use ATP to pump cations such as Cd^{2+}, Zn^{2+}, or Cu^{+} out of the cytosol (Ranjbar & Malcata, 2022).

In microalgae, HMAs analogous to those in plants have been identified. For example, heterologous overexpression of AtHMA4 in *Chlamydomonas reinhardtii* significantly increased the tolerance and accumulation of Cd^{2+} and Zn^{2+} (Ibuot et al., 2020). Similarly, transcriptomic analyses of *Dunaliella acidophila* exposed to Cd revealed upregulation of the ZIP, NRAMP1, and CTR (copper transporter) genes, suggesting their role in metal uptake and detoxification (Puente-Sánchez et al., 2018). Metal entry may occur via direct active routes—specific transporters driven by ATP or electrochemical gradients—or indirectly via the internalization of metal–organic ligand complexes (Yang et al., 2025). Toxic metals often enter the cell unintentionally via transporters for essential micronutrients (e.g., Cd^{2+} can enter via Zn^{2+} or Ca^{2+} transporters). Once in the cytosol, these ions may interfere with cellular functions, prompting the cell to initiate sequestration responses.

6.2.3 Intracellular Sequestration and Biotransformation

To mitigate cellular damage, microalgae sequester metals into inert internal compartments or chemically neutralize them. A common destination is the vacuole: various tonoplast transporters are induced under Cd stress and sequester toxic cations into acidic vacuoles (Ranjbar & Malcata, 2022). For example, overexpression of the vacuolar antiporter CrMTP4 increased Cd accumulation and tolerance in *Chlamydomonas* sp. (Ibuot et al., 2017). Simultaneously, the cell synthesizes chelating molecules, notably phytochelatins (PCs)—small cysteine-rich peptides enzymatically derived from glutathione—and metallothioneins (MTs), which are cytosolic proteins rich in thiol-containing residues. Upon exposure to heavy metals (e.g., Cd, As, and Hg), the enzyme phytochelatin synthase polymerizes glutathione into phytochelatins (γ-Glu-Cys)_n-Gly, which contain multiple thiol groups that efficiently coordinate metal cations (Yang et al., 2025). Virtually all heavy metals induce PCs to some extent, although responses vary by metal and algal species (Balzano et al., 2020). MTs also sequester metals via cysteine residues and facilitate their transport to vacuoles (Penen et al., 2017). Both PCs and MTs reduce the concentration of free ions in the cytoplasm, thereby alleviating enzyme inhibition and oxidative stress.

Additionally, many microalgae exhibit enhanced antioxidant defenses in response to metal stress. Increases in glutathione levels and the activity of enzymes such as superoxide dismutase (SOD) and catalase (CAT) are common. For example, *Scenedesmus obliquus* showed significant increases in SOD and CAT activities at 5–10 mg L^{-1} Cd^{2+} (Xu et al., 2024), whereas *Chlorella pyrenoidosa* exposed to Cr (III) or Cr(VI) presented 1.5- to 3-fold increases in these enzymatic activities (Liu et al., 2024). In some cases, algae can biotransform contaminants: species of *Chlorella* have been shown to reduce Cr(VI) to Cr(III), with the reduced form stored intracellularly (Zhou et al., 2024). This valence shift facilitates the precipitation or complexation of Cr(III), followed by cellular storage.

6.2.4 Process Drivers Modulating Cellular Fate

The performance of algal bioremediation depends not only on the intrinsic biology of the microalgae but also on the operational conditions of the medium and cultivation system. Key factors include pH, ionic strength/salinity, the relative availability of nutrients (particularly the nitrogen-to-phosphorus ratio (N:P)), light intensity and quality, and the design of the reactor in which the microalgae are cultivated. These factors can either enhance or inhibit the cellular mechanisms described, ultimately affecting the efficiency of removing heavy metals (e.g., Cd^{2+}) and nutrients (e.g., PO_4^{3-}) from treated water. Their principal effects are summarized below (see Table 6.1 for a synthesis of the impact and references).

Table 6.1 Comparative synthesis of plant-scale algal systems

Configuration	Principal advantages	Key limitations	Scale-up levers	References
High-rate algal ponds	Low energy demand and consistent N and P removal in real effluents; mature design windows	Sensitivity to seasonality and land-area requirements; diurnal pH oscillations	Year-round validation by controlling HRT, surface loading, and CO_2 addition to stabilize pH and productivity	Li et al. (2023)
Rotating algal biofilms	High areal productivity and simplified solids capture via attached growth	Mechanical maintenance and biofouling control; need for stable hydraulics	Fix rotation, shear, and irradiance over multi-month campaigns to stabilize harvest cost and quality	Nguyen et al. (2024)
Trains of closed photobioreactors with P recovery	Robust phosphorus removal and recovery in secondary effluents with fine control at plant flow rates	Higher capital expenditure (CAPEX) and instrumentation/ control requirements	Transfer pH, light, and flow setpoints from pilot and validate around 568 m^3 day^{-1} with stable biomass capture	Molitor et al. (2024)
Algal turf systems in channels	Effective interception of dissolved loads with periodic harvest and flexible hydraulic integration	Sensitivity to suspended solids and channel maintenance	On-site tuning of slope, velocity, and harvest frequency; integration with ponds to buffer seasonality	Adey et al. (2013)

This is arguably the most influential factor. The environmental pH affects both the speciation chemistry of contaminants and the ionization of functional groups on the algal surface. In general, highly acidic pH protonates ligands (–COOH → –$COOH_2^+$), reducing the negative surface charge and thereby diminishing the adsorption of metal cations. At extremely low pH, biosorption decreases sharply due to competition from protons for binding sites (Yang et al., 2025). Conversely, a slightly neutral to alkaline pH favors the deprotonation of carboxyl and phosphate groups, enhancing metal binding; however, above a certain threshold (pH >~ 8–9), many heavy metals precipitate as hydroxides (e.g., $Cr(OH)_3$ and $Zn(OH)_2$), making them unavailable for cellular uptake. Additionally, high pH promotes phosphate removal via abiotic precipitation with Ca^{2+} or Mg^{2+}, forming compounds such as hydroxyapatite ($Ca_5(PO_4)_3OH$) or struvite, thereby reducing the soluble fraction accessible to algae (Tango et al., 2023). An optimal pH range, therefore, exists. Many studies place the optimal range for metal removal by algae in the slightly acidic to neutral region (pH ~5–7), which balances high adsorption with minimal chemical precipitation (Villen-Guzman et al., 2021; Aneja et al., 2010). For example, in *Spirulina* sp., maximum Pb^{2+} biosorption was reported at pH ~4–5 (82% at pH 4), whereas for Zn^{2+}, the optimum was near pH ~8 (Aneja et al., 2010), highlighting metal-specific chemistry. In any case, pH control in algal bioreactors is essential (especially since photosynthesis tends to increase the pH through CO_2 consumption) to maintain favorable conditions for both metal capture and nutrient assimilation. Most microalgae grow well at pH 7–9 (Mahlangu et al., 2024), which coincides with high nitrogen and phosphorus removal efficiencies during secondary treatment.

The presence of high concentrations of competing ions in the medium can mask or displace binding sites on the algal biomass. Elevated ionic strength (e.g., in brackish or concentrated wastewater) typically reduces heavy metal biosorption due to the shielding effect of cations such as Na^+, K^+, and Ca^{2+}, which compete for negatively charged cell wall sites (Villen-Guzman et al., 2021). Studies with *Spirulina* (*Arthrospira*) have shown that increasing the ionic strength (via added chlorides) decreases the Pb^{2+} adsorption capacity, confirming the relevance of ion-exchange mechanisms. In highly ionic media, inert cations occupy binding sites, displacing target metals (Villen-Guzman et al., 2021). Consequently, the removal efficiency of metals such as Cd^{2+} is often lower in saline or hard water than in soft freshwater. Nonetheless, some marine microalgae tolerate salinity and can still remove metals in hypersaline environments, albeit with slower kinetics. Regarding PO_4^{3-} removal, research indicates that high ionic strength does not significantly hinder active phosphate uptake by microalgae but may favor chemical precipitation with divalent cations at elevated pH. For example, in high-alkalinity systems (pH > 8.5), phosphate reacts with Ca^{2+} to form precipitates such as hydroxyapatite, reducing the soluble fraction available for algal uptake (Tango et al., 2023; Fernandes et al., 2017).

The nitrogen-to-phosphorus (N:P) ratio in the medium modulates algal metabolism and, in turn, the capacity for contaminant removal. A balanced N:P ratio near the optimal range for algal growth (classically suggested by the Redfield ratio of ~16:1 molar, although it varies by species) promotes abundant, metabolically active biomass, which maximizes nutrient uptake and metal removal (via both biosorption and bioaccumulation) owing to increased cellular surface area and nutritional demand (Tango et al., 2023). Conversely, highly imbalanced ratios lead to nutrient limitation. For example, if the N:P ratio is too high (excess N, low P < 5:1), phosphorus becomes limiting, restricting algal growth and resulting in lower removal of both N and metals (as insufficient biomass is produced). In contrast, moderately high N:P ratios (10:1 to ~20:1) are optimal in various studies, achieving nearly 100% phosphate removal and >90% nitrogen removal, as they provide sufficient P for growth while maintaining a slight N excess to support protein synthesis (Choi & Lee, 2015). One study with *Chlorella vulgaris* reported that an N:P ratio of 10:1 maximized both productivity and nutrient removal from wastewater (Tango et al., 2023). Another study reported 100% phosphate removal in a high-load algal lagoon with N:P = 17:1. In our own analysis, optimal PO_4^{3-} removal occurred at N:P = 20:1 (with complete phosphate consumption). At the same time, extremely low or high ratios reduced the efficiency. Furthermore, certain algae under phosphate deficiency (very high N:P) have shown increased uptake of metals such as arsenate due to the use of high-affinity phosphate transporters that inadvertently absorb the arsenate analog (Ranjbar & Malcata, 2022). Overall, maintaining proper nutritional balance (including supplementation with N or P in wastewater if needed) enhances the simultaneous removal of multiple contaminants.

Light drives photosynthesis and, in turn, microalgal growth in autotrophic systems. Suboptimal light intensity limits growth rates and nutrient/contaminant uptake, whereas excessive light intensity can cause photoinhibition and oxidative stress. An optimal light range is generally defined for each species—typically ~1850–14,800 lux (≈25–200 μmol photons m^{-2} s^{-1})—to ensure maximal cell proliferation (Mahlangu et al., 2024). Within this range, increased light enhances nitrate and phosphate uptake and the production of metabolites (e.g., phycocyanin and antioxidants) involved in metal detoxification (Elgarahy et al., 2021).

A study on *Scenedesmus obliquus*, *Dunaliella salina*, and *Botryococcus braunii* evaluated different photoperiods and spectra, reporting that intensities of 50–150 μmol photons m^{-2} s^{-1}, with a red–blue light ratio, maximized both growth and nutrient uptake. In contrast, higher intensities induced photoinhibition and oxidative damage. Spectral quality also affects metabolite production: wavelengths in the blue or moderate UV range have been shown to stimulate the synthesis of carotenoids and polyphenols with chelating properties, increasing metal tolerance. Algal cultivation systems range from open ponds to advanced closed bioreactors, and their design significantly influences the aforementioned factors. High-rate algal ponds (HRAPs) are shallow channels that are stirred by paddlewheels, where algae receive direct sunlight. These systems often operate at high pH levels during peak photosynthetic hours, enabling cost-effective removal of nutrients and metals. Compared with conventional unmixed lagoons, HRAPs can increase metal removal rates by up to tenfold (Halder, 2014) owing to improved light penetration and reduced stratification. One study reported ~74% nitrogen and 92% phosphorus removal from urban leachate via HRAPs (Villar-Navarro et al., 2018) (notably higher than that in passive systems). However, HRAPs are subject to diurnal pH and temperature fluctuations, which must be monitored to prevent issues such as excessive phosphate precipitation (which, while removing P from water, can reduce its bioavailability to algae).

Closed photobioreactors (FBRs), such as bubble columns, flat panels, or tubular systems, enable strict control over parameters such as pH, CO_2, light, and sterility. By supplying additional CO_2, these systems can maintain pH within the optimal neutral range, thereby enabling continuous nitrate and phosphate assimilation without chemical losses. Moreover, biomass concentrations can be much higher, increasing the overall metal adsorption capacity. For example, a flat-plate photobioreactor using *Chlorella* achieved >95% Cu^{2+} removal at 0.1 mg/L within 3 days—an outcome that is difficult to achieve in open ponds lacking precise control (Jayaraman et al., 2024). The main drawbacks are energy and operational costs (e.g., for pumps and artificial lighting). Nevertheless, optimizing light, temperature, pH, and nutrient conditions in closed reactors has been shown to increase both biomass productivity and metal bioremediation efficiency (Mahlangu et al., 2024). Finally, hybrid algal membrane bioreactors (MBRs) integrate algal cultivation with membrane filtration, allowing for cell retention and longer biomass residence times. This enhances effluent clarification while simultaneously removing contaminants (Jayaraman et al., 2024). In algal MBRs, microalgae have demonstrated removal efficiencies of >99% for ammonium and ~100% for phosphate, as well as metal absorption ranging from 13% to 100%, depending on the element (Nedaei & Shokrkar, 2025). The use of membranes prevents algal loss from the effluent, increasing the exposure time to contaminants. Some designs also incorporate light–dark cycles to promote heterotrophic biodegradation of organic pollutants. An additional advantage is that metal-enriched algal biomass can be easily harvested via the membrane for disposal or valorization (e.g., conversion into metal-sorbing biochar) (Guan et al., 2023).

6.3 Fate of Environmental Pollutants in Algal Cells

6.3.1 Trace Metals (Cd, Pb, and Cr) and Their Intracellular Distribution

Heavy trace metals such as Cd^{2+}, Pb^{2+}, and Cr(VI) follow distinct pathways within microalgal cells. Initially, they adsorb onto the cell wall through interactions with negatively charged functional groups, including phosphates, amines, hydroxyls, and carboxyls. These groups attract metal cations via electrostatic forces, ion-exchange mechanisms, or complexation (Yang et al., 2025). This interaction can lead to the formation of inorganic precipitates: Pb^{2+} and Cd^{2+} ions, for example, react with environmental anions to form compounds such as lead phosphate ($Pb_3(PO_4)_2$), cadmium phosphate ($Cd_3(PO_4)_2$), or cadmium sulfide (CdS), which tend to accumulate in the periplasmic space or within the cell wall matrix (Yang et al., 2025). Simultaneously, bioaccumulation processes commence as metal ions cross the plasma membrane via either specific transporters or passive diffusion, resulting in their distribution into the cytoplasm and organelles. The identified mechanisms include both active and indirect transport routes. Once inside the cytosol, the metal ions bind to organic ligands and metal-binding proteins before being sequestered into vacuoles (Golnaraghi Ghomi et al., 2020).

Upon internalization, algae activate detoxification systems. The vacuoles, chloroplasts, and mitochondria serve as key metal-storage compartments, where metals form stable complexes with organic acids or phosphates, effectively isolating them from the cytosol (Balzano et al., 2020). Chelating peptides, such as phytochelatins, and metal-binding proteins, such as metallothioneins—rich in cysteine residues—are synthesized. These biomolecules coordinate Cd, Pb, and Cr ions, significantly reducing their reactivity (source: pmc.ncbi.nlm.nih.gov). The synthesis and induction of these molecules depend on the specific metal and algal species; their binding results in less toxic complexes that are subsequently transported into vacuoles for sequestration (Balzano et al., 2020).

In addition to accumulation and chelation, certain microalgae can biotransform metals. A representative example is *Chlorella* sp. MQ 1, which reduces Cr(VI) to Cr (III) via light-dependent pathways, storing the resulting insoluble chromium within intracellular compartments (Zhou et al., 2024). Similar detoxification pathways, including the methylation and conversion of arsenic or mercury into less toxic organic species, have also been described. A trace metal within an algal cell can partition among several fractions: surface-adsorbed, cytoplasmic-bound to ligands, vacuolar-sequestered, and biotransformed species. The relative distribution among these compartments is highly dependent on the metal type and the algal species involved (Yang et al., 2025; Balzano et al., 2020). This differential partitioning is essential for tolerance: by immobilizing metals at the cell wall or within vacuoles and converting them into less reactive forms, microalgae safeguard their vital processes while actively removing pollutants from their environment.

6.3.2 Ammonium, Phosphate (Dissolved Nutrients)

Algal cells assimilate inorganic nutrients such as NH_4^+ and PO_4^{3-}, which are incorporated into primary metabolic pathways. Ammonium assimilation occurs through the glutamine synthetase-glutamate synthase (GS-GOGAT) pathway in *Oocystis lacustris*. In this pathway, NH_4^+ is reduced to an active form, and it combines with α-ketoglutarate via GS to produce glutamine, which is then converted to glutamate via GOGAT. These amino acids are used for the synthesis of proteins and nucleic acids (Guan et al., 2023). The activity of GS increases at moderate NH_4^+ concentrations ($\approx$10 mg L^{1}) but decreases under excess ammonium (>50 mg L^{-1}); this inhibition suggests that high nitrate concentrations can even inhibit its own assimilation (Tian et al., 2021). Nonetheless, there is species-specific tolerance, with some organisms, such as *Tetraselmis tetrathele*, able to grow at 0.31–0.87 g L^{-1} before substantial inhibition occurs (Tian et al., 2021), whereas other diatoms are affected at 3 mg L^{-1} (Farahin et al., 2021). These factors included increased oxidative damage, reduced activity of the photosynthesis apparatus, and suppression of lipid biosynthesis in response to high ammonium concentrations. The adverse effects of colonizing maize plants are very likely controlled by the efficiency of the GS-GOGAT pathway and alternate mechanisms, including glutamate dehydrogenase (GDH) activity (Zhou et al., 2024). Phosphate is taken up by microalgae via high-affinity transporters and then incorporated into essential biomolecules such as ATP, $NADP^+$, phospholipids, and nucleic acids, which are critical for energy metabolism and cellular replication (Bossa et al., 2024). In the presence of high phosphate concentrations, microalgae can exhibit "luxurious uptake," with excess phosphate bound within cells as polyphosphate (PolyP). This process is driven by enzymatic complexes such as VTC4, which polymerize phosphate, and depositions are made in the acidocalcisomes of these vacuolar bodies. Organelle reserves of 4–8% of cell dry weight can be achieved under high-phosphate conditions (compared with ~1% at natural levels), a noteworthy storage level (Molitor et al., 2024). PolyP, as a reserve of phosphorus, has been shown to function as an intracellular energy buffer in metabolism (Magalhães et al., 2024). In the presence of abundant phosphate, ATP-dependent synthesis of PolyP is followed by the release of inorganic phosphate upon hydrolysis to sustain metabolism and cell division in the context of nutrient scarcity (Plouviez & Brown, 2024). Recently, we discovered strains in biofilms or high-density cultures that can accumulate polyphosphate, accounting for up to 14% of their dry weight, exhibiting significant biotechnological value for phosphorus recovery. Finally, acidocalcisomes also assist in cellular detoxification: negatively charged polyphosphates can chelate cations, including Ca^{2+}, Mg^{2+}, and heavy metals, thereby increasing metal–phosphate precipitate formation. Microencapsulation reduces cytotoxicity and protects microalgal cells against pollutant-induced damage (Molitor et al., 2024).

6.3.3 Metabolism of Aromatic Hydrocarbons (BTEX) in Microalgae

Aromatic hydrocarbons such as benzene, toluene, ethylbenzene, and xylenes—collectively known as BTEX—are major pollutants present in petroleum spills and various industrial effluents. Emerging evidence indicates that certain microalgae possess the metabolic capacity to biotransform and eliminate these compounds, either as isolated cultures or in symbiotic consortia with specialized bacteria. In axenic systems, several microalgal species have demonstrated a remarkable capacity to degrade BTEX. For example, a 2025 meta-analysis on the degradation of aromatic contaminants reported that *Thalassiosira* sp. could remove up to 97% of the initial benzene concentration (100 mg L^{-1}) within 7 days. Similarly, the chlorophyte *Parachlorella kessleri* eliminated 63% of toluene, 62% of ethylbenzene, and 40% of xylenes within just 2 days (Eregie et al., 2025). These results were supported by a 2023 study involving the marine microalga *Rhinomonas reticulata*, which achieved degradation efficiencies of 72% for n-propylbenzene and 56% for iso-propylbenzene over 7 days. In that case, degradation followed zero-order kinetics and was enhanced at moderate inoculum densities (Du et al., 2023). The mechanisms underlying these processes suggest that microalgae not only adsorb BTEX compounds onto their cell surfaces but can also enzymatically modify them. By inducing specific oxidative enzymes, such as monooxygenases and dioxygenases, aromatic rings undergo hydroxylation or oxidation, producing intermediates such as catechols and phenols, which are subsequently routed into central catabolic pathways. This metabolic versatility positions microalgae as promising agents for the primary degradation of volatile organic pollutants in aquatic systems.

However, the efficiency of BTEX degradation increases significantly when microalgae form consortia with aromatic hydrocarbon-degrading bacteria. A 2024 study demonstrated that a phototrophic consortium comprising *Chlorella sorokiniana, Rhodococcus erythropolis,* and *Pseudomonas putida* could remove approximately 95% of benzene and 93% of toluene within 7 days at initial concentrations of ~100 mg L^{-1}. This synergistic configuration is highly effective: while microalgae supply oxygen and organic nutrients via photosynthesis, bacteria carry out specialized enzymatic reactions—such as those catalyzed by monooxygenases and catechol 1,2-dioxygenases—that cleave aromatic rings and transform toxic intermediates into less harmful metabolites (Cai et al., 2024; Urbina-Suarez et al., 2025). Compared with monocultures, this mutualistic interaction greatly accelerates the biodegradation of BTEX compounds (Li et al., 2022).

Additional studies have shown that coculture systems can outperform individual strains even under high pollutant loads. For example, a coculture of *Dunaliella salina* and *Halomonas mongoliensis* grown under saline conditions completely degraded 500 mg/L phenol in 8 days, whereas *Dunaliella* alone removed only 78% during the same period. This highlights the advantages of microbial coevolution: not only is the degradative performance enhanced, but both organisms also show increased tolerance to toxic compounds. Furthermore, the extracellular polymeric substances (EPS) secreted by microalgae aid in emulsifying hydrocarbons and increasing their bioavailability, thereby facilitating bacterial access and degradation (Cai et al., 2024).

The synergistic potential of these consortia extends to the removal of aromatic compounds other than BTEX. In the aforementioned *Dunaliella-Halomonas* system, the use of an adaptively evolved *Dunaliella* strain led to a marked improvement in phenol degradation efficiency at 3% NaCl, achieving 500 mg L^{-1} elimination within 8 days. In comparison, the evolved algal strain alone achieved 78% degradation over 7 days, substantially outperforming the nonadapted variant (Cai et al., 2024). Other reports have shown that *Chlorella*-based consortia can degrade phenol at concentrations up to 1200 mg L^{-1} within 60 h (Li et al., 2022). These findings suggest that microalgae enhance bacterial degradation by providing continuous oxygenation and nutrient capture, while bacteria metabolize compounds that microalgae alone cannot efficiently process. The result is a highly effective, complementary degradation system with significant potential for biotechnological applications in contaminated water treatment.

6.4 Valorization of Algal Biomass Post-treatment

Bioremediation generates a biomass stream that serves as the feedstock for an algal biorefinery, and the routing depends on the contaminant profile, the biomass composition, and operational stability, consistent with recent frameworks that map technologies, economics, and circular outcomes in microalgal biorefineries (Geng et al., 2025). When residual metals remain below safety thresholds and intracellular polyphosphate is significant, the biomass can be directed to nutrient recovery and soil inputs, supported by recent advances in polyphosphate accumulation and phosphorus upcycling with microalgae and cyanobacteria (Plouviez & Brown, 2024). When carbonate nucleation is favored by dissolved inorganic carbon, calcium availability, and pH, conversion to carbonate biominerals with stable carbon capture becomes feasible under conditions that are transferable to scale (Fazal et al., 2025). When the operation delivers robust phosphorus removal and recovery from real secondary effluents at plant-relevant flow rates, the captured biomass can consistently supply downstream valorization streams, as shown for photobioreactor trains operating at about 568 m^3 day^{-1} (Molitor et al., 2024). When metals or persistent organics exceed limits, stabilization routes such as hydrothermal carbonization lower bioavailability and enable the safe use of the material (Oliveira et al., 2025).

Within this biorefinery perspective, the resulting algal biomass is not a waste stream. It is a resource whose destination is defined by measurable quality attributes and residual contaminants so that the same platform can support carbonate biominerals, polyphosphate-enriched fertilizers, or lipid products, depending on indicators and site conditions (Geng et al., 2025). Routing relies on a compact set of indicators that include total and speciated metals in the biomass, the polyphosphate fraction, and stability markers such as pH control, light regime, and areal productivity, which are reported as practical levers for reliable operation under real effluents (Molitor et al., 2024). Among the routes studied, carbonate biominerals, polyphosphate-based fertilizers, and lipid products are prioritized based on biomass quality indicators and demonstrated operating windows (Fazal et al., 2025).

6.4.1 Carbonate Biomineralization ($CaCO_3$)

Some microalgae precipitate calcium carbonate ($CaCO_3$) as a natural byproduct of their photosynthetic metabolism, thereby contributing to the stable sequestration of inorganic carbon. During photosynthesis, microalgae consume dissolved CO_2 and release hydroxide ions (OH^-), which increase the local pH and may exceed the solubility threshold for $CaCO_3$ in the presence of calcium ions (Ca^{2+}), leading to the spontaneous precipitation of this mineral. In cultures of *Acutodesmus obliquus*, biomass has been shown to act as an effective nucleation site for carbonate crystallization, increasing precipitation rates by up to 75% under light compared with dark conditions. This capacity is further enhanced in dried biomass relative to live cells, likely due to a higher concentration of nucleation sites or structural changes induced by desiccation (Solovchenko et al., 1834).

Studies with *Nannochloropsis oceanica* IMET1 have also demonstrated that algal growth and carbonate precipitation can be simultaneously optimized by increasing pH and supplementing the medium with sodium bicarbonate at a concentration near 0.02 M. In pilot-scale photobioreactors (500 L), these conditions enable stable carbon capture via $CaCO_3$ formation, up to 60% greater than in unmodified systems, highlighting the potential for industrial-scale carbon sequestration (Solovchenko et al., 1834). This process is critically dependent on the interplay among the Ca^{2+} concentration, dissolved inorganic carbon, pH, and availability of nucleation sites on the algal surface (Zuorro et al., 2025). Moreover, certain cyanobacteria and green algae can produce extracellular enzymes, such as urease and carbonic anhydrase, that modulate local pH and promote the formation and stabilization of $CaCO_3$ (Li et al., 2022). Some algae also form intracellular amorphous carbonate inclusions, known as micropearls, which serve as calcium reservoirs, ballast for cellular equilibrium, and pH buffers. Thus, algal biomineralization not only enhances carbon capture but also yields a mineral coproduct with potential applications in ecological restoration, sustainable construction materials, and agriculture.

6.4.2 Polyphosphate-Based Fertilizers

Another promising valorization route involves using nutrient-rich algal biomass as a slow-release biofertilizer. Microalgae store phosphorus in the form of polyphosphates within specialized vacuoles known as acidocalcisomes, where these polymers are stabilized as dense granules complexed with divalent cations (Bossa et al., 2024). Under luxury uptake conditions, cellular phosphorus content can increase from ~1% to 4–6% of dry weight (Bossa et al., 2024). When this biomass is applied to soil, the polyphosphates undergo gradual hydrolysis, releasing orthophosphate that plants can assimilate, thereby functioning as a controlled-release fertilizer.

In addition to phosphorus, microalgae contribute nitrogen, potassium, micronutrients, and phytohormones, collectively enhancing soil fertility and plant growth (Miranda et al., 2024). Field experiments have validated the efficacy of these biofertilizers. In a Chinese hawthorn orchard, the application of live microalgae increased fruit yield by 15.7–29.6%, depending on the dosage and application method. It also improved the soluble sugar content and increased the soil carbon and nitrogen levels without increasing greenhouse gas emissions (Ma et al., 2024). Other studies have shown that microalgae–microorganism consortia provide a broader spectrum of nutrients (N, P, K) than conventional biofertilizers do, thereby reducing reliance on synthetic alternatives (Ren et al., 2025). Furthermore, recent reviews on biofertilizers and biostimulants report that microalgae improve nutrient bioavailability, produce bioactive compounds, and contribute to the restoration of degraded soils, positioning them as sustainable alternatives to chemical fertilizers (Miranda et al., 2024; Contreras-Ropero et al., 2024). These findings support the use of posttreatment algal biomass as a polyphosphate-based, slow-release fertilizer—particularly when the heavy metal content is adequately controlled.

6.4.3 Biofuels and Lipid-Derived Products

Under controlled stress conditions—especially nitrogen (N) and phosphorus (P) limitation—many microalgae redirect their metabolism toward the massive accumulation of lipids, which are key precursors for the production of biodiesel and other renewable biofuels. In *Monoraphidium braunii*, for example, reducing N and P concentrations by 75% led to more than a threefold increase in lipid productivity, highlighting nutrient stress as a potent trigger for lipid accumulation (Solovchenko et al., 1834). Salinity stress (e.g., exposure to 250 mM NaCl) has also been shown to significantly increase the lipid content in this species, indicating the versatility of strategies for metabolic modulation. In *Tetradesmus obliquus*, exposure to heavy metal stress resulted in a lipid content of approximately 180 mg per gram of dry biomass when supplemented with optimal concentrations of cobalt (0.04 mM Co^{2+}). Metal-induced stress also shifted the fatty acid profile toward higher proportions of saturated and monounsaturated fatty acids—traits that improve biodiesel quality by increasing cetane number, viscosity, and flash point, all of which are favorable for fuel performance (Solovchenko et al., 1834).

In diatoms such as *Phaeodactylum tricornutum*, manipulating light conditions (specifically, exposure to blue light at an intensity of 100 μmol photons m^{-2} s^{-1}) doubled lipid productivity to 539 mg g^{-1} of dry weight while increasing total biomass to 1.6 g L^{-1}. Moreover, this diatom synthesizes high-value omega-3 fatty acids, further expanding the portfolio of products derived from algal cultivation (Li et al., 2022). With such strategies, certain strains can yield up to 0.3 kg of biodiesel per kg of dry biomass, along with valuable coproducts such as glycerol. Although the main barrier to commercial-scale algal biodiesel production remains the high energy cost associated with harvesting and lipid extraction, integrating phytoremediation systems with biofuel production offers an auspicious approach. Wastewater treatment not only provides essential nutrients for algal growth but also generates additional revenue streams, thereby mitigating the environmental impact and enhancing the overall economic viability of the process (Molitor et al., 2024; Solovchenko et al., 1834).

6.5 Advantages, Limitations, and Scale-Up of Algal Systems

Algal configurations with demonstrated plant-scale performance can be grouped into four archetypes that balance operational control, energy demand, biomass capture, thickening and dewatering, and the feasibility of routing toward product pathways. High-rate algal ponds sustain consistent nitrogen and phosphorus removal in real effluents when hydraulic retention time (HRT), surface loading rate, and carbon dioxide (CO_2) supply are adjusted to stabilize pH and productivity throughout the year; they exhibit refined design windows that facilitate adoption in municipal and industrial tertiary treatment (Li et al., 2023). Rotating algal biofilms increases areal productivity and simplifies solid–liquid separation via attached growth, which stabilizes harvesting costs when rotation, shear, and irradiance are controlled during extended campaigns; recent evidence in complex matrices includes field-scale intensification and scale-up analyses (Nguyen et al., 2024). Trains of closed photobioreactors oriented to polishing and biological phosphorus recovery demonstrate fine control of process variables with secondary effluents, with documented operation at around 568 m^3 day^{-1} and biomass capture compatible with valorization routes, while keeping the effluent within strict limits under plant conditions (Molitor et al., 2024). Algal turf systems (ATS) deployed in channels and flow-ways intercept dissolved loads and stabilize water quality through periodic harvesting, with on-site adjustment of slope, velocity, and harvest frequency providing hydraulic flexibility and reproducible performance under field conditions (Adey et al., 2013).

Comparisons across archetypes should consider cross-cutting operational determinants that condition plant-level adoption. Biomass capture with thickening and dewatering concentrates increases operating costs and governs variance in biomass quality; therefore, selection of the separation train must align with the intended end use to avoid rework and off-specification losses. Recent evidence converges on reducing energy per unit of solids captured, ensuring floc stability under process hydraulics, and aligning the capture-equipment set with the target quality of the product stream—measures that relieve bottlenecks and stabilize revenue in valorization schemes (Kendler et al., 2025; Vázquez-Romero et al., 2024). Under these premises, configuration assessment goes beyond peak rates and focuses on predictable mass balances over annual cycles, with reproducible operational control in real effluents.

The transition from laboratory and pilot to plant operation is structured around validations with real influents across complete seasonal cycles, tracking community stability and process control, and extended trials that consolidate separation-train behavior in terms of specific capture energy, solids content, and reproducibility of biomass quality. This approach prioritizes the governance of variables under site-specific disturbances and coupling with operational logistics, while reserving the definition of end-use criteria and coproduct acceptance for Sect. 6.4, where routing indicators and thresholds are established. Evidence from photobioreactors for phosphorus recovery shows that transferring setpoints from pilot to plant—controlling pH, light, and flow—supports flow rates of hundreds of cubic meters per day and delivers biomass suitable for valorization, with documented operational consistency (Molitor et al., 2024). The techno-economic linkage is expressed directly in three operational fronts: circulation or aeration energy, use of supplemental light where applicable, and biomass capture with thickening and dewatering. Revenues, in turn, are associated with regulatory compliance for nitrogen and phosphorus, as well as with the stability of coproduct streams. Balance improvements are observed when facilities are co-located with existing assets, when energy per unit of solids captured is reduced, and when biomass quality is maintained within end-use specifications—

measures that simultaneously reduce cost and revenue variance under real operating conditions (Geng et al., 2025; Vázquez-Romero et al., 2024).

6.6 Future Perspectives

The enhancement of cellular detoxification pathways in microalgae through genetic engineering is an emerging field with significant potential to expand the natural capabilities of these microorganisms. While microalgae inherently possess mechanisms to cope with heavy metals and organic pollutants, biotechnology aims to strengthen these systems or introduce novel metabolic pathways through metabolic engineering strategies. For example, overexpression of genes encoding chelating proteins, such as phytochelatins or heterologous metallothioneins, could substantially increase intracellular sequestration capacity for toxic cations, such as Cd^{2+} and Hg^{2+} (Ranjbar & Malcata, 2022). Similarly, the introduction of high-affinity transporters—such as ZIP transporters for Zn and Co or improved phosphate permeases—can optimize the initial uptake of metals and nutrients in contaminated environments (Krishnan et al., 2018). A proven approach to developing more robust strains involves the selection and directed evolution of strains under environmental stress. For example, Yang et al. (2025) described the genetic manipulation of acidophilic microalgae tailored for efficient biosorption of Cr(VI) and Cd^{2+} in acid mine drainage, a crucial advancement for treating low-pH effluents that are inhospitable to other organisms (Hassanien et al., 2023). These strains exhibit adaptive modifications that increase metal resistance and accumulation capacity. In the field of synthetic biology, progress has been made in incorporating complete degradation pathways for complex organic pollutants, including organophosphate pesticides and aromatic compounds. For example, the introduction of bacterial gene clusters encoding aromatic-ring dioxygenases into model microalgal species (*Chlamydomonas reinhardtii* and *Phaeodactylum tricornutum*) is laying the groundwork for the design of transgenic algae capable of mineralizing organic contaminants through photosynthesis, potentially significantly broadening their bioremediation spectrum (Webster et al., 2024).

The use of precision gene-editing tools such as CRISPR/Cas9 and TALENs has revolutionized these possibilities. These technologies allow the silencing of regulatory genes that divert metabolic resources into undesirable pathways and redirect metabolism toward increased production of protective molecules, such as antioxidants (superoxide dismutase, catalase) and chelators, thereby increasing algal tolerance to contaminants (Ranjbar & Malcata, 2022). Furthermore, the stable integration of exogenous genes into algal chloroplasts and nuclei has enabled the creation of robust expression vectors—essential for establishing transgenic bioremediation strains (Roushan et al., 2023). Omics technologies—genomics, transcriptomics, proteomics, and metabolomics—form the backbone of these efforts, helping to identify genetic targets and metabolic pathways activated in response to contaminant stress. For example, transcriptomic analyses in diatoms exposed to BTEX compounds revealed the induction of unique enzymes involved in previously unknown degradation pathways (Sattayawat et al., 2021). This knowledge is critical for rational engineering and the design of functional algal consortia, where different strains—or even mixtures of microalgae and cyanobacteria—are programmed to act cooperatively in the sequential degradation of complex pollutants.

In the future, the next generation of "on-demand" microalgae could incorporate inducible genetic switches that regulate the expression of efflux pumps and other detoxification mechanisms only when contaminant concentrations exceed specific thresholds, optimizing energy use and maximizing cellular efficiency (Krishnan et al., 2018). Nonetheless, several technical challenges persist, including the efficient genetic transformation of non-model species, the development of effective biological containment measures to prevent the environmental release of modified algae, and securing regulatory approval for commercial deployment. Despite these hurdles, the integration of synthetic biology with omics technologies is advancing toward the development of resistant, fast-acting, and selective microalgae capable of functioning as cellular biofactories for environmental remediation and sustainable resource recovery (Ranjbar & Malcata, 2022).

6.7 Regulatory Frameworks, Economic-Environmental Feasibility, and Adoption Barriers

The industrial deployment of microalgae-based bioremediation technologies depends not only on scientific advances but also on the establishment of appropriate regulatory frameworks and the demonstration of economic and environmental feasibility through integrated life-cycle assessment (LCA) and technoeconomic analysis (TEA). In recent years, regulatory agencies have begun to formally recognize nutrient biorecovery processes, such as phosphorus recovery. For example, the European Union has set ambitious targets for 2029, including recovering at least 50% of phosphorus from sludge and 80% from incineration ash, prompting wastewater treatment plants to adopt innovative technologies—including microalgal cultivation—to extract nutrients and reintegrate them into the production chain as sustainable fertilizers (Krishnan et al., 2018). Regulations also focus on the quality of biofertilizers derived from algal biomass, with ongoing revisions to ensure compliance with stringent limits on heavy metals, pathogens, and organic contaminants.

However, regarding the removal of hazardous pollutants, current environmental regulations—such as those from the U.S. Environmental Protection Agency (EPA) and the European Water Framework Directive—do not yet explicitly recognize genetically modified microalgae or algal consortia as authorized "treatment agents." Thus, it is imperative to update biosafety policies and discharge permit regulations to enable the safe, large-scale adoption of these technologies (El-Sheekh et al., 2025). The use of transgenic algae in open systems remains a sensitive issue; it is anticipated that regulation will require strict containment measures, such as the use of closed photobioreactors or effective postprocessing biomass inactivation systems, to prevent environmental release (Krishnan et al., 2018).

From an economic standpoint, numerous TEA studies conclude that integrating multiple value streams is essential for financial viability. Producing biodiesel from microalgae alone remains economically unfeasible with current technologies. However, combining the simultaneous removal of nutrients and metals—which constitute a valued environmental service—with the sale of bioproducts significantly improves the economic balance. For example, integrated facilities treating tertiary wastewater can remove more than 90% of nitrogen and phosphorus, generate revenue by valorizing residual biomass as biofertilizer, and thereby reduce net treatment costs (Soares et al., 2023). Despite this potential, significant barriers remain: capital investment in large-scale algal cultivation systems—whether open ponds or photobioreactors—is high. Additionally, the operational cost of harvesting diluted biomass remains a challenge, as conventional techniques (e.g., flotation, bioflocculation) entail substantial energy consumption, accounting for more than 30% of total costs in some schemes. The development of more efficient harvesting technologies is thus key to improving economic competitiveness (Su et al., 2023).

Life cycle assessments (LCAs) highlight potential environmental benefits. Microalgae not only remove pollutants but also fix CO_2 during growth, partially offsetting the process's carbon footprint. A comparative study between conventional chemical precipitation and a microalgal cultivation system revealed greenhouse gas emission reductions of 30–40%, provided that the energy used for pumping and lighting originates from renewable or clean sources. However, a critical issue is the safe final disposal of contaminants concentrated in the biomass, particularly heavy metals. If this biomass is not reused properly or disposed of, some of its environmental benefits could be negated. Consequently, recent studies have explored methods to stabilize these contaminants via biomineralization into calcium carbonate or encapsulation into biochar through hydrothermal carbonization, transforming waste into inert forms suitable for subsequent use or safe disposal (Soares et al., 2023; Su et al., 2023).

Regarding industrial acceptance, barriers include the need to demonstrate scalability. Many processes encounter complications when scaled up to pilot or commercial levels due to issues such as contamination by other algae or bacteria, seasonal variability in solar radiation, and logistical challenges with managing large volumes. In open systems, maintaining dominant monocultures is difficult, and spontaneous consortia often form. While this may not be inherently negative—as mixed communities are usually robust and efficient—it complicates process control. Conversely, closed systems such as tubular or flat-panel photobioreactors offer greater control but significantly increase construction and operational costs (Soares et al., 2023).

Ultimately, commercial success will depend on achieving a favorable cost-benefit ratio, wherein microalgae must offer flexibility—capable of simultaneously treating complex mixtures of contaminants (nutrients, metals, and organic compounds) in a single step—something rarely feasible with conventional technologies that require multiple treatment stages. Public perception and governmental support are decisive factors: initiatives aligned with a circular economy and "green" treatment strategies tend to enjoy strong societal acceptance, enabling incentives such as carbon credits for CO_2 fixation or subsidies for nutrient removal that help prevent eutrophication (Krishnan et al., 2018).

6.8 Operational and Design Guidelines for Scale-Up

Plant-scale implementation should begin with an influent characterization that captures seasonal variability and the chemical speciation relevant to process control. It is advisable to run campaigns in dry and wet seasons that measure trace metals and BTEX (benzene, toluene, ethylbenzene, and xylene), together with bioavailable fractions of nitrogen (N) and phosphorus (P), and to translate these profiles into setpoints for pH, alkalinity, and carbon dioxide (CO_2) dosing. The goal is to maintain a near-neutral window that favors assimilation and reduces abiotic precipitation under real operating conditions. Evidence from high-rate algal ponds indicates that tuning hydraulic retention time (HRT), surface loading, and CO_2 stabilizes productivity and removal efficiencies in municipal and industrial effluents, supporting the fixation of these setpoints with site data before scaling up operating shifts and flow rates (Li et al., 2023).

Cultivation should be validated under actual influent conditions and the site-specific photoperiod, with tracking of areal productivity, dissolved oxygen, and microalgal community stability to operate within measurable envelopes rather than laboratory peak rates. For rotating algal biofilm configurations, rotation, shear, and irradiance should be controlled over campaigns lasting weeks to months, as these parameters stabilize solids capture and simplify solid–liquid separation in complex matrices. Recent reviews and reports consolidate their potential and detail intensification margins that are transferable to field conditions (Nguyen et al., 2024). The separation train should be selected based on specific energy per kilogram of solids and the preservation of floc integrity, as these metrics govern operating expenditure (OPEX) and the consistency of biomass quality for downstream routing. Recent techno-economic assessments converge on initial capture, thickening, and dewatering as the most cost-sensitive determinants in algal tertiary treatment. Consequently, it is prudent to compare on-site alternatives using uniform indicators—capture efficiency at the target flow, cake solids, and consumption of auxiliaries—before committing to equipment procurement (Kendler et al., 2025; Deepa et al., 2023).

Operational control should be linked to valorization through a compact panel of process indicators, audited per batch or on a weekly basis, depending on the harvesting regime. In plant-scale systems with biological phosphorus recovery, maintaining pH, illumination, and flow at pilot-validated setpoints has sustained flows of 568 m^3 day^{-1} while keeping effluents within strict limits and producing biomass suitable for coproducts. This justifies institutionalizing these indicators as routing gates and, where appropriate, as diversion alarms that trigger stabilization measures (Molitor et al., 2024). For biomineral carbonation, it is recommended to verify the availability of dissolved inorganic carbon and calcium to ensure pH control conducive to nucleation. Additionally, it is necessary to certify the mineral phase, crystallinity, and trace inclusions to ensure fitness for construction use or soil amendment. Such certification supports both the claim of stable carbon sequestration and regulatory acceptance of the coproduct. For polyphosphate-based fertilizers, quantify polyphosphate (PolyP) via orthophosphate release, benchmark each batch against the most stringent metal standards in the target market, and define blending strategies that maintain specification despite seasonal variability. These decisions depend on the biomass quality delivered by the cultivation and separation trains and should therefore be embedded in the operational sampling plan and batch traceability (Molitor et al., 2024). When routing targets lipids, formalize windows of nutritional stress and light regimes that increase neutral lipid production without breaching effluent limits, and track the fatty acid profile in parallel with removal performance to ensure fuel specifications are met before allocating extraction capacity. This approach minimizes reprocessing and anchors the valorization claim under plant conditions (Nobre et al., 2024).

Techno-economic integration becomes operational when the system is co-located with existing pumping, CO_2, and power infrastructure; when the capture train is sized to the most frequent flow regime rather than the historical maximum; and when field measurements are instrumented for circulation or aeration energy, the fraction of supplemental illumination (where applicable), and the specific energy of capture and thickening. Techno-economic analysis (TEA) models that simultaneously incorporate the compliance value for N and P, carbon storage potential, and coproduct pricing best reflect real plant performance and enable early deviation management. Methodological details for TEA and life-cycle assessment (LCA) are developed in the feasibility and regulatory framework section (Nobre et al., 2024). Finally, quality management should close the loop with batch certificates that include metal speciation in biomass, the polyphosphate fraction, or carbonate purity, as well as moisture or lipid content, depending on the product route, along with the retention of countersamples for audits. Experience at the municipal scale indicates that consolidating this quality-assurance scheme accelerates regulatory acceptance and stabilizes revenues in valorization scenarios, while facilitating the transfer of performance from pilot to commercial practice (Molitor et al., 2024; Alam et al., 2024).

6.9 Conclusion

Microalgae-based remediation is emerging as an advanced biotechnological platform that integrates contaminant capture, intracellular transformation, and valorization within a single modular system. At the subcellular level, passive biosorption, active transmembrane transport, and vacuolar sequestration mechanisms mitigate the toxicity of trace metals, nutrients, and persistent aromatic compounds through highly specific metabolic pathways. However, the absence of standardized protocols for quantifying the intracellular fate of pollutants limits interstudy comparability, hampers the development of robust kinetic models, and constrains the formulation of regulatory criteria. Consequently, large-scale implementation requires not only the optimization of operational and environmental variables but also the reinforcement of methodological frameworks that validate the functional effectiveness of these systems under real-world conditions.

From a circular bioeconomic perspective, the valorization of algal biomass post-remediation is not a collateral benefit but rather a structural pillar that defines the economic viability of such systems. The production of controlled-release fertilizers, lipid-based biofuels, and carbonated biominerals transforms treated biomass into a strategic input for the agricultural, energy, and sustainable construction sectors. Nevertheless, persistent technological challenges—including the high energy demand of harvesting processes, susceptibility to contamination in open systems, and the absence of specific regulations for genetically modified algal cultures—continue to limit industrial scalability. The integration of precision gene-editing tools, rational design of functional algal consortia, and multiomic analyses outlines a clear roadmap toward consolidating microalgae as intelligent cellular biofactories capable of operating under criteria of metabolic efficiency, contaminant traceability, and systemic profitability.

References

Adey, W. H., Laughinghouse, H. D., Miller, J. B., Hayek, L. C., Thompson, J. G., Bertman, S., Hampel, K., & Puvanendran, S. (2013). Algal turf scrubber (ATS) Floways on the Great Wicomico River, Chesapeake Bay: Productivity, algal community structure, substrate and chemistry. *Journal of Phycology, 49*, 489–501. https://doi.org/10.1111/jpy.12056

Alam, M. M., Hodaei, M., Hartnett, E., Gincley, B., Khan, F., Kim, G.-Y., Pinto, A. J., & Bradley, I. M. (2024). Community structure and function during periods of high performance and system upset in a full-scale mixed microalgal wastewater resource recovery facility. *Water Research, 259*, 121819. https://doi.org/10.1016/j.watres.2024.121819

Alharbi, R. M., Abdel-Raouf, N., Mohamed, M. S., Fathy, W. A., Ibraheem, I. B. M., & Hozayen, W. G. (2025). Phycomediation of cadmium contaminated aqueous solutions using *Chlamydomonas* Sp.: Process optimization and adsorption characterization. *Frontiers in Bioengineering and Biotechnology, 13*. https://doi.org/10.3389/fbioe.2025.1558757

Aneja, R. K., Chaudhary, G., Ahluwalia, S. S., & Goyal, D. (2010). Biosorption of Pb2+ and Zn2+ by non-living biomass of spirulina Sp. *Indian Journal of Microbiology, 50*, 438–442. https://doi.org/10.1007/s12088-011-0091-8

Bagasariya, A., Upadhayay, D., Marchawala, F., Bhattacharya, I., & Andhare, P. (2021). Application of microalgae for nutrient recovery from wastewater. *International Journal of Biology, Pharmacy and Allied Sciences, 10*. https://doi.org/10.31032/IJBPAS/2021/10.4.1002

Balzano, S., Sardo, A., Blasio, M., Chahine, T. B., Dell'Anno, F., Sansone, C., & Brunet, C. (2020). Microalgal metallothioneins and phytochelatins and their potential use in bioremediation. *Frontiers in Microbiology, 11*. https://doi.org/10.3389/fmicb.2020.00517

Bossa, R., Di Colandrea, M., Salbitani, G., & Carfagna, S. (2024). Phosphorous utilization in microalgae: Physiological aspects and applied implications. *Plants, 13*, 2127. https://doi.org/10.3390/plants13152127

Cai, Z., Karunakaran, E., & Pandhal, J. (2024). Bottom-up construction and screening of algae-bacteria consortia for pollutant biodegradation. *Frontiers in Microbiology, 15*. https://doi.org/10.3389/fmicb.2024.1349016

Choi, H. J., & Lee, S. M. (2015). Effect of the N/P ratio on biomass productivity and nutrient removal from municipal wastewater. *Bioprocess and Biosystems Engineering, 38*, 761–766. https://doi.org/10.1007/s00449-014-1317-z

Contreras-Ropero, J. E., Barajas-Solano, A. F., García-Martínez, J. B., Barajas-Ferrerira, C., & Machuca-Martínez, F. (2024). Production of industrial-interest colorants in microalgae and cyanobacteria: Leveraging nutrient dynamics and photoperiod optimization. *Ingeniería y Competitividad, 26*. https://doi.org/10.25100/iyc.v26i2.13679

Deepa, P., Sowndhararajan, K., & Kim, S. (2023). A review of the harvesting techniques of microalgae. *Water (Basel), 15*, 3074. https://doi.org/10.3390/w15173074

Du, S., Cui, J., Meng, F., Li, H., Cui, H., & Xia, Y. (2023). Bioremediation of Propylbenzenes by a novel marine microalga Rhinomonas Reticulata S6A isolated from Daya Bay: Acute toxicity, growth kinetics and biodegradation performance. *Frontiers in Marine Science, 10*. https://doi.org/10.3389/fmars.2023.1171944

Elgarahy, A. M., Elwakeel, K. Z., Mohammad, S. H., & Elshoubaky, G. A. (2021). A critical review of biosorption of dyes, heavy metals and metalloids from wastewater as an efficient and green process. *Clean Eng Technol, 4*, 100209. https://doi.org/10.1016/j.clet.2021.100209

El-Sheekh, M. M., El-Kassas, H. Y., & Ali, S. S. (2025). Microalgae-based bioremediation of refractory pollutants: An approach towards environmental sustainability. *Microbial Cell Factories, 24*, 19. https://doi.org/10.1186/s12934-024-02638-0

Eregie, S. B., Sanusi, I. A., & Ademola, O. O. (2025). Current status and future prospects of microalgae-based degradation of spent lubricant oil hydrocarbon towards environmental sustainability: A mini review and bibliometric analysis. *Archives of Microbiology, 207*, 149. https://doi.org/10.1007/s00203-025-04332-0

Farahin, A. W., Natrah, I., Nagao, N., Yusoff, F. M., Shariff, M., Banerjee, S., Katayama, T., Nakakuni, M., Koyama, M., Nakasaki, K., et al. (2021). Tolerance of Tetraselmis Tetrathele to high ammonium nitrogen and its effect on growth rate, carotenoid, and fatty acids productivity. *Frontiers in Bioengineering and Biotechnology, 9*. https://doi.org/10.3389/fbioe.2021.568776

Fayemiwo, O. M., Daramola, M. O., & Moothi, K. (2017). BTEX compounds in water - future trends and directions for water treatment. *Water SA, 43*, 602. https://doi.org/10.4314/wsa.v43i4.08

Fazal, T., Wang, Y., Zhang, Y., Hou, S., & Zhang, C. (2025). Evaluating microalgal-induced carbonate precipitation for marine carbon sequestration using chlorella species. *Journal of Environmental Management, 394*, 127245. https://doi.org/10.1016/j.jenvman.2025.127245

Fernandes, T. V., Suárez-Muñoz, M., Trebuch, L. M., Verbraak, P. J., & Van de Waal, D. B. (2017). Toward an ecologically optimized N:P recovery from wastewater by microalgae. *Frontiers in Microbiology, 8*. https://doi.org/10.3389/fmicb.2017.01742

Fujie, T., Muraoka, A., Ito, K., Ozaki, Y., Yamamoto, C., & Kaji, T. (2022). Lead induces a metal transporter, ZIP8, via activation of the NF-KB signaling pathway and the induction is involved in the protection against Lead cytotoxicity by intracellular Lead accumulation independent mechanisms in cultured vascular endothelial cells. *The Journal of Toxicological Sciences, 47*, 493–501. https://doi.org/10.2131/jts.47.493

Gan, X., Klose, H., & Reinecke, D. (2022). Optimizing nutrient removal and biomass production of the algal turf scrubber (ATS) under variable cultivation conditions by using response surface methodology. *Frontiers in Bioengineering and Biotechnology, 10*. https://doi.org/10.3389/fbioe.2022.962719

Geng, Y., Shaukat, A., Azhar, W., Raza, Q.-U.-A., Tahir, A., Abideen, M. Z. u., Zia, M. A. B., Bashir, M. A., & Rehim, A. (2025). Microalgal biorefineries: A systematic review of technological trade-offs and innovation pathways. *Biotechnology for Biofuels and Bioproducts, 18*, 93. https://doi.org/10.1186/s13068-025-02694-7

Golnaraghi Ghomi, A., Asasian-Kolur, N., Sharifian, S., & Golnaraghi, A. (2020). Biosorpion for sustainable recovery of precious metals from wastewater. *Journal of Environmental Chemical Engineering, 8*, 103996. https://doi.org/10.1016/j.jece.2020.103996

Guan, C.-Y., Kao, Y.-L., Pham, V. T., Wu, P.-H., & Yu, C.-P. (2023). Valorization of heavy metal-adsorbed microalgae from a membrane bioreactor for Levulinic acid production. *Journal of Environmental Chemical Engineering, 11*, 110852. https://doi.org/10.1016/j.jece.2023.110852

Halder, S. (2014). Bioremediation of heavy metals through fresh water microalgae: A review. *Scholars Academic Journal of Biosciences (SAJB), 2*, 825–830. https://doi.org/10.36347/sajb.2014.v02i11.016

Hariz, H. B., Montemezzani, V., Shim, Y., Rendle, D., Picken, C., Park, J. B. K., & Craggs, R. J. (2025). Nutrient removal performance of novel filamentous algae nutrient scrubber (FANS) configurations. *Algal Research, 86*, 103937. https://doi.org/10.1016/j.algal.2025.103937

Hassanien, A., Saadaoui, I., Schipper, K., Al-Marri, S., Dalgamouni, T., Aouida, M., Saeed, S., & Al-Jabri, H. M. (2023). Genetic engineering to enhance microalgal-based produced water treatment with emphasis on CRISPR/Cas9: A review. *Frontiers in Bioengineering and Biotechnology, 10*. https://doi.org/10.3389/fbioe.2022.1104914

Heisler, J., Glibert, P. M., Burkholder, J. M., Anderson, D. M., Cochlan, W., Dennison, W. C., Dortch, Q., Gobler, C. J., Heil, C. A., Humphries, E., et al. (2008). Eutrophication and harmful algal blooms: A scientific consensus. *Harmful Algae, 8*, 3–13. https://doi.org/10.1016/j.hal.2008.08.006

Ibuot, A., Dean, A. P., McIntosh, O. A., & Pittman, J. K. (2017). Metal bioremediation by CrMTP4 over-expressing *Chlamydomonas Reinhardtii* in comparison to natural wastewater-tolerant microalgae strains. *Algal Research, 24*, 89–96. https://doi.org/10.1016/j.algal.2017.03.002

Ibuot, A., Webster, R. E., Williams, L. E., & Pittman, J. K. (2020). Increased metal tolerance and bioaccumulation of zinc and cadmium in *Chlamydomonas Reinhardtii* expressing a AtHMA4 C-terminal domain protein. *Biotechnology and Bioengineering, 117*, 2996–3005. https://doi.org/10.1002/bit.27476

Janpum, C., Pombubpa, N., Monshupanee, T., Incharoensakdi, A., & In-na, P. (2022). Advancement on mixed microalgal-bacterial cultivation systems for nitrogen and phosphorus recoveries from wastewater to promote sustainable bioeconomy. *Journal of Biotechnology, 360*, 198–210. https://doi.org/10.1016/j.jbiotec.2022.11.008

Jayaraman, J., Kumaraswamy, J., Rao, Y. K. S. S., Karthick, M., Baskar, S., Anish, M., Sharma, A., Yadav, A. S., Alam, T., & Ammarullah, M. I. (2024). Wastewater treatment by algae-based membrane bioreactors: A review of the arrangement of a membrane reactor, physico-chemical properties, advantages and challenges. *RSC Advances, 14*, 34769–34790. https://doi.org/10.1039/D4RA04417G

Jomova, K., Alomar, S. Y., Nepovimova, E., Kuca, K., & Valko, M. (2025). Heavy metals: Toxicity and human health effects. *Archives of Toxicology, 99*, 153–209. https://doi.org/10.1007/s00204-024-03903-2

Kendler, S., Magnanelli, E., Bless, M., & Nordtvedt, T. S. (2025). A review of dewatering and drying energy requirements in microalgae production: Pathways towards industrial uptake and bioeconomy integration. *Cleaner and Circular Bioeconomy, 12*, 100184. https://doi.org/10.1016/j.clcb.2025.100184

Krishnan, A., Qian, X., Ananyev, G., Lun, D. S., & Dismukes, G. C. (2018). Rewiring of cyanobacterial metabolism for hydrogen production. In *Synthetic biology approaches and challenges* (pp. 171–213). Springer.

Li, H., Watson, J., Zhang, Y., Lu, H., & Liu, Z. (2020). Environment-enhancing process for algal wastewater treatment, heavy metal control and hydrothermal biofuel production: A critical review. *Bioresource Technology, 298*, 122421. https://doi.org/10.1016/j.biortech.2019.122421

Li, Z., Li, S., Li, T., Gao, X., & Zhu, L. (2022). Physiological and transcriptomic responses of chlorella Sorokiniana to ciprofloxacin reveal molecular mechanisms for antibiotic removal. *iScience, 25*, 104638. https://doi.org/10.1016/j.isci.2022.104638

Li, M., Wang, Y., Zhang, J., Liu, B., Xue, H., Wu, L., & Li, Z. (2023). Knowledge mapping of high-rate algal ponds research. *Water (Basel), 15*, 1916. https://doi.org/10.3390/w15101916

Li, C., Wu, X., Wu, J., & Li, P. (2026). Enhancing nitrogen and phosphorus removal from aquaculture waste water via mechanical harvesting of rotating algal-bacterial biofilm system. *Aquaculture, 611*, 743036. https://doi.org/10.1016/j.aquaculture.2025.743036

Liu, T., Guo, H., Yu, Q., Wang, Y., Liu, H., Zeng, Y., Wang, Y., Liu, C., & Li, J. (2024). The impact of Cr(III) and Cr(VI) on lipid accumulation in chlorella Pyrenoidosa. *Processes, 12*, 905. https://doi.org/10.3390/pr12050905

Ma, F., Li, Y., Han, X., Li, K., Zhao, M., Guo, L., Li, S., Wang, K., Qin, K., Duan, J., et al. (2024). Microalgae-based biofertilizer improves fruit yield and controls greenhouse gas emissions in a hawthorn orchard. *PLoS One, 19*, e0307774. https://doi.org/10.1371/journal.pone.0307774

Magalhães, I. B., Pereira, A. S. A. d. P., Silva, T. A., Ferreira, J., Braga, M. Q., Couto, E. A., Assemany, P. P., & Calijuri, M. L. (2024). Advancements in high-rate algal pond technology for enhanced wastewater treatment and biomass production: A review. *Journal of Water Process Engineering, 66*, 105929. https://doi.org/10.1016/j.jwpe.2024.105929

Mahlangu, D., Mphahlele, K., De Paola, F., & Mthombeni, N. H. (2024). Microalgae-mediated biosorption for effective heavy metals removal from wastewater: A review. *Water (Basel), 16*, 718. https://doi.org/10.3390/w16050718

Miranda, A. M., Hernandez-Tenorio, F., Villalta, F., Vargas, G. J., & Sáez, A. A. (2024). Advances in the development of biofertilizers and biostimulants from microalgae. *Biology-Basel, 13*, 199. https://doi.org/10.3390/biology13030199

Molitor, H. R., Kim, G.-Y., Hartnett, E., Gincley, B., Alam, M. M., Feng, J., Avila, N. M., Fisher, A., Hodaei, M., Li, Y., et al. (2024). Intensive microalgal cultivation and tertiary phosphorus recovery from wastewaters via the EcoRecover process. *Environmental Science & Technology, 58*, 8803–8814. https://doi.org/10.1021/acs.est.3c10264

Mrowiec, B., & Suschka, J. (2009). Presence and effects of aromatic hydrocarbons on sewage treatment efficiency. Proceedings of the Annual International Conference on Soils, Sediments, Water and Energy: Vol. 14

Nedaei, L., & Shokrkar, H. (2025). Investigating the removal of pollutants from wastewater using microalgae. *Chemical Review and Letters, 8*, 426–440.

Ng, A., Weerakoon, D., Lim, E., & Padhye, L. P. (2019). Fate of environmental pollutants. *Water Environment Research, 91*, 1294–1325. https://doi.org/10.1002/wer.1225

Nguyen, V.-T., Le, V.-A., Do, Q.-H., Le, T.-N.-C., & Vo, T.-D.-H. (2024). Emerging revolving algae biofilm system for algal biomass production and nutrient recovery from wastewater. *Science of the Total Environment, 912*, 168911. https://doi.org/10.1016/j.scitotenv.2023.168911

Nobre, M. L. F., Tavares, D., Fraga, C., Oliveira, B., Dias, M., Mesquita, S., Oliveira, C. M., & Pires, J. C. M. (2024). Techno-economic analysis of a circular microalgal approach for enhanced wastewater treatment and resource recovery in northern Portugal. *Journal of Cleaner Production, 434*, 140389. https://doi.org/10.1016/j.jclepro.2023.140389

Oliveira, A. P., Assemany, P. P., Jackeline de Siqueira, C., de Jesus Júnior, M. M., Rodrigues, F. D., de Oliveira, L. F., Campos, M. T., Oliveira Carneiro, A. D., & Calijuri, M. L. (2025). Hydrothermal carbonization of microalgae biomass from wastewater treatment: Effects of acid pretreatment. *ACS Omega*. https://doi.org/10.1021/acsomega.5c02582

Penen, F., Isaure, M. P., Dobritzsch, D., Bertalan, I., Castillo-Michel, H., Proux, O., Gontier, E., Le Coustumer, P., & Schaumlöffel, D. (2017). Pools of cadmium in Chlamydomonas Reinhardtii revealed by chemical imaging and XAS spectroscopy. *Metallomics, 9*, 910–923. https://doi.org/10.1039/C7MT00029D

Plouviez, M., & Brown, N. (2024). Polyphosphate accumulation in microalgae and cyanobacteria: Recent advances and opportunities for phosphorus upcycling. *Current Opinion in Biotechnology, 90*, 103207. https://doi.org/10.1016/j.copbio.2024.103207

Puente-Sánchez, F., Díaz, S., Penacho, V., Aguilera, A., & Olsson, S. (2018). Basis of genetic adaptation to heavy metal stress in the acidophilic green alga *Chlamydomonas Acidophila*. *Aquatic Toxicology, 200*, 62–72. https://doi.org/10.1016/j.aquatox.2018.04.020

Ranjbar, S., & Malcata, F. X. (2022). Is genetic engineering a route to enhance microalgae-mediated bioremediation of heavy metal-containing effluents? *Molecules, 27*, 1473. https://doi.org/10.3390/molecules27051473

Ren, C.-G., Kong, C.-C., Li, S.-M., Wang, X.-J., Yu, X., Wang, Y.-C., Qin, S., & Cui, H.-L. (2025). Symbiotic microalgae and microbes: A new frontier in saline agriculture. *Frontiers in Microbiology, 16*. https://doi.org/10.3389/fmicb.2025.1540274

Roushan, M. R., Chen, C., Ahmadi, P., & Ward, V. C. A. (2023). Agrobacterium tumefaciens-Ingeniería Genética Mediada Por Microalgas Verdes, Chlorella vulgaris. *Journal of Visualized Experiments*. https://doi.org/10.3791/65382

Saravanan, P., Saravanan, V., Rajeshkannan, R., Arnica, G., Rajasimman, M., Baskar, G., & Pugazhendhi, A. (2024). Comprehensive review on toxic heavy metals in the aquatic system: Sources, identification, treatment strategies, and health risk assessment. *Environmental Research, 258*, 119440. https://doi.org/10.1016/j.envres.2024.119440

Sattayawat, P., Yunus, I. S., Noirungsee, N., Mukjang, N., Pathom-Aree, W., Pekkoh, J., & Pumas, C. (2021). Synthetic biology-based approaches for microalgal bio-removal of heavy metals from wastewater effluents. *Frontiers in Environmental Science, 9*. https://doi.org/10.3389/fenvs.2021.778260

Sbihi, K., Elhamji, S., Lghoul, S., Aziz, K., El Maallem, A., Mabrouki, J., El-Sheekh, M., & Aziz, F. (2024). Biosorption of hexavalent chromium by freshwater microalgae Craticula Subminuscula from aqueous solutions. *Sustainability, 16*, 918. https://doi.org/10.3390/su16020918

Slocombe, S. P., Zúñiga-Burgos, T., Chu, L., Wood, N. J., Camargo-Valero, M. A., & Baker, A. (2020). Fixing the broken phosphorus cycle: Wastewater remediation by microalgal polyphosphates. *Frontiers in Plant Science, 11*. https://doi.org/10.3389/fpls.2020.00982

Soares, E. J., de Meneses, A. M., Silva, N. F., dos Santos, W. B., de Almeida Lopes, T. S., de Sousa, L. C., & Ferreira, W. B. (2023). Potencial de geração de biocombustíveis e biorremediação de microalgas cultivadas em efluente doméstico tratado. *Revista DAE, 71*, 141–152. https://doi.org/10.36659/dae.2023.044

Solovchenko, A., Plouviez, M., & Khozin-Goldberg, I. (2024). Getting grip on phosphorus: Potential of microalgae as a vehicle for sustainable usage of this macronutrient. *Plants, 13*, 1834. https://doi.org/10.3390/plants13131834

Su, M., Bastiaens, L., Verspreet, J., & Hayes, M. (2023). Applications of microalgae in foods, pharma and feeds and their use as fertilizers and biostimulants: Legislation and regulatory aspects for consideration. *Food, 12*, 3878. https://doi.org/10.3390/foods12203878

Tango, M. D., Zanetoni Filho, J. A., Daniel, L. A., Leite, L. D. S., Hoffmann, M. T., & Moutinho, F. H. M. (2023). Effects of bicarbonate addition and N:P ratio on microalgae growth and resource recovery from domestic wastewater. *Agriengineering, 5*, 1178–1195. https://doi.org/10.3390/agriengineering5030075

Tian, X., Fang, Y., Jin, Y., Yi, Z., Li, J., Du, A., He, K., Huang, Y., & Zhao, H. (2021). Ammonium detoxification mechanism of ammonium-tolerant duckweed (Landoltia Punctata) revealed by carbon and nitrogen metabolism under ammonium stress. *Environmental Pollution, 277*, 116834. https://doi.org/10.1016/j.envpol.2021.116834

Urbina-Suarez, N. A., Salcedo-Pabón, C. J., Contreras-Ropero, J. E., López-Barrera, G. L., García-Martínez, J. B., Barajas-Solano, A. F., & Machuca-Martínez, F. (2025). Biotechnological strategy for tannery wastewater treatment: Bicarbonate/H2O2 oxidation integrated with microalgae cultivation. *Case Studies in Chemical and Environmental Engineering, 11*, 101060. https://doi.org/10.1016/j.cscee.2024.101060

Vázquez-Romero, B., Villar-Navarro, E., Perales, J. A., Garrido-Pérez, C., & Ruiz, J. (2024). Techno-economic analysis of using microalgae to treat streams from fish RAS farming and replace fish meal: A case study. *Journal of Water Process Engineering, 59*, 104904. https://doi.org/10.1016/j.jwpe.2024.104904

Villar-Navarro, E., Baena-Nogueras, R. M., Paniw, M., Perales, J. A., & Lara-Martín, P. A. (2018). Removal of pharmaceuticals in urban wastewater: High rate algae pond (HRAP) based technologies as an alternative to activated sludge based processes. *Water Research, 139*, 19–29. https://doi.org/10.1016/j.watres.2018.03.072

Villen-Guzman, M., Jiménez, C., & Rodriguez-Maroto, J. M. (2021). Batch and fixed-bed biosorption of Pb (II) using free and alginate-immobilized spirulina. *Processes, 9*, 466. https://doi.org/10.3390/pr9030466

Vo, T. P., Danaee, S., Chaiwong, C., Pham, B. T., Poddar, N., Kim, M., Kuzhiumparambil, U., Songsomboon, C., Pernice, M., Ngo, H. H., et al. (2024). Microalgae-bacteria consortia for organic pollutants remediation from wastewater: A critical review. *Journal of Environmental Chemical Engineering, 12*, 114213. https://doi.org/10.1016/j.jece.2024.114213

Vo, T.-D.-H., Nguyen, V.-T., Le, V.-A., Do, Q.-H., Nguyen, T.-Y.-P., Nguyen, P.-T., Lin, C., You, S.-J., Visvanathan, C., & Bui, X.-T. (2025). Simultaneous organic and nutrient removal in wastewater using a revolving algae biofilm reactor. *Environmental Technology and Innovation, 37*, 103949. https://doi.org/10.1016/j.eti.2024.103949

Wang, Q., Jin, W., Zhou, X., Guo, S., Gao, S.-H., Chen, C., Tu, R., Han, S.-F., Jiang, J., & Feng, X. (2019). Growth enhancement of biodiesel-promising microalga chlorella Pyrenoidosa in municipal wastewater by polyphosphate-accumulating organisms. *Journal of Cleaner Production, 240*, 118148. https://doi.org/10.1016/j.jclepro.2019.118148

Webster, L. J., Villa-Gomez, D., Brown, R., Clarke, W., & Schenk, P. M. (2024). A synthetic biology approach for the treatment of pollutants with microalgae. *Frontiers in Bioengineering and Biotechnology, 12*. https://doi.org/10.3389/fbioe.2024.1379301

Wei, C. (2024). Growth and phosphate uptake of microalgae under different phosphate conditions. *E3S Web of Conferences, 573*, 01004. https://doi.org/10.1051/e3sconf/202457301004

Whitton, R., Ometto, F., Pidou, M., Jarvis, P., Villa, R., & Jefferson, B. (2015). Microalgae for municipal wastewater nutrient remediation: Mechanisms, reactors and outlook for tertiary treatment. *Environmental Technology Reviews, 4*, 133–148. https://doi.org/10.1080/21622515.2015.1105308

Xu, P., Tu, X., An, Z., Mi, W., Wan, D., Bi, Y., & Song, G. (2024). Cadmium-induced physiological responses, biosorption and bioaccumulation in Scenedesmus Obliquus. *Toxics, 12*, 262. https://doi.org/10.3390/toxics12040262

Yang, X., Wu, X., Hao, H., & He, Z. (2008). Mechanisms and assessment of water eutrophication. *J Zhejiang Univ Sci B, 9*, 197–209. https://doi.org/10.1631/jzus.B0710626

Yang, X.-Y., Wei, Y.-X., Su, Y.-Q., Zhang, Z.-W., Tang, X.-Y., Chen, Y.-E., Yuan, M., & Yuan, S. (2025). The strategies microalgae adopt to counteract the toxic effect of heavy metals. *Microorganisms, 13*, 989. https://doi.org/10.3390/microorganisms13050989

Zhou, T., Xie, Z., Jiang, X., Zou, X., Cheng, J., Chen, C., Kuang, C., Ye, J., Wang, Y., & Liu, F. (2024). Efficient solar-powered bioremediation of hexavalent chromium in contaminated waters by *Chlorella* Sp. MQ-1. *Water (Basel), 16*, 3315. https://doi.org/10.3390/w16223315

Zuorro, A., Contreras-Ropero, J. E., Parada-Solano, R. J., García-Martínez, J. B., López-Barrera, G. L., Urbina-Suarez, N. A., & Barajas-Solano, A. F. (2025). Development of a biotechnological strategy for CO2 capture in coke plant emissions using microalgae. *Processes, 13*, 2121. https://doi.org/10.3390/pr13072121

The Dual Role of Algae-Based Microbial Fuel Cells in Wastewater Treatment and Bioenergy Generation

7

Ishita Mukherjee, Satadal Sahoo, Sanhita Maity,
Vishal Kumar Parida, and Anirban Pradhan

Abstract

In recent times, industrialization and globalization have driven the global economy, but they have also led to significant environmental harm. The environmental degradation caused by human energy consumption and the inevitable depletion of fossil fuels is driving the demand for a new, sustainable, eco-friendly, and reliable energy source. Recently, novel bio-based strategies with intriguing potential for generating bioenergy and treating wastewater have garnered widespread attention from researchers. Specifically, algae-based microbial fuel cells (A-MFCs) offer several advantages, which include carbon dioxide (CO_2) fixation, bioenergy generation, and photosynthetic oxygenation for power recovery and wastewater treatment. A-MFCs possess the ability to produce bioelectricity due to their sustainable long-term power generation and the ability to generate more value-added products from microalgal biomass. These systems are efficient in removing nitrogen, phosphorus, and CO_2 from wastewater, and they have been utilized to remove pollutants from both industrial and domestic wastewater sources. Despite their potential, fuel cells face several challenges, including low power output, electrode fouling, and high material costs. This chapter comprises four sections: wastewater treatment at the cathode of A-MFCs, a promising approach to bioelectricity production using A-MFCs, the role of microalgae in the anodic

I. Mukherjee · S. Sahoo · A. Pradhan (✉)
Department of Chemistry, Birla Institute of Technology Mesra, Ranchi, Jharkhand, India
e-mail: anirbanpradhan@bitmesra.ac.in

S. Maity
Amity Institute of Applied Sciences, Amity University Jharkhand, Ranchi, Jharkhand, India

V. K. Parida
Amity School of Engineering and Technology, Amity University Jharkhand, Ranchi, Jharkhand, India

L. Kumar et al. (eds.), *Algal Bioremediation*,
https://doi.org/10.1007/978-981-95-8793-3_7

compartment, and the interplay between the compartments that affects bioelectricity production. With the ongoing developments, A-MFCs open the door and pave the way for a cleaner and greener future.

Keywords

Microbial fuel cells · Wastewater treatment · Bio-energy · Algae-based MFCs

7.1 Introduction

The increasing demand for efficient wastewater treatment and clean energy worldwide has sparked interest in sustainable technologies, which address both concerns simultaneously. Consequently, a growing research interest in alternative renewable energy sources is emerging to address worldwide concerns about environmental sustainability and energy security. The production of renewable biofuel using green technology while lowering the greenhouse gas (GHG) emissions can meet (Yap et al., 2021) the future energy demands. According to a report by the International Energy Agency, liquid biofuels have been utilized in the transportation industry for several years, with the aim of reducing greenhouse gas emissions and enhancing energy security. First-generation biofuels, primarily extracted from food and oil crops, are projected to experience growth in production and consumption of liquid biofuels. However, meeting overall energy demands remains limited due to constrained market structures and a shortage of agricultural methods in emerging economies. Second-generation biofuels are produced from energy crops; however, the process of commercialization has yet to advance, and extensive areas of land are still required. Biofuels derived from microalgae are considered the third generation of biofuel, which can significantly meet primary energy demands by utilizing non-arable land. Microalgae can flourish in adverse conditions, producing large amounts of biomass and sequestering carbon (Cheah et al., 2016) through the process of photosynthesis and wastewater treatment. In comparison to other conventional crops, microalgae may be the best biomass candidates for producing bioenergy (Hussain et al., 2021) and other value-added products. Meanwhile, the water treatment industry is an electricity-intensive sector (Khatri et al., 2020) due to high electricity consumption and GHG emissions. Therefore, improving the operational efficiency and energy management of the wastewater plant to reduce carbon emissions through the synergy of microalgae cultivation and bioremediation in wastewater treatment for biofuel production (Batista et al., 2015) is an effective strategy for a sustainable bioenergy future. For an integrated and sustainable solution to the aforementioned challenges, the application of microbial fuel cells (MFCs) has garnered considerable attention for simultaneously treating wastewater (Logan et al., 2006) and generating renewable energy.

MFCs are a type of bio-electrochemical system that utilizes the metabolic activity of the microorganisms to convert the chemical energy of organic substrates into electrical energy. In standard MFCs, organic substances in wastewater undergo oxidation by microorganisms at the anode, which releases electrons that proceed to the cathode via an external circuit to produce electricity. Algae can produce oxygen through photosynthesis when exposed to light (Li et al., 2020), which suggests the cathodic oxygen reduction reaction (ORR) and eliminates the need for external aeration. Moreover, algae help eliminate nutrients and purify the water by assimilating nutrients like phosphorus and nitrogen (Sutherland et al., 2015) from the effluent. A-MFCs are ideal for incorporation into wastewater treatment systems that aim for energy neutrality or positivity due to their capabilities. In addition to supplying oxygen and removing nutrients, growing algae in MFC systems produces valuable biomass that can be converted into biofuels such as biogas, biodiesel, or bioethanol. This gives energy recovery a third dimension (Rawat et al., 2011), which could make A-MFCs economically attractive and environmentally sustainable. Despite the above advantages, several obstacles hinder the actual implementation of A-MFCs. Light availability, temperature, CO_2 content, and reactor design all affect the algal culture's growth conditions, which in turn impact the system's performance. Maintaining equilibrium between microbial activity and algal photosynthesis can be challenging, particularly in large-scale systems, under changing environmental conditions. Furthermore, technical problems restrict power output and system stability, including oxygen crossing to the anode, biofilm control, electrode fouling, and internal resistance. In this chapter, the potential of A-MFCs has been explored for both wastewater treatment and bioenergy generation. It discusses the role of algae in nutrient removal, removal of heavy metals, production of bioethanol and biodiesel, and the pretreatment methods, including sedimentation, flotation, and filtration, while examining the operational challenges and future prospects of this technology.

7.2 Design Considerations for Algae-Based MFCs

MFCs are a novel and intriguing technology that generates electricity from renewable biomass via microbial catalytic reactions at the anode end. MFCs enable the removal of specific pollutants and nutrients in wastewater, thereby facilitating bioremediation. MFCs are also utilized to recover heavy metals, decolorize dyes, and produce bioenergy, including biomass, biomethane, and biohydrogen. Thus, MFCs offer the dual advantages of treating wastewater and generating power, making the overall process both eco-friendly and economically feasible. A-MFC systems are advantageous because they have the ability to act as effective electron donors from the anodic end or electron acceptors from the cathodic end during photosynthetic reaction, and are also capable of removing organic matter. The core performance of A-MFCs depends on the design and selection of materials. The electrodes used must be biocompatible with microalgae, conductive, stable in aqueous environments, and provide a large surface area for electron transfer. Carbon-based electrodes, including carbon cloth, graphite rods, carbon nanotubes, and graphene-based composites, are widely used due to their high conductivity, chemical stability, and non-toxic nature. Metal-based electrodes, such as stainless-steel mesh, nickel foam, or copper-based materials, may be used; however, they can leach toxic ions that are harmful to algae, thereby reducing long-term stability. Hence, carbon-based electrodes are generally preferred, although metal oxides (e.g., manganese dioxide (MnO_2) and titanium dioxide (TiO_2)-coated surfaces) can sometimes enhance catalytic activity. Nafion 117 is the most widely used proton exchange membrane (PEM) due to its high proton conductivity, but it is expensive and susceptible to biofouling. Other sustainable options, such as cation exchange membranes, ultrafiltration membranes, or even naturally derived materials (e.g., chitosan-based membranes), are being investigated, as these can reduce cost and improve long-term stability. The synergy between microbial activity in the anode and algal activity in the cathode is essential for maximizing electricity generation and biomass accumulation.

7.2.1 Single-Chamber Microbial Fuel Cells

Single-chamber (membrane-less) MFCs (Fig. 7.1) have been thoroughly studied. A typical single-chamber MFC has both the cathode and the anode connected through an electric circuit. The anode is submerged in wastewater, where degradation of organic pollutants causes the release of protons and electrons. At the cathode, algae generate oxygen, which serves as the electron acceptor. This process enables the simultaneous generation of bioelectricity and wastewater treatment. *Spirulina platensis*, a type of blue-green algae (Fu et al., 2010), produces electric power

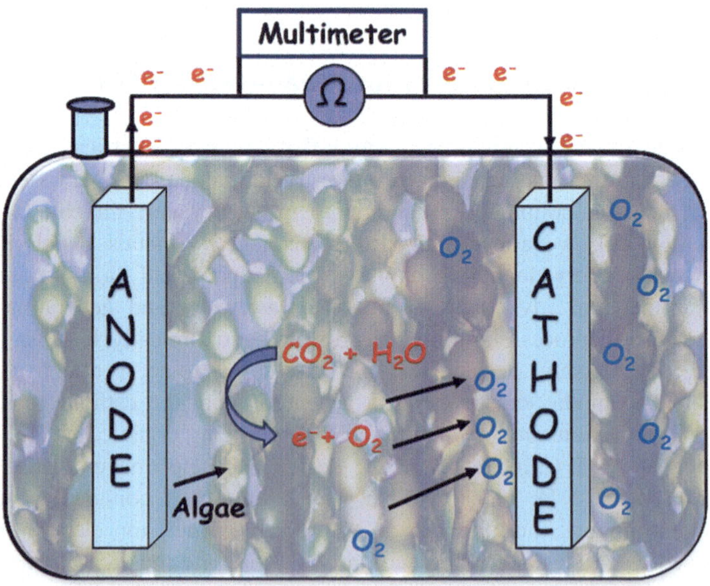

Fig. 7.1 Single-chamber algae-based microbial fuel cell

with a power density output of 0.132 mW m^{-2} in the presence of light and with an output of 1.64 mW m^{-2} in the dark. Single-chambered MFCs can run for longer periods of time as they generate more power in dark conditions. When Nishio et al. used algae-based single-chamber MFC bioreactors with *Lactobacillus* and *Geobacter* to produce energy from photosynthetically growing *Chlamydomonas reinhardtii* (Nishio et al., 2013), they found that their system might generate a power density of 0.078 W m^{-2}. Caprariis and his coworkers (Caprariis et al., 2014) have developed a bio-photovoltaic cell that produces sustainable energy by utilizing the activity of the green microalgae *Chlorella vulgaris*.

7.2.2 Dual-Chamber Microbial Fuel Cells

In this type of MFC, both the cathode and anode (Fig. 7.2) are separated by a PEM. The electroactive bacteria reside in the anode chamber, and the algae occupy the cathode chamber. This configuration offers researchers more control over each chamber, but separate chambers make the system more challenging and expensive. In 2015, Gajda et al. developed an MFC (Gajda et al., 2015) in which the phototrophic biofilm at the cathodic end provided oxygen through the oxido-reduction reaction and the growth of algal biomass, while the anaerobic biofilms at the anode could produce current. This technology produces biomass in addition to generating electricity and cleaning up wastewater. Zhang and coworkers utilized green algae in the cathodic chamber with a 1000 Ω resistor (Zhang et al., 2011), exhibiting good nutrient removal and power output at 68 ± 5 mW m^{-2}. A mediator-less photosynthetic algal microbial fuel cell was used by Strik and co-workers (Strik et al., 2008) to produce electricity in an open system for 100 days. They reported the MFC's maximum power output capability was 110 mW m^{-2} of photobioreactor surface area.

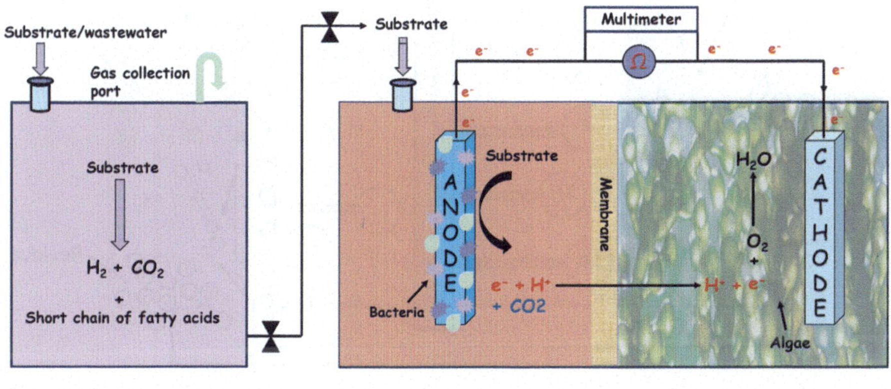

Fig. 7.2 Double-chamber algae-based microbial fuel cell

7.2.3 Photosynthetic Sediment Microbial Fuel Cells

To make this MFC, an anode is placed in a sediment chamber, and a cathode chamber containing microalgae (Fig. 7.3) is placed on top of the sediment. The CO_2 evolved by the anodic bacterial activity is consumed by the algae cells present in the cathode compartment. This is followed by the production of oxygen, and power is also generated. He et al. built a sediment-type independent phototrophic MFC (He et al., 2009), which, after 145 days of operation, generated a maximum current of 0.054 ± 0.002 mA at a resistance of 1 kΩ. In 2014, Commault and colleagues developed a membraneless sediment-type MFC (Commault et al., 2014) using a photosynthetic biocathode composed of cyanobacteria and microalgae. Throughout 180 days without feeding, this generated a maximum power density of 11 mW m^{-2}.

7.3 Wastewater Treatment and Generation of Value-Added Products

Microalgae are attractive for wastewater treatment due to their ability to rapidly assimilate excess nutrients, such as nitrogen and phosphorus, thereby improving water quality. At the same time, the accumulated biomass serves as a sustainable feedstock, rich in bioactive compounds and suitable for conversion into biofuels. This dual role makes microalgae highly promising for integrated wastewater remediation and bioresource generation. The following sub-sections focus on the role of

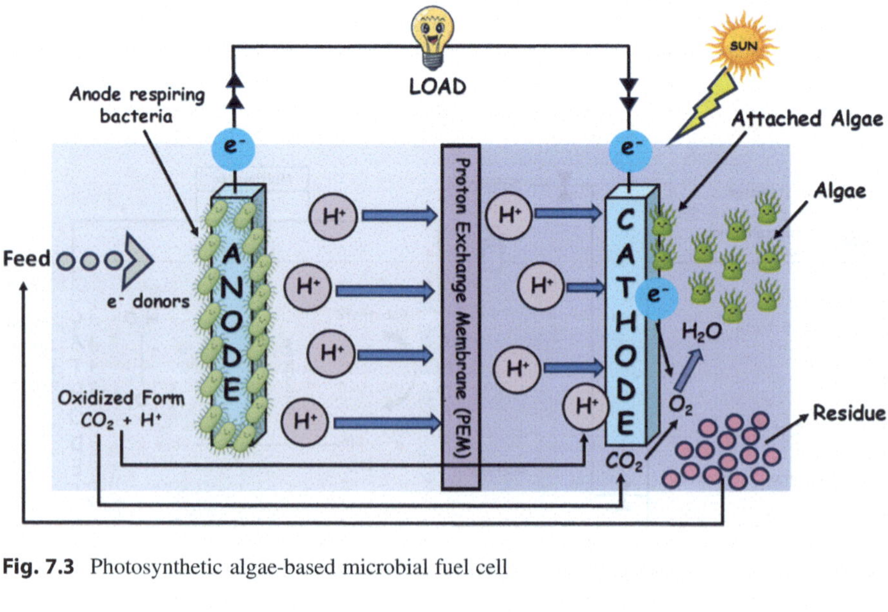

Fig. 7.3 Photosynthetic algae-based microbial fuel cell

microalgae in algal cultivation, nutrient removal, heavy metal removal, and treating EC-polluted wastewater during wastewater treatment.

7.3.1 Algal Cultivation in Wastewater

The cultivation of algae in wastewater is a novel and environmentally friendly approach to growing algae while also purifying the wastewater. The cultivation of algae addresses two major challenges: treating wastewater and generating bioresources, specifically algal biomass. Wastewater is a rich blend of organic matter, nitrogen, and phosphorus, providing an ideal environment for algal growth without the need for additional fertilizers. Algae aid in the purification of water by absorbing nutrients and eliminating pollutants, such as heavy metals and pathogens. Algal growth also helps in decreasing the biological oxygen demand (BOD). The algae growth also helps improve the water quality by ingesting heavy metals, organic contaminants, and pharmaceutical residues. It generates oxygen through photosynthesis, which promotes aerobic microbial breakdown of organic substrates in wastewater and helps in CO_2 fixation, reducing greenhouse gas emissions. This technique is a prevalent approach in both municipal and industrial environments as a sustainable and eco-friendly alternative.

7.3.2 Algae for Nutrient Removal from Wastewater

In an aquatic ecosystem, algae are fast-growing photosynthetic organisms that have an innate ability to accumulate nutrients (nitrogen and phosphorus) to create bioactive substances such as proteins, lipids, and carbohydrates (Khoo et al., 2019; Liu et al., 2020) for use in commercial applications from various marine environments. As a photosynthetic organism, algae carry out the process of photosynthesis, assimilating CO_2 and water into oxygen and biomass. For the removal of nutrients in wastewater, algae undergo the process of nitrogen assimilation and phosphorylation. Nitrogen assimilation is the process of converting inorganic nitrogen (such as nitrate, nitrite, ammonia, etc.) into its organic form (Barsanti & Gualtieri, 2005), which includes genes like ribonucleic acid (RNA) and deoxyribonucleic acid (DNA), proteins, peptides, enzymes, and energy transfer molecules like adenosine diphosphate (ADP) and adenosine triphosphate (ATP). Nitrate and nitrite reductase aid in the reduction of nitrate and nitrite to ammonium during the assimilation process. Ammonium is being incorporated into the intracellular amino acid glutamine (Gonçalves et al., 2017) with the help of glutamate and ATP. Phosphorylation is the process by which intracellular organic molecules (Su, 2021; Mohsenpour et al., 2021), including proteins, lipids, and nucleic acids, are formed from the inorganic phosphorus (H_2PO^{4-} and $HPO_4{}^{2-}$). The removal of nutrients is facilitated by MFCs through the utilization of algae to degrade organic matter and absorb excess nutrients. This enhances bioelectricity generation, making A-MFCs a sustainable solution for both nutrient removal and the production of renewable energy.

7.3.3 Algae for Heavy Metal Removal in Wastewater

The development of industrialization and civilization has raised the level of heavy metal pollution in the environment. Heavy metals may occur in the water ecosystem dissolved or in molecular form. The ions, including lead (Pb), cadmium (Cd), arsenic (As), chromium (Cr), mercury (Hg), etc., have the ability to accumulate on or in living organisms. This poses an ecological threat to the ecosystem due to its carcinogenic and toxic properties. The majority of the conventional methods (chemical precipitation, ion exchange, adsorption, and electrochemical processes) (Mata et al., 2008) are costly, cause inconvenience, and generate hazardous waste. Biological methods, such as biosorption and bioremediation, focus on removing inorganic pollutants from wastewater by binding metals in water with dead or living biological material. The concept of utilizing microorganisms as biosorbents for heavy metal ions has garnered significant attention due to their biological origin and low cost. The removal of heavy metals using microorganisms (Klimiuk & Łebkowska, 2005) is a rapid process; researchers have demonstrated that 85%–90% of all removed metals can be achieved in 15–20 min. Algae are a class of microorganisms with the highest sorption capacities, available in an unlimited supply (Romera et al., 2007; Klimmek et al., 2001), making them an effective biosorbent for heavy metals. Algae offer an infinite number of binding sites, high affinity for metal ions, and potential for recovery. In the sorption process, living biomass is more advantageous due to the continuous multiplication of microorganisms and simultaneous bioaccumulation (Bădescu et al., 2017), but dead biomass is also used to adsorb metal ions.

7.3.4 Algae for Treating EC-Polluted Wastewater

Algae have demonstrated significant potential in treating wastewater that contains novel pollutants, such as microplastics, endocrine-disrupting substances, pharmaceuticals, and personal care products. At low concentrations, these pollutants, which are frequently resistant to traditional treatment methods, pose serious threats to human health and the environment. Algae help remove harmful pollutants through processes such as biosorption, biodegradation, enzymatic breakdown, and photocatalytic activity when exposed to light. Bioremediation is a sustainable, solar-powered, and environmentally friendly reclamation method for treating emerging contaminant (EC) water using algae. The two primary techniques for removing EC are sorption and biodegradation. The sorption mechanism by algae is highly specific to the EC structure, the tendency to absorb EC, and the surrounding conditions. According to a study, ECs typically absorb activated wastewater more effectively than algal biomass. The study by Norvill et al. (2016) speculates that microalgae can use extracellular enzymes or heterotrophic biodegradation to break down specific EC contaminants. In a recent study that evaluated the removal of estrogens (Hom-Diaz et al., 2015) by live and dead algae (as a control), biodegradation was responsible for 20%–54% of the 60%–100% clearance. Another study supports (Liu et al., 2015) the detoxification response of microalgae biodegrading antibiotics.

7.4 Treatment Methods for the Separation and Dewatering of Microalgae Biomass

Algal biomass is valued for its potential in producing biofuels, but algae growth (0.02%–0.06% dry solids) renders it challenging to maintain a sustainable balance in the algal process. Due to the small size of algae (<30 μm) and high water content, the separation and dewatering process becomes technically challenging. The cell walls of healthy algae carry negative surface charges, which help keep a steady suspension. Microalgae are inherently difficult to extract from solution. One of the challenging areas in producing biofuel is the sustainable harvesting of microalgae, which limits the commercial use of algae. Filtration, flocculation, flotation, sedimentation, and a combination of these methods are a few of the separation and dewatering procedures. An outline of microalgal harvesting techniques and a summary of the advantages and disadvantages of each strategy are intended to be provided in this section.

7.4.1 Sedimentation

Sedimentation is a gravity-based separation process that causes the liquid or solid particles to separate from a liquid of different density. Typically, the sedimentation process is not used for harvesting algae. Researchers recommend this step as a pre-concentration step, in conjunction with the use of other harvesting techniques. It is one of the simplest, low-energy-consumption, and inexpensive pieces of equipment used as a treatment method. The limitations of this method include a slow process and a low efficiency for the small or motile species like microalgae.

7.4.2 Flocculation

Flocculation occurs when algae cells clump together in flocs, either naturally or as a result of the addition of a flocculant. It is an essential pretreatment step prior to other harvesting methods, as it increases the size of the particles, which speeds up the flotation or settling process. Limestone and multiple metallic salts (such as ferric chloride, ferric sulphate, and aluminum chloride) are used to eliminate the presence of suspended solids from wastewater. These salts are effective at eliminating microalgae from wastewater. These inorganic flocculants hinder the growth media and negatively affect microalgal viability, making them unusable. Cationic polyelectrolytes (positively charged, water-soluble polymers) are used as flocculants for the recovery of microalgae. Based on research, metal salts at lower concentrations (25 mg/L) can produce up to 35 times less biomass (Granados et al., 2012) than cationic polyelectrolytes. Microalgae are also recovered using non-ionic polymers at a lower concentration of 0.5–1 mg/L. Along with microalgae, microorganisms can cause flocculation and generate bio-flocculants. It has been demonstrated that the bacterium *Paenibacillus* sp. AM49 produces a bio-flocculant (Oh et al., 2001) that is efficient in harvesting *Chlorella vulgaris*. Every flocculation technique is not effective for every microalga species and habitat, considering the numerous flocculating agents available for algal harvesting. The decreased energy consumption is a clear advantage over other harvesting techniques.

7.4.3 Flotation

Flotation is a technique that elevates microalgae to the water or medium surface using tiny air bubbles that attach to the algal cells, causing them to float on the surface. Flotation is a process that is classified by the technique of producing bubbles. Dissolved air flotation (DAF), in which pressurized water that is fully air saturated is released into a flotation container at an ambient pressure, producing tiny particles that range in size from 10 to 100 μm. Lagoons that accumulate microalgal biomass are one of the most popular techniques for treating wastewater. According to a study by Edzwald, DAF is more effective than sedimentation when combined with chemical flocculation. The significant energy needed to pressurize the water is one of the disadvantages of using DAF. Dispersed air flotation, also referred to as foam or froth flotation, is a process where floating algae are present in a reactor with a high-speed mechanical rotator, where a steady stream of air is passed. The ensuing bubbles have a diameter of approximately 1 mm (Garg et al., 2012), which brings the algae cells to the surface, where they accumulate as foam. The efficiency of this process is dependent on the microalgal species and growth conditions, and it highly relies on hydrophobic interactions. Harvesting of microalgae can be accomplished efficiently by combining flotation and flocculation. Flocculation aggregates the cells and enhances bubble attachment, while flotation rapidly removes the formed flocs from the liquid. When compared to sedimentation (Sharma et al., 2013), this method is rapid and can eliminate 95% of the algae in less than 20 min. This process incurs significant operating expenses, as the tiny bubbles are essential for the process to function. The cost of flotation may be comparable to or higher than that of centrifugation, considering the expenses associated with flocculants, surfactants, and energy costs. It is a fast and scalable method for removing microalgae from wastewater; however, the high energy and equipment costs, especially for DAF systems, limit the feasibility of the flotation process.

7.4.4 Filtration

Filtration is considered a simpler and more cost-effective physical separation method for removing algae from wastewater. In this medium, the liquid is passed through a porous medium that retains the algae cells while allowing the treated water to pass through. Microfiltration (pore size: 0.1–10 μm) is the most common filtration method for algae recovery; however, large or flocculated cells might be treated using the macrofiltration method. Limitations include maintenance of the membrane, fouling, and pumping; the method of membrane filtration (Sharma et al., 2013) is expensive for large-scale operations. The wastewater sector has researched belt filters and rotary vacuum filters for microalgae harvesting. In a study, Mohn and co-workers showed that a rotary vacuum filter can be used for microalgae species like *Coelastrum* to 18% dry weight (Mohn, 1988), but harvesting smaller microalgae using belt or rotary vacuum filters would remain ineffective. Forward osmosis (FO) has been recently proven to be an effective separation process for the production of biofuel. By applying the osmotic pressure generated by an ionic strength gradient to drive the process, this approach uses less energy than conventional filtration methods. FO has been proposed as a cost-effective method in dewatering freshwater microalgae by the NASA OMEGA project and other research studies. Low flow rates (4 $L/h.m^{-2}$) and limitation to freshwater cultivation are two drawbacks of this method (Buckwalter et al., 2013). Filtration is often used as a polishing step after techniques like flocculation (to remove aggregated algae), sedimentation (to clarify the effluent), and filtration (to remove residual suspended algae) have been completed. It is a reliable method for the removal of microalgae; however, it requires good filter selection, maintenance, and possible integration with other steps to overcome fouling and cost issues.

7.4.5 Drying

It is the final dewatering step that helps in the removal of water for long-term processing and storage. Due to the high enthalpy of water (Sharma et al., 2013), other dewatering methods are preferred (as mentioned above) before the drying step. Some of the prevalent techniques for drying microalgae include spray drying, drum drying, freeze drying, and solar drying. Among these, spray and freeze-drying techniques are expensive. The simplest and lowest-cost method is the sun-drying method, but it requires a large area of land. Drying the algal biomass can be converted to biofuels or used as biofertilizers. In the wastewater treatment process, drying ensures safe and efficient use of harvested microalgae.

7.5 Bioenergy Generation

The pretreatment of the algal biomass before its processing is a crucial step in enhancing the efficiency of processes such as biofuel production, bioethanol fermentation, and biogas generation using algal biomass. The cell walls of most microalgae are resistant, which lowers the conversion efficiency of biofuel. Therefore, pretreatment technologies are used to break or disrupt the cell wall, thereby increasing the accessibility of intracellular compounds and improving bioconversion yields. These techniques can be broadly categorized into three categories: physical (thermal and mechanical), chemical, and biological. The most effective pretreatments for disrupting microalgae cells are considered to be the physical methods. By using heat or mechanical agitation (such as microwaves and sonication), the crystalline structures within the cell wall break down. Although heat pretreatment has been extensively studied, its effects differ based on the microalgae species. Physical methods, including sonication and microwave pretreatments (Passos et al., 2014), require more energy, and they are usually less dependent on microalgae species. Repeated freeze-thaw cycles cause the formation of ice crystals, which rupture the cell walls of the microalgal species. Chemical pretreatments utilize acid and alkali reagents to solubilize or hydrolyze components of the algal cell wall, such as cellulose, hemicellulose, and polysaccharides. Chemical pretreatments (Passos et al., 2014) have been found to be highly effective when combined with heat; however, their commercial application is limited by chemical contamination. Biological pretreatments, or the use of enzymes (cellulases, hemicellulases, and proteases), break down the components of the cell wall, but the research is limited. Biohydrogen is primarily produced through biological routes, such as dark fermentation, photofermentation, and photobiological processes, which utilize a wide range of readily degradable substrates, including carbohydrates, organic waste, and simple sugars. In these processes, microorganisms (e.g., *Clostridium*, *Enterobacter*, or photosynthetic bacteria) metabolize the substrates under anaerobic or light-driven conditions to release hydrogen gas as a byproduct. In contrast to bioethanol, biomethane, and biodiesel production, biohydrogen generation does not require any pretreatment process. Overall, pretreatment technologies are crucial for unlocking the full potential of algal biomass in bioenergy and bioproduct applications. Selecting an appropriate pretreatment method can significantly enhance conversion efficiency, product yield, and process sustainability.

7.5.1 Biodiesel Production from Microalgae

Microalgae have emerged as a promising resource for biodiesel production due to their high lipid content (20%–50% [wt/wt]), rapid growth rates, and ability to thrive on non-arable land using wastewater or saline water. Lipid productivity is a crucial factor when selecting algal species for biofuel production. Although microalgae like *Botryococcus braunii* have a lipid content of up to 75% of their dry biomass weight, a higher lipid content is linked to poor growth and low efficiency. In comparison to freshwater, microalgae isolated from industrial wastewater produced 3 to 10 times better biomass and lipid productivity when supplemented with various organic carbon substrates. To improve the quality and quantity of biodiesel production, the role of pretreatment techniques, such as lipid extraction and transesterification, comes into play. Transesterification, also known as an ester exchange reaction, of lipid feedstock (such as vegetable or animal fats) produces biodiesel, a mixture of fatty acid alkyl esters. These raw materials are primarily made up of triglycerides (90%–98%), with trace amounts of free fatty acids, monoglycerides, and diglycerides. It is a process that helps in the conversion of triglycerides into esters.

In 2021, Singh and co-workers cultivated *Chlorella minutissima* (a microalgae species) in a 1500 L open pond (Sharma et al., 2021) using commercially available fertilizers and explored the microwave-assisted transesterification process. They observed a 90.21% biodiesel yield at 69.93 °C with a 6-min reaction time. The species *Spirulina maxima* was transesterified in two phases, with methanol (Rahman et al., 2017) being used in the first step and potassium hydroxide (KOH) in the second. As a result, 86.1% biodiesel was produced. A wet algal paste produced from *Microchloropsis gaditana* (*N. gaditana*) B3 was trans-esterified using lipase (López et al., 2016) Novozyme 435 from *Cinachyra antarctica*, showing a 99.5% rate of conversion to biodiesel. To achieve high biodiesel production, it is necessary to optimize the parameters for biomass pretreatment. Recent developments and process intensification are pushing this technology closer to commercialization. The future of green energy highly depends on microalgal-based biodiesel production.

7.5.2 Bioethanol from Algal Metabolites

Bioethanol is a renewable biofuel derived from sugar-rich crops, such as sugarcane. However, algae species have recently received increasing attention as a third-generation feedstock. Bioethanol can be produced from a range of biomass feedstocks, including cheap lignin-based biomass linked to second-generation feedstock or easily fermentable starches and sugars paired to first-generation feedstock. Since microalgae have a high lipid content and are rich in carbohydrates, which can be fermented into ethanol, they are considered a source of biofuel. The fermentation of bioethanol produces CO_2 in large amounts as a byproduct. This drawback can be resolved by combining the production of carbohydrate-rich microalgae (Ho et al., 2011) with bioethanol fermentation. In 2023, Yirgu and co-workers found that when *Scenedesmus* sp. is grown in anaerobically digested brewery wastewater, it achieves the maximum production of carbohydrates (222.59 ± 3.16 mg g^{-1}). When the microwave pretreatment method is employed, the yield for reducing sugars is 150.52 ± 5.57 mg g^{-1}. Within 24 hrs of the fermentation period, this produced the highest bioethanol (Yirgu et al., 2023) yield (0.1 gg^{-1} of lipid-extracted biomass). In another study by Condor et al. (2024), wastewater was used as a healthy medium to produce Chlorella FSP-E, and under optimal conditions, the maximum bioethanol output was 0.22 ± 0.01 g ethanol g-biomass-1. Simultaneous saccharification and fermentation (SSF) and separate hydrolysis and fermentation (SHF) are two processes used to convert microalgal hydrolysates into bioethanol. SHF offers ideal conditions, such as pH, revolutions per minute (rpm), and temperature, for both fermentation and hydrolysis. SHF provides benefits such as cost-effective chemicals and equipment (Lee et al., 2017), as the hydrolysis and fermentation stages are conducted in two separate systems. In accordance with a study by Chng et al., bioethanol (Chng et al., 2018) produced from *Scenedesmus dimorphus UTEX 1234* and *Saccharomyces cerevisiae subsp. diastaticus* (*S. diastaticus*) using SSF in a single step produced roughly 0.0214 g g^{-1} of bioethanol. Additionally, a study comparing SSF and SHF was conducted by Kim and coworkers, which showed that the SSF process (Kim et al., 2017) produced approximately 2.7 mg mL^{-1} of bioethanol from *Porphyridium cruentum*, whereas the SHF method produced 0.61 mg mL^{-1} of bioethanol. With continued growing research, algal bioethanol is moving closer to becoming an environmentally friendly energy solution.

7.5.3 Biomethane Production by Microalgae

As microalgae species are enriched with carbohydrates, they make them a suitable feedstock for biomethane production by fermentation. Biomethane is a renewable biofuel primarily composed of methane (CH_4) and produced through anaerobic digestion (AD) of organic matter. Several challenges are faced in the conversion of biomethane from microalgae, including rigid cell walls (such as those of *Chlorella vulgaris*), which limit digestibility; lower C/N ratios (6 to 10), which lead to ammonia inhibition, high water content, and a slow biodegradation process, *resulting in* poor methane yields. In the year 2007, Yen and Brune studied the AD of *Scenedesmus* and *Chlorella* species (Yen & Brune, 2007) and reported methane yields of 0.2–0.3 m^3 CH_4/kg volatile solids. In 2011, Ehimen et al. demonstrated that lipid-extracted algae residues (Ehimen et al., 2011) could produce 60%–70% of the methane compared to raw biomass. Ward et al. (2014) investigated the anaerobic digestion of *Scenedesmus* and *Chlorella vulgaris*, which were grown as part of an integrated wastewater pond system. The results showed that biomethane fermentation from these microalgae species requires less energy than biodiesel production, even if they produce less methane (Ward et al., 2014) than regular freshwater microalgae (high N concentrations in wastewater). The approach of co-digestion with carbon-rich waste (food waste) improves the C/N ratio. In 2011, Ras and co-workers co-digested *Chlorella* with sludge (Ras et al., 2011) and achieved a 60% increase in methane yield. Pretreatment techniques, including ultrasonication, enzymatic treatment, etc., help break down the tough cell walls of algae and improve digestibility. Biomethane production is a viable and sustainable pathway for generating renewable energy. When integrated with wastewater treatment, this approach holds tremendous potential for a circular, low-carbon bioeconomy.

7.5.4 Microalgal Hydrogen Production

Green algae can be used to produce molecular hydrogen (H_2) through a process known as fermentative metabolism. Algae (especially green microalgae) utilize special enzymes to convert sunlight and water into hydrogen during photosynthesis under certain conditions. In anaerobic conditions, microalgae species such as *Scenedesmus* sp., *Chlorella pyrenoidosa*, and *Chlamydomonas moewusii* have demonstrated the ability to produce H_2 (Vijayaraghavan et al., 2010). The ability of freshwater algae species to generate hydrogen (Gaffron & Rubin, 1942) was studied under various conditions (2–4 h and alternating light and dark periods), and

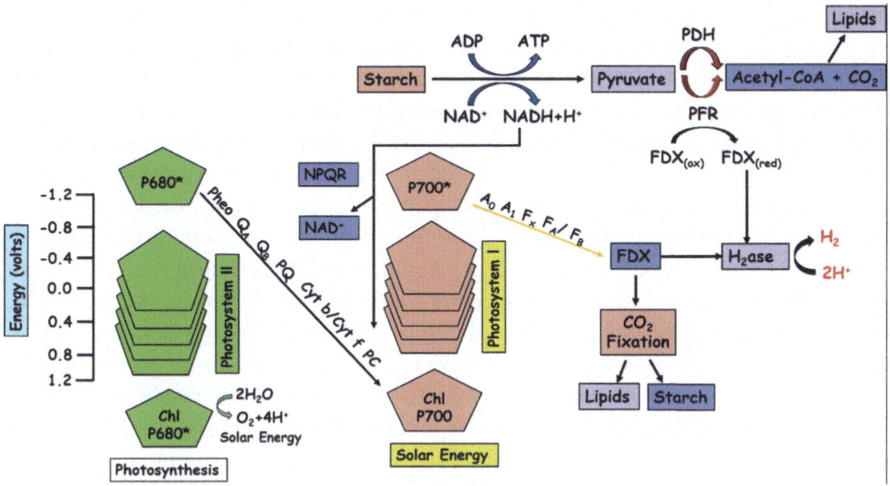

Fig. 7.4 A simplified illustration (photosynthetic and glycolytic pathways) of the pathways used for lipid, starch, and H_2 production in eukaryotic microalgae. The abbreviations mentioned in the above figure are discussed herein [(i) ADP adenosine diphosphate, (ii) ATP adenosine triphosphate, (iii) NAD^+ nicotinamide adenine dinucleotide (+ indicates it is in its oxidized form), (iv) NADH nicotinamide adenine dinucleotide (with hydrogen) (reduced form), (v) PDH pyruvate dehydrogenase complex, (vi) CO_2 carbon dioxide, (vii) Acetyl-CoA acetyl group attached to a co-enzyme A, (viii) PFR pyruvate-ferredoxin oxidoreductase, (ix) H_2ase hydrogenase, (x) Pheo pheophytin, (xi) FDX ferredoxin, (xii) FDX(ox) oxidized ferredoxin, (xiii) FDX(red) reduced ferredoxin, (xiv) NPQR NAD(P)H-plastoquinone oxidoreductase,(xv) Q_A and Q_B plastoquinone electron acceptors in photosystem (II), (xvi) Chl P700 chlorophyll pigment 700 of photosystem II, (xvii) Chl P680 chlorophyll pigment 680 of photosystem I, (xviii) PQ plastoquinone, (xix) PC plastocyanin, (xx) Cyt b/Cyt f cytochrome b6f complex, (xxi) A_0 chlorophyll a, (xxii) A_1 phylloquinone, (xxiii) F_x iron-sulfur clusters (intermediate electron acceptor), (xxiv) F_A/F_B iron-sulfur clusters (terminal electron acceptors)]

it was found that the species produced 49%, 85%, and 88% hydrogen content, respectively.

The biological mechanism of converting light energy into chemical energy is discussed in Fig. 7.4. In the thylakoid membranes, this photosynthetic process is carried out, which begins with light absorption by pigment molecules (carotenoids, phycobilins, and chlorophylls) that interact with light-harvesting protein complexes. These complexes are connected to two multimembrane protein complexes: Photosystem I (PSI) and Photosystem II (PSII). PS I and PS II have been identified as P700 and P680 (P means pigment) for their respective chlorophyll. The light energy is absorbed by the pigments, exciting electrons in P680, where water molecules split into oxygen ($2H2O \rightarrow O2 + 4H^+ + 4e^-$). This process releases oxygen, and electrons are transferred along the photosynthetic electron-transport chain by plastoquinone (PQ), the cytochrome *b6/f* complex (*Cyb6/f*), plastocyanin (PC), PS I, and ferredoxin (FDX). Oxygenic phototrophs (green algae, cyanobacteria, etc.) extract electrons along with protons, which are used in the reduction of PQ and NAD^+ and serve as metabolic energy sources. Compared to other internal processes, they are capable of producing H_2 in anaerobic environments by hydrogenase-mediated proton reduction (or nitrogenase). Ferredoxin/NADH then transduces the protons and electrons, obtained from water oxidation, to hydrogenase. As a result, the photosynthetically reduced ferredoxin (or NADH), which connects hydrogenase (or nitrogenase) to the electron transport chain (Prince & Kheshgi, 2005), may serve as an electron donor for hydrogenase. The hydrogenase present in the chloroplast is oxygen-sensitive (PS II releases oxygen); the rate of H_2 generation in photosynthetic species is relatively low. Enhancement of respiration, photochemical reduction of oxygen by PS I, and reversible suppression of oxygen evolution in PS II (Kruse et al., 2005) are some of the mechanisms that can reduce the concentration of oxygen. Among these, a sulfur-control mechanism is commonly employed to deplete oxygen. Melis et al. introduced the method of sulfur deprivation to produce hydrogen in green algae. A reversible decrease in photosynthetic rate has been observed, resulting in PS II becoming inactive. This drives cellular respiration to "anaerobiosis," which initiates the evolution of H_2 by hydrogenase. However, sulfur control is difficult in the case of wastewater. According to a study by Hwang et al., microalgae instantly produced oxygen when anaerobic effluent's acetate concentration was above the critical level (<15 mM). This study hypothesized that anaerobic conditions (Laurinavichene et al., 2008) could be achieved in actual wastewater, even in the absence of sulfur control, by maintaining acetate concentrations above 15 mM. This suggests that fermenter effluent may be utilized as an oxygen regulator and growth medium for the synthesis of hydrogen by microalgae. The species *Chlorella vulgaris*, which exhibits hydrogenase activity in relation to atmospheric oxygen levels, was studied by Hwang and colleagues in 2014. The finding suggested that an oxygen-tolerant [FeFe] hydrogenase (Hwang et al., 2014) has been identified in eukaryotic microalgae. This might offer a possibility to develop an artificial hydrogenase that is resistant to oxygen.

7.6 Challenges of Algae-Based MFC Design and Operation

Despite the growing interest in A-MFCs as an eco-friendly approach to coupling wastewater treatment with bioelectricity generation, several significant challenges must be addressed before large-scale implementation is feasible. To provide a consolidated overview of recent progress in this field, a summary of studies related to algae-based microbial fuel cells is presented in Table 7.1, highlighting their system configurations, electrode and membrane materials, key findings, and references. A major technical constraint is the undesired diffusion of oxygen from the algal biocathode into the anodic compartment. Since the anode chamber requires strict anaerobic conditions for optimal activity of electrogenic bacteria, oxygen intrusion can result in a loss of electrons to aerobic respiration pathways, thereby decreasing coulombic efficiency and power output. Additionally, maintaining robust algal growth within the system is operationally demanding, as it requires consistent light exposure, optimal temperature, and a reliable supply of carbon dioxide, which are difficult to control in open or large-scale reactor configurations. Limited light penetration in turbid or high-strength wastewater further restricts algal

Table 7.1 Studies related to algal-based microbial fuel cell for wastewater treatment and bioenergy generation

System study	Electrode material	Membrane	Key findings	Reference
Photosynthetic MFC with algae in cathode chamber	Carbon veil anode and carbon cloth cathode	Not reported	Stable power output; algae oxygenated cathode and sustained system.	Gajda et al. (2017)
Fresh algal-biomass MFC to produce energy	Carbon fiber veil anode and carbon fiber veil cathode	Terracotta membrane	A theoretical 42 W per cubic meter of fresh culture (6–10^5 cells mL^{-1}) was achieved. The algal biomass does not need any pretreatment.	Walter et al. (2015)
Photosynthetic algae microbial fuel cell for bioenergy generation	Carbon felt anode and carbon fiber cloth cathode	Nafion 117	Urea as nitrogen source promoted the power generation and CO2 sequestration. B-PAMFC is an energy-positive system with a maximum net energy of 1.824 kWh m^{-3}.	Li et al. (2019)
Photosynthetic microbial fuel cell for wastewater treatment	The cathode and anode chambers were made of acrylic sheets.	Cation exchange membrane	Under continuous illumination, PMFC with UDW (untreated domestic water) achieved a maximum working voltage 33% higher than that of WTW (wetland-treated wastewater).	Ullah (2024)
Single-chamber and double-chamber-microbial fuel cell for energy conversion	H-type Plexiglass identical bottles for both cathode and anode.	Polyethersulfone (PES)	The cathode-based algal double chamber fuel cells generated the highest power density along with the best	Mahmoud et al. (2021)

(continued)

Table 7.1 (continued)

System study	Electrode material	Membrane	Key findings	Reference
			removal of COD content.	
Algae-based microbial fuel cell was developed to enhance cathodic reactions.	Stainless steel mesh as anode and carbon felt as cathode.	Exterior wall of earthen pots was used as a separator.	MFC with biocathode efficiently removed COD (>75%) of waste stream. MFC with bio-cathode exhibited higher power density of 54.48 mW m^{-2}.	Yadav et al. (2020)
Single-chamber air cathode MFC	The plain graphite felt and platinum-coated carbon cloth served as the anode and cathode electrodes.	Pre-treated proton exchange membrane	MFCs supplemented with raw algae and raw algae with acetate clearly showed higher power density, greater current generation, and improved removal of COD (chemical oxygen demand).	Kondaveeti et al. (2019)
Microalgal-based photoautotrophic microbial fuel cell (PMFC) for bioenergy recovery	Carbon brushes were used as electrodes in both anode and cathode.	Nafion 117	Microalgae in the cathodic chamber greatly affected nutrients removal and/or recovery, with 27.7%–50.0% and 37.1%–67.9% of N and P removal amounts in the PMFC, respectively.	Wang et al. (2019)
Microbial fuel cell and a membrane photobioreactor.	The cathode electrode was a piece of carbon cloth coated with activated carbon and carbon brush used as an anode electrode.	Cation exchange membrane	The highest energy production of 0.205 kWh m^{-3} was obtained with the highest algal biomass production.	Tse et al. (2016)

(continued)

Table 7.1 (continued)

System study	Electrode material	Membrane	Key findings	Reference
Photosynthetic microbial fuel cell	Both anode and cathode are made of bare carbon felt.	The wall of the clayware cylinder as proton exchange membrane	Cu(II) dosed algal biomass yielded 1.2 times higher lipid with 14% lower biomass growth than control algal biomass.	Das et al. (2024)

photosynthetic efficiency, which in turn affects oxygen availability at the cathode. Another significant challenge lies in the selection and coexistence of compatible algal and bacterial consortia.

7.7 Conclusion

Wastewater contains a diverse and dynamic microbiome, along with potentially inhibitory substances, which can disrupt the stability and functional synergy between algae and electrogenic microbes. Moreover, biofilm formation on electrodes, although necessary for microbial colonization, can become detrimental if it becomes overgrown, leading to increased internal resistance and decreased electron transfer rates. Fouling and clogging of electrodes during long-term operation can further impair system performance and increase maintenance requirements. High internal resistance remains a critical barrier in A-MFC systems, often attributed to suboptimal electrode spacing, poor ionic conductivity of the electrolyte, and the use of low-efficiency electrode materials. These factors collectively reduce the overall power density and energy recovery from the system. Furthermore, scaling up A-MFCs from laboratory setups to pilot or industrial-scale reactors introduces complex engineering challenges. Ensuring homogeneous distribution of light, nutrients, and electrochemical gradients becomes increasingly difficult, affecting both treatment efficiency and energy output. Economically, the cost of high-performance materials, such as carbon-based electrodes, light sources, and reactor infrastructure, is currently a limiting factor, especially in developing regions where cost-effective treatment options are most needed. In addition, the operational sustainability of A-MFCs is threatened by seasonal and environmental fluctuations. Changes in temperature, light intensity, and wastewater composition can result in inconsistent system performance. To address these limitations, ongoing research is exploring advanced materials, such as nanostructured and conductive biofilms, as well as synthetic biological approaches to engineer more resilient algal-bacterial communities. Future efforts should also focus on integrating A-MFCs with other renewable technologies and circular bioeconomy models to enhance their feasibility and commercial potential.

References

Bădescu, I. S., Bulgariu, D., & Bulgariu, L. (2017). Alternative utilization of algal biomass (Ulva sp.) loaded with Zn (II) ions for improving of soil quality. *Journal of Applied Phycology, 29*, 1069–1079.

Barsanti, L., & Gualtieri, P. (2005). *Algae: Anatomy, biochemistry, and bio technology*. CRC Press.

Batista, A. P., Ambrosano, L., Graça, S., Sousa, C., Marques, P. A. S. S., Ribeiro, B., Botrel, E. P., Castro Neto, P., & Gouveia, L. (2015). Combining urban wastewater treatment with biohydrogen production– An integrated microalgae-based approach. *Bioresource Technology, 184*, 230–235.

Buckwalter, P., Embaye, T., Gormly, S., & Trent, J. D. (2013). Dewatering microalgae by forward osmosis. *Desalination, 312*, 19.

Caprariis, B. D., Filippis, P. D., Battista, A. D., Palma, L. D., & Scarsella, M. (2014). Exoelectrogenic activity of a green microalgae, *Chlorella vulgaris*, in a bio−photovoltaic cells (BPVs). *Chemical Engineering Transactions, 38*, 523–528.

Cheah, W. Y., Ling, T. C., Show, P. L., Juan, J. C., Chang, J.-S., & Lee, D.-J. (2016). Cultivation in wastewaters for energy: A microalgae platform. *Applied Energy, 179*, 609–625.

Chng, L. M., Teo, K. S., Chan, D. J. C., Lee, K. T., & Toh, P. Y. (2018). Fermentation of microalgae biomass through mild acid pretreatment for bioethanol production. *Journal of Energy Safety Technology, 2*, 15–22.

Commault, A. S., Lear, G., & Novis, P. (2014). Photosynthetic biocathode enhances the power output of a sediment−type microbial fuel cell. *New Zealand Journal of Botany, 52*, 48–59.

Condor, B. E., de Luna, M. D. G., Lacson, C. F. Z., Acebu, P. I. G., Abarca, R. R. M., Nagarajan, D., Lee, D.-J., & Chang, J.-S. (2024). Effects of carbon dioxide concentration and swine wastewater on the cultivation of Chlorella vulgaris FSP-E and bioethanol production from microalgae biomass. *Applied Energy, 369*, 123617.

Das, S., Kumar, S., Mehta, A. K., & Ghangreka, M. M. (2024). Heavy metals removal by algae and usage of activated metal-enriched biomass as cathode catalyst for improving performance of photosynthetic microbial fuel cell. *Bioresource Technology, 406*, 131038.

Ehimen, E. A., Sun, Z. F., Carrington, C. G., Birch, E. J., & Eaton-Rye, J. J. (2011). Anaerobic digestion of microalgae residues resulting from the biodiesel production process. *Applied Energy, 88*, 3454–3463.

Fu, C.-C., Hung, T.-C., Wu, W.-T., Wen, T.-C., & Su, C.-H. (2010). Current and voltage responses in instant photosynthetic microbial cells with *Spirulina platensis*. *Biochemical Engineering Journal, 52*, 175–180.

Gaffron, H., & Rubin, J. (1942). Fermentation and photo chemical products of hydrogen in algae. *The Journal of General Physiology, 26*, 219.

Gajda, I., Greenman, J., Melhuish, C., & Ieropoulos, I. (2015). Self−sustainable electricity production from algae grown in a microbial fuel cell system. *Biomass Bioenergy, 82*, 87–93.

Gajda, I., Greenman, J., Melhuish, C., & Ieropoulos, I. (2017). Photosynthetic cathodes for microbial fuel cells. *Energy & Environmental Science, 10*(3), 818–827.

Garg, S., Li, Y., Wang, L., & Schenk, P. M. (2012). Flotation of marine microalgae: Effect of algal hydrophobicity. *Bioresource Technology, 121*, 471.

Gonçalves, A. L., Pires, J. C. M., & Simões, M. (2017). A review on the use of micro algal consortia for wastewater treatment. *Algal Research, 24*, 403–415.

Granados, M., Acie'n, F., Gomez, C., Fernandez-Sevilla, J., & Grima, E. M. (2012). Evaluation of flocculants for the recovery of freshwater microalgae. *Bioresource Technology, 118*, 102.

He, Z., Kan, J., Mansfeld, F., Angenent, L. T., & Nealson, K. H. (2009). Self−sustained phototrophic microbial fuel cells based on the synergistic cooperation between photosynthetic microorganisms and heterotrophic bacteria. *Environmental Science & Technology, 43*, 1648–1654.

Ho, S.-H., Chen, C.-Y., Lee, D.-J., & Chang, J.-S. (2011). Perspectives on microalgal CO2-emission mitigation systems—A review. *Biotechnology Advances, 29*, 189.

Hom-Diaz, A., Llorca, M., Rodríguez-Mozaz, S., Vicent, T., Barceló, D., & Blánquez, P. (2015). Microalgae cultivation on wastewater digestate: B-estradiol and 17a-ethynylestradiol degradation and transformation products identification. *Journal of Environmental Management, 155*, 106.

Hussain, F., Shah, S. Z., Ahmad, H., Abubshait, S. A., Abubshait, H. A., Laref, A., Manikandan, A., Kusuma, H. S., & Iqbal, M. (2021). Microalgae an ecofriendly and sustainable wastewater treatment option: Biomass application in biofuel and bio fertilizer production. A review. *Renewable and Sustainable Energy Reviews, 137*, 110603.

Hwang, J. H., Kabra, A. N., Kim, J. R., & Jeon, B.-H. (2014). Photoheterotrophic microalgal hydrogen production using acetate-and butyrate-rich wastewater effluent. *Energy, 78*, 887.

Khatri, N., Khatri, K. K., & Sharma, A. (2020). Enhanced energy saving in wastewater treatment plant using dissolved oxygen control and hydrocyclone. *Environmental Technology & Innovation, 18*, 100678.

Khoo, C. G., Dasan, Y. K., Lam, M. K., & Lee, K. T. (2019). Algae biorefinery: Review on a broad spectrum of downstream processes and products. *Bioresource Technology, 292*, 121964.

Kim, H. M., Oh, C. H., & Bae, H. J. (2017). Comparison of red microalgae (*Porphyridium cruentum*) culture conditions for bioethanol production. *Bioresource Technology, 233*, 44–50.

Klimiuk, E., & Łebkowska, M. (2005). *Biotechnology in environmental protection*. PWN. (in Polish).

Klimmek, S., Stan, H. J., & Wilke, A. (2001). Comparative analysis of the biosorption of cadmium, lead, nickel and zinc by alga. *Environmental Science & Technology, 35*, 4283–4288.

Kondaveeti, S., Mohanakrishna, G., Pagolu, R., Kim, I. W., Kalia, V. C., & Lee, J. K. (2019). Bioelectrogenesis from raw algal biomass through microbial fuel cells: Effect of acetate as co-substrate. *Indian Journal of Microbiology, 59*, 22–26.

Kruse, O., Rupprecht, J., Bader, K.-P., Thomas-Hall, S., Schenk, P. M., Finazzi, G., & Hankamer, B. (2005). Improved photobiological H_2 production in engineered green algal cells. *The Journal of Biological Chemistry, 280*, 34170.

Laurinavichene, T. V., Kosourov, S. N., Ghirardi, M. L., Seibert, M., & Tsygankov, A. A. (2008). Prolongation of H2 photo production by immobilized, sulfur-limited *Chlamydomonas reinhardtii* cultures. *Journal of Biotechnology, 134*, 275.

Lee, S. Y., Cho, J. M., Chang, Y. K., & Oh, Y. K. (2017). Cell disruption and lipid extraction for microalgal biorefineries: A review. *Bioresource Technology, 244*(Pt 2), 1317–1328.

Li, M., Zhou, M., Luo, J., Tan, C., Tian, X., Su, P., & Gu, T. (2019). Carbon dioxide sequestration accompanied by bioenergy generation using a bubbling-type photosynthetic algae microbial fuel cell. *Bioresource Technology, 280*, 95–103.

Li, M., Zhou, M., Tian, X., Tan, C., & McDaniel, C. T. (2020). Algae-based microbial fuel cells for sustainable energy generation and wastewater treatment: A review. *Bioresource Technology, 313*, 123708.

Liu, Y., Wang, F., Chen, X., Zhang, J., & Gao, B. (2015). Cellular responses and biodegradation of amoxicillin in Microcystis aeruginosa at different nitrogen levels. *Ecotoxicology and Environmental Safety, 111*, 138.

Liu, J., Pemberton, B., Lewis, J., Scales, P. J., & Martin, G. J. O. (2020). Wastewater treatment using filamentous algae - A review. *Bioresource Technology, 298*, 22556.

Logan, B. E., Hamelers, B., Rozendal, R., Schröder, U., Keller, J., Freguia, S., & Rabaey, K. (2006). Microbial fuel cells: Methodology and technology. *Environmental Science & Technology, 40*(17), 5181–5192.

López, E. N., Medina, A. R., Cerdán, L. E., Moreno, P. A., Sánchez, M. D., & Grima, E. M. (2016). Fatty acid methyl ester production from wet microalgal biomass by lipase-catalyzed direct transesterification. *Biomass and Bioenergy, 93*, 6–12.

Mahmoud, R. H., Samhan, F. A., Ibrahim, M. K., Ali, G. H., & Hassan, R. Y. A. (2021). Waste to energy conversion utilizing nanostructured algal-based microbial fuel cells. *Electrochemical Science Advances, 2*(6), e2100071.

Mata, Y. N., Blázquez, M. L., Ballester, A. M., González, F. R., & Muñoz, J. A. (2008). Characterization of the biosorption of cadmium, lead and copper with the brown alga Fucus vesiculosus. *Journal of Hazardous Materials, 158*, 316–323.

Mohn, F. H. (1988). Harvesting of microalgal biomass. In M. A. Borowitzka & L. J. Borowitzka (Eds.), *Microalgal bio technology* (p. 395). Cambridge University Press.

Mohsenpour, S. F., Hennige, S., Willoughby, N., Adeloye, A., & Gutierrez, T. (2021). Integrating micro-algae into wastewater treatment: A review. *Science of the Total Environment, 752*, 142168.

Nishio, K., Hashimoto, K., & Watanabe, K. (2013). Light/electricity conversion by defined cocultures of *Chlamydomonas* and *Geobacter*. *Journal of Bioscience and Bioengineering, 115*, 412–417.

Norvill, Z. N., Shilton, A., & Guieysse, B. (2016). Emerging contaminant degradation and removal in algal wastewater treatment ponds: Identifying the research gaps. *Journal of Hazardous Materials, 313*, 291.

Oh, H.-M., Lee, S. J., Park, M.-H., Kim, H.-S., Kim, H.-C., Yoon, J.-H., Kwon, G.-S., & Yoon, B.-D. (2001). Harvesting of Chlorella vulgaris using a bio-flocculant from *Paenibacillus* sp. AM49. *Biotechnology Letters, 23*, 1229.

Passos, F., Uggetti, E., Carrere, H., & Ferrer, I. (2014). Pretreatment of microalgae to improve biogas production: A review. *Bioresource Technology, 72*, 403.

Prince, R. C., & Kheshgi, H. S. (2005). The photobiological production of hydrogen: Potential efficiency and effective ness as a renewable fuel. *Critical Reviews in Microbiology, 31*, 19.

Rahman, M. A., Aziz, M. A., Al-khulaidi, R. A., Sakib, N., & Islam, M. (2017). Biodiesel production from microalgae Spirulina maxima by two step process: Optimization of process variable. *Journal of Radiation Research and Applied Science, 10*(2), 140–147.

Ras, M., Lardon, L., Bruno, S., & Steyer, J. P. (2011). Experimental study on a coupled process of production and anaerobic digestion of *Chlorella vulgaris*. *Bioresource Technology, 102*(1), 200–206.

Rawat, I., Ranjith Kumar, R., Mutanda, T., & Bux, F. (2011). Dual role of microalgae: Phycoremediation of domestic wastewater and biomass production for sustainable biofuels production. *Applied Energy, 88*(10), 3411–3424.

Romera, E., González, F., Ballester, A., Blázquez, M. L., & Muñoz, J. A. (2007). Comparative study of biosorption of heavy metals using different types of alga. *Bioresource Technology, 98*, 3344–3353.

Sharma, K. K., Garg, S., Li, Y., Malekizadeh, A., & Schenk, P. M. (2013). Critical analysis of current microalgae dewatering techniques. *Biofuels, 4*, 397.

Sharma, A. K., Sharma, A., Singh, Y., & Chen, W.-H. (2021). Production of a sustainable fuel from microalgae Chlorella minutissima grown in a 1500 L open raceway ponds. *Biomass and Bioenergy, 149*, 106073.

Strik, D. P. B. T. B., Terlouw, H., Hamelers, H. V. M., & Buisman, C. J. N. (2008). Renewable sustainable biocatalyzed electricity production in a photosynthetic algal microbial fuel cell (PAMFC). *Applied Microbiology and Biotechnology, 81*, 659–668.

Su, Y. (2021). Revisiting carbon, nitrogen, and phosphorus metabolisms in microalgae for wastewater treatment. *Science of the Total Environment, 762*, 144590.

Sutherland, D. L., Turnbull, M. H., & Craggs, R. J. (2015). Increased pond depth improves algal productivity and nutrient removal in wastewater treatment high-rate algal ponds. *Water Research, 70*, 9–19.

Tse, H. T., Luo, S., Li, J., & He, Z. (2016). Coupling microbial fuel cells with a membrane photobioreactor for wastewater treatment and bioenergy production. *Bioprocess and Biosystems Engineering, 39*, 1703–1710.

Ullah, Z. (2024). Effect of catholyte on performance of photosynthetic microbial fuel cell for wastewater treatment and energy recovery. *Renewable Energy, 221*, 119810.

Vijayaraghavan, K., Karthik, R., & Nalini, S. K. (2010). Hydrogen generation from algae: A review. *Journal of Plant Sciences, 5*, 1.

Walter, X. A., Greenman, J., Taylor, B., & Ieropoulos, I. A. (2015). Microbial fuel cells continuously fuelled by untreated fresh algal biomass. *Algal Research, 11*, 103–107.

Wang, Y., Lin, Z., Su, X., Zhao, P., Zhou, J., He, Q., & Ai., H. (2019). Cost-effective domestic wastewater treatment and bioenergy recovery in an immobilized microalgal-based photoautotrophic microbial fuel cell (PMFC). *Chemical Engineering Journal, 372*, 956–965.

Ward, A. J., Lewis, D. M., & Green, F. B. (2014). Anaerobic digestion of algae biomass: A review. *Algal Research, 5*, 204.

Yadav, G., Sharma, I., Ghangrekar, M., & Sen, R. (2020). A live bio-cathode to enhance power output steered by bacteria-microalgae synergistic metabolism in microbial fuel cell. *Journal of Power Sources, 449*, 227560.

Yap, J. K., Sankaran, R., Chew, K. W., Munawaroh, H. S., Ho, S. H., Banu, J. R., & Show, P. L. (2021). Advancement of green technologies: A comprehensive review on the potential application of microalgae biomass. *Chemosphere, 281*, 130886.

Yen, H. W., & Brune, D. E. (2007). Anaerobic co-digestion of algal sludge and waste paper to produce methane. *Bioresource Technology, 98*(1), 130–134.

Yirgu, Z., Leta, S., Hussen, A., Khan, M. M., & Aragaw, T. (2023). Pretreatment of lipid- extracted biomass of *Scenedesmus* sp. grown in wastewater for bioethanol production. *Biomass Conversion and Biorefinery, 14*(15), 16867–16878.

Zhang, Y., Noori, J. S., & Angelidaki, I. (2011). Simultaneous organic carbon, nutrients removal and energy production in a photomicrobial fuel cell (PFC). *Energy & Environmental Science, 4*, 4340–4346.

Algae in Circular Bioeconomy: Valorization of Algal Biomass Using Pyrolysis, Hydrothermal Liquefaction, and Gasification Techniques

8

Rojalini Samanta, Monika Kumari, Priyadarshini Banerjee, Kaushal Kant Verma, Anant Nag, and Kishanta Kumar Pradhan

Abstract

The transition toward a circular bioeconomy necessitates sustainable resource utilization, waste valorization, and renewable energy production. Algal biomass has emerged as a promising feedstock due to its rapid growth rate, ability to thrive in nonarable lands and wastewaters, and high biochemical composition, making it an ideal candidate for biofuel and biochemical production. However, to fully harness its potential, efficient conversion technologies must be implemented. This chapter explores the utilization of algal biomass through thermochemical conversion techniques, including pyrolysis, hydrothermal liquefaction (HTL), and gasification. The chapter provides a comparative assessment of these techniques based on their process parameters, product yields, environmental impact, and economic feasibility. Additionally, it highlights the role of algal biomass valorization in advancing a sustainable bioeconomy by integrating with existing biorefineries and reducing dependency on fossil-based resources. At the same time, this upgradation holds great promise; several technical, economic, and regulatory challenges remain, including high production costs, feedstock variability, and scalability issues. The chapter concludes by discussing potential future advancements in process intensification, biorefinery approaches, and policy frameworks that could facilitate the commercialization of algal biofuels and chemicals. Overall, the integration of algal biomass conversion

R. Samanta
Department of Pharmacy, Usha Martin University, Ranchi, Jharkhand, India

M. Kumari · P. Banerjee · K. K. Verma · A. Nag · K. K. Pradhan (✉)
Department of Pharmaceutical Sciences and Technology, Birla Institute of Technology - Mesra, Ranchi, India
e-mail: kkpradhan@bitmesra.ac.in

L. Kumar et al. (eds.), *Algal Bioremediation*,
https://doi.org/10.1007/978-981-95-8793-3_8

into the circular bioeconomy presents a viable pathway toward sustainable energy and resource management.

Keywords

Circular bioeconomy · Algal biomass · Pyrolysis · Hydrothermal liquefaction (HTL) · Gasification · Waste valorization · Sustainable energy · Environmental impact

8.1 Introduction

8.1.1 Overview of Circular Bioeconomy

The circular bioeconomy represents an integrated and transformative approach to sustainable development by combining the principles of the bioeconomy, which relies on renewable biological resources for producing energy, materials, and chemicals, with those of the circular economy, which emphasizes resource efficiency, waste reduction, and environmental regeneration. This model is gaining global attention as a critical pathway to address pressing socioeconomic and ecological challenges such as climate change, resource depletion, and pollution (Strategy, 2018). The circular bioeconomy can be defined as an economic system that sustainably utilizes renewable biological resources, recycles and reuses bio-based products, and returns nutrients to the environment in a way that mimics natural ecological cycles. It promotes closed loop use of biomass and encourages the adoption of technologies such as green chemistry, industrial symbiosis, and biotechnology to extract maximum value from resources while minimizing waste and emissions. A particularly promising aspect within this model is the integration of algae, especially microalgae, as a sustainable solution to multiple environmental and industrial challenges. Algae are versatile and highly productive organisms that can convert sunlight, carbon dioxide, and nutrients often derived from waste into valuable biomass. Their role in the circular bioeconomy is most prominent in areas such as wastewater treatment, nutrient recovery, and the generation of bioproducts. Microalgae are highly effective in recovering nutrients like nitrogen and phosphorus from municipal and industrial wastewater, both of which are essential for algal growth and biomass production (Ngo et al., 2022; Lens & Khandelwal, 2023). Algae-based wastewater treatment not only offers a sustainable and low-cost alternative to conventional methods but also contributes to carbon mitigation, with estimates suggesting the sequestration of approximately 1.83 kg of CO_2 per kg of dry algal biomass (Khan et al., 2018). Additionally, these systems can remove microplastics, heavy metals, and other contaminants, thereby enhancing the reusability of water and improving environmental safety (Lens & Khandelwal, 2023).

Beyond environmental remediation, algae are an invaluable feedstock for biorefineries, which can convert algal biomass into a diverse range of high-value bioproducts. These include biofuels such as biodiesel and bioethanol, bioplastics, biofertilizers, pigments, vitamins, omega-3 fatty acids, therapeutic agents, and nutraceuticals (Jasiūnas et al., 2021; Papadaki et al., 2024). Marine algae, in particular, are known to be rich in bioactive compounds and fine chemicals, making them highly suitable for pharmaceutical and food industry applications (Papadaki et al., 2024). The algal biorefinery concept aligns seamlessly with circular bioeconomy principles by ensuring that waste streams are repurposed and the entire biomass is utilized efficiently. This holistic approach enhances both the environmental and economic sustainability of the process. However, the commercial-scale adoption of algae-based systems still faces several challenges. These include the need to optimize cultivation conditions (e.g., light, temperature, and nutrient availability), reduce energy-intensive downstream processes (e.g., harvesting, drying, and extraction), and improve overall cost-effectiveness (Papadaki et al., 2024; Satya et al., 2023). Addressing these limitations requires ongoing investment in research and innovation, particularly in fields like metabolic engineering, synthetic biology, and process integration.

Key principles underpinning the circular bioeconomy include sustainable resource use, where biomass is sourced from agriculture, forestry, marine ecosystems, and organic waste; waste minimization, which involves reusing and converting biowaste into new products; resource efficiency, achieved by designing products that are recyclable, repairable, or biodegradable; and environmental regeneration, through practices that restore soil fertility, enhance biodiversity, and support ecosystem services (Strategy, 2018; De Schoenmakere et al., 2018). Algae-based systems naturally embody these principles, as they not only recycle nutrients and carbon but also contribute to food and energy security without competing for arable land. Core elements of the circular bioeconomy encompass a wide array of biological feedstocks, including crops, wood, algae, and organic waste; bioproducts such as biofuels, bioplastics, biochemicals, and biofertilizers; enabling technologies like anaerobic digestion, fermentation, enzymatic processing, and biorefineries; and systems integration, which aligns multiple sectors including agriculture, aquaculture, forestry, waste management, and manufacturing to create synergies and close resource loops. The benefits of such a model are multidimensional. Environmentally, it reduces dependence on fossil fuels, cuts greenhouse gas emissions, and converts waste materials into usable products. Economically, it fosters innovation, creates green jobs, and opens new markets for bio-based industries. Socially, it supports rural economies and enhances resilience by decentralizing production systems. It expedites the advancement of cleaner and more efficient processes and materials through technology (Strategy, 2018; Gawel et al., 2019).

Practical applications of the circular bioeconomy are already underway in several regions. Examples include biorefineries that convert agricultural residues into bioethanol and bioplastics, containers made from biodegradable materials derived from starch or cellulose, bioenergy production from algae or food waste, and circular agriculture systems that utilize composted food waste as an organic fertilizer. In the algal domain specifically, innovative projects are exploring integrated aquaculture systems where algae clean aquaculture wastewater while providing feed or bioactive extracts, thus creating a zero-waste, multi-output system (Jasiūnas et al., 2021;

Papadaki et al., 2024). On the global stage, the European Union's Bioeconomy Strategy (2018) explicitly incorporates circularity in the use of biomass and promotes sustainable production systems. The United Nations Sustainable Development Goals (SDGs), particularly SDG 12 (responsible consumption and production), SDG 13 (climate action), and SDG 7 (affordable and clean energy), align strongly with the objectives of the circular bioeconomy. International organizations such as the OECD and the Biofuture Platform are also advocating for cross-border cooperation, policy support, and public–private partnerships to scale up circular bio-based solutions (De Schoenmakere et al., 2018; Gawel et al., 2019). Despite its promise, the circular bioeconomy still faces significant hurdles. These include technological and infrastructural gaps, especially in the developing regions; the need for harmonized regulatory frameworks; market competition with conventional fossil-based products; and public awareness and consumer acceptance. Algae-based approaches, while innovative, must also overcome issues of scalability, economic feasibility, and standardization. Nonetheless, future directions are promising. With ongoing advancements in biotechnologies, the emergence of innovative circular farming systems, and the strengthening of international networks, the circular bioeconomy is poised to become a cornerstone of sustainable global development. In conclusion, the circular bioeconomy offers a comprehensive and forward-thinking strategy for transitioning away from the traditional linear, fossil-based economy toward a regenerative, resilient, and bio-based model. By integrating biological resource management with circular design principles and leveraging the immense potential of organisms like algae, it supports long-term environmental stewardship, economic prosperity, and social well-being. Continued innovation, investment, and cooperation across sectors and borders will be key to realizing the full potential of this transformative economic paradigm.

8.1.2 Role of Algae in Sustainable Bioresource Management

Algal biomass holds immense promise for advancing a circular bioeconomy, offering an innovative solution to modern environmental and economic challenges. With its rapid growth, ability to thrive in diverse environments, and capacity to sequester carbon dioxide, algae present a multifaceted opportunity to produce sustainable bioproducts while addressing critical issues such as greenhouse gas emissions, wastewater pollution, and solid waste management. One of the most compelling environmental benefits of algal cultivation is its ability to absorb carbon dioxide during photosynthesis, effectively reducing atmospheric CO_2 levels. This not only contributes to mitigating climate change but also enhances the sustainability profile of algal-based bioproducts (Chen et al., 2023). Algae can also play a pivotal role in wastewater treatment. They utilize nutrients such as nitrogen and phosphorus from wastewater, thereby improving water quality while simultaneously generating biomass for further use (Jasiūnas et al., 2021; Vellaiyan, 2024). This dual function supports both environmental remediation and resource recovery.

Algae are particularly rich in lipids and carbohydrates, making them an excellent feedstock for a variety of biofuels, including biodiesel, bioethanol, and biomethane. Their ability to grow in saline or wastewater environments means they don't compete with traditional crops for freshwater or arable land, further boosting their sustainability credentials (Geng et al., 2025; Sangtani et al., 2022). Beyond fuels, algae are a source of high-value compounds such as pigments, vitamins, antioxidants, and even therapeutic agents. These biochemicals have applications in pharmaceuticals, cosmetics, and the food industry, making algal biomass a versatile input in bio-based manufacturing (Vishwakarma et al., 2022; Kaushik et al., 2023). Once the valuable compounds are extracted, the residual biomass can still be utilized. It serves effectively as animal feed or organic fertilizer, contributing to agricultural sustainability and minimizing waste (Jasiūnas et al., 2021; Chen et al., 2023). To ensure the commercial feasibility of algal technologies, integrated biorefinery models have been proposed. These systems aim to maximize economic returns by using every component of the algal biomass to produce multiple outputs like fuels, chemicals, feed, and fertilizers, in one cohesive process (Vishwakarma et al., 2022; Kaushik et al., 2023). Moreover, by cultivating algae using waste nutrients from industrial effluents or wastewater, production costs can be significantly reduced. This makes the entire process more economically viable and ecologically sound (Vellaiyan, 2024). Emerging research is exploring how algae can be used to treat and valorize solid waste. By integrating algal systems into waste management, organic waste can be converted into valuable biomass, thus supporting waste reduction and resource circularity (Leong & Chang, 2023). This aligns with global goals of sustainable development and waste-to-resource strategies.

8.1.3 Importance of Biomass Valorization for Energy and Material Recovery

Biomass valorization plays a crucial role in advancing sustainable development by enabling the recovery of both energy and materials from renewable biological resources. This process helps reduce our dependence on fossil fuels and mitigates environmental impacts by converting biomass into valuable end products such as biofuels, chemicals, and sustainable materials. The following sections outline the key aspects of biomass valorization. In the realm of energy recovery, biofuels such as biobutanol emerge as promising, eco-friendly alternatives to conventional fossil fuels, contributing to lower greenhouse gas emissions and addressing concerns about fossil fuel depletion (Gupta et al., 2023). Additionally, innovative electrochemical processes enable the direct valorization of biomass-derived feedstocks, such as lignocellulose and glycerol, by converting them into high-performance fuels and organic chemicals through paired electrolysis, thereby enhancing both energy efficiency and economic viability (Chandrasekhar et al., 2021). On the material recovery front, biomass residues, such as ashes produced from thermochemical conversion, can be repurposed for valuable applications, including fertilizers and soil amendments, thereby reinforcing the principles of a circular economy (Adeniyi et al., 2024). A hierarchical approach to biomass valorization further ensures the prioritization of methods that generate the highest environmental and economic returns while maximizing resource efficiency (Cansado et al., 2025). However, despite its many advantages, the widespread adoption of biomass valorization still faces challenges related to technological scalability, cost-effectiveness, and potential environmental trade-offs. Overcoming these barriers through continued innovation and policy support is essential for harnessing the full potential of biomass in achieving long-term sustainability goals (Zografa kis et al., 2010).

8.2 Algal Biomass: A Renewable Resource

8.2.1 Composition and Biochemical Properties of Algal Biomass

Algal biomass is gaining increasing attention for its diverse applications in food, feed, biofuels, and bioproducts. Its biochemical composition, particularly the content of proteins, carbohydrates, lipids, and bioactive compounds, is shaped by several factors, including the algal species, environmental conditions, and nutrient availability. A deep understanding of these variables is crucial for tailoring algal cultivation to meet specific industrial or ecological objectives. Different algal species naturally possess distinct biochemical profiles, making species selection a critical step in biomass utilization. For example, *Chlorella sorokiniana* is known to contain around 40% protein, 30% carbohydrates, and 18% lipids under optimal growth conditions, highlighting its potential for both nutritional and energy applications (Lacroux et al., 2021). Freshwater microalgae, such as *Nannochloris bacillaris* and *Tetracystis* species, also exhibit promising biochemical traits. These species can accumulate lipid levels as high as 32–36 g per 100 g of dry weight, and they also exhibit favorable essential amino acid profiles, making them suitable for both biofuel production and high-quality feed supplements (Microalgae to bioenergy production, 2024).

The environment in which algae are cultivated plays a fundamental role in shaping their biochemical makeup. Parameters such as temperature, light intensity, and pH can significantly influence the balance of macronutrients within the biomass. For instance, optimal temperature conditions are known to enhance the accumulation of lipids and carbohydrates, both of which are crucial for bioenergy applications (Hussain & Rittmann, 2023). Light intensity, meanwhile, directly impacts photosynthetic activity, which in turn affects biomass productivity and the concentration of valuable biochemical compounds (Lacroux et al., 2021). The availability and balance of nutrients, especially carbon, nitrogen, and phosphorus, are critical for algal growth and composition. These nutrients not only support basic cellular processes but also influence the synthesis of target compounds. Under nutrient-rich conditions, algae tend to prioritize protein synthesis, whereas nutrient limitation (particularly nitrogen deprivation) can trigger increased lipid accumulation, a desirable trait for biodiesel production (Hussain & Rittmann, 2023). However, while nutrient management can be used strategically to shift biomass composition, over-fertilization or imbalanced nutrient supply may have negative ecological consequences, including harmful algal blooms and eutrophication.

8.2.2 Growth Conditions and Cultivation Strategies for Enhanced Biomass Yield

Maximizing biomass yield in crop species is a multifaceted challenge that involves striking the right balance between biological, environmental, and agronomic factors. From planting density to ecological adaptability and photosynthetic efficiency, several key variables influence the amount of biomass a crop can produce. Understanding and optimizing these factors is essential not only for improving agricultural productivity but also for ensuring that biomass cultivation remains economically viable and environmentally sustainable. Planting density is one of the most fundamental factors affecting biomass yield. Research indicates that, up to a certain point, increasing planting density yields a linear increase in biomass. However, beyond this threshold, yield starts to decline due to intensified competition among plants for sunlight, water, and nutrients (Shepherd et al., 2023). For example, field studies have demonstrated that many annual crops follow similar patterns of growth scaling, where the maximum potential size at maturity is a critical determinant of optimal planting density (Shepherd et al., 2023). Finding this density "sweet spot" is crucial to ensure plants have enough space to thrive without underutilizing available land.

Environmental conditions, especially tolerance to abiotic stresses such as drought and salinity, play a significant role in crop productivity. The variability in stress tolerance among different germplasms makes genotype selection a key strategy for maximizing biomass yield in diverse climates. The EU OPTIMISC project, which focused on optimizing Miscanthus as a biomass crop, found that certain hybrids significantly outperformed conventional varieties when exposed to varying environmental conditions (Batista-Silva et al., 2020). This highlights the importance of breeding and selecting genotypes that are not only high-yielding but also resilient to the specific stresses of their growing regions. At the physiological level, photosynthesis and respiration are fundamental to biomass production. Improvements in photosynthetic efficiency, particularly the rate of CO_2 fixation, can significantly enhance the conversion of solar energy into plant matter. Likewise, optimizing respiration processes ensures that more energy is directed toward growth rather than maintenance. Recent research has demonstrated that targeted genetic modifications can enhance the efficiency of these fundamental biological processes, offering a promising approach to increase biomass yields across various crops (Jaiswal et al., 2023). This is particularly critical in the context of rising global food and energy demands.

8.2.3 Potential Applications of Algal Biomass in Bioeconomy

As the world seeks sustainable alternatives to fossil fuels and environmentally harmful industrial practices, algal biomass emerges as a promising solution within the circular bioeconomy. Thanks to its rapid growth, high photosynthetic efficiency, and ability to thrive on nonarable land, algae offer multiple environmental benefits. From reducing greenhouse gas emissions to improving water quality and producing renewable biofuels, algae are uniquely positioned to address key ecological challenges. One of the most impactful environmental benefits of algae is its ability to sequester carbon dioxide. Microalgae are particularly efficient at this, with the capacity to capture approximately 1.3 kg of CO_2 for every 1 kg of biomass produced (Plöhn et al., 2021). This makes algae a valuable tool for mitigating climate change, especially when integrated into industrial systems that emit large volumes of CO_2. Moreover, the use of algal biofuels such as biodiesel and biogas produces significantly lower emissions of greenhouse gases, nitrogen oxides, and sulfur oxides compared to conventional fossil fuels (Plöhn et al., 2021). Their photosynthetic capabilities allow algae to continuously convert atmospheric CO_2 into valuable biomass, contributing to a sustainable and low-carbon energy future (Bhatt et al., 2022). Beyond carbon capture, algae can also play a transformative role in wastewater treatment. Algae are capable of utilizing wastewater as a nutrient source, thereby reducing the need for freshwater inputs and simultaneously removing pollutants such as nitrogen and phosphorus from waste streams (Bhatt et al., 2022). When integrated into wastewater treatment systems, algae not only purify the water but also generate biomass that can be harvested for further use (Morillas-España et al., 2022; Ravanipour et al., 2021). This dual-purpose function makes algal cultivation a compelling approach to water management, especially in regions facing water scarcity and pollution issues.

The biofuel potential of algae is another significant environmental advantage. Due to their high lipid content and rapid growth rates, algae are considered a superior feedstock for producing a range of renewable fuels, including biodiesel, bioethanol, and biogas (Saad et al., 2019). Unlike traditional biofuel crops, algae can be grown year-round and do not require fertile land or freshwater. This not only avoids competition with food production but also supports the development of decentralized, locally produced energy sources, enhancing national and regional energy security (Saad et al., 2019). Algae's versatility goes beyond energy and environmental services. Their ability to thrive on nonarable or marginal lands means they can be cultivated without displacing food crops or reducing soil fertility. In fact, their productivity per unit area far exceeds that of most terrestrial biomass sources (Bhatt et al., 2022). This makes algal cultivation a desirable option for sustainable land management and bio-based industries, enabling the efficient production of bioproducts in areas that are otherwise underutilized.

8.3 Thermal Conversion Techniques for Algal Biomass Valorization

Pyrolysis is a thermochemical conversion process in which organic material (such as algal biomass) is decomposed under oxygen-limited or inert conditions to yield bio-oil, syngas, and biochar. It is a crucial method for converting algae into energy-rich fuels and chemicals (Naaz et al., 2023).

8.3.1 Pyrolysis

The thermal breakdown of algal biomass essentially causes pyrolysis. When exposed to elevated temperatures (typically between 300 °C and 600 °C) in an inert atmosphere (usually nitrogen), the temperature used breaks the chemical bonds in the carbohydrates, lipids, and proteins of algal biomass. The thermal degradation will result in byproducts, including volatile vapors, non-condensable gases, and a solid biochar residue of carbon-rich material. Because the pyrolytic reactions are endothermic, heat must be constantly supplied to maintain the process and facilitate conversion (Choudhary et al., 2020). A central characteristic of pyrolysis is that it occurs in the absence of oxygen. This is a critical aspect of this process. The presence of oxygen would allow the organic feedstock to combust, producing carbon dioxide and water as it oxidizes the organic material into its simplest forms. By excluding oxygen, pyrolysis thermally decomposes molecules without combusting organic compounds, yielding intermediate products rich in energy, such as bio-oil. This is a key difference from other thermal treatments, such as combustion or gasification, which cannot occur in the absence of oxygen or air (Saravanan et al., 2023). The chemical reactions that occur during pyrolysis largely depend on the specific type of algal biomass used. Lipids will decompose mostly into fatty acids, hydrocarbons, and ketones, making lipids ideal for producing bio-oil. Proteins will tend to break down into ammonia, amines, and nitriles, producing nitrogen species to the vapor phase. Carbohydrates, such as starch, decompose into furans, levoglucosan, and gases. The pigments and pigment-like compounds in the biomass generate aromatic species and phenol. Unique activation energies, characterize each of these reactions and the dominant decomposition pathway will be influenced by a multitude of factors, like temperature, heating rate, and the specific type of biomass (Saravanan et al., 2023; Behera et al., 2022). Rapid and uniform heat transfer within the algal biomass particles is essential for efficient pyrolysis. Smaller particles reach the optimum temperature more quickly; thus, the rapid production of volatile compounds, such as bio-oil, is favored. On the other hand, larger particles require a longer time to reach target temperatures, resulting in greater amounts of char being produced. Initially, as biomass is heated, moisture is removed through drying up to a temperature of about 150 °C, before devolatilization occurs, producing volatile products over a range of approximately 300–600 °C. Above 500 °C, carbonization of the remaining solid typically occurs, resulting in the formation of char (Leong et al., 2021).

8.3.1.1 Kinetics and Reaction Time

The pyrolysis process and product yield vary widely, depending on the reaction timescale and the composition of the algal feedstock. Fast pyrolysis is on the order of milliseconds to seconds and is designed to maximize the collection of the condensable vapors (bio-oils) via rapid heating of the biomass. Slow pyrolysis allows the reaction to occur over a longer timescale, favoring the formation of char and more stable gas products. The reaction kinetics typically exhibit Arrhenius-like behavior, where the decomposition rates increase with rising temperature. However, there is a caveat regarding temperature; if these vapors are overheated, cracking occurs, and they become non-condensable gases. The overall composition of the algal biomass (lipids, proteins, carbohydrates) will also importantly define the reaction pathways and yields of pyrolysis products. Algae are distinct from woody or lignocellulosic biomass. The composition of algal biomass is the most important aspect of pyrolysis. Algal biomass with a higher lipid content also yields higher bio-oil and hydrocarbon-rich vapors, making it preferable for liquid fuel production. Algal biomass with high protein content will produce nitrogenous compounds, which have implications for the quality and stability of pyrolysis products when the biomass is pyrolyzed. Algal biomass also generally includes an abundance of inorganic salts, which may catalyze reactions influencing other reaction pathways or may inhibit the formation of bio-oil entirely. In summary, the pyrolysis of algal biomass is unpredictable and depends on the exact algae species, growing conditions, and harvesting or processing methods (Leong et al., 2021).

8.3.1.2 Energy Balance and Efficiency

Due to pyrolysis being an endothermic process, the thermal decomposition of biomass must have a reliable external heat source. This heat is often produced by burning a fraction of non-condensable gases, like syngas produced from the reaction. However, in terms of energy efficiency, pyrolysis reactor operators can implement energy integration in reactor design, such as hot gas recirculation, to help achieve the temperature requirement while minimizing total energy consumption. The product yield and distribution in pyrolysis of algal biomass are significantly influenced by several process parameters that can be controlled. All of them have a significant influence on the quantity and quality of bio-oil, non-condensable gases, and char (Thaha et al., 2025). In the pyrolysis process, temperature is the most important parameter, as the pyrolysis reaction typically proceeds within a temperature range of 300 °C to 600 °C, and its value significantly impacts the degree of organic matter breakdown and the distribution of the final products. If the pyrolysis process is conducted at low temperatures (e.g., less than approximately 400 °C), the primary outcome will be biochar products. Moderate pyrolysis temperatures (between 450 °C and 550 °C) are generally regarded as optimal for maximizing bio-oil yield. At pyrolysis temperatures above 600 °C, there is an increased production of non-condensable gases and a decreased yield of bio-oil. Thus, to optimize the pyrolysis process stages and to potentially control the outcome for desired products, the temperature must be carefully controlled. Algae with a high lipid content are particularly favorable for pyrolysis at approximately 500 °C because they will produce more bio-oil at this temperature. The optimal temperature range for the thermal degradation of lipids and proteins in algal biomass typically falls between 450 °C and 550 °C. Therefore, if temperatures were to rise above them, the benign vapours created through pyrolysis are subject to cracking into smaller gaseous molecules, thus reducing both the quantity and quality of the produced bio-oil. Accordingly, it is advantageous and important to continue conducting pyrolysis at moderate temperatures to obtain more liquid and less gas (Thaha et al., 2025; Devi & Chaudhuri, 2024). Heating rate—defined as the rate of temperature increase inside the pyrolysis reactor (usually reported in °C min^{-1})—is a significant factor in determining product distribution. When heating rates are high (generally higher than 100 °C/min), volatiles can quickly escape the reactor as vapour; these higher heating rates lead to greater vapour production and bio-oil yield forces, but minimum secondary reactions. Conversely, at low heating rates (typically lower than 10 °C/min), volatiles have more time to interact with hot surfaces, which encourages secondary cracking and leads to higher levels of char and non-condensable gases, but with a reduced yield of bio-oil (Dutta et al., 2023). Due to the high volatile content in algae, a high heating rate facilitates rapid vaporization and prevents degradation of heat-sensitive compounds, such as lipids.

Residence time is the time that volatile compounds or vapours stay in the hot zone of the pyrolysis reactor. A shorter vapor residence time, under 2 s, can reduce secondary cracking reactions, conserve higher molecular weight vapours, and improve bio-oil yield and quality. Longer residence times increase the possibility of vapor cracking into lower molecular weight molecules, resulting in the production of more non-condensable gases, and a decrease in the overall yield and quality of bio-oil. Residence time is a crucial variable in controlling the desired pyrolysis products (Dutta et al., 2023; Amalapridman et al., 2025). A short residence time is necessary to maintain bio-oil precursors and minimize the degradation of nitrogenous compounds, which can yield unwanted NO gases. The particle size of the algal biomass sent into the pyrolysis reactor can significantly impact the efficiency and completeness of the pyrolysis process. The smaller the particle size (<1 mm), the better the heat transfer, and with heat transfer comes faster and more uniform pyrolysis. With improved heat transfer and a suitable particle size, volatiles can be released, resulting in a higher yield of bio-oil and other desired products. Larger particle sizes incur the issues associated with heat transfer; therefore, gradual or no pyrolysis will ensue, meaning vapours may not be released as efficiently, thus contributing to lower overall product output. Therefore, particle size must be optimized to create efficient thermal decomposition and higher overall product output from the pyrolysis process.

8.3.1.3 Application to Algal Biomass

Algal biomass needs to be dried and pulverized into fine powder or slurry. It permits even heat treatment, which is necessary for regulated vaporization. The moisture level of algal biomass before pyrolysis is important in an overall sense, as well as in terms of safety and quality. Biomass with a high moisture content over 20% requires more energy to dry the samples, which detracts from the thermal efficiency of the entire system. High levels of water in bio-oil products can also create an emulsion, which can cause quality and stability issues. Low moisture content (preferably <10%) is advantageous for pyrolysis, allowing for high-quality, cleaner vaporization (Javed et al., 2022). Algae naturally contain high water (up to 90%). Effective dewatering and drying processes are essential before pyrolysis. The design and functioning of a pyrolysis reactor influence the manner in which the heat is transferred and the subsequent interaction with the algal biomass. Fixed-bed reactors contain a simple design but suffer from poor heat distribution, which can impede the overall uniformity of the pyrolysis reaction. Fluidized-bed reactors offer excellent heat transfer and good performance for small particles, such as algae. Rotary kilns facilitate the continuous transfer of biomass, enabling precise control over residence time, which is ideal for large-scale processing. Microwave-assisted pyrolysis (MAP) employs a unique approach, providing heat from the inside out, which improves the speed of pyrolysis and promotes uniformity and efficiency throughout the entire process and its products (Ganesan et al., 2024). Fluidized-bed and microwave reactors are highly efficient due to algae's small particle size and high water content. In pyrolysis, an inert gas, generally nitrogen or argon, is used to inhibit biomass oxidation and transport the formed vapors to the condensation units. The inert gas flow rate can have a substantial impact on reaction results. A lower inert gas flow rate will increase the vapor residence time in the reactor, which increases the possibility of secondary cracking, potentially decreasing the yield and quality of bio-oil. Conversely, a higher gas flow rate will decrease residence time and thus limit secondary reactions, although there are some caveats. Obtaining very high flow rates can unintentionally cool the reactor, and biomass may not completely vaporize. It is essential not to overlook the importance of choosing the best, i.e., the optimal inert gas flow rate, which balances both thermal efficiency and vapor residence time (Ganesan et al., 2024; Rout et al., 2023). A moderate flow rate of inert gas (typically nitrogen) is ideal for pyrolysis, as it provides effective vapor sweeping while preventing the oxidation of reactive intermediates and oxygenated compounds. The use of catalysts during pyrolysis can also significantly impact the subsequent chemical reactions and the quality of the bio-oil. Catalytic pyrolysis facilitates important transformations such as deoxygenation, dehydration, and denitrogenation, promoting the reduction of acidic, oxygenated, and nitrogenated compounds in the bio-oil. These modifications improve the stability, heating value, and flammability of the fuel produced, thereby potentially increasing its applicability as an energy source (Wicker et al., 2021). Since algae contain high levels of nitrogen (due to their proteins), catalytic pyrolysis (e.g., with zeolites or CaO) can minimize the production of toxic NOx compounds and enhance the quality of the bio-oil.

8.3.1.4 Products

Following the pyrolysis process, which removes volatile compounds from biomass, biochar is a stable, carbon-rich solid residue that remains. Due to its chemical stability and porous structure, this leftover material is renowned for its numerous applications. Biochar is a valuable byproduct of the pyrolysis process, playing a crucial role in soil improvement, carbon sequestration, and environmental remediation. The three primary byproducts of pyrolysis—biochar, bio-oil, and syngas—each have special benefits and uses. A porous substance with a large surface area and a high carbon content, biochar is frequently enhanced with vital minerals such as calcium, magnesium, potassium, and, depending on the algal source, phosphorus and nitrogen. It is frequently added to soil to increase fertility and water retention, acts as a sorbent for environmental remediation processes, such as heavy metal adsorption, and serves as a long-term carbon sink by storing atmospheric CO_2 for centuries. Water, organic acids, aldehydes, ketones, phenols, and other oxygenated hydrocarbons combine to form bio-oil, also referred to as pyrolysis oil, a renewable liquid fuel. Although it can be directly utilized in boilers and turbines to generate heat and electricity, upgrading is frequently required due to its high acidity, water content, and thermal instability. The valuable chemical components of bio-oil, such as furans, phenols, and acetic acid, can be extracted for use in solvents, polymers, and pharmaceuticals. Bio-oil can also be hydrotreated or catalytically cracked to produce green diesel, jet fuel, or petrol. A flexible energy source, syngas is a flammable gas mixture primarily composed of carbon monoxide (CO), hydrogen (H_2), and methane (CH_4), with trace amounts of CO_2 and light hydrocarbons. It can be burned directly to produce heat, converted into synthetic fuels such as methanol, dimethyl ether (DME), or hydrocarbons through Fischer-Tropsch synthesis, or used in internal combustion engines or turbines to generate electricity. Syngas is also utilized in the industrial synthesis of ammonia, methanol, and other useful chemicals, and it is a major source of hydrogen for fuel cells.(Teri et al., 2018).

8.3.1.5 Applications in Energy and Material Sectors

Three main products are yielded by pyrolysing algal biomass: syngas, biochar, and bio-oil. Each of these products possesses distinctive and growing applications in the material and energy sectors. By converting biological waste into valuable, added-value products, these products not only offer renewable alternatives to fossil fuels and resources, but they also promote circularity. A liquid carrier of energy with high heating value (typically 15–20 MJ/kg) is bio-oil from algal pyrolysis. It may be used as a refinery co-processing feedstock with crude oil or directly in furnaces and boilers to produce heat. Bio-oil can be processed into drop-in transportation fuels, such as diesel, petrol, and jet fuel, that can coexist with existing infrastructure by upgrading (e.g., catalytic hydrotreating). Use of bio-oil helps achieve energy security and diversity by reducing dependence on petroleum. Solid oxide fuel cells (SOFCs), internal combustion engines, and gas turbines are capable of burning syngas to provide power and heat. It aids in distributed energy systems, particularly in rural or off-grid settings. The fuel cell and ecological production of hydrogen are facilitated by its hydrogen-rich structure, which enables it to integrate into the hydrogen economy as well. Activated biochar can be utilized to produce high-surface-area carbon materials for supercapacitors and battery electrodes. Especially in pollution control equipment and bio-refineries (e.g., tar reforming or catalytic cracking in gasification operations), it serves as a low-cost catalyst support material (Teri et al., 2018).

8.3.2 Hydrothermal Liquefaction (HTL)

Hydrothermal liquefaction (HTL) is a thermochemical process that converts wet biomass into bio-crude oil, syngas, aqueous products, and solid residues under subcritical water conditions (typically 250–374 °C and 10–25 MPa). The process mimics the natural geological transformation of biomass into fossil fuels but accelerates it to occur within minutes to hours (Gu et al., 2020). In HTL, water acts both as a reactant and a reaction medium. The high pressure maintains water in the liquid state, enabling hydrolysis, depolymerization, and deoxygenation reactions that break down macromolecules, such as lipids, proteins, and carbohydrates, into smaller organic compounds and ultimately bio-crude. Lipid-rich algae favor fatty acid degradation into hydrocarbons, while proteins lead to nitrogenous compounds, and carbohydrates primarily yield oxygenates (Yin et al., 2023). Catalysts such as alkali salts, transition metals, or zeolites may be used to enhance product selectivity and reaction rates. Key operating parameters influencing HTL efficiency include temperature, residence time, biomass concentration, catalyst presence, and reactor configuration. For instance, increasing the temperature enhances bio-crude yield and quality but also promotes gasification and char formation beyond optimal levels (Haider et al., 2020). A typical operating range of 280–350 °C is used for 30–60 min in continuous or batch systems.

A major advantage of HTL over pyrolysis and gasification is its ability to process high-moisture feedstocks, such as algal slurries, without the need for energy-intensive drying. Algae, which can contain over 80% moisture, are thus ideal candidates for HTL. This results in improved energy efficiency and reduced processing costs (Alptekin & Ince, 2022a). Furthermore, HTL bio-crude contains higher energy density and lower oxygen content compared to pyrolysis oils, making it more suitable for upgrading into transportation fuels. The aqueous phase can be further utilized for nutrient recovery or biogas generation via anaerobic digestion (Zhou et al., 2020). HTL also results in fewer tars and particulates compared to gasification, simplifying downstream processing. HTL-derived bio-crude typically contains 60–75% carbon, 8–15% hydrogen, 10–20% oxygen, and 3–6% nitrogen, with a heating value around 30–37 MJ/kg. However, it also contains heteroatoms (N, S, O) and heavy compounds that require upgrading. Upgrading strategies include hydrotreating, catalytic cracking, and emulsification. Hydrotreating is the most widely used process, where hydrogen is used in the presence of catalysts (e.g., $NiMo/Al_2O_3$) to remove oxygen (deoxygenation), nitrogen (denitrogenation), and sulfur (desulfurization) (Jayanarasimhan et al., 2024). However, nitrogen removal is particularly challenging due to the formation of recalcitrant heterocyclic compounds from algal proteins.

Both subcritical (250–374 °C, 10–25 MPa) and supercritical (>374 °C, >22 MPa) operating conditions are possible for HTL. Supercritical conditions encourage the production of gas, whereas subcritical conditions are typically more energy-efficient and appropriate for producing bio-crude (Faizan et al., 2023). Reduced nitrogen/oxygen content, along with enhanced selectivity towards higher-quality oils, has been demonstrated by catalytic HTL (utilizing transition metals, alkali salts, or zeolites). Reactor configurations vary from industrial practice-type continuous-flow systems to semi-continuous ones for intermediate tests, and batch systems for bench-scale studies. For large quantities of algal slurries with uniform quality, continuous HTL offers special promise (Gu et al., 2020).

HTL faces numerous financial and technological challenges despite potential benefits. The high concentration of nitrogen in algal biomass is a major concern because it creates nitrogenous compounds that make downstream hydrotreating more challenging. Additionally, the incorporation of heteroatoms, i.e., those that include oxygen and sulfur, compromises fuel stability and necessitates more advanced upgrading techniques (Yin et al., 2023). The cost of operations rises when foulants, poisons, or cooked catalysts make them inactive. The occurrence of salts, nitrogen moieties, and organic acids in the aqueous phase byproduct requires energy-intensive processing or valorization schemes. Lastly, the requirement for high-pressure systems makes scalability more challenging, resulting in higher capital and maintenance costs (Haider et al., 2020). Recently published work includes integrated hydrothermal liquefaction (HTL) systems where the aqueous phase is recycled for nutrient reuse or undergoes anaerobic digestion to enhance carbon efficiency. Heterogeneous catalyst development, specifically bifunctional zeolites and Ni-Mo sulfides, is facilitating cost reductions in upgrading and improving oil quality (Zhou et al., 2020). Techno-economic assessments and life cycle analyses suggest that integrating HTL with waste heat utilization and infrastructure developments will enhance overall viability. Near-term commercialization opportunities are reinforced by demonstrations from pilot scales, like operating HTL plants continuously in the United States and Europe (Alptekin & Ince, 2022b).

8.3.3 Gasification

Gasification is a high-temperature thermochemical process (700–1200 °C) conducted in the presence of a controlled number of oxidizing agents (air, oxygen, or steam) to convert carbonaceous materials into syngas (a mixture of CO, H_2, CO_2, CH_4, and light hydrocarbons) and solid residues (char and ash) (Jayanarasimhan et al., 2024). The key stages in algal biomass gasification include drying, pyrolysis, oxidation, and reduction. The choice of gasifying medium has a significant impact on the syngas composition. Steam gasification promotes hydrogen production, while oxygen and air produce syngas with different calorific values. Algal biomass, due to its high ash and nitrogen content, presents specific challenges in gasification, including slagging, fouling, and NOx emissions. However, its low lignin content and high reactivity make it more amenable to gasification than lignocellulosic feedstocks. Temperature is the most critical parameter. Higher temperatures favor syngas yield and reduce tar formation but can increase operational costs. The type of gasifier (fixed bed, fluidized bed, or entrained flow) also impacts conversion efficiency. Steam-to-biomass ratio (SBR), equivalence ratio (ER), and particle size are important factors for syngas composition optimization (Geng et al., 2025).

Syngas is a versatile intermediate that can be converted into various fuels and chemicals through catalytic processes such as Fischer–Tropsch synthesis (FTS), methanol synthesis, or mixed alcohol synthesis. FTS converts syngas into hydrocarbons (C_1–C_{20}), which can be refined into gasoline, diesel, or jet fuel (Wang et al., 2020). Methanol and dimethyl ether (DME) production from syngas is also gaining momentum as alternative fuel pathways. Additionally, syngas fermentation by acetogenic bacteria offers routes to bioethanol or biobutanol with high selectivity under milder conditions (Ağbulut et al., 2023). Gasification can be differentiated into several types based on the type of oxidizing agent. Air gasification offers economic benefits in the process but is hindered by high nitrogen dilution, resulting in syngas with a low calorific value. Although the cost incurred in producing oxygen is quite high, gasification of oxygen yields syngas of improved quality, suitable for chemical synthesis (Chernova et al., 2022). Steam gasification reduces the yields of tar and increases the production of hydrogen. Despite such huge energy requirements, plasma gasification procedures produce cleaner synthesis gas and minimize tar production by utilizing high-intensity plasma torches that achieve extremely high temperatures. As it does not cause drying out, wet biomass such as algae is particularly suited to gasification by supercritical water (SCWG). The process produces hydrogen-rich syngas but requires corrosion-resistant materials for reactor components [70].

Tar production resulting in difficulty in cleaning gas and decreased efficiency is among the significant problems. Algae having high levels of ash and alkalis cause reactor slagging, fouling, and sintering problems. Additionally, the high concentration of nitrogen and sulfur in algal biomass emissions leads to the production of NO_x and SO_x, necessitating downstream cleaning. For commercial-scale systems, stable operation is not straightforward due to variability in feedstock (particle size, moisture levels, and biochemical composition). Furthermore, without heat integration, the energy consumed in gasification and syngas cleaning tends to reduce system efficiency [71]. To achieve maximum tar cracking and maximize hydrogen yields, recent research has focused on catalytic gasification using alkali-metal and nickel-based catalysts. Gasification, when employed alongside carbon capture and storage (CCS) and integrated gasification combined cycle power plants (IGCC), defines integrated systems that have shown promise in reducing emissions while enhancing efficiency [72]. Furthermore, to enhance syngas quality and economics, algae co-gasification with coal, lignocellulosic biomass, or municipal solid waste is being investigated. To minimize ash-related problems, research is underway on specific pre-treatment methodologies applicable to microalgae, such as torrefaction and pelletization. Future configurations of biorefineries will likely depend significantly on algal gasification, as the focus remains on producing carbon-neutral fuels and renewable hydrogen [73].

Table 8.1 Comparative analysis of pyrolysis, HTL, and gasification [74]

Aspect	Pyrolysis	HTL	Gasification
Process	Thermal degradation without oxygen	High-temperature and high-pressure water process	Partial oxidation with limited oxygen
Products	Bio-oil, syngas, and biochar	Bio-crude oil, aqueous phase, and solid residues	Syngas and char
Efficiency	High bio-oil yield and energy-intensive	High yield from wet algae and capital-intensive	Efficient syngas production and lower yields from algae
Environmental impact	Sustainable (biochar sequestration) requires VOC management	Low carbon footprint and no drying required	Cleaner than incineration and carbon capture potential
Circular bioeconomy fit	Strong and versatile product use	Strong, multiple, and valuable products	Strong energy generation and industrial use of byproducts

8.4 Comparative Analysis of Pyrolysis, HTL, and Gasification

Compared to different aspects, all the methods have advantages and some limitations based on the utilization of algal biomass, as depicted in Table 8.1.

8.5 Conclusion

Thermochemical decomposition of algal biomass through pyrolysis, HTL, and gasification has effectively been valorized in the bioeconomy by producing biofuels, biochemicals, etc., which helps sustainable development with good product yield, positive impact on nature, and human needs. Pyrolysis effectively contributes to the production of bio-oil, syngas, and biochar for energy generation through thermal utilization. In contrast, HTL processes wet biomass without requiring intentional energy consumption. Gasification can be utilized for the production of fuels and chemicals, although it presents some challenges, including high ash and nitrogen content in algal feeds. To conclude, Algal biomass can be transformed into valuable products that strengthen the bioeconomy by closing the carbon loop through thermochemical conversion methods such as pyrolysis, HTL, and gasification, which yield bio-oil, syngas, and biochar. Another promising route is its integration with existing biorefineries, such as sugar-based facilities, to enhance the production of fertilizers, nutraceuticals, fuels, and other products. Moreover, supportive policy measures, including incentives, regulatory frameworks, and public–private partnerships, can shape industrial perspectives while driving research, innovation, and scalability for future advancements.

Key Takeaways

Algal biomass can be converted into various substances that can enhance the bioeconomy by the following approaches:

1. Closing the carbon loop through thermochemical conversion in carbon emissions controlled by processes like pyrolysis, HTL, and gasification, which produce bio-oil, syngas, and biochar.
2. Another approach is integrating existing biorefineries, such as sugar-based biorefineries, enhancing the production of fertilizers, nutraceuticals, fuels, etc.
3. Finally, policy changes can modify the industrial perspective by providing incentives, establishing a regulatory framework, and fostering public–private partnerships that can drive R&D and scalability.

References

Adeniyi, A. G., Iwuozor, K. O., Emenike, E. C., Ajala, O. J., Ogunniyi, S., & Muritala, K. B. (2024). Thermochemical co-conversion of biomass-plastic waste to biochar: A review. *Green Chemical Engineering, 5*(1), 31–49.

Ağbulut, Ü., Sirohi, R., Lichtfouse, E., Chen, W.-H., Len, C., Show, P. L., Le, A. T., Nguyen, X. P., & Hoang, A. T. (2023). Microalgae bio-oil production by pyrolysis and hydrothermal liquefaction: Mechanism and characteristics. *Bioresource Technology, 376*, 128860. https://doi.org/10.1016/j.biortech.2023.128860

Alptekin, F. M., & Ince, M. (2022a). Review on catalytic biomass gasification for hydrogen production as a sustainable energy form and social, technological, economic, environmental, and political analysis of catalysts. *ACS Omega, 7*(29), 24918–24941. https://doi.org/10.1021/acsomega.2c0153

Alptekin, F. M., & Ince, M. (2022b). Review on catalytic biomass gasification for hydrogen production as a sustainable energy form and social, technological, economic, environmental, and political analysis of catalysts. *ACS Omega, 7*(29), 24918–24941. https://doi.org/10.1021/acsomega.2c01538

Amalapridman, V., Ofori, P. A., & Abbey, L. (2025). Valorization of algal biomass to biofuel: A review. *Biomass, 5*(2), 26.

Batista-Silva, W., da Fonseca-Pereira, P., Martins, A. O., Zsögön, A., Nunes-Nesi, A., & Araujo, W. L. (2020). Engineering improved photosynthesis in the era of synthetic biology. *Plant Communications, 1*(2), 100032.

Behera, B., Selvam, S. M., & Balasubramanian, P. (2022). Hydrothermal processing of microalgal biomass: Circular bio-economy perspectives for addressing food-water-energy nexus. *Bioresource Technology, 359*, 127443.

Bhatt, P., Bhandari, G., Turco, R. F., Aminikhoei, Z., Bhatt, K., & Simsek, H. (2022). Algae in wastewater treatment, mechanism, and application of biomass for production of value-added product. *Environmental Pollution, 309*, 119688.

Cansado, I. P. D. P., Mourão, P. A. M., Castanheiro, J. E., Geraldo, P. F., Suero, S. R., & Cano, B. L. (2025). A review of the biomass valorization hierarchy. *Sustainability, 17*(1), 335.

Chandrasekhar, K., Kumar, A. N., Raj, T., Kumar, G., & Kim, S. H. (2021). Bioelectrochemical system-mediated waste valorization. *Systems Microbiology and Biomanufacturing, 1*, 432–443.

Chen, H., Jiang, Y., Zhu, K., Yang, J., Fu, Y., & Wang, S. (2023). A review on industrial CO_2 capture through microalgae regulated by phytohormones and cultivation processes. *Energies, 16*(2), 897.

Chernova, N. I., Grigorenko, A. V., Kiseleva, S. V., Larina, O. M., Kumar, V., & Vlaskin, M. S. (2022). Comparative evaluation of pyrolysis and hydrothermal liquefaction for obtaining biofuel from a sustainable consortium of microalgae Arthrospira platensis with heterotrophic bacteria. *Processes, 10*(11), 2202.

Choudhary, P., Assemany, P. P., Naaz, F., Bhattacharya, A., de Siqueira Castro, J., do Couto Couto, E. D. A., et al. (2020). A review of biochemical and thermochemical energy conversion routes of wastewater grown algal biomass. *Science of the Total Environment, 726*, 137961.

De Schoenmakere, M., Hoogeveen, Y., Gillabel, J., & Manshoven, S. (2018). *The circular economy and the bioeconomy: Partners in sustainability.*

Devi, N. D., & Chaudhuri, A. (2024). Valorization of algal blooms and their residues into renewable energy. In *Biodegradable waste processing for sustainable developments* (pp. 257–271). CRC Press.

Dutta, N., Kundu, P., Lee, J. T. E., & Bhattacharya, S. (2023). Implementation and optimization of algal biomass in value-added products recovery: A step towards algae-based green economy. *Hydrobiology, 2*(2), 326–346.

Faizan, M., et al. (2023). Critical review on catalytic biomass gasification: State-of-Art progress, technical challenges, and perspectives in future development. *Journal of Cleaner Production, 408*, 137224.

Ganesan, J. J., Nagarajan, D., Rathinam, B., & Chien, J. R. C. (2024). Low-carbon biofuels from macroalgae towards a sustainable circular bioeconomy and green future. *Biomass and Bioenergy, 190*, 107389.

Gawel, E., Pannicke, N., & Hagemann, N. (2019). A path transition towards a bioeconomy—The crucial role of sustainability. *Sustainability, 11*(11), 3005.

Geng, Y., Shaukat, A., Azhar, W., Raza, Q.-U.-A., Tahir, A., Abideen, M. Z., Zia, M. A., Bashir, M. A., & Rehim, A. (2025). Microalgal biorefineries: A systematic review of technological trade-offs and innovation pathways. *Biotechnology for Biofuels and Bioproducts, 18*, 93. https://doi.org/10.1186/s13068-025-02694-7

Gu, X., Martinez-Fernandez, J. S., Pang, N., Fu, X., & Chen, S. (2020). Recent development of hydrothermal liquefaction for algal biorefinery. *Renewable and Sustainable Energy Reviews, 121*, 109707. https://doi.org/10.1016/j.rser.2020.109707

Gupta, V. K., Tuohy, M., Nguyen, Q. D., Bhat, R., & Ramteke, P. W. (Eds.). (2023). *Valorization of biomass to bioproducts: Organic acids and biofuels*. Elsevier.

Haider, M. S., Castello, D., & Rosendahl, L. A. (2020). Two-stage catalytic hydrotreatment of highly nitrogenous biocrude from continuous hydrothermal liquefaction: A rational design of the stabilization stage. *Biomass and Bioenergy, 139*, 105658.

Hussain, J., & Rittmann, B. E. (2023). Algae as a source of renewable energy: Opportunities, challenges, and recent developments. *Sustainable Energy & Fuels, 7*(11), 2515–2544.

Jaiswal, K. K., Dutta, S., Banerjee, I., Pohrmen, C. B., & Kumar, V. (2023). Photosynthetic microalgae–based carbon sequestration and generation of biomass in biorefinery approach for renewable biofuels for a cleaner environment. *Biomass Conversion and Biorefinery, 13*(9), 7403–7421.

Jasiūnas, J., Lund, P. D., & Mikkola, J. (2021). Energy system resilience–A review. *Renewable and Sustainable Energy Reviews, 150*, 111476.

Javed, M. U., Mukhtar, H., Hayat, M. T., Rashid, U., Mumtaz, M. W., & Ngamcharussrivichai, C. (2022). Sustainable processing of algal biomass for a comprehensive biorefinery. *Journal of Biotechnology, 352*, 47–58.

Jayanarasimhan, A., Pathak, R. M., Shivapuji, A. M., & Rao, L. (2024). Tar formation in gasification systems: A holistic review of remediation approaches and removal methods. *ACS Omega, 9*(2), 2060–2079. https://doi.org/10.1021/acsomega.3c04425

Kaushik, A., Sangtani, R., Parmar, H. S., & Bala, K. (2023). Algal metabolites: Paving the way towards new generation antidiabetic therapeutics. *Algal Research, 69*, 102904.

Khan, M. I., Shin, J. H., & Kim, J. D. (2018). The promising future of microalgae: Current status, challenges, and optimization of a sustainable and renewable industry for biofuels, feed, and other products. *Microbial Cell Factories, 17*, 1–21.

Lacroux, J., Seira, J., Trably, E., Bernet, N., Steyer, J. P., & van Lis, R. (2021). Mixotrophic growth of Chlorella sorokiniana on acetate and butyrate: Interplay between substrate, C: N ratio and pH. *Frontiers in Microbiology, 12*, 703614.

Lens, P. N., & Khandelwal, A. (2023). *Algal systems for resource recovery from waste and wastewater*. IWA Publishing.

Leong, Y. K., & Chang, J. S. (2023). Waste stream valorization-based low-carbon bioeconomy utilizing algae as a biorefinery platform. *Renewable and Sustainable Energy Reviews, 178*, 113245.

Leong, Y. K., Chen, W. H., Lee, D. J., & Chang, J. S. (2021). Supercritical water gasification (SCWG) as a potential tool for the valorization of phycoremediation-derived waste algal biomass for biofuel generation. *Journal of Hazardous Materials, 418*, 126278.

Microalgae to bioenergy production. (2024). Recent advances, influencing parameters, utilization of wastewater—A critical review. *Science of the Total Environment, 946*, 174230. https://doi.org/10.1016/j.scitotenv.2024.174230

Morillas-España, A., Lafarga, T., Sánchez-Zurano, A., Acién-Fernández, F. G., & González-López, C. (2022). Microalgae based wastewater treatment coupled to the production of high value agricultural products: Current needs and challenges. *Chemosphere, 291*, 132968.

Naaz, F., Samuchiwal, S., Dalvi, V., Bhattacharya, A., Pant, K. K., & Malik, A. (2023). Hydrothermal liquefaction could be a sustainable approach for valorization of wastewater grown algal biomass into cleaner fuel. *Energy Conversion and Management, 283*, 116887.

Ngo, H. H., Nguyen, T. T., Guo, W., Nguyen, D. D., Pandey, A., Bui, X. T., et al. (2022). Circular bioeconomy for resource recovery from wastewaters using algae-based technologies. In *Biomass, biofuels, and biochemicals* (pp. 217–236). Elsevier.

Papadaki, S., Tricha, N., Panagiotopoulou, M., & Krokida, M. (2024). Innovative bioactive products with medicinal value from microalgae and their overall process optimization through the implementation of life cycle analysis—An overview. *Marine Drugs, 22*(4), 152.

Plöhn, M., Spain, O., Sirin, S., Silva, M., Escudero-Oñate, C., Ferrando-Climent, L., et al. (2021). Wastewater treatment by microalgae. *Physiologia Plantarum, 173*(2), 568–578.

Ravanipour, M., Hamidi, A., & Mahvi, A. H. (2021). Microalgae biodiesel: A systematic review in Iran. *Renewable and Sustainable Energy Reviews, 150*, 111426. https://doi.org/10.1016/j.rser.2021.111426

Rout, P. R., Goel, M., Mohanty, A., Pandey, D. S., Halder, N., Mukherjee, S., et al. (2023). Recent advancements in microalgal mediated valorisation of wastewater from hydrothermal liquefaction of biomass. *Bioenergy Research, 16*(1), 45–60.

Saad, M. G., Dosoky, N. S., Zoromba, M. S., & Shafik, H. M. (2019). Algal biofuels: Current status and key challenges. *Energies, 12*(10), 1920.

Sangtani, R., Sonbhadra, S., Nogueira, R., & Kiran, B. (2022). Algal biorefinery: A paradigm for a sustainable circular bioeconomy. In *Zero waste biorefinery* (pp. 295–323). Springer Nature Singapore.

Saravanan, A., Kumar, P. S., Badawi, M., Mohanakrishna, G., & Aminabhavi, T. M. (2023). Valorization of micro-algae biomass for the development of green biorefinery: Perspectives on techno-economic analysis and the way towards sustainability. *Chemical Engineering Journal, 453*, 139754.

Satya, A. D. M., Cheah, W. Y., Yazdi, S. K., Cheng, Y. S., Khoo, K. S., Vo, D. V. N., et al. (2023). Progress in microalgae cultivation for wastewater bioremediation and a circular bioeconomy. *Environmental Research, 218*, 114948.

Shepherd, J. G., Clifton-Brown, J. C., Hastings, A., Long, S. P., & Lovett, A. A. (2023). Novel Miscanthus hybrids: Modelling productivity on marginal land in Europe using dynamics of canopy development determined by light interception. *GCB Bioenergy, 15*(2), 249–267. https://doi.org/10.1111/gcbb.13029

Strategy, U. B. (2018). *A sustainable bioeconomy for Europe: Strengthening the connection between economy, society, and the environment*. European Commission. 2018. https://doi.org/10.2777/478385

Teri, G., Luo, H., Savage, P. E., & Mahadevan, R. (2018). Biochemical valorization of aqueous-phase products from hydrothermal liquefaction of algal biomass. *Green Chemistry, 20*(10), 2301–2310. https://doi.org/10.1039/C8GC00045A

Thaha, A. N., Ghamari, M., Jothiprakash, G., Velusamy, S., Karthikeyan, S., Ramesh, D., & Sundaram, S. (2025). High impact biomass valorization for second generation biorefineries in India: Recent developments and future strategies for sustainable circular economy. *Biomass, 5*(1), 16.

Vellaiyan, S. (2024). An integrated approach for wastewater treatment and algae cultivation: Nutrient removal analysis, biodiesel extraction, and energy and environmental metrics enhancement. *Journal of Environmental Management, 354*, 120410.

Vinson, D. W., & Elgowainy, A. (2021). Life-cycle analysis of fuels from algae via thermochemical conversion pathways. *Renewable and Sustainable Energy Reviews, 139*, 110702. https://doi.org/10.1016/j.rser.2020.110702

Vishwakarma, R., Dhaka, V., Ariyadasa, T. U., & Malik, A. (2022). Exploring algal technologies for a circular bio-based economy in rural sector. *Journal of Cleaner Production, 354*, 131653.

Wang, W., Chen, W. T., & Savage, P. E. (2020). Upgrading of HTL bio-crude from algae via hydroprocessing: A review. *Renewable and Sustainable Energy Reviews, 133*, 110103. https://doi.org/10.1016/j.rser.2020.110103

Wicker, R. J., Kumar, G., Khan, E., & Bhatnagar, A. (2021). Emergent green technologies for cost-effective valorization of microalgal biomass to renewable fuel products under a biorefinery scheme. *Chemical Engineering Journal, 415*, 128932.

Yin, S., Shao, Y., Tian, B., & Zhu, J. (2023). Review on nitrogen transformation during microalgae thermochemical liquefaction: Recent advances and future perspectives. *Energy & Fuels, 37*(3). https://doi.org/10.1021/acs.energyfuels.2c03300

Zhou, Y., et al. (2020). Catalytic thermochemical conversion of algae and catalytic upgrading of algal oil/biocrude: A review. *Catalysts, 10*(2), 145. https://doi.org/10.3390/catal10020145

Zografa kis, N., Sifaki, E., Pagalou, M., Nikitaki, G., Psarakis, V., & Tsagarakis, K. P. (2010). Assessment of public acceptance and willingness to pay for renewable energy sources in Crete. *Renewable and Sustainable Energy Reviews, 14*(3), 1088–1095.

9 Application of Microalgae for Treating Reverse Osmosis Reject Water: Prospects and Challenges

K. M. Meera Sheriffa Begum and Prakash Binnal

Abstract

Although reverse osmosis is an efficient technique for treating brackish and seawater, it suffers from the disadvantage of generating huge quantities of reject water. Microalgae-based treatment of reverse osmosis reject water is attracting wide attention recently. In this regard, the present chapter aims at reviewing: (i) species of marine microalgae employed for ROR treatment, (ii) optimization of cultivation conditions, (iii) type of photobioreactors used for desalination, (iv) biomass productivities and lipid productivities obtained during desalination, (v) biochemical and elemental composition of microalgae cultivated in ROR, and (vi) efficiency of treatment of ROR. Additionally, we describe the perspectives and challenges associated with ROR treatment by microalgae, the scale-up of technology, and the current status of technology at an industrial scale.

Keywords

Reverse Osmosis Reject Water · Microalgae-based Desalination · Biochar · Photobioreactor · Pyrolysis

K. M. Meera Sheriffa Begum
Department of Chemical Engineering, National Institute of Technology, Tiruchirappalli, Tamil Nadu, India

P. Binnal (✉)
Department of Chemical Engineering, Siddaganga Institute of Technology, Tumakuru, Karnataka, India
e-mail: pb@sit.ac.in

L. Kumar et al. (eds.), *Algal Bioremediation*,
https://doi.org/10.1007/978-981-95-8793-3_9

9.1 Introduction

Currently, RO-based desalination plants account for a significant portion of the total demand for desalinated water (Matos et al., 2017a). However, one of the major drawbacks of this system is the production of a large amount of reject stream called "Reverse Osmosis Reject (ROR)," which contains concentrated nutrients and presents challenges for disposal. ROR is highly concentrated in terms of nutrients and potentially harmful organic compounds (Patel et al., 2021). Therefore, there is concern about the discharge of untreated ROR into the environment, as it can pose a potential long-term risk to ecosystems and human health (Bhandari & Prajapati, 2022).

Various technologies, such as adsorption, advanced oxidation processes (AOP) [i.e., ozonation and ozone-based advanced oxidation], Fenton oxidation, photocatalysis, UV/H2O2, and electrochemical oxidation, as well as forward osmosis (FO), have been extensively developed and tested for the treatment of ROR (Rana et al., 2021). Biological treatments using fungi, bacteria, and marine microalgae are attracting attention as low-cost alternatives to conventional methods. In particular, microalgae-based treatment technology is currently a crucial emerging field due to its high potential in removing nitrogen (N), phosphorus (P), and other organic contaminants. Marine microalgae are capable of growing rapidly in ROR media enriched with nutrients (Shirazi et al., 2018). Additionally, the algal biomass recovered after ROR treatment serves as a feedstock for the production of various biofuels through thermochemical conversions, such as gasification and pyrolysis.

Reverse osmosis (RO) is a widely used desalination technology that employs a semipermeable membrane to eliminate salts and other impurities from hyper-saline water (Wei et al., 2020). The share of RO-based desalination plants toward generation of desalinated water is 70%, and this trend is expected to grow exponentially in the near future (Miller et al., 2015). Although the technology is suitable for several applications, the high energy demand (an amount of electrical energy of 3–4 kWh/m^3) is a significant concern and challenge for it. Furthermore, the large amount of rejected water produced as the undesired by-product from the RO desalination unit creates many environmental and ecological issues (Chen et al., 2010). The reject generated during the RO desalination is referred to as reverse osmosis reject (ROR), the safe disposal of which is a major challenge in the process. Approximately 0.1–0.5 L of ROR is generated for each liter of purified water in a typical industrial RO unit, when the source is seawater or brackish water, respectively (Rantanen, 2008). The ROR is enriched with phosphorus, nitrogen, minerals, including calcium, sodium, chloride, and trace elements, such as potassium, magnesium, iron, and silica. Due to high concentrations of minerals and nutrients, direct discharge into the environment can lead to eutrophication in surface water bodies. Furthermore, ROR is one of the fastest-growing waste streams worldwide (Satthong et al., 2019).

9.1.1 Photo-Bio-Desalination of ROR Using Microalgae

Microalgal systems coupling brackish water treatment with simultaneous biomass production are attracting attention recently as a sustainable, yet being a low-cost solution to address the task of disposing of ROR. Photo-bio-desalination can be defined as an emerging and innovative approach that utilizes the unique photosynthetic ability of microalgae to desalinate ROR with simultaneous production of algal biomass (Wei et al., 2020). Microalgae utilize sunlight and chlorophyll to convert carbon dioxide and water into organic compounds (glucose), and release oxygen in the process. Salt uptake by microalgae from the surrounding water occurs through biosorption and bioaccumulation, thereby desalinating the water by decreasing the concentration of dissolved salts and also producing biomass (Miller et al., 2015). Thus, photo-bio-desalination is an integrated, sustainable, and low-cost approach to addressing water scarcity issues, reducing the environmental and ecological impact of desalination processes, and most importantly, providing an economically viable system for desalination of ROR (Chen et al., 2010). Furthermore, being a rich source of proteins and vitamins (B1, B2, B6, and B12), the algal biomass obtained post-desalination is an important byproduct that can be used for the extraction of several food supplements (Satthong et al., 2019). Some authors have reviewed the scientific works on photo-bio-desalination using microalgae (Saranya et al., 2025; Hanifa et al., 2025; Hasnain et al., 2025). In contrast, this chapter exclusively focuses on a review of studies conducted in the domain of bio-desalination of ROR using microalgae.

9.1.2 Characteristics of RO Reject Water

The characteristics of RO reject water, including total nitrogen, total phosphorus, salinity, conductivity, pH, and other parameters, are summarized in Table 9.1.

The characteristics of ROR were dependent on the type and characteristics of feed water employed to the RO unit. Bhandari and Prajapati (2022) used two different samples of ROR, from a domestic RO unit (ROR-DU) and from a commercial drinking water RO plant (ROR-CU). Do et al. (2021) used municipal wastewater, while Bhandari et al. (2023) and Arash Mohseni et al. (2021) used ROR from a drinking water treatment plant. Ângelo P. Matos et al. (2017b), Hyoungmin Woo (2019), and Mohseni et al. (2020) prepared synthetic ROR. Almutairi et al. (2021) employed both original rejected water and used reject water for the cultivation of *Chlorella vulgaris*. Maeng et al. (2018a) utilized concentrated synthetic ROR. Chang et al. (2020) employed municipal wastewater. The ROR in their studies was obtained from Fengsheng Environmental Protection Co., Ltd. (Chongqing, China) and had the highest TN and TP (246 ppm and 63.8 ppm, respectively). Mohseni et al. (2021) used extremely concentrated ROR in their study. The ROR was collected from a local wastewater treatment plant in Victoria, Australia and contained high TDS of 5500 mg/L and COD of 176 ppm.

Table 9.1 Characteristics of ROR as reported by various authors

TN[a] (mg/L)	TP[a] (mg/L)	Conductivity (μS/cm)	Salinity (mg/L)	TDS[a] (mg/L)	pH	COD (ppm)	Ref.
6.7	2.51	714	400	487	7.6	–	Bhandari and Prajapati (2022) (ROR-DU)
5.67	2.71	1151	600	806	7.4		Bhandari and Prajapati, (2022) (ROR-CU)
58.49	0.87	–	–	–	7.06	–	Do et al. (2021)
14.69	8.16	–	400	717	7.75	–	Bhandari et al. (2023)
61.8	20.3	**11,200**	–	**5500**	7.5	**175.5**	Mohseni et al. (2021)
–	–	3000	0.02#	1823	7.3		Matos et al. (2017b)
29–34	10–13	–	–	–	7.5	97–120	Woo et al. (2019)
43.2	13.1	11.1	–	5.5	7.7	165	Mohseni et al. (2020)
39	42	–	–	67.59	7.5	–	Almutairi et al. (2021)
33–39	10–11	–	–	–	7.6	96–123	Maeng et al. (2018a)
246	**63.8**	–	–	–	8.3	540	Chang et al. (2020)

[a]TN-Total nitrates, TP-Total phosphorus, COD-Chemical oxygen demand, # Molarity, $ Synthetic ROR

9.1.3 Mechanisms of Bio-Desalination

The basic mechanism of salt removal by microalgae is biosorption (adsorption) and bioaccumulation (absorption) (Patel et al., 2021). Figure 9.1 depicts the principles of bio-desalination.

Biosorption is quite common in the bio-desalination process. It is a metabolic independent path that involves quick bonding of ions or molecules to living or nonliving algae cells. It occurs due to ion exchange or complexation. Wi et al. (Wei et al., 2020) showed that the (–COOH, –NH, –OH, –CHO) of pectin and protein (primary, secondary, and tertiary amides) were responsible for biosorption of Na^+ and Cl^- via electrostatic attraction. For Cl^-, the attachment site is provided by an amide functional group (with positive ionic charge), which also assists in surface complexation with cell wall, while other functional groups with negative ionic charge provide sites for Na^+ ions (Fig. 9.1).

Rajfur et al. (2014) investigated the competitiveness of biosorption of different cations on the algal surface and suggested that Na^+ can replace Mn^{2+} to be bound on

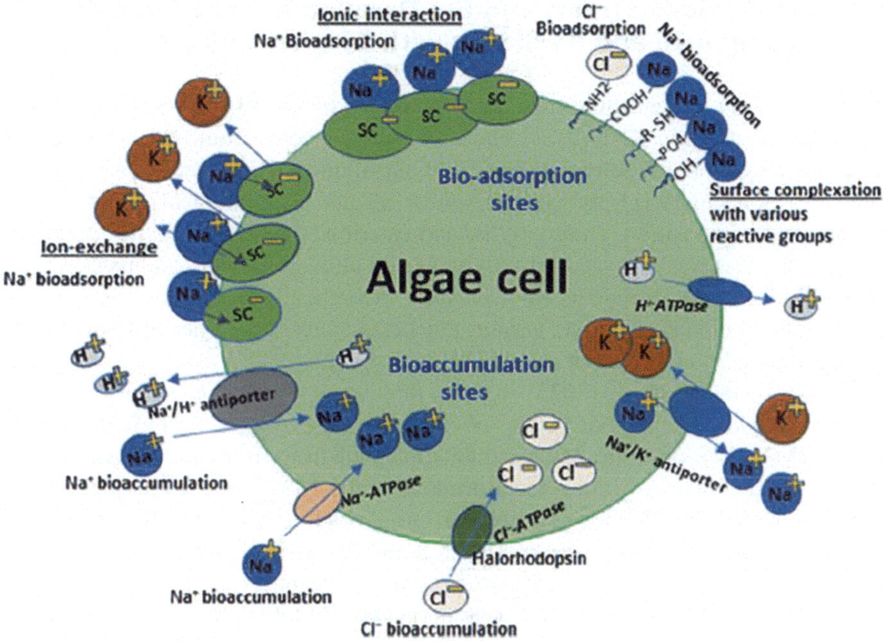

Fig. 9.1 Type of interactions involved in bioadsorption and bioaccumulation of Na^+ and Cl^-. (Reproduced with permission from Springer) (Patel et al., 2021)

the algal surface. Wei et al. (2020) showed that functional groups on *S. obliquus* included: –OH or –NH, –CHO, and – COOH. As these groups are negatively charged, the effectiveness of biosorption of Na^+ through electrostatic attraction increases.

On the other hand, bioaccumulation is an energy-dependent active biological process that occurs in living cells involving salt uptake and accumulation. It is completed in two steps and is comparatively a slow process. Initially, the adsorption of salt on the outer cell wall occurs, followed by its steady diffusion intracellularly (Timková et al., 2018). Blumwald et.al (1983) illustrated the salt adaptation mechanism of *cyanobacterium Synechococcus 6311* and suggested that the osmotic shock inhibits the sodium pump and the ATPase, which further powers the sodium pump. Thus, it becomes difficult for the Na^+ pump to overcome the permeability of the plasmalemma to NaCl. This results in a net uptake of NaCl after the salt shock, and salt bioaccumulation occurs.

However, the salt removal ability varies greatly depending on type of algae species, and their salt removal capacities are affected by other external factors, such as pH, temperature, contact time, ratio of algae cells to salts.

9.2 Microalgae Strains and Bio-Desalination Experiments Using ROR and Its Blends with Synthetic Media

Do et al. (2021) utilized two microalgal strains *Desmodesmus* sp. KNUA024 and *Chlorella sorokiniana* KNUA071. The ROR was collected from a local municipal wastewater treatment facility and used without dilution. Desalination experiments were also done in BG11 for comparison of results. Estimation of growth rates, biochemical composition, chlorophylls, and caterionds were done. After desalination, the biomass was analyzed for proximate and ultimate analysis and these results were employed to determine its calorific value theoretically. The spent biomass was transformed to biodiesel and the various physicochemical properties were estimated through fatty acid methyl ester (FAME) composition.

Mamta Bhandari et al. (2023) utilized three pure microalgal strains, namely, *C. sorokiniana* (NCIM 5561), *S. obliquus* (NCIM 5526), *and Scenedesmus* sp. (NCIM 5712), and one native strain (obtained from a nearby drainage line). The ROR was obtained from a local drinking water RO plant. Batch experiments were conducted in 250 mL photobioreactors (PBR), with an illumination of 4500–5000 lux, light:dark cycle of 16 h:8 h and 25 °C. Two blends of ROR with BG11 were studied (50% and 75% ROR). At regular intervals, the samples were collected from PBR and analyzed for biomass yield, chlorophyll-a content, specific growth rates, and treatment efficiency of ROR (removal rates of TN and TP).

Bhandari and Prajapati (2022) demonstrated *Chlorella pyrenoidosa* (NCIM 2738) for the treatment of ROR. ROR was collected from a commercial RO plant located in Uttarakhand, India. Desalination experiments were performed in various blends of synthetic medium (BG11 medium) and ROR (25%, 50%, 75%), along with 100% BG11 and 100% ROR mediums. Experiments were performed in 250 mL flasks with 50 mL working volume, and observations were recorded. The experiments were carried out in a triplicate manner. During desalination, the variations in chlorophyll-a, elemental composition, and biochemical composition (relative lipid, protein, and carbohydrate contents) of algal biomass were evaluated. Lipid%, biomass productivity [BP], and lipid productivity [LP] were calculated.

Matos et al. (2017b) used ROR from the Community of Uruçu (semiarid region of Paraíba state, Brazil). The ROR was directly used for desalination studies without blending with synthetic medium. The influence of utilizing ROR on lipid and fatty acid methyl ester (FAME) of microalgae was evaluated. Woo et al. (2019) used a combined treatment strategy that involved pretreatment of ROR with ozone followed by microalgae treatment. In this study, synthetic ROR was prepared (Table 9.1). Various dosage O_3 (0, 1, and 2 mg of O_3 per mg of C) were tested before treating ROR with microalgae-assisted desalination. The ozonated ROR was treated with fresh algal biomass for 24 h. Following the algae treatment, the spent biomass was separated, and the filtrate was used for dead-end filtration tests. This combined strategy was found to be more efficient in removing both caffeine and carbamazepine, as well as removing organic matter and inorganic nutrients from ROR in a single bioreactor.

Mohseni et al. (2021) used four common microalgal species (*Scenedesmus abundans*, *Chlorella vulgaris*, *Chlamydomonas reinhardtii*, and *Coelastrum microporum)*. Further, two marine microalgae, *Nannochloropsis salina* and *Dunaliella tertiolecta,* were tested in batch treatment. The ROR was collected from a wastewater reclamation facility located in Victoria, Australia. For batch experiments, 400 ml of ROR was used. The cultivation conditions were: Light intensity—180 μmol/m^2/s, temperature—23 °C, cultivation time—10 days. For semi batch operation, the biomass was separated from the treated ROR by centrifugation and reused for ROR treatment.

Mohseni et al. (2020) used *Chlorella vulgaris* and a marine microalga *Nannochloropsis salina* in suspended and alginate-immobilized cultures for batch and semicontinuous treatment of the ROR. The source of ROR was the same as the one used in (Mohseni et al., 2021). *C. vulgaris* and *N. salina* were cultivated in MLA medium and f/2 medium, respectively. The cultivation period 10–14 h, and the spent biomass was separated by centrifugation. The cells were washed with demineralized water and reused for the treatment of ROR. For immobilized algal beads preparation, 4% sodium alginate solution and 2% $CaCl_2$ solution were used. The desalination experiments were conducted using both suspended and alginate-immobilized cultures, in batch and semicontinuous operation. For experiments on immobilized cultures, the algal suspensions were added to ROR.

Almutairi et al. (2021) used freshwater microalga *C. vulgaris* (Chlorophyceae) from the Algal Biotechnology Unit, National Research Centre, Cairo, Egypt. ROR water from a reverse osmosis (RO) treatment plant (with an initial salinity of 67.61 g L^{-1}) was utilized for the growth of acclimatized cells of *Chlorella vulgaris*. Growth studies were conducted in 200 L vertical photobioreactor and gradually subjected to hypersaline conditions by adding 2 g NaCl and 4.5 ppm of $MgSO.7H_2O$ for 28 days. The light intensity used in PBR was 120 mmol m^{-2} s^{-1}, and the desalination experiments were conducted for 15 days. Desalination experiments `using the acclimatized alga were performed using two varieties of ROR, the original and treated rejected water (ORW and TRW, respectively). Following the bio-desalination, algal samples were subjected to oil extraction in a Soxhlet apparatus using a mixed solvent of n-hexane and isopropanol (volume ratio of 3:2).

Maeng et al. (2018a) studied the bio-desalination of ROR using *Scenedesmus quadricauda.* The synthetic ROR was prepared, and batch experiments were conducted with 100% ROR in 250 ml flasks with continuous illumination. For a few trials, the flasks were aerated with CO_2-enriched air at a flow rate of 40 mL/min.

Wang et al. (2016) demonstrated the performance of two microalgae strains, *Chlorella* sp. ZTY4 and *Scenedesmus* sp. *LX1* for the treatment of ROR obtained from two local municipal wastewater treatment plants of Beijing (plants A and B). These plants adopted a combined strategy of treating wastewater involving microfiltration followed by RO. Desalination experiments were conducted in 500 mL flasks, using 250 ml of medium inoculated with 1% (v/v) of cell culture. The optimum parameters were: light intensity—55-60 μmol/m^2/s, light to dark cycle ratio—14 h:10 h, and temperature 25 °C. The growth characteristics, lipid, and TAG accumulation ability, and the mechanisms of removal of Ca^{+2}, Mg^{+2}, TN, and TP were discussed.

Bhandari et al. (2024) discussed the performance of *Chlorella pyrenoidosa*, *Scenedesmus* sp., *Scenedesmus obliquus*, and *Chlorella sorokiniana* on desalination of ROR supplemented with bicarbonate. The authors demonstrated that the bicarbonate-enriched ROR had a significant influence on PUFA accumulation of *C. pyrenoidosa,* while there was no effect on *Scenedesmus* sp. Moreover, the presence of bicarbonate in the RO reject initiated the synthesis of biofuel precursor. Hence, the carbohydrate and lipid contents of *Scenedesmus obliquus* and *Chlorella sorokiniana* were reported as 340 mg L^{-1} and 1456 mg L^{-1}, at a dosage of 0.5 and 1.0 g L^{-1} bicarbonate, respectively.

9.3 Biomass Growth Rates, Lipid Content, Biomass and Lipid Productivities of Microalgae Cultivated in ROR and Blends

In this section, we describe the consolidated results of specific growth rate, doubling time, biomass concentration, biomass productivity, and lipid productivity of microalgae cultivated in ROR and their blends (Table 9.2). Wang et al. (2016) reported the highest biomass productivity of 320.5 mg/L.day for *Scenedesmus* sp. *LX1*. However, the highest lipid productivity of 49.5 mg Lipid /(day.L) was reported by Chang et al. (2020). Lipid productivity and biomass productivity are valuable tools to access the efficiency of algal based system. The calculation of lipid productivity considers both lipid% and biomass productivity and hence used as a yardstick to rank the microalgae. Biomass concentrations as high as 1.49 g/L were reported by Almutairi et al. (2021) and lipid content of 31.25% were reported by Chang et al. (2020). These factors indicated that, ROR can significantly reduce the requirements of fresh nutrient medium and improve the economy of RO plants. A low lipid content of 4.5% was reported by Matos et al. (2017b) (4.5%) and the significantly high specific growth rate of 0.771 day^{-1} was reported by Do et al. (2021).

9.4 Desalination Performance of ROR Treatment by Microalgae

Table 9.3 lists the desalination ability of various microalgae in ROR. Do et al. (2021) reported the highest TN and TO removal ability of *C. sorokiniana KNUA071* and *Desmodesmus* sp. KNUA024 were 91.9%, 97%, 51%, and 82% respectively. They also reported the reduction levels of cations and anions. Among cations, the sodium ions removal rate was highest (60.38%), while among anions, the chloride ion removal rate was 74.54% and 76.74%, respectively. Bhandari et al. (2023) reported that, among three species tested, *Chlorella sorokiniana* was most effective in removal of TDS (85.24%), while *Scenedesmus obliquus* was efficient in removal of TN and TP (77.59% and 82.71%).

Table 9.2 Growth rate and lipid accumulation characteristics of microalgae cultivated in ROR

Species	Growth rate (day^{-1})	Doubling time (day)	Biomass conc (g/L)	Lipid content (% w/w)	Biomass productivity (mg/(L-day)	Lipid productivity (mg/(L-day)	Ref.
C. sorokiniana KNUA071	0.771	0.899	0.9	13.3	NA (not available)	NA (not available)	Do et al. (2021)
Desmodesmus sp. KNUA024	0.5	1.386	0.76	29.3	NA (not available)	NA (not available)	
Scenedesmus obliquus	0.209	3.31	1.36	28.85	84.8	6.71	Bhandari et al. (2023)
Chlorella sorokiniana	0.176	3.93	1.3	16.59	86.59	6.45	
Scenedesmus sp	0.277	2.502	1.33	24.57	80.81	6.08	
Chlorella pyrenoidosa	NA	NA	0.86	10.0	53.33	5.33	Bhandari and Prajapati (2022)
C. vulgaris (25% ROR)	0.59	NA	NA	12.5	NA (not available)	7.37	Matos et al. (2017b)
S. platensis (50% ROR)	1.55	NA	NA	4.5	NA	6.97	
N. gaditana (75% ROR)	0.96	NA	NA	12.6	NA	12.1	
S. quadricauda strain (AG 10003)	NA	NA	NA	NA	NA	NA	Woo et al. (2019)
C. vulgaris	0.27	NA	NA	NA	320	NA	Mohseni et al. (2020)
N. salina	0.25	NA	NA	NA	299	NA	
Chlorella vulgaris	NA	6.2	**1.49**	13.2	0.11	14.3	Almutairi et al. (2021)
	NA	NA	1.27	31.25		**49.5**	Chang et al. (2020)
Chlorella sp. *ZTY4*	NA	NA	NA	NA	318.7	30.6	Wang et al. (2016)
Scenedesmus sp. *LX1*	NA	NA	0.76	NA	**320.5**	31.5	
Chlorella pyrenoidosa	0.17	4.1	1.02	NA	88	NA	Bhandari et al. (2024)

Table 9.3 Performance of microalgae in treatment of ROR

Species	% TN removal	% TP removal	DIC/DOC (mg/(L. day))	% TDS Removal	Cations	Anions	Metal ions	Ref.
C. sorokiniana KNUA071	91.9	97	NA	NA	Na^{+}-60.38 Ca^{+2}–14.59 Mg^{+2}–75.4 K^{+}-24.6	Cl-74.54	Mn^{+2}–98 Zn^{+2}–64 Co^{+2}–62 Ni^{+2}–50	Do et al. (2021)
Desmodesmus sp. KNUA024	51	82	NA	NA	NA^{+}-NA Ca^{+2}–37.08 Mg^{+2}–2.67 K^{+}-1.12	Cl-76.74	Mn^{+2}-NA Zn^{+2}–62.6 Co^{+2}–58.4 Ni^{+2}–45.68	
Scenedesmus obliquus	77.59	82.71	NA	79.69	NA	NA	NA	Bhandari et al. (2023)
Chlorella sorokiniana	75.36	80.48	NA	85.24	NA	NA	NA	
Scenedesmus sp	67.48	79.07	NA	84.36	NA	NA	NA	
C. vulgaris	3.4	NA	DOC-8.1		NA	NA	NA	Mohseni et al. (2020)
N. salina	3.1	NA	DOC-9.5		NA	NA	NA	
C. vulgaris	10.6	NA	DOC-35.5		NA	NA	NA	
N. salina	10.0	NA	DOC-35		NA	NA	NA	
S. quadricauda	85	92	NA	86% COD	NA	NA	NA	Maeng et al. (2018b)

Chlorella sp. *ZTY4*	89.8	89.7	NA	37.2% COD	Ca^{+2}–55.9 Mg^{+2}–56	NA	NA	Wang et al. (2016)
Scenedesmus sp. *LX1*	89.7	92.4	NA	33.7% COD	Ca^{+2}–58.7 Mg^{+2}–28.7	NA	NA	
S. abundans	11.5	7.1	DOC-8.6	NA	NA	NA	NA	Mohseni et al. (2021)
N. salina	18	8.2	DOC-12.4	NA	NA	NA	NA	
S. quadricauda strain (AG 10003)	89	94	COD-70% Carbamazepine-94% Caffeine-93%	NA	NA	NA	NA	Woo et al. (2019)
N. gaditana	80	86	NA	NA	NA	NA	NA	Matos et al. (2017b)

Mohseni et al. (2020) reported that among three species tested, *C. vulgaris* was most efficient in removal of DOC (35.5 mg/(L.day)) through the biotic pathway. The highest COD removal of ROR was 37.2% by the *Chlorella* sp. *ZTY4* (Wang et al., 2016). There was no significant difference in the desalination rates of immobilized cells and suspended cells. In semicontinuous mode, microalgae removed >50% TN and >80% of TP, while generating a biomass of 335–360 mg DCWL^{-1} day^{-1}. The organic matter of ROR also reduced considerably (>65%).

Mohseni et al. (2021) showed that, the DOC removal rate of 12.4 mg/(L.day) was achieved by *N. salina*. *S. abundans* and *N. salina* were efficient in reducing the organic matter (11.6–18 mg/L/d TN, 7.2–8.1 mg/L/d TP, and 8.5–12.5 mg/L/d DOC, respectively). At higher salinity, nitrogen uptake reduced but no significant effect on TP removal was observed.

As explained under Sect. 9.2, Woo et al. (2019) adopted combined strategy involving ozone treatment followed by algal treatment for ROR. Following the algal treatment, fluorescence intensity of ROR reduced by 25%, while, combined strategy of ozone treatment with algae treatment reduced the fluorescence by 75–82%. The COD reduced by 70% in algal membrane reactor when operated at 300 mmol photons m^{-2} s^{-1}. At this optimized light intensity, the TN and TP reduced by 89% and 94%, respectively. Furthermore, the authors reported that the combined strategy was able to achieve the caffeine content reduction and carbamazepine content reduction by 93% and 94%, respectively.

Matos et al. (2017b) reported that the ROR (75%) medium was able to be recycled thrice for the successive cultivation *N. gaditana*, in which each individual cycle was of 7 days of cultivation. In the first cultivation cycle, *N. gaditana* cells reduced the total N (initial concentration 415 mg L^{-1}) by 60% and total P (initial concentration 22.5 mg L^{-1}) by 71.1%. After three cultivation cycles, the TN and TP were reduced by 80% and 86%, respectively.

9.5 Biochemical and Elemental Composition of Microalgae After Bio-Desalination

Post desalination, the algae cells are harvested for further processing and transformation into valuable products. The biochemical and elemental analyses are key characteristics for understanding the further application of residual biomass. Various authors have reported these results (Table 9.4).

9.6 Conversion of Microalgal Biomass Cultivated in ROR to Valuable Products

The results of biochemical analysis, elemental analysis of algal biomass described previously in this report, clearly suggest that the algal biomass can be separated from treated ROR through solid–liquid separating unit operations such as filtration/centrifugation and converted to valuable products. This step further enhances the

Table 9.4 Biochemical and elemental analysis of various microalgae cultivated in ROR

Species	Carbohydrate (%, w/w)	Protein (%, w/w)	%C	%H	%N	%S	C/N	Ref.
C. sorokiniana KNUA071	30.39	19.78	36.98	5.00	1.84	0.47	NA	Do et al. (2021)
Desmodesmus sp. KNUA024	18.66	21.11	52.94	7.85	3.17	0.23	NA	
Scenedesmus obliquus	27.5	12.41	36.94	5.62	2.77	0.08	13.4	Bhandari et al. (2023)
Chlorella sorokiniana	26.56	9.45	41.75	5.54	2.66	0.22	18.28	
Scenedesmus sp.	29.83	13.24	32.34	4.19	1.82	0.28	19.96	
Chlorella pyrenoidosa	28.41	29.75	46.08	6.67	2.67	0.22	7.37	Bhandari and Prajapati (2022)
S. obliquus	32.89	62.41	25.50	41.57	1.39	NA	31.52	Bhandari et al. (2024)
Scenedesmus sp.	42.35	55.12	25	38.97	1.37	NA	34.65	
Chlorealla pyrenoidosa	34.58	58.74	27.88[a]	47.39[a]	1.41[a]	NA	23.23[a]	

[a]The results are calculated based on the empirical formula of microalgal biomass provided in the article

feasibility of the process. Several authors have addressed this issue, and the key results of which are described here.

9.6.1 Conversion of Residual Biomass to Biodiesel

Do et al. (2021) extracted the lipids from residual biomass and transformed them to biodiesel using a method modified by Breuer et al. (2013). The properties of biodiesel were calculated using the data of fatty acid methyl ester (FAMEs) and are reported in Table 9.5. Almutairi et al. (2021) extracted the oil from residual biomass of *Chlorella* using Soxhlet apparatus using 750 ml of a nonpolar solvent mixture (n-hexane:isopropanol, 3:2, v:v). FAMEs were obtained using acid hydrolysis followed by a GC system (GC Perkin Elmer Auto System XL). Bhandari et al. (2024) used microwave pretreatment and modified Bligh and Dyer's method (Rana et al., 2020) for lipid extraction and quantification. The lipid was subjected to transesterification to produce FAMEs using the protocol described by Rana and Prajapati (2021).

9.6.2 Conversion of Residual Biomass to Biogas

Bhandari et al. (2024) assessed the potential of residual microalgae of *C. pyrenoidosa, C. sorokiniana, Scenedesmus* sp., and *S. obliquus* biomass to biogas. At a bicarbonate concentration of 1 g/L, the theoretical methane potential (TMP) of ROR was 542 mL CH_4 g^{-1} VS for *C. pyrenoidosa*, while 508 mL CH_4 g^{-1} VS for *C. sorokiniana*. No significant improvement in TMP was observed for *Scenedesmus* spp. It was demonstrated that 500 m^3 ROR supplemented with 500 kg of sodium bicarbonate could generate 21.7 kg day^{-1} of *C. pyrenoidosa* biomass and 29.8 kg day^{-1} of *C. sorokiniana* biomass, which had a TMP of 11.8 m^3 day^{-1} (421.3 MJ energy) and 14.28 m^3 day^{-1} (511.6 MJ energy), respectively.

9.6.3 Conversion of Residual Biomass of *D. salina* Grown in ROR to β-Carotene

Zhu et al. (2018) designed a low-cost floating photobioreactor to cultivate *Dunaliella salina*, using ROR from seawater desalination as culture medium and extracted β-carotene from residual biomass. The culture medium was bubbled with CO_2, to generate bicarbonate, which enhanced total inorganic carbon to 0.254 mol L^{-1}. A pilot-scale floating PBR having a surface area of 1 m^2 was used for cultivation. From 1000 L of ROR, 300 g of biomass containing 14.5 g β-carotene was extracted, which had a selling price of more than $40. This could significantly enhance the economics of the desalination industry.

Table 9.5 Physicochemical properties of biodiesel (FAMEs) produced through residual algal biomass

Species	Physicochemical properties						
	Saponification value (mg KOH/g oil)	Density @20 °C (g/cc)	Kinematic viscosity at 40 °C (mm^2/s)	Cold filter plug-going point (°C)	Oxidative stability (h)	Iodine value G I_2/100 g oil	Cetane number
C. sorokiniana KNUA071 (Do et al., 2021)	183.3	0.85	3.5	−8.5	5.8	135.1	45.7
Desmodesmus sp. KNUA024 (Do et al., 2021)	190.9	0.88	3.80	−6.5	5.8	129.3	45.8
Chlorella vulgaris (Almutairi et al., 2021)	194.41	NA	NA	1.1675	NA	94.68	53.0
Chlorealla pyrenoidosa (Almutairi et al., 2021)	174.56	0.87	4.29	–15.64	Nd-	42.90	68.52
Chlorella sorokiniana (Bhandari et al., 2024)	196.79	0.98	4.54	−15.62	20.45	52.39	62.25

9.6.4 Conversion of *S. platensis* Grown in ROR to Phycocyanin

Matos et al. (2021) used ROR from brackish groundwater RO membranes (FILMTEC™ TW30 4040, Midland, USA) desalination equipment, located in the community of Urucu, Sao Joao do Cariri, Paraiba State, Brazil. Outdoor studies were carried out using two concrete raceway ponds of total capacity 4 m^3 and inoculated with 2 m^3 of fresh culture medium. These ponds were operated in a batch mode for 24 days, following which, the cells were separated from treated ROR and Phycocyanin concentration (PC) was extracted from dried *S. platensis* biomass in phosphate buffer (pH 7.0). It was demonstrated that 60% ROR was the optimum concentration at which *S. platensis* exhibited a biomass concentration of 2.9 g L^{-1}, while the phycocyanin concentration was 9.0%. Furthermore, the biomass productivity was 10.3 g m^{-2} day^{-1} with 45.0% of protein content, along with production of amino acids, pigments, and fatty acids.

9.6.5 Further Scope of Utilization of Algal Biomass

The microalgae biomass cultivated in ROR can be alternatively utilized directly for biochar production using pyrolysis technology. Microalgal biochar has several applications. Due to its high nutritional content and ion exchange characteristics, it can be applied in sustainable agriculture by partially substituting artificial fertilizers, which over time deplete the soil's nutritional value (Mona et al., 2021). Due to its high surface area, it can be used in industrial effluents by adsorbing heavy metals and organic pollutants. Biochar from microalgae can be used for efficient ammonia removal in sustainable wastewater treatment due to its nanoporous structure and high adsorption capacity (Zhou et al., 2019). Nickel-adsorbed algal biochar has been successfully utilized as a cost-effective catalyst for the oxygen reduction reaction in microbial carbon-capture cells, achieving a power density 3.5 times higher than commercial alternatives (Neethu et al., 2024). Furthermore, Lu et al. (2023) examined the physiochemical characteristics of *Nannochloropsis* microalgae biochar, suggesting that it could be a viable addition to blends of microalgae-based biodiesel and a potential. Microalgae biochar exhibits potential as a material for the storage of energy. Sun et al. (2023) proposed a method for recovering phosphorus from algae biomass while enhancing the biochar's electrochemical capacitance for use in supercapacitors. Several studies in the literature have shown that biochar produced from algal biomass has excellent properties such as high carbon content (72.39% (Azizi et al., 2020) and low ash content (4.72% (Yu et al., 2020). Choi et al. (2020) demonstrated that biochar with a low concentration of oxygen was produced from *Chlorella* sp. A high surface area of 117 m^2/g was reported by Arun et al. (2020). Shi et al. (2021) showed that, with KOH modification in a molar ratio of 1:6, the BET surface area of biochar from *Chlorella* sp. and *Spirulina* sp. increased from 4.95 to 312 m^2 g^{-1} and 5.8 to 382 m^2 g^{-1}, respectively. The above results show that, a high-quality biochar can be produced from microalgal biomass. However, reports in utilization of residual biomass obtained post desalination are not so far addressed in literature. Hence, significant scope exists in this direction of research. Furthermore, algal biochar can be produced through several techniques as Torrefaction, pyrolysis, hydrothermal process (Hydrothermal carbonization, Hydrothermal liquefaction, gasification) substitute fuel for the energy industry.

9.7 Economics and Feasibility Assessment of Mass Cultivation of Microalgae in ROR of Commercial RO Plant

Bhandari and Prajapati (2022) showed that the RO reject from a commercial RO plant (ROR-CU) was tested to evaluate the feasibility and economics of mass algae cultivation in ROR. The salinity of ROR-CU was higher than ROR-DU (600 mS). For the studies, two concentrations of ROR (50% and 75%) were chosen, while 100% BG11 and ROR-CU served as positive and negative controls, respectively. It was observed that the performance of *C. pyrenoidosa* was poor at 75% and 100% ROR (inhibited growth), whereas better results were obtained at 50% ROR. At this concentration, highest biomass concentration and biomass productivity of 1.38 g/L and 86 mg L^{-1} day^{-1}, lipid content of 33.32% were observed, respectively. Additionally, the Chl-a content was 13.19 mg. L^{-1} (which was lower than the positive control). In addition, a remarkably high lipid-containing biomass (28.98 mg L^{-1} day¯1) could be obtained in ROR-CU media, which was approximately 2.3 times higher than that in the positive control. The theoretical calculations showed that, for the production of 1000 kg of dry algal biomass of *C. pyrenoidosa*, approximately 743 m^3 of freshwater was required. However, a 50% blend with ROR-CU reduced the quantity of water to 371.5 m^3. Further, it was demonstrated that if 100% ROR was used, the quantity of water required was 1230.45 m^3 of ROR-CU.

In a report by Bhandari et al. (2023), the authors further analyzed the cost economics of using ROR for mass cultivation of algae. The basis of calculation was 100 kg/day of dried biomass of *S. obliquus* using RO reject as nutrient medium, with/without supplementation. The cost of freshwater was assumed to be 0.77 USD per m^3. The costs of ROR were considered as zero. It was shown that the total cost of freshwater and nutrients would be $9259.71 and $4908.34, respectively, in 50% and 75% RO reject. However, in 50% and 75% ROR media, the cost was reduced by 41% and 56%, respectively. Furthermore, for the cultivation of *Scenedesmus sp*, using 75% ROR could reduce the cost by 72.88%. Hence, integration of microalgae cultivation with ROR was proved to be economically feasible. However, the authors do not recommend 100% ROR usage due to the challenges of lipid productivity. The above studies illustrate that post desalination algal biomass can be employed for several applications, thus improving the overall economics of an algal-based desalination plant.

9.8 Challenges and Limitations of Microalgae-Mediated Bio-Desalination Technology

Although the microalgae-based bio-desalination system offers several advantages, certain challenges and limitations hinder its implementation on a larger scale. Some of these limitations include:

(i) Poor performance of algae strains: Selection of strains with excellent growth characteristics and desalination ability.
(ii) Complicated and expensive pretreatment: In the case of treatment of ROR from seawater desalination plant, simple and effective pretreatment methods are required to reduce the load on the algal desalination system.
(iii) Improper N/P ratio of ROR: The composition of ROR indicates a lower N/P ratio, high salinity, high TDS, and potential toxicity from ammonia and metals.
(iv) Biomass separation after desalination: The separation of spent biomass from treated water after desalination offers several challenges. Although flocculation using alum is a simple option, it introduces the metal ions into the treated water. On the other hand, membrane separation operations increase the cost of technology. Hence, there is a necessity for a low-cost biomass separation system following the desalination.

9.9 Conclusion

This book chapter summarizes the potential of microalgae in treating RO-rejected water. The characteristics of ROR (as reported by various researchers), potential algae strains employed, the performance of the algal strains in bio-desalination process (as depicted by parameters such as biomass concentration, lipid yield, extent of reduction in salinity, and TDS), and the techniques to handle the spent algal biomass obtained after desalination were discussed in detail. The analysis of results reported illustrates that significant potential exists for the microalgal desalination technology. It is a sustainable and novel approach for handling large amounts of ROR, encouraging the development of low-cost and efficient photobioreactor designs for industrial-scale implementation. Furthermore, industries on the extraction of phytochemicals can employ the ROR for the growth of microalgae (*Spirulina platensis*, for instance) and perform the extraction of valuable phytochemicals. However, further data generation in pilot-scale studies and validation of the idea are critical before implementation at large scale.

References

Almutairi, A. W., El-Sayed, A. E., & Reda, M. M. (2021). Evaluation of high salinity adaptation for lipid bio-accumulation in the green microalga Chlorella vulgaris. *Saudi Journal of Biological Sciences., 28*(7), 3981–3988.

Arun, J., Gopinath, K. P., Vigneshwar, S. S., & Swetha, A. (2020). Sustainable and eco-friendly approach for phosphorus recovery from wastewater by hydrothermally carbonized microalgae: Study on spent bio-char as fertilizer. *Journal of Water Process Engineering., 38*, 101567.

Azizi, K., Moraveji, M. K., Arregi, A., Amutio, M., Lopez, G., & Olazar, M. (2020). On the pyrolysis of different microalgae species in a conical spouted bed reactor: Bio-fuel yields and characterization. *Bioresource Technology., 311*, 123561.

Bhandari, M., & Prajapati, S. K. (2022). Use of reverse osmosis reject from drinking water plant for microalgal biomass production. *Water Research, 210*, 117989.

Bhandari, M., Kharkwal, S., & Prajapati, S. K. (2023). Recycling drinking water RO reject for microalgae-mediated resource recovery. *Resources, Conservation and Recycling., 188*, 106699.

Bhandari, M., Kharkwal, S., & Prajapati, S. K. (2024). Bicarbonate-assisted microalgae cultivation for drinking water RO reject recycling and bioproduct generation. *Bioresource Technology Reports., 25*, 101756.

Blumwald, E., Mehlhorn, R. J., & Packer, L. (1983). Ionic osmoregulation during salt adaptation of the cyanobacterium Synechococcus 6311. *Plant Physiology, 73*(2), 377–380.

Breuer, G., Evers, W. A., de Vree, J. H., Kleinegris, D. M., Martens, D. E., Wijffels, R. H., & Lamers, P. P. (2013). Analysis of fatty acid content and composition in microalgae. *Journal of Visualized Experiments: JoVE, 80*, 50628.

Chang, H., Hu, R., Zou, Y., Quan, X., Zhong, N., Zhao, S., & Sun, Y. (2020). Highly efficient reverse osmosis concentrate remediation by microalgae for biolipid production assisted with electrooxidation. *Water Research, 174*, 115642.

Chen, J. P., Chian, E. S., Sheng, P. X., Nanayakkara, K. N., Wang, L. K., & Ting, Y. P. (2010). Desalination of seawater by reverse osmosis. In *Membrane and desalination technologies* (pp. 559–601). Humana Press.

Choi, Y. K., Choi, T. R., Gurav, R., Bhatia, S. K., Park, Y. L., Kim, H. J., Kan, E., & Yang, Y. H. (2020). Adsorption behavior of tetracycline onto spirulina sp.(microalgae)-derived biochars produced at different temperatures. *Science of the Total Environment., 710*, 136282.

Do, J. M., Jo, S. W., Yeo, H. T., Shin, D. H., Oh, H., Hong, J. W., & Yoon, H. S. (2021). Biological treatment of reverse osmosis concentrate by microalgae cultivation and utilization of the resulting algal biomass. *Journal of Water Process Engineering., 42*, 102157.

Hanifa, N. M., Thevarajah, B., Liyanaarachchi, V. C., Nimarshana, P. H., Boopathy, R., & Ariyadasa, T. U. (2025). Simultaneous bioremediation, resource recovery and natural dye production via textile wet processing wastewater-integrated microalgae cultivation: A review. *Current Pollution Reports., 11*(1), 38.

Hasnain, M., Zainab, R., Ali, F., & Abideen, Z. (2025). An overview of biosorption, remediation, and desalination potential of algae to remove wastewater toxic pollutants for environmental safety. *Environmental Monitoring and Assessment., 197*(8), 853.

Lu, H., Xie, R., Almoallim, H. S., Alharbi, S. A., Jhanani, G. K., Praveenkumar, T. R., Anderson, A., & Xia, C. (2023). Utilization of the Nannochloropsis microalgae biochar prepared via microwave assisted pyrolysis on the mixed biomass fuel pellets. *Environmental Research., 231*, 116078.

Maeng, S. K., You, S. H., Nam, J. Y., Ryu, H., Timmes, T. C., & Kim, H. C. (2018a). The growth of Scenedesmus quadricauda in RO concentrate and the impacts on refractory organic matter, Escherichia coli, and trace organic compounds. *Water Research, 134*, 292–300.

Maeng, S. K., Khan, W., Park, J. W., Han, I., Yang, H. S., Song, K. G., Choi, W. J., Kim, S., Woo, H., & Kim, H. C. (2018b). Treatment of highly saline RO concentrate using Scenedesmus quadricauda for enhanced removal of refractory organic matter. *Desalination, 430*, 128–135.

Matos, Â. P., Moecke, E. H., & Sant'Anna, E. S. (2017a). The use of desalination concentrates as a potential substrate for microalgae cultivation in Brazil. *Algal Research, 24*, 505–508.

Matos, Â. P., Moecke, E. H., & Sant'Anna, E. S. (2017b). The use of desalination concentrate as a potential substrate for microalgae cultivation in Brazil. *Algal Research, 24*, 505–508.

Matos, Â. P., da Silva, T., & Sant'Anna, E. S. (2021). The feasibility of using inland desalination concentrate (DC) as an alternative substrate for Spirulina platensis mass cultivation. *Waste and Biomass Valorization., 12*(6), 3193–3203.

Miller, S., Shemer, H., & Semiat, R. (2015). Energy and environmental issues in desalination. *Desalination, 366*, 2–8.

Mohseni, A., Kube, M., Fan, L., & Roddick, F. A. (2020). Potential of Chlorella vulgaris and Nannochloropsis Salina for nutrient and organic matter removal from municipal wastewater reverse osmosis concentrate. *Environmental Science and Pollution Research., 27*(21), 26905–26914.

Mohseni, A., Fan, L., & Roddick, F. A. (2021). Impact of microalgae species and solution salinity on algal treatment of wastewater reverse osmosis concentrate. *Chemosphere, 285*, 131487.

Mona, S., Malyan, S. K., Saini, N., Deepak, B., Pugazhendhi, A., & Kumar, S. S. (2021). Towards sustainable agriculture with carbon sequestration, and greenhouse gas mitigation using algal biochar. *Chemosphere, 275*, 129856.

Neethu, B., Ihjas, K., Chakraborty, I., & Ghangrekar, M. M. (2024). Nickel adsorbed algae biochar based oxygen reduction reaction catalyst. *Bioelectrochemistry, 159*, 108747.

Patel, A. K., Tseng, Y. S., Singhania, R. R., Chen, C. W., Chang, J. S., & Di Dong, C. (2021). Novel application of microalgae platform for biodesalination process: A review. *Bioresource Technology, 337*, 125343.

Rajfur, M., Jozwiak, M. A., & Klos, A. (2014). The impact of various cations on the sorption of manganese in the thallus of freshwater algae spirogyra sp. and sea algae palmaria palmata. *Ecological Chemistry and Engineering., 21*(1), 35.

Rana, M. S., & Prajapati, S. K. (2021). Stimulating effects of glycerol on the growth, phycoremediation and biofuel potential of Chlorella pyrenoidosa cultivated in wastewater. *Environmental Technology & Innovation, 24*, 102082.

Rana, M. S., Bhushan, S., Sudhakar, D. R., & Prajapati, S. K. (2020). Effect of iron oxide nanoparticles on growth and biofuel potential of Chlorella spp. *Algal Research, 49*, 101942.

Rana, M. S., Sharma, A. K., Parambil, J. V., & Prajapati, S. K. (2021). Potential of reverse osmosis reject water as a growth medium for the production of algal metabolites–A state-of-the-art review. *Journal of Water Process Engineering., 40*, 101849.

Rantanen, M. (2008). Efficient use and consumption of water in power generation. *Wärtsilä Technical Journal.*

Saranya, S., Dhayanithi, S., & Chellapandi, P. (2025). Sustainable biogas-powered desalination using marine microalgae: A review. *Renewable and Sustainable Energy Reviews., 219*, 115886.

Satthong, S., Saego, K., Kitrungloadjanaporn, P., Nuttavut, N., Amornsamankul, S., & Triampo, W. (2019). Modeling the effects of light sources on the growth of algae. *Adv. Difference Equ., 2019*(1), 170.

Shi, S., Ochedi, F. O., Yu, J., & Liu, Y. (2021). Porous biochars derived from microalgae pyrolysis for CO2 adsorption. *Energy & Fuels, 35*(9), 7646–7656.

Shirazi, S. A., Rastegary, J., Aghajani, M., & Ghassemi, A. (2018). Simultaneous biomass production and water desalination concentrate treatment by using microalgae. *Desalination and Water Treatment, 135*, 101–107.

Sun, J., Benavente, V., Jansson, S., & Mašek, O. (2023). Comparative characterisation and phytotoxicity assessment of biochar and hydrochar derived from municipal wastewater microalgae biomass. *Bioresource Technology, 386*, 129567.

Timková, I., Sedláková-Kaduková, J., & Pristaš, P. (2018). Biosorption and bioaccumulation abilities of actinomycetes/streptomycetes isolated from metal contaminated sites. *Separations., 5*(4), 54.

Wang, X. X., Wu, Y. H., Zhang, T. Y., Xu, X. Q., Dao, G. H., & Hu, H. Y. (2016). Simultaneous nitrogen, phosphorous, and hardness removal from reverse osmosis concentrate by microalgae cultivation. *Water Research, 94*, 215–224.

Wei, J., Gao, L., Shen, G., Yang, X., & Li, M. (2020). The role of adsorption in microalgae biological desalination: Salt removal from brackish water using Scenedesmus obliquus. *Desalination, 493*, 114616.

Woo, H., Yang, H. S., Timmes, T. C., Han, C., Nam, J. Y., Byun, S., Kim, S., Ryu, H., & Kim, H. C. (2019). Treatment of reverse osmosis concentrate using an algal-based MBR combined with ozone pretreatment. *Water Research, 159*, 164–175.

Yu, K. L., Chen, W. H., Sheen, H. K., Chang, J. S., Lin, C. S., Ong, H. C., Show, P. L., Ng, E. P., & Ling, T. C. (2020). Production of microalgal biochar and reducing sugar using wet torrefaction with microwave-assisted heating and acid hydrolysis pretreatment. *Renewable Energy, 156*, 349–360.

Zhou, N., Wang, Y., Yao, D., Li, S., Tang, J., Shen, D., Zhu, X., Huang, L., Zhong, M. E., & Zhou, Z. (2019). Novel wet pyrolysis providing simultaneous conversion and activation to produce surface-functionalized biochars for cadmium remediation. *Journal of Cleaner Production., 221*, 63–72.

Zhu, C., Zhai, X., Jia, J., Wang, J., Han, D., Li, Y., Tang, Y., & Chi, Z. (2018). Seawater desalination concentrate for cultivation of Dunaliella salina with floating photobioreactor to produce β-carotene. *Algal Research, 35*, 319–324.

Microalgae-Mediated Microbial Fuel Cells for Wastewater Treatment and Bioenergy: Insights and Perspectives

10

Sabeela Beevi Ummalyma and B. R. Sreelekhmy

Abstract

Algae are photosynthetic organisms that can fix CO_2 and produce biomass faster than their terrestrial counterparts. Recently, the application of algae in microbial fuel cells (MFCs) has garnered interest in sustainable electricity generation, wastewater treatment, and biofuel production. Algae produce oxygen during photosynthesis, reducing operational costs by eliminating the need for air sparging. The microalgae in MFCs will enhance the system's performance, providing a cost-effective and sustainable process. Algae-mediated microbial fuel cells (A-MFCs) have been proven to be more beneficial in various applications, including carbon sequestration, resource recovery, bioremediation of wastewater, power generation, biofuel production, and the creation of value-added products. The performance of these fuel cells depends on several operational parameters, such as electrode material types, substrates, microbial consortia, and electrochemical reactions. In this chapter, we highlight the potential application of microalgae in MFCs for efficient power generation and sustainable utilization, aligning with SDG goals such as 6, 7, and 13. The application of A-MFCs in wastewater treatment, bioenergy production, and energy security for communities is highlighted, along with the factors influencing A-MFCs. It can be concluded that A-MFCs are paving the way for futuristic, sustainable solutions in wastewater treatment and bioenergy production.

S. B. Ummalyma (✉) · B. R. Sreelekhmy
Division of Environmental Biotechnology, Department of Biosciences, Rajagiri College of Social Sciences (Autonomous), Kochi, India
e-mail: sabeela@rajagiri.edu

L. Kumar et al. (eds.), *Algal Bioremediation*,
https://doi.org/10.1007/978-981-95-8793-3_10

Keywords

Microalgae · Biomass · Microbial fuel cells · Wastewater treatment · Biofuels · Sustainable process

10.1 Introduction

Currently, energy demands are increasing, and fossil fuel-based energy sources create numerous environmental issues, including global warming-related calamities resulting from the release of excess greenhouse gases and CO_2. It has directed the worldwide research to focus on alternative energy sources such as renewable energies (wind, solar, and bioenergy). Renewable energy is a sustainable, carbon-neutral energy source but still more research is required for lowering the production cost, installation, storage, energy yield, and efficiencies. Microbial fuel cells (MFCs) are alternative energy systems for bioelectricity generation. The application of algae in MFCs facilitates carbon sequestration, reduces the system's cost, and achieves high conversion efficiencies (Arun et al., 2020). Bioelectrochemical systems (BES) are the basic principle of MFCs. This system comprises major components, including an anode where the oxidation reaction occurs, a cathode where the reduction reaction takes place, and an ion exchange membrane separating the two electrodes. Bioelectrochemical systems provide avenues for wastewater treatment, resource recovery from waste streams, and sustainable energy generation. BES systems harness the potential of microorganisms to enable electron transfer in electrochemical reactions through the biocatalytic potential of electroactive microorganisms (EABs). Electroactive bacteria can be grouped into two categories: electro-exporting bacteria, which are capable of accepting electrons from organic feedstocks and donating them to the anode, and electron-accepting bacteria, which take up electrons from the cathodes, reducing CO_2 and other byproducts (Baek & Lee, 2024).

Microalgal bioelectrochemical systems (MBES) are employed for removing nutrients and pollutants, as well as resource recovery from wastewater. MES are simple MFCs, sediment-type microalgal fuel cells (SMFCs), microalgae carbon capture cells (MCCCs), and photosynthetic algal microbial fuel cells (PAMFCs). Microalgae-based bioelectrochemical reaction can reduce the cost of aeration (mechanical) due to oxygen release as a result of photosynthesis by microalgae along with concurrent uptake of N, P, and CO_2 during light reaction at the cathode reaction and fresh or pretreated algal biomass at the anode as substrates. The application of algae in MFCs offers several advantages, including the internal generation of electron acceptors (oxygen) through photosynthetic processes for cathode reactions, electron transfer via electroactive proteins, and carbon capture and sequestration, as well as low-cost wastewater treatment and energy generation (Ummalyma et al., 2019; Arun et al., 2020). The chapter discusses how the potential application of microalgae in MFCs for efficient power generation and sustainable utilization aligns with SDG goals such as 6, 7, and 13. The application of A-MFCs in wastewater treatment, bioenergy production, and energy security for communities is highlighted, along with the factors influencing A-MFCs.

10.2 Microalgae-Microbial Fuel Cells

Microalgae-microbial fuel cells (mMFC) is a device that converts solar energy into electrical energy through biological pathways (Tay et al., 2022). In these, microalgae serve multiple roles. At the anode: (1) microalgal biomass acts as a biocatalyst that supports the breakdown of organic pollutants and generates electrons for the anode, and (2) biomass can be utilized as a substrate for bacterial oxidative degradation to donate electrons to the anode. At the cathode: (1) to supply oxygen for cathode reduction for MFC functioning and (2) CO_2 released during the oxidative breakdown of organic molecules at the anode compartment is used for the photosynthesis of microalgae. It is a combined process of wastewater bioremediation, CO_2 sequestration, and biomass production, along with electricity generation in a self-sustainable way. The ideal representation of the biochemical reactions in the anode and cathode chambers of mMFC is as follows (Lee et al., 2015):

At anode:

$$\text{Organic substrates} + 2H_2O \rightarrow CO_2 + H^+ \text{ (to cathode)} + e^- \text{ (external circuit)} \tag{10.1}$$

At cathode:

$$nCO_2 + nH_2O + \text{light} \rightarrow (CH_2O)_n \text{ (algae biomass)} + nO_2 \tag{10.2}$$

$$2O_2 + 8e^- + 8H^+ \rightarrow 4H_2O \tag{10.3}$$

The overall reaction can be written as:

$$\text{Organics} + \text{light} \rightarrow \text{biomass} + \text{power} \tag{10.4}$$

When all the carbon dioxide produced can be consumed by the algae in the presence of light, the oxygen released can act as an electron acceptor.

MFC has many advantages and challenges compared to traditional MFC. However, CO_2 sequestration happens in autotrophic growth; the rate is limited by the algal cells, light intensity, and source. High cell density inhibits the light penetration, which largely decelerates cell growth. The mMFC requires a large surface area for light harvesting, which makes the downstream processing of the biomass expensive. Excessive light intensity can, however, hinder the growth of cells. Since algae release a sufficient amount of oxygen at the cathode chamber, this reduces the cost of mechanical aeration. Moreover, the possible use of algal biomass as feed or for biorefinery purposes can realize the zero-carbon discharge scheme (Lee et al., 2015).

10.2.1 Role of Microalgae at Anode Chamber

Microalgae in the anode chamber serve as electron donors by either oxidatively degrading organic pollutants or acting as a substrate for bacterial oxidative degradation, which also donates electrons to the anode.

(a) *Algae as EEA in the Anodic Compartment*

Certain photosynthetic cyanobacteria and other green microalgae, such as *Chlorella pyrenoidosa and Nitzschia palea* (Xu et al., 2015; Khan et al., 2022), *act as* bioanode catalysts for higher electrogenic activity without O_2 production (Mohan et al., 2014). It provides protons and electrons to the cathode chamber. This photosynthetic MFC can minimize operating costs by operating under anaerobic conditions, producing biomass that can be utilized as resources for biofuels, pigments, proteins, and other value-added products. *Chlorella pyrenoidosa* was applied in the anode of an MFC system as an electron donor. Under optimized conditions of dissolved oxygen, algal cell populations density, and the incident light, the maximum power density of 6030 mW m^{-2} is reported (Xu et al., 2015). Other MFC types, such as cyanobacteria, are used as photosynthetic MFC for electron transport, and mediators are required for further transport from them (Nishio et al., 2013). But the major disadvantage is that the electron mediators are harmful to MFCs, unstable, and unsuitable for long-term operation.

Sometimes, especially in the case of single-chambered microalgae microbial fuel cells (SCmMFC), both microalgae and bacteria are synergistically grown in a single chamber (Chandra et al., 2012). This configuration has several advantages, including a simpler configuration, convenient operation, low setup cost, and ease of industrial scale-up. However, this system has bottlenecks, including low coulombic efficiency caused by substrate crossover and oxygen diffusion, resulting in high oxygen consumption by both algae and bacteria. Here, both autotrophic and heterotrophic microorganisms are grown synchronously, resulting in 100% consumption of the CO_2 produced by the bacteria.

(b) *Biomass as Feed at the Anodic Compartment*

Microalgal biomass can be used as a substrate in the anode chamber of microbial fuel cells, to boost bioelectricity generation (Mekuto et al., 2020; Tay et al., 2022). Algal biomass is rich in fats, sugars, proteins, and vitamins, making it a valuable source of organic material for the anode half-cell, which can be utilized to generate bioelectricity without requiring any preparation. For example, the application of 5 g/L of dry algal biomass produced the highest power density of 1.78 W/m^2 compared to acetate-fed systems (0.661 W/m^2) (Min et al., 2005). This enhanced performance is attributed to the gradual release of electrons from the complex algal matrices. Velasquez-Orta et al. (2009) tested dry *powders made from Chlorella vulgaris and Ulva lactuca in their MFC design, achieving* maximum power densities of 0.98 W/m^2 and 0.76 W/m^2, respectively. The thick cell wall of microalgae is difficult for microorganisms to break down directly in the anode chamber of MFCs. However, pretreatment of the algal biomass is preferred for enhancing the power output by sonication (Rashid et al., 2013), thermal treatment (Kondaveeti et al., 2014), or microwave treatment (Gadhamshetty et al., 2013). The activated sludge, along with microalgae *Scenedesmus* biomass used as a nutrient source at the anode, and sonicated and thermal pretreated algal biomass showed higher microbial digestibility of biomass, which further enhanced the performance of the MFC (Rashid et al., 2013). This type of MFC can utilize different algal biomass produced from the cathode compartment, including fresh, untreated algae cake after lipid extraction, algal powder, and pretreated biomass as an anodic substrate. This approach sowed dual benefits, including wastewater treatment and low-cost substrates for MFC processing.

10.2.2 Role of Microalgae at the Cathode Chamber

In the cathode chamber, through photosynthesis, microalgae produce O_2 in situ, thus serving as the natural electron acceptor in the cathode and eliminating the need for mechanical aeration. They consume CO_2 released from the anode, helping to close the carbon loop and reduce emissions. Under illumination, algae enhance the cathodic reduction reactions. MFCs are categorized into three types based on how algae interact with electrodes and electrolytes: sediment-type algae MFCs (SMFCs), microbial carbon capture cells (MCCs), and photosynthetic algae MFCs (PAMFCs).

10.2.2.1 Photosynthetic Algae MFC (PAMFCs)

Integrating microalgae at the cathode chamber of MFCs offers a sustainable and energy-efficient alternative to traditional methods that rely on mechanical aeration or chemical electron acceptors, which can account for up to 50% of total operating expenses (del Campo et al., 2015). Dissolved oxygen from the algal biofilm has been proven to be an influential factor in the performance of the electrochemical system (Rago et al., 2017). During photosynthesis, they generate dissolved oxygen in situ, acting as a natural electron acceptor, thus reducing the need for external aeration systems. Thus, reducing CO_2 and converting it back into algal biomass and water. pH is detrimental to algae in the cathode, as it affects the oxygen reduction reaction (ORR) in MFCs. Though mild acidic pH in the range of 6.2—6.8 is suitable for the growth of microalgae, neutral to slightly higher pH is suitable for ORR, and results in enhanced mfc performance (Reddy et al., 2019). The design for the PAMFCs is crucial, as the requirement of dissolved oxygen in the cathodic chamber drives the cathodic oxygen-reduction reactions and thus the MFC functioning. PAMFCs are primarily designed to synchronize the supply of oxygen (for electron acceptance) with the uptake of CO_2 during photosynthesis, rather than to enhance microalgal activity. Thus, the configuration of PAMFCs should allow for light penetration. Thus, during the light phase, the DO and cell voltage gradually increase, and once the dark phase starts, the DO level and cell voltage decrease. DO influences the generation of cell voltages at the cathode, as oxygen serves as the electron acceptor

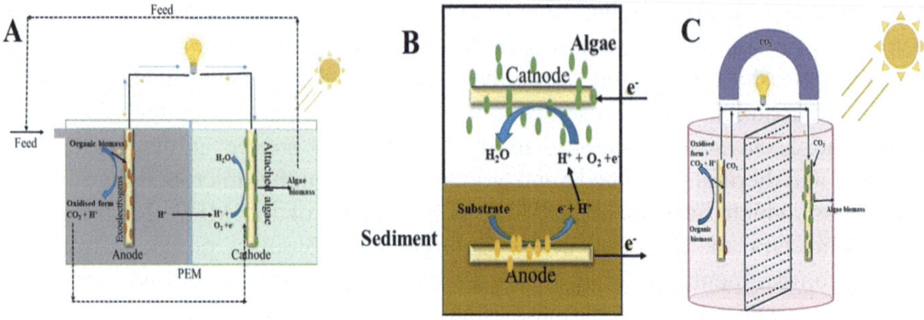

Fig. 10.1 Schematic representation of: (**a**) photosynthetic algal microbial fuel cell (PAMFC), (**b**) sediment type algae MFCs (SMFCs), and (**c**) microbial carbon capture cells (MCC)

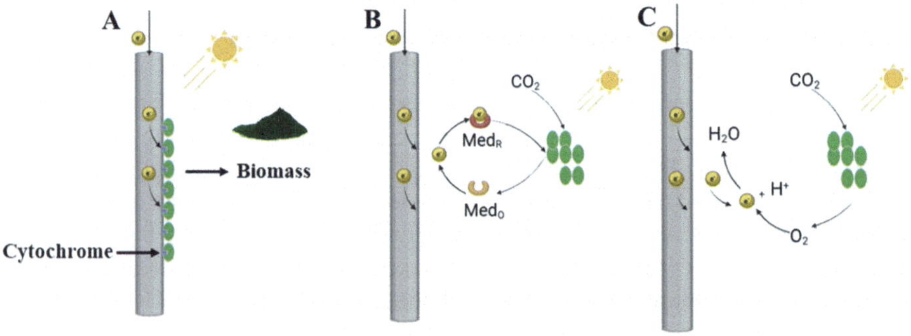

Fig. 10.2 Mechanism of electron transfer among algae and the electrode in the MFC reactor system

(Sarma et al., 2024). Sarma et al. (2024) reported that the maximum DO concentration of 10.7 ± 0.26 mg L^{-1} in the microalgae bio-cathode leads to a 49% increase in power generation compared to the control. The schematic representation of the PAMFC is shown in Fig. 10.1a. The cathodic chamber's algae growth is a self-sustaining cycle. The various electron transfer of algae and the electrode are shown in Fig. 10.2. As time progresses, microalgae in suspension can form a biofilm on the electrode surface. This biofilm directly accepts electrons, transferring toward the MFC circuit, and these electrons enter the algal cell. Biofilm at the cathode acts as a direct mediator in electron transfer, minimizing both ohmic and charge transfer resistances in the MFC (Kakarla & Min, 2014; Saba et al., 2017). In this case, self-supported mediators like c-type cytochromes from the outer membrane of algal cells facilitate electron transfer from the cathode to the algae (Fig. 10.2a). For algal suspensions, intermediate mediators can accept electrons from the cathode and transfer it to the suspended algae (Fig. 10.2b). These reduced mediators enter algal cells, release electrons and become oxidized, and then exit the algal cells back into the catholyte. Most cases of algae release O_2 during their photosynthesis, and this O_2 acts as a natural electron acceptor from the cathode and produces water (Fig. 10.2c).

10.2.2.2 Sediment Type Algae MFCs (SMFCs)

Photosynthetic-sediment MFC is a modified version of PAMFCs. In SMFCs, the anode is arranged in the sediment to create better contact between the electrode and the electrolyte, and the cathode compartment, filled with microalgae, is placed on top of the sediment (Jeon et al., 2012; Taşkan et al., 2021). Figure 10.1b shows the diagrammatic representation of SMFCs. The anodic bacterial activity leads to CO_2 production, which is utilized by the algal cell at the cathode compartment, resulting in oxygen release and power generation. A recent innovation involves a membrane-free, SMMFC incorporating a photosynthetic biocathode enriched with microbial consortium including microalgae and cyanobacteria, which achieved a sustained peak power density of around 11 mW/m^2 over a period of 180 days without any additional feeding (Commault et al., 2014). However, the development of membrane-free SMMFC reduces the complexity and cost; however, the chance of oxygen diffusion to the anode is unavoidable, and this adversely affects its performance, as the diffused oxygen hinders the growth and bioactivity of the anaerobic bacteria in the anode (Sarma & Mohanty, 2023). The use of common membranes, such as Nafion, ultrafiltration, and ion exchange membranes, is limited in MFCs nowadays due to their high cost, oxygen leakages, substrate losses, and biofouling. Thus, much research is emphasizing their replacement (Sarma & Mohanty, 2023; Mehrotra et al., 2021).

10.2.2.3 Microalgae Carbon Capture Cells

Microalgae autotrophic cells are capable of fixing CO_2 for their growth. In microalgae carbon capture cells (MCCs), CO_2 produced at the anode is directed into the cathode chamber, where algae consume it during photosynthesis and generate oxygen in the process. MCCs differ from PAMFCs mainly due to the minimal CO_2 emissions from the anode compartment. It can also utilize flue gases from fossil fuel combustion and fermentation industries (Chi et al., 2011; Arun et al., 2020), and helps reduce CO2 emissions through the efforts of bacteria and algae (Gajda et al., 2015). This system can be used for efficient power generation, carbon capture, and wastewater treatment simultaneously, without the need for mechanical aeration or biorefinery applications. A notable feature of MCCs is their ability to sustain high dissolved oxygen (DO) levels in the cathode chamber, reaching up to 7.6 mg/L, which supports efficient oxygen reduction reactions essential for power generation (Wang et al., 2010). The presence of DO higher than optimum could affect the electron transfer rate and electricity generation (Xu et al., 2015). A synergetic association is utilized for the sustainable production of MCCs by applying algal biomass as an electron donor in the anodic compartment and utilizing CO2 from the anodic compartment as a carbon source for algal biomass production, which is mutually beneficial in terms of simultaneously producing electricity and capturing CO_2.

10.3 Factors Influencing Microalgae Microbial Fuel Cells

Several factors influence the growth and performance of mMFCs, including microalgal strains, light intensity, temperature, pH, dissolved oxygen, and carbon dioxide. The detailed discussion is as follows:

10.3.1 Microbial Strains

mMFCs mainly rely on the range of both microalgae and bacteria, their inoculum size for electrogenesis, and voltage output. The inoculum used for the anodic chamber will be a pure bacterium or a microbial consortium from activated and anaerobic sludge, municipal wastewater, and bioreactor effluent (Saba et al., 2017). Pure culture is helpful for understanding the electron transfer mechanism and behavior of the specific species in MFCs. Commonly preferred organisms in MFCs are *Shewanella* and *Geobacter* (Nishio et al., 2013; Walter et al., 2013). In addition to this, other reported bacteria that act as electrogenes are *B. substilis* and *Klebsiella aerogenes* (Doyle & Marsili, 2018). The most commonly studied microalgae in the cathode chamber is *Chlorella* sp. (Anandapadmanaban et al., 2025). Power generation in M-MFCs depends on the O_2 concentration at the cathode. The application of *Chlorella* sp. at the cathode of MFCs produced a high-power density of 54.48 mW/m^2 (Yadav et al., 2020). Using *C. vulgaris* in the cathode chamber achieved a maximum power density of 122.5 mW/m^2 while cleaning hydroponic wastewater, with a COD removal efficiency of 93.7%. However, the use of potent exoelectrogens, such as Shewanella and Geobacter, in the anode, along with microalgal species in the cathode chamber, could enhance power density in mMFCs.

10.3.2 pH

pH is a vital parameter that influences electrogenic microorganisms and the overall performance of the systems, and consequently, power generation. The optimum pH for m-MFCs is reported to be between 6 and 8; an imbalance in ion concentrations leads to a pH gradient, disturbing the reaction within the cells and ultimately decreasing electricity generation (Sharma et al., 2022). The anode chamber of m-MFCs prefers a neutral pH, which is optimal for the growth of exoelectrogenic bacteria (Elshobary et al., 2020). The microalgae species exhibited better growth in the pH range of 6.8–7.2 in synthetic media. In wastewater media, the pH increases to 8.9 (Ummalyma & Bhaskar, 2024; Reddy et al., 2019). The pH increase in m-MFCs will increase the salinity; high salinity can impede the growth of microalgae in the cathode chamber. However, the selection of stress-tolerant microalgae species in MFCs can enable them to survive in extreme niches, such as those characterized by high salt, temperature, and pH levels. The mMFCs required mild operating conditions for both anode bacteria and cathode microalgae, such as temperature

(25–30 °C) and pH (6–8). pH in the cathode plays a crucial role in the cathode reaction. According to the Nernst equations, the cathode potential of ORR depends on the pH. It is reported that a neutral to slightly alkaline pH in the cathode is optimum for ORR for enhanced power generation (Reddy et al., 2019; Sharma et al., 2024a, b).

10.3.3 Temperature

The activation of exoelectrogens and the efficiency of substrate degradation depend on the operating temperature of the system, which in turn influences internal resistance, electrode potential, and voltage output. High temperatures affect the conductivity of proton exchange membranes (PEMs). A study has shown that extreme temperatures decrease the conductivity of the membrane (Ummalyma et al., 2019; Li et al., 2013). A study was conducted in two chambered MFCs separated by PEM to investigate the influence of a wide range of temperatures from 10–55 °C on their performance. Data show that maximum power density is attained at 37 °C, which is further decreased up to 21% when the temperature rises to 43 °C, at 55 °C, no steady power generation is observed. This is mainly due to the internal resistance within the cells (Li et al., 2013). It has been reported that, in most wastewater treatment using mMFCs, the optimum temperature ranges from 30 °C to 35 °C, which depends on the behavior of microbes in the cathode and anode chambers (Sharma et al., 2022).

10.3.4 Light Intensity

Light intensity is a crucial parameter that affects microalgae growth and photosynthesis, thereby enhancing oxygen generation and improving the overall performance of the cathode chamber in M-MFCs. Higher light intensity leads to improved system performance. During daylight, algae produce more oxygen through photosynthesis, which supports oxidation–reduction reactions that enhance power generation. During dark conditions, oxygen is utilized for respiration, which causes a decrease in DO at the cathode and lowers the performance of MFCs (Sharma et al., 2022). The growth of microalgae is increased in the light intensity range between 3500 lux and 10,000 lux, after which it is saturated in the MFCs. When light intensity increases beyond 10,000 lux and the lower light intensity is 3500–5000 lux, photoinhibition of algal biomass occurs. However, careful attention is given to selecting the ideal light intensity for the mMFCs. Microalgae growth at the cathode chamber can be improved by applying an artificial light system, such as light-emitting diodes, which improves the performance of MFCs.

10.3.5 Carbon Dioxide and Dissolved Oxygen

CO_2 is essential for photosynthesis, microalgal biomass production, and oxygen evolution. CO_2 can be supplied either in situ or ex situ. In situ, the carbon content available in wastewater can be utilized by microalgae as a substrate for biomass production (Ahirwar et al., 2023). It has been reported that 2.79 g/L of biomass is produced by *C. sorokiniana* under mixotrophic conditions by assimilating 2% CO_2, glucose, and acetic acids at 7000 lux light intensity (Nair & Chakraborty, 2020). The O_2 generated after anaerobic digestion in the anode chamber can be directly used as a carbon source for algae in the cathode. Although it is cost-effective, the process control is challenging as it depends on the performance of the anode. In contrast, CO_2 gas or bicarbonate form can be externally purged into the catholyte to enhance MFC performance. Tang et al. (2011) studied the different concentrations of CO_2 at the cathode chamber of photosynthetic MFCs using *C. pyrenoidosa* and *S. obliquus*. Data showed that both microalgae sequestered a maximum of 1.55—1.84 g/L of CO_2, respectively. This method is costly, but controlled, and better algal growth can be expected. CO_2 fixation, photosynthesis, and dissolved oxygen are interconnected, which depend on the parameters inside the MFC's cells. The optimum dissolved oxygen concentration required for the mMFCs is 7.8—9.5 mg/L. Researchers have reported a decrease in power density of up to 53.4%, as high DO concentration in the system causes diffusion of O_2 towards the anode, and declines the energy output. It has been reported that 6.8 mg/L of DO produces a maximum 282 mV voltage output and power density of 149.76 mW/m^2 in dual-chambered MFCs. The high DO concentration receives more electrons, which increases potential in the cathode and produces more electricity (Sharma et al., 2022). High DO in the cathode affects the microalgae multiplication; however, it is vital to optimize the DO concentration in each microalga-based MFC.

10.4 mMFCs for Wastewater Treatment

Microalgae have attracted attention for their dual ability to remove nutrients from wastewater and efficiently fix atmospheric CO_2. Studies have shown that using an integrated photo-biochemical system combining *Chlamydomonas reinhardtii* and *Pseudokirchneriella subcapitata* can achieve remarkable nutrient removal, up to 98% of nitrogen (in the form of ammonium) and 82% of phosphorus (as phosphate) from municipal wastewater (Xiao et al., 2012). Here, nutrient removal happens at the anode and cathode chambers of the system. Approximately 55% of phosphate removal was attributed to algal activity in the cathode chamber, while the remaining 27% was due to bacterial action in the anode. The microalgae utilized nitrogen and phosphorus for growth, resulting in increased biomass production, which holds potential for further use in biorefinery applications. Additionally, microalgae-based biocathodes support wastewater treatment through cathodic reduction and the sequestration of CO_2, thereby enhancing biomass production. The produced biomass can be further used for biofuel generation and other value-added products.

Table 10.1 Integrated wastewater treatment and electricity generation by microalgal species in mMFCs

Wastewater	Microalage species	Type of mMFCs	COD removal (%)	Power generation (mW/m^2)	References
Tapioca wastewater	*Spriulina platensis*	DCmMFC	66.6	14.5	Hadiyanto et al. (2023)
Industrial wastewater	*Chlorella vulgaris*	DCmMFC	78.6	327	Huarachi-Olivera et al. (2018)
Domestic sludge	Blue green algae	SCmMFC	78	114	Yuan et al. (2011)
Anaerobic digestor wastewater	*Spirulina maxima*	DCmMFC	20.5	67	Inglesby and Fisher (2013)
Textile wastewater	*Chlorella vulgaris*	SCmMFC	98	123.2	Logroño et al. (2017)
Domestic wastewater	*Chlorella vulgaris*	DCmMFC	19.45	–	Wang et al. (2010)
Municipal wastewater	*Dunaliella tertiolecta*	DCmMFC	16.8	5.3	Lakaniemi et al. (2012)
Domestic wastewater	*Scenedesmus quadricauda*	ABMFC	80.2	62.9	Yang et al. (2018)
Anaerobic digester sludge	*Chlorella vulgaris*	DCmMFC	93.7	112.5	Yolanda et al. (2025)
Anaerobic sludge	*Chlorella vulgaris*	PMMFCs	80.41%	1.70 $W m^{-3}$	Qin et al. (2024)
Synthetic wastewater	*Scenedesmus obliquus*	ABM	92.52%	13.24 mW/m^3	Bhadra et al. (2024)

Note: *DCmMFC* Double chambered microalgae-microbial fuel cell, *SCmMFC* Single chambered microalgae-microbial fuel cell, *ABMFC* Algal biofilm assisted microbial fuel cell, *PMMFCs* Photosynthetic microbial fuel cell, *ABM* Algal biocathode MFC

Additionally, sequential treatment of wastewater, initially in the anode compartment using bacteria and subsequently in the cathode compartment using algae, can effectively remove nutrients from wastewater and significantly reduce chemical oxygen demand (COD). Integrated wastewater treatment and electricity generation by different mMFCs are represented in Table 10.1.

10.5 Role in Bioenergy Production

Other than the generation of bioelectricity, microalgal biomass produced at the cathode can be exploited for other bioenergy conversion. Wastewater treatment, combined with bioelectricity generation and microalgal biomass productivity, is crucial for producing low-cost biomass for bioenergy conversions. Microalgal biomass enriched with lipids is used for biodiesel conversion through transesterification reactions (Ummalyma et al., 2024). Fermentation of microalgal carbohydrates produces bioethanol. The sugar content of the algal biomass varies depending on the conditions of MMFC systems and the type of wastewater and substrate available for assimilation by microalgae. Spent biomass after lipid extraction contains 54% reducing sugars, which are further used in fermentation to produce bioethanol with a yield of 92–116 mg/g biomass (Hemalatha et al., 2019). *Chlorella vulgaris* enriched with carbohydrates is hydrolyzed using enzymes and fermented with recombinant yeast, resulting in an ethanol yield of 8.01 g/L (de Carvalho Silvello et al., 2023).

Another approach to utilizing biomass for bioenergy conversion is thermochemical processes. In this process, biomass is thermally depolymerized and then repolymerized for conversion into various products suitable for use as energy and biorefinery chemicals (Ummalyma et al., 2024). Pyrolysis, gasification, combustion, and hydrothermal liquefaction are the various techniques adopted for thermochemical conversions. Biomass derived from MMFCs is typically wet in nature and serves as a suitable substrate for the production of biochar and bio-oil through the hydrothermal liquefaction process (Fan et al., 2020). Dry biomass is used in the pyrolytic process at various temperature ranges, from 250 °C to 700 °C, to produce syngas, bio-oils, and biochar. Microalgal biomass obtained from *Messastrum gracile* SVM11CT7 is used for hydrothermal liquefaction to produce 29.6% bio-oil, enriched with hydrocarbons containing nitrogen- and oxygen-cyclic compounds, and with a high calorific value of 37.19 MJ/kg (Kiran et al., 2024). MMFC systems are also suitable for producing biohydrogen, in addition to generating electricity. Hydrogen is a clean energy source; water is only a by-product of combustion. Different processes are adopted for biohydrogen conversions, including direct and indirect photolysis (Ummalyma et al., 2024; Marbelia et al., 2024). Biohydrogen has a high energy density and efficiency (142 MJ/kg), making it the most efficient green energy source (Marbelia et al., 2024).

10.6 Future Scope

Bioenergy and value-added products from microalgae-based MFCs using wastewater are attractive in a circular bioeconomy approach. However, the scale-up of MFCs remains challenging. Hence, the commercialization of mMFCs has some barriers and limitations. Microalgal biomass production is dependent on the climatic conditions and seasonal variations. It is dependent on the microalgal interaction with microbes and its electrogenic potential. The role of microalgae-associated bacteria in their potential for electrogenicity needs to be investigated. Symbiotic microorganisms are beneficial for the proper functioning of fuel cell systems; however, extensive research is needed in this area (Ummalyma & Bhaskar, 2024). In addition to this, the selection of robust algal strains for anode and cathode compartments, control of cathodic reactions, CO_2 uptake for power generation, and modeling and simulation of algae-based MFC, along with artificial intelligence and machine learning application tools. Sustainability of mMFCs depends on the anodic and cathodic reactions. MMFC applications are not only for bioelectricity generation; they can be used for the complete utilization of biomass and resources recovered from the wastewater in a zero-waste biorefinery approach. Applications promise cost-effective, eco-friendly technology for renewable energy production.

10.7 Conclusion

mMFCs are potential dual-application devices that synergistically couple microalgae and exoelectrogens, enabling simultaneous wastewater treatment and sustainable renewable energy generation. Microalgae have a role in the anode and cathode chambers. In the anode chamber, microalgae serve as electron donors by either oxidatively degrading organic pollutants or acting as a substrate for bacterial oxidative degradation, which also donates electrons to the anode. In the cathode chamber, oxygen availability is boosted by the photosynthetic activity of microalgae, which then function as the natural electron acceptor at the cathode and replace the need for mechanical aeration. It also supports pH stabilization and contributes to carbon dioxide sequestration, thereby improving overall system efficiency and reducing operational expenses compared to conventional MFCs. The growth of microalgae is controlled by various operational parameters, which, in turn, improve the performance of mMFC. Within a circular economy framework, the generated algal biomass can serve as a technological intervention for other bioenergy and bioproduct conversions.

References

Ahirwar, A., Das, S., Das, S., Yang, Y. H., Bhatia, S. K., Vinayak, V., & Ghangrekar, M. M. (2023). Photosynthetic microbial fuel cell for bioenergy and valuable production: A review of circular bio-economy approach. *Algal Research, 70*, 102973. https://doi.org/10.1016/j.algal.2023.102973

Anandapadmanaban, B. H., Liu, S. H., & Lin, C. W. (2025). Prospects of microalgae in the cathode chamber of microbial fuel cells: From sequestration to bioproduct production. *Biomass and Bioenergy, 194*, 107616. https://doi.org/10.1016/j.biombioe.2025.107616

Arun, S., Sinharoy, A., Pakshirajan, K., & Lens, P. N. (2020). Algae based microbial fuel cells for wastewater treatment and recovery of value-added products. *Renewable and Sustainable Energy Reviews, 132*, 110041.

Baek, G., & Lee, J. (2024). Algae-derived electrodes in bioelectrochemical systems. *Journal of Environmental Chemical Engineering, 12*, 112535. https://doi.org/10.1016/j.jece.2024.112535

Bhadra, S., Nayak, S., & Sevda, S. (2024). Simultaneous organic wastewater treatment and bioelectricity production in a dual chamber microbial fuel cell with Scenedesmus obliquus biocathode. *Energy Conversion and Management, 316*, 118849.

Chandra, R., Subhash, G. V., & Mohan, S. V. (2012). Mixotrophic operation of photo-bioelectrocatalytic fuel cell under anoxygenic microenvironment enhances the light dependent bioelectrogenic activity. *Bioresource Technology, 109*, 46–56.

Chi, Z., O'Fallon, J. V., & Chen, S. (2011). Bicarbonate produced from carbon capture for algae culture. *Trends in Biotechnology, 29*(11), 537–541.

Commault, A. S., Lear, G., Novis, P., & Weld, R. J. (2014). Photosynthetic biocathode enhances the power output of a sediment-type microbial fuel cell. *New Zealand Journal of Botany, 52*(1), 48–59.

de Carvalho Silvello, M. A., Gasparotto, G. A., & Goldbeck, R. (2023). Enzymatic hydrolysis of carbohydrate-rich *Chlorella vulgaris* for third-generation bioethanol production by cellulase-recombinant yeast. *Cleaner Chemical Engineering, 6*, 100111. https://doi.org/10.1016/j.clce.2023.100111

del Campo, A. G., Perez, J. F., Cañizares, P., Rodrigo, M. A., Fernandez, F. J., & Lobato, J. (2015). Characterization of light/dark cycle and long-term performance test in a photosynthetic microbial fuel cell. *Fuel, 140*, 209–216.

Doyle, L. E., & Marsili, E. (2018). Weak electricigens: A new avenue for bioelectrochemical research. *Bioresource Technology, 258*(2018), 354–364.

Elshobary, M. E., Zabed, H. M., Yun, J., Zhang, G., & Qi, X. (2020). Recent insights into microalgae-assisted microbial fuel cells for generating sustainable bioelectricity. *International Journal of Hydrogen Energy, 46*, 3135–3159.

Fan, L., Zhang, H., Li, J., et al. (2020). Algal biorefinery to value-added products by using combined processes based on thermochemical conversion: A review. *Algal Research, 47*, 101819.

Gadhamshetty, V., Belanger, D., Gardiner, C. J., Cummings, A., & Hynes, A. (2013). Evaluation of Laminaria-based microbial fuel cells (LbMs) for electricity production. *Bioresource Technology, 127*, 378–385.

Gajda, I., Greenman, J., Melhuish, C., & Ieropoulos, I. (2015). Self-sustainable electricity production from algae grown in a microbial fuel cell system. *Biomass Bioenergy, 82*, 87–93.

Hadiyanto, H., Christwardana, M., & da Costa, C. (2023). Electrogenic and biomass production capabilities of a microalgae–microbial fuel cell (MMFC) system using tapioca wastewater and Spirulina platensis for COD reduction. *Energy Sources, Part A: Recovery, Utilization, and Environmental Effects, 45*(2), 3409–3420.

Hemalatha, M., Sravan, J. S., Min, B., & Mohan, S. V. (2019). Microalgae-biorefinery with cascading resource recovery design associated to dairy wastewater treatment. *Bioresource Technology, 284*, 424–429. https://doi.org/10.1016/j.biortech.2019.03.106

Huarachi-Olivera, R., Dueñas-Gonza, A., Yapo-Pari, U., Vega, P., Romero-Ugarte, M., Tapia, J., & Esparza, M. (2018). Bioelectrogenesis with microbial fuel cells (MFCs) using the microalga *Chlorella vulgaris* and bacterial communities. *Electronic Journal of Biotechnology, 31*, 34–43.

Inglesby, A. E., & Fisher, A. C. (2013). Downstream application of a microbial fuel cell for energy recovery from an *Arthrospira maxi*ma fed anaerobic digester effluent. *RSC Advances, 3*(38), 17387–17394.

Jeon, H. J., Seo, K. W., Lee, S. H., Yang, Y. H., Kumaran, R. S., Kim, S., et al. (2012). Production of algal biomass (*Chlorella vulgaris*) using sediment microbial fuel cells. *Bioresource Technology, 109*, 308–311.

Kakarla, R., & Min, B. (2014). Photoautotrophic microalgae Scenedesmus obliquus attached on a cathode as oxygen producers for microbial fuel cell (MFC) operation. *International Journal of Hydrogen Energy, 39*(19), 10275–10283.

Khan, M. J., Das, S., Vinayak, V., Pant, D., & Ghangrekar, M. M. (2022). Live diatoms as potential biocatalyst in a microbial fuel cell for harvesting continuous diafuel, carotenoids and bioelectricity. *Chemosphere, 291*, 132841.

Kiran, B. R., Singh, P., Kuravi, S. D., Mohanty, K., & Mohan, S. V. (2024). Modulating cultivation regimes of *Messastrum gracile* SVMIICT7 for biomass productivity integrated with resource recovery via hydrothermal liquefaction. *Journal of Environmental Management, 356*, 120458.

Kondaveeti, S., Choi, K. S., Kakarla, R., & Min, B. (2014). Microalgae Scenedesmus obliquus as renewable biomass feedstock for electricity generation in microbial fuel cells (MFCs). *Frontiers of Environmental Science & Engineering, 8*, 784–791.

Lakaniemi, A. M., Tuovinen, O. H., & Puhakka, J. A. (2012). Production of electricity and butanol from microalgal biomass in microbial fuel cells. *Bioenergy Research, 5*, 481–491.

Lee, D. J., Chang, J. S., & Lai, J. Y. (2015). Microalgae–microbial fuel cell: A mini review. *Bioresource Technology, 198*, 891–895.

Li, L. H., Sun, Y. M., Yuan, Z. H., Kong, X. Y., & Li, Y. (2013). Effect of temperature change on power generation of microbial fuel cell. *Environmental Technology, 34*, 1929–1934.

Logroño, W., Pérez, M., Urquizo, G., Kadier, A., Echeverría, M., Recalde, C., & Rákhely, G. (2017). Single chamber microbial fuel cell (SCMFC) with a cathodic microalgal biofilm: A preliminary assessment of the generation of bioelectricity and biodegradation of real dye textile wastewater. *Chemosphere, 176*, 378–388.

Marbelia, L., Bilad, M. R., Passaris, I., Discart, V., Vandamme, D., Beuckels, A., et al. (2024). Membrane photobioreactors for integrated microalgae cultivation and nutrient remediation of membrane bioreactors effluent. *Bioresource Technology, 163*, 228–235. https://doi.org/10.1016/j.biortech.2014.04.012

Mehrotra, S., Kumar, V. K., Gajalakshmi, S., & Pathak, B. (2021). Bioelectrogenesis from ceramic membrane-based algal-microbial fuel cells treating dairy industry wastewater. *Sustainable Energy Technologies and Assessments, 48*, 101653.

Mekuto, L., Olowolafe, A. V., Huberts, R., Dyantyi, N., Pandit, S., & Nomngongo, P. (2020). Microalgae as a biocathode and feedstock in anode chamber for a selfsustainable microbial fuel cell technology: A review. *South African Journal of Chemical Engineering, 31*(1), 7–16.

Min, B., Kim, J., Oh, S., Regan, J. M., & Logan, B. E. (2005). Electricity generation from swine wastewater using microbial fuel cells. *Water Research, 39*(20), 4961–4968.

Mohan, S. V., Srikanth, S., Chiranjeevi, P., Arora, S., & Chandra, R. (2014). Algal biocathode for in situ terminal electron acceptor (TEA) production: Synergetic association of bacteria–microalgae metabolism for the functioning of biofuel cell. *Bioresource Technology, 166*, 566–574.

Nair, A., & Chakraborty, S. (2020). Synergistic effects between autotrophy and heterotrophy in optimization of mixotrophic cultivation of *Chlorella sorokiniana* in bubble column photobioreactors. *Algal Research, 46*, 101799.

Nishio, K., Hashimoto, K., & Watanabe, K. (2013). Light/electricity conversion by defined cocultures of Chlamydomonas and Geobacter. *Journal of Bioscience and Bioengineering, 115*(4), 412–417.

Qin, L., Qin, Y., Cui, N., Han, X., Lu, H., Yang, T., & Liang, W. (2024). Photosynthetic microalgae microbial fuel cells for bioelectricity generation and microalgae lipid recovery using Gd-Co@N-CSs/NF as cathode. *Chemical Engineering Journal, 490*, 151647.

Rago, L., Cristiani, P., Villa, F., Zecchin, S., Colombo, A., Cavalca, L., & Schievano, A. (2017). Influences of dissolved oxygen concentration on biocathodic microbial communities in microbial fuel cells. *Bioelectrochemistry, 116*, 39–51.

Rashid, N., Cui, Y. F., Rehman, M. S. U., & Han, J. I. (2013). Enhanced electricity generation by using algae biomass and activated sludge in microbial fuel cell. *Science of the Total Environment, 456*, 91–94.

Reddy, C. N., Nguyen, H. T., Noori, M. T., & Min, B. (2019). Potential applications of algae in the cathode of microbial fuel cells for enhanced electricity generation with simultaneous nutrient removal and algae biorefinery: Current status and future perspectives. *Bioresource Technology, 292*, 122010.

Saba, B., Christy, A. D., Yu, Z., & Co, A. C. (2017). Sustainable power generation from bacterio-algal microbial fuel cells (MFCs): An overview. *Renewable and Sustainable Energy Reviews, 73*, 75–84.

Sarma, P. J., & Mohanty, K. (2023). Development and comprehensive characterization of low-cost hybrid clay based ceramic membrane for power enhancement in plant based microbial fuel cells (PMFCs). *Materials Chemistry and Physics, 296*, 127337.

Sarma, P. J., Malakar, B., & Mohanty, K. (2024). Self-sustaining bioelectricity generation in plant-based microbial fuel cells (PMFCs) with microalgae-assisted oxygen-reducing biocathode. *Biomass Conversion and Biorefinery, 14*(15), 16973–16986.

Sharma, M., Salama, E. S., Zhang, P., Zhang, L., Xing, X., Yue, J., Song, Z., Nan, L., Yujun, S., & Li, X. (2022). Microalgae-assisted microbial fuel cells for electricity generation coupled with wastewater treatment: Biotechnological perspective. *Journal of Water Process Engineering, 49*, 102966. https://doi.org/10.1016/j.jwpe.2022.102966

Sharma, M., Jalalah, M., Alsareii, S. A., Harraz, F. A., Xue, W., Thakur, N., et al. (2024a). Microalgal cycling in the cathode of microbial fuel cells (MFCs) induced oxygen reduction reaction (ORR) and electricity: A biocatalytic process for clean energy. *Chemical Engineering Journal, 479*, 147431.

Sharma, J., Kumar, M., Ahlawat, A., Mishra, S., Smita, S., & Sharma, P. (2024b). Chapter 3: Progress and prospects of algae-based microbial fuel cells. In D. M. Mahapatra, S. S. Kumar, & L. Singh (Eds.), *Bioelectrochemical systems: The way forward algae based bioelectrochemical systems for carbon sequestration, carbon storage, bioremediation and bioproduct generation* (Vol. 3, pp. 33–49). Academic Press. https://doi.org/10.1016/B978-0-323-91023-1.00003-X

Tang, D., Han, W., Li, P., Miao, X., & Zhong, J. (2011). CO_2 biofixation and fatty acid composition of *Scenedesmus obliquus* and *Chlorella pyrenoidosa* in response to different CO_2 levels. *Bioresource Technology, 102*(3), 3071–3076.

Taşkan, B., Bakır, M., & Taşkan, E. (2021). Enhanced power generation from algal biomass using multi-anode membrane-less sediment microbial fuel cell. *International Journal of Energy Research, 45*(2), 2011–2022.

Tay, Z. H. Y., Ng, F. L., Ling, T. C., Iwamoto, M., & Phang, S. M. (2022). The use of marine microalgae in microbial fuel cells, photosynthetic microbial fuel cells and biophotovoltaic platforms for bioelectricity generation. *3 Biotech, 12*(7), 148.

Ummalyma, S. B., & Bhaskar, T. (2024). Recent advances in the roles of biocatalyst in biofuel cells and its applications: An overview. *Biotechnology and Genetic Engineering Reviews, 40*, 2051–2089.

Ummalyma, S. B., Sahoo, D., Pandey, A., & Prajeesh, K. P. (2019). Microalgae–microbial fuel cell. *Materials Research Foundations, 46*, 1–20.

Ummalyma, S. B., Udayan, A., & Sreekumar, N. (2024). Phycoremediation of emerging contaminants and heavy metals from industrial wastewater: A sustainable green approach for bioeconomy. *Bioresource Technology Reports, 27*, 101920. https://doi.org/10.1016/j.biteb.2024.101920

Velasquez-Orta, S. B., Curtis, T. P., & Logan, B. E. (2009). Energy from algae using microbial fuel cells. *Biotechnology and Bioengineering, 103*(6), 1068–1076.

Walter, X. A., Greenman, J., & Ieropoulos, I. A. (2013). Oxygenic phototrophic biofilms for improved cathode performance in microbial fuel cells. *Algal Research, 2*, 183–187.

Wang, X., Feng, Y., Liu, J., Lee, H., Li, C., Li, N., & Ren, N. (2010). Sequestration of CO_2 discharged from anode by algal cathode in microbial carbon capture cells (MCCs). *Biosensors and Bioelectronics, 25*(12), 2639–2643.

Xiao, L., Young, E. B., Berges, J. A., & He, Z. (2012). Integrated photo-bioelectrochemical system for contaminants removal and bioenergy production. *Environmental Science & Technology, 46*(20), 11459–11466.

Xu, C., Poon, K., Choi, M. M., & Wang, R. (2015). Using live algae at the anode of a microbial fuel cell to generate electricity. *Environmental Science and Pollution Research, 22*, 15621–15635.

Yadav, G., Sharma, I., Ghangrekar, M., & Sen, R. (2020). A live bio-cathode to enhance power output steered by bacteria-microalgae synergistic metabolism in microbial fuel cell. *Journal of Power Sources, 449*, 227560.

Yang, Z., Pei, H., Hou, Q., Jiang, L., Zhang, L., & Nie, C. (2018). Algal biofilm-assisted microbial fuel cell to enhance domestic wastewater treatment: Nutrient, organics removal and bioenergy production. *Chemical Engineering Journal, 332*, 277–285.

Yolanda, Y. D., Kim, S., Sohn, W., Shon, H. K., Yang, E., & Lee, S. (2025). Simultaneous nutrient-abundant hydroponic wastewater treatment, direct carbon capture, and bioenergy harvesting using microalgae–microbial fuel cells. *Desalination and Water Treatment, 321*, 100941. https://doi.org/10.1016/j.dwt.2024.100941

Yuan, Y., Chen, Q., Zhou, S., Zhuang, L., & Hu, P. (2011). Bioelectricity generation and microcystins removal in a blue-green algae powered microbial fuel cell. *Journal of Hazardous Materials, 187*(1–3), 591–595.

Metagenomics and Meta-Transcriptomics for the Prospective Bioremediation of Microplastics Using Algae–Bacteria Consortium

11

Sana Parveen, Simran Maratha, Ruchika Agarwal, and Shailesh Kumar Patidar

Abstract

Microplastics have become a significant environmental challenge as they are ubiquitous across ecosystems, enter the food chain, and persist in the environment. Plants, algae, and their associated microbiome can effectively bioremediate the microplastics by immobilizing, accumulating, and degrading them. They can even reuse them as a potential source of carbon. Algae–bacteria consortia have gained significant recognition for their potential in bioremediating emerging contaminants. While being exposed to microplastics, the host algae recruited several bacteria (from the phycosphere) to alter chemical functionalities and deform polymer structure to degrade microplastics in nature. Metagenomics elucidates the structural and functional capabilities of microbial communities that play a significant role in the degradation of microplastics. High-throughput sequencing techniques, functional gene annotations, and comparative metagenomics provide necessary insights into microbial diversity and metabolic pathways. Integrating metagenomics and meta-transcriptomics into bioremediation strategies using an alga–bacteria system offers a promising approach to addressing microplastic pollution. RNA sequencing and expression profiling reveal active biochemical pathways and investigate the adaptive responses of microbial communities to microplastic exposure. These omics-based methods not only harness the genetic and functional diversity of microbial populations but could also integrate with machine learning and artificial intelligence to improve predictive modelling for optimized bioremediation strategies. This chapter examines the current strategies and mechanisms by which algae–bacteria

S. Parveen · S. Maratha · R. Agarwal · S. K. Patidar (✉)
Department of Environmental Science, School of Earth Sciences, Central University of Rajasthan, Ajmer, Rajasthan, India
e-mail: shailesh.patidar@curaj.ac.in

L. Kumar et al. (eds.), *Algal Bioremediation*,
https://doi.org/10.1007/978-981-95-8793-3_11

consortia facilitate microplastic biodegradation, utilizing metagenomics and meta-transcriptomics approaches.

Keywords

Algae–Bacteria Consortium · Metagenomics · Microplastics · Meta-transcriptomics · Bioremediation

11.1 Introduction

Microplastic (MP) pollution is a pervasive environmental issue with significant implications for ecosystems and human health. These particles, smaller than 5 mm, originate from both primary sources, such as cosmetics and industrial processes, and secondary sources, like the degradation of larger plastic items. They have invaded diverse environments, posing serious risks to plants, marine life, and humans. Biodegradable plastics, such as poly-3-hydroxybutyrate, are generally biocompatible and nontoxic; however, under certain conditions (e.g., high concentrations, microplastic formation, or the presence of additives), they may indirectly affect organism survival and growth. If found in excess, they increase metabolic burden, reduce nutrient availability, and create osmotic pressure (Song et al., 2024). MPs can accumulate in the food chain, leading to altered metabolism, reduced growth, and increased mortality rate in various species. They also show risks of immunotoxicity and neurotoxicity in humans. Due to their large surface area, they serve as vectors to transport heavy metals and other pollutants, leading to synergistic toxic effects (Madiraju et al., 2024). MPs are highly durable and resistant to natural degradation due to their strong carbon–carbon bonds, creating an urgent need for sustainable solutions. While significant efforts are underway to mitigate microplastic pollution, challenges remain in fully understanding their ecological impacts and developing comprehensive strategies for effective management. Conventional methods such as microfiltration, adsorption, and photodegradation often fall short in tackling the scale and complexity of microplastic pollution (Bubu-Davies & Anwuri, 2022). As a result, biological approaches are gaining attention. Microbial communities at the plastic–environment interface have shown promise in breaking down these resistant materials. Algae (*Chlamydomonas* and *Chlorella*), bacteria (*Klebsiella*, *Ralstonia*, and *Achromobacter*), diatoms (*Navicula* and *Nitzschia*), and fungi (Aspergillus, Fusarium, and Cladosporium) have shown MP-degrading properties. Degradation of MPs using algae–bacteria consortia is being recognized as an effective and eco-friendly strategy (Chandel et al., 2025). Such consortia utilize the synergistic interactions between microalgae and bacteria to colonize the plastic surface, form biofilms, and release extracellular enzymes capable of degrading the complex polymers that cleave or oxidize them. Key enzyme groups include hydrolases, oxidoreductases, dehalogenases, and urethanases, among others. Several microalgae and cyanobacteria secrete laccase-like enzymes in addition to contributing oxygen, photosensitizers, and reactive oxygen species, which enhance the activity of bacterial enzymes (Ren et al., 2025). There is further production of exopolysaccharide, which aids in altering the polymer structure to improve degradation. These consortia overcome metabolic bottlenecks compared to single-species systems, increasing degradation efficiency (Chettri et al., 2023). Additionally, photosynthetic microorganisms utilize sunlight and CO_2 to produce useful biomolecules such as carbohydrates and proteins.

The metagenomics and meta-transcriptomics are advanced scientific tools that can unlock the full potential of consortia. The use of metagenomics is useful in identifying and characterizing microbial communities, allowing us to understand the diversity of these communities and their potential functional roles. Researchers who use next-generation sequencing (NGS) approaches have identified diverse microorganisms capable of degrading plastic. Metagenomic approaches are used to decipher the microbiome of the plastic (plastisphere) for a better understanding of the role of each member in microplastic degradation. This involves the taxonomy of the abundant microbe and its functional characteristics available on different forms of plastics, such as polyethylene (PE), polystyrene (PS), polypropylene (PP), and low-density polyethylene (LDPE) (Purohit et al., 2020). Hu et al. (2024) have also identified, through these studies, key genes and enzymes, such as carbohydrate-active enzymes (CAZymes) and plastic-degrading enzymes (PDZymes), that are involved in microplastic degradation. Comparative metagenomics is applied to the analysis of microbial communities in polluted versus pristine sites, and degraders such as *Rhodococcus* can be pinpointed and thus targeted (Dvořák et al., 2017).

Through RNA sequencing and meta-transcriptomics, gene activity can be captured in real-time during microbial responses to microplastic stress, which significantly reveals activated enzymes during the process (Gambarini et al., 2024). For instance, bacteria may upregulate hydrolase genes in the presence of PE, while algae activate stress response pathways in response to MPs, thus gaining knowledge to optimize bioremediation strategies. This chapter discusses some of the individual and integrated omics approaches, as well as tools and techniques, that can be utilized for a comprehensive understanding of microbial communities and their functional roles in the degradation of plastic. By using advanced genomic tools (metagenomics and meta-transcriptomics) to shed light on metabolic pathways of such microbial consortia, it contributes to the development of innovative biotechnological solutions, such as tailored microbial consortia for the development of enhanced MP-degrading solutions. When integrated with artificial intelligence (AI) and machine learning (ML), these technologies enhance bioremediation efficiency by enabling real-time data analysis, proactive environmental adjustments, and accurate forecasting of remediation outcomes by predictive modelling. AI and ML also reduce production costs by reducing the need for manual intervention (Akintola, 2024). Yet, challenges persist in maintaining environmental variables, such as salinity and pH, which affect microbial efficiency and the scaling of lab-scale systems to real-world scenarios. Ethical and regulatory concerns regarding the use of genetically modified microorganisms (GMOs) for environmental applications persist. The challenges in using metagenomics and meta-transcriptomics stem from the complexity of microbial communities, massive data sets that demand advanced bioinformatics skills, the lack of exhaustive databases to fully understand the microbial communities, and the limitations of current methodologies (Barone et al., 2024). Still, these hurdles inspire creative solutions that blend algae, bacteria, nanotechnology, and omics approaches. This chapter explores the potential of algae–bacteria consortia enhanced by omics approaches to tackle MP pollution. It delves into the degradation mechanisms, the collaborative dynamics within the plastosphere, and the role of AI in optimizing these processes while also addressing the technical and scalability challenges. As microplastics continue to pose a serious threat to environmental health, these omics-guided microbial partnerships represent a promising pathway toward a cleaner and more sustainable future.

11.2 Algae–Bacteria Consortia in the Bioremediation of Microplastics

The wastewater treatment plant is a potential point source of land-based microplastic pollution, with reported particle concentrations ranging from $0.28–3.14 \times 10^4$ particles L^{-1} (Liu et al., 2021). As a sustainable approach in the remediation of environmental microplastic pollution, bioremediation has emerged as a break-through in the field. As microalgae are capable of utilizing photosynthesis and other metabolic processes and possess a large surface area that facilitates effective pollutant absorption, they have proven to be highly efficient biological agents. Solar energy is harnessed by microalgae to grow and also interact with contaminants, thereby becoming a potential tool for removing microplastics, especially in various environmental settings. Previously, studies showed that microalgae help in the recovery of biofuel from the microplastic *Chlamydomonas reinhardtii* and *Chlorella vulgaris*, which were applied to remove and transform different types of microplastics (HDPE, LDPE, PP, and PVC). All four microplastics show greater than 90% removal efficiency highest being served by polypropylene, with 98% energy recovery (Sponza & Öztekin, 2023). Bacteria individually play an important role in the disintegration of MPs by forming biofilms at different stages of develop-ment. Among microorganisms, Pseudomonas species are recognized as effective degraders of polyethylene (PE). A comparative study on the biodegradability of low-density polyethylene (LDPE) tested different Pseudomonas strains, including *P. putida* KT2440 (ATCC 47054), *P. syringae* DC3000 (ATCC 10862), *P. aeruginosa* PAO1 (ATCC 15729), and *P. aeruginosa* (ATCC 15692). The findings revealed that *P. aeruginosa* PAO1 demonstrated superior degradation performance compared to the other strains examined (Rambabu et al., 2023).

There are many ways algae and bacteria interact from symbiotic to parasitic. Algae and bacteria fulfill complementary yet interdependent roles within aquatic ecosystems. Algae act as photosynthetic producers assimilating CO_2, releasing O_2, and taking up inorganic nutrients, while bacteria decompose and recycle organic matter, regenerating essential nutrients and supplying growth-promoting factors. When combined, their interactions form a self-sustaining and resilient system in which algal exudates fuel bacterial metabolism, and bacterial recycling and detoxification enhance both algal productivity and pollutant removal. This synergy significantly outperforms single-species approaches by enhancing biomass yield, improving nutrient removal, and promoting ecological stability. Recent studies reinforce these advantages from enhanced nutrient removal efficiencies in wastewater treatment (Fallahi et al., 2021). Suitable substrates with light allow the formation of algal–bacterial consortia, exchanging vitamins, carbon, nitrogen, and phytohormones. This combination eliminates pollutants, especially Phthalate esters (PAEs), more efficiently than using algae or bacteria alone. These interactions promote effective microplastic mitigation (Chettri et al., 2023).

11.2.1 Mechanism of Microplastic Degradation by Plants, Algae, Bacteria, and Fungi

According to recent studies, a variety of biological entities, including bacteria, algae, and plants, employ different yet complementary mechanisms to help mitigate microplastic contamination.

(i) *Bacteria*: The most explored among these for microplastic biodegradation are probably bacteria because of their shorter doubling times, huge metabolic potential, and environmental adaptability. The depolymerization of synthetic polymers is triggered by extracellular enzymes secreted by bacteria that colonize plastic surfaces, including *Pseudomonas*, *Bacillus*, *Rhodococcus*, and *Ideonella sakaiensis* (Yoshida et al., 2016). Assimilation, mineralization, biodegradation, and biodeterioration are the four steps that usually comprise the microbial degradation process. Initially, microplastics undergo physical and chemical changes due to bacteria adhering to their surface and creating biofilms, or biodeterioration (Wang et al., 2024a, b). Enzymatic cleavage of polymer chains into smaller oligomers or monomers (biofragmentation) is facilitated by enzymes, such as PETase, MHETase, laccase, monooxygenase, and peroxidases. Afterward, these monomers enter the cell, participating in pathways such as the TCA cycle and β-oxidation cycle, and are subsequently assimilated by the microbial cell, resulting in complete mineralization to CO_2 and H_2O under aerobic conditions or CH_4 under anaerobic conditions (Gao et al., 2024). Bacteria involved in the degradation of microplastics and their degradation efficiency are shown in Table 11.1.

(ii) *Algae*: Microalgae have been used in several studies to break down and bioremediate microplastics. They are particularly interesting, environmentally benign, and sustainable when it comes to controlling the carbon source from consuming microplastics (Barone et al., 2020). Microalgae facilitate the biodegradation of plastic waste through enzymatic reactions that destabilize the chemical bonds of plastic polymers. Consequently, the potential of microalgae for converting microplastics can be characterized as a photosynthetic microorganism capable of utilizing carbon sources and sunlight to promote biomass

Table 11.1 Bacteria involved in degradation of microplastics and their degradation efficiency

Microorganism	Degrading plastic	Degradation efficiency	References
A. radioresistens	Styrofoam	16.7 ± 0.6%	Xiang et al. (2023)
S. maltophilia and B. velezensis	Polystyrene	43.5 ± 0.8%	Xiang et al. (2023)
Comamonas testosteroni NCIMB 8955, *Bacillus firmus* NCTC 10335	High-density polyethylene	15.30%, 13.00%	Newrick et al. (2025)
C. testosteroni NCIMB 8955	Polythene	21.81%	Newrick et al. (2025)
Bacillus anthracis str. and Bacillus cereus ATCC 14579.	polyester	2.43% and 1.15%	Rosariastuti et al. (2024)
Alcaligenes faecalis	Polyolefins	3.5%weight loss	Tareen et al. (2022)

production. Microplastics interact with microalgae in various ways, including adherence to their surfaces or the formation of aggregates. These interactions are contingent upon factors such as the size and surface properties of the microplastics, as well as the specific type of microalgae involved. Although certain microplastics may be entrapped within the substances produced by microalgae, their absorption as a carbon source is infrequent and primarily reliant on their size. Another important role played by microalgae concerning plastic materials is linked to their capacity to alter the density of the colonized polymer, which consequently affects the vertical fluxes of plastics (Nava & Leoni, 2021). Algae are involved in the degradation of microplastics, and their degradation efficiency is shown in Table 11.2.

(iii) *Plants*: Recent research has included a look at how plants interact with microplastics and nanoplastics, investigating whether some plant species can absorb and transport such pollutants. As a result, plants can be utilized to remove microplastics and nanoplastics from polluted environments. Additionally, in addition to taking in and moving these pollutants, other factors related to plants, including root exudates and mycorrhiza, may help immobilize or break down microplastics and nanoplastics. These pollutants can be trapped in plant roots, thereby rendering them immobile and reducing their availability to other parts of the plant, which helps minimize damage to surrounding soil organisms. Furthermore, such pollutants may be stabilized by plants through attachment to their large leaf surfaces. The attachment of these pollutants to leaf surfaces is due to various interactions, including electrostatic and Van der Waals forces, hydrogen bonding, micropore filling, and interactions between microplastics and nano plastics and polysaccharides, as well as other components like lipids, proteins, cellulose, lignin, phenolic compounds, surface-active compounds, and minerals found on plant leaves (Thapliyal et al., 2024). A previous study showed that water hyacinth acts as a potential phytoremediator for MPs.

Table 11.2 Algae involved in the degradation of microplastics, and their degradation efficiency

Microorganism	Degrading plastic	Degradation efficiency	References
Synechocystis sp.	Polystyrene	23.2 ± 0.21%	Gowthami et al. (2025)
Chlorella vulgaris	polyethylene	84%	Lotfigolsefidi et al. (2025)
Scenedesmus dimorphus	Low-density polyethylene	3.74%	Muhonja et al. (2018)
Uronema africanum Borge	Low-density polyethylene	19% weight loss	Sanniyasi et al. (2021)
Chlorella vulgaris	polyethene	84%	Esmaeili Nasrabadi et al. (2023)
C. vulgaris	polypropylene (PP) and polyethylene terephthalate (PET)	55.7% for PP & 95.0% for PET	Hadiyanto et al. (2025)
Chlorella sp. and *Cyanobacteria* sp.	LDPE	37.91% reduction in carbon weight	Bhuyar et al. (2021)
S. platensis	Styrofoam	81% reduction in weight	Eydi Gabrabad et al. (2024)
Spirulina sp.	Terylene and propylene	48.61% for terylene and 36.7% for PP	Khoironi et al. (2019)

Results demonstrated a significant reduction of MPs in treated water (up to ~70–80%), with smaller MPs (<100 μm) removed more effectively due to stronger adhesion on root surfaces (Yin et al., 2025).

(iv) *Fungi*: Fungi surround plastic and consume it as food, which is influenced by several environmental factors like heat and physiochemical conditions like pH, etc. Several enzymes, like cutinase, lipase, proteases, carboxylesterases, esterases, and lignocellulolytic enzymes, are involved in the oxidation and hydrolysis of these polymers (Srikanth et al., 2022). The effects of fungi on the physicochemical properties of plastics include changes in crystallinity, molecular weight, tensile properties, extent of fragmentation, and functional groups present on the plastic surface. Different changes occur in the physicochemical properties of MPs by degradation through fungi, such as crystal structure, molecular mass, elastic nature, and type of functional group present (Sánchez, 2020). Earlier, *Aspergillus flavus* PEDX3 was identified as a potential PE-degrading microorganism from the gut contents of *Galleria mellonella* larvae. Among the 25 isolates, the *A. flavus* strain proved to be the most efficient at degrading both LDPE and HDPE (Zhang et al., 2020).

11.2.2 Algae–Bacteria Consortium for the Bioremediation of Microplastics and Other Emerging Contaminants

The algal–bacterial symbiotic system is a biological purification system that initially integrates for sewage treatment and resource utilization, while simultaneously having the corresponding effect of carbon sequestration and pollution reduction. A well-documented coexistence of algae and bacteria has been observed; however, only a few studies have successfully synthesized a symbiotic alga–bacterium system for wastewater treatment. For the removal of pollutants, co-cultivation of microalgae with bacteria emerges as a promising approach in which the photosynthetic capacity of microalgae is used to develop a symbiotic relationship with bacteria based on the exchange of O_2 and CO_2. Various microalgae cultivated with bacteria, such as *Rhizobium* or *Azospirillum*, lead to higher biomass and the capacity to degrade pollutants. An intermediate compound is transformed by algae and further shaped to the final product by bacteria. Previously, a great symbiosis between the two microorganisms, characterized by a balanced CO_2/O_2 exchange, was produced by C. vulgaris, a microalga with high tolerance to numerous organic pollutants and rapid growth rates, and *R. opacus*, a bacterium that can withstand and biodegrade high concentrations of organic pollutants. This innovative system can be investigated as a potential method for bioremediation of wastewater effluent with elevated levels of organic contaminants (León-Vaz et al., 2025).

Previously, research conducted by Afonso et al. (2024) found that the removal of microplastics ranges from 25% to 85%, demonstrating that algae–bacteria consortia are best suited for the remediation of microplastics. Microalgae secrete enzymes and exopolysaccharides (EPS), which promote the degradation of microplastics into simpler and less toxic compounds. The most common monosaccharide compositions of polysaccharides are pentose, hexose, methyl pentose, methyl hexose, uronic acid, sulfate, and monosaccharide components, including glucose, fucose, arabinose, galactose, mannose, xylose, glucuronic acid, and galacturonic acid. The polysaccharide of EPS contains hydroxyl, carboxylic, and sulfate groups due to the presence of these monosaccharides and monosugars. Because of the breakdown of functional groups like carboxyl and sulfate at the cell surface, the cells of microalgae are negatively charged and form hetero-aggregates with positively charged plastic particles (Das et al., 2023). It was highlighted in previous research that the role of the phycosphere in the degradation of microplastics is significant, noting that phycosphere-derived dissolved organic matter (DOM) creates spatial gradients of various organic components, such as aromatic proteins and humic acid-like substances. This expansion of niche-width for microbial communities is crucial for enhancing their degradation capabilities (Fan et al., 2024). It was found that *Chaetoceros neoracile and Rhodomonas* can be a promising sink for microplastic reduction in deep-sea water. *C. vulgaris*, an algae recognized for its rapid growth and biodegradability, shows a high absorption capability for microplastic degradation because of its cell walls, which are rich in polysaccharides and proteins (Long et al., 2015). Finally, the decomposition of this microalga does not create toxic residues, maintaining clean and safe treatment processes, which was experimentally proven to

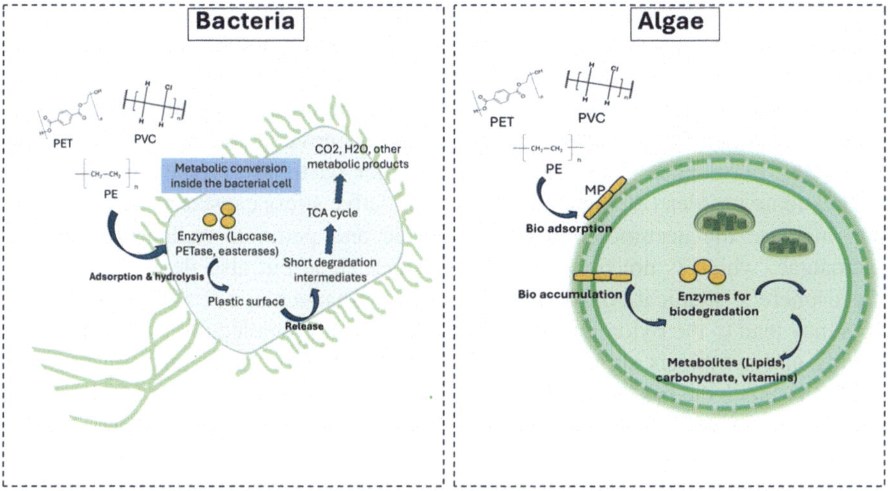

Fig. 11.1 Mechanism of microplastic degradation by bacteria and algae

be the case (Lotfigolsefidi et al., 2025). In a similar study of *Pseudomonas mendocina*, considered the most effective bacterium for degrading plastic, it degrades plastic while removing CO_2, which can be used to promote biomass production in microalgae. Therefore, degradation occurs in a more sustainable and economical manner. While most studies have focused on laboratory scale, several pilot-scale findings have been conducted for wastewater treatment. Previously, cyanobacteria were used for wastewater treatment at the secondary level, showing removal efficiencies of 78.26%, 76%, 79.55%, 4.77%, and 58.74% for COD, total chemical oxygen demand (tCOD), BOD, and nutrients such as nitrates and total phosphorus, respectively. There are still gaps in the study of algae–bacteria consortia for the remediation of microplastic degradation. This can be achieved by deploying a modular photobioreactor, utilizing real-time monitoring with machine learning, or employing IoT-based sensors, which can facilitate setup at an industrial scale. The mechanism of microplastic degradation by bacteria and algae is shown in Fig. 11.1.

11.2.3 Phycosphere Assemblage and Alteration of Chemical Functionalities Under Microplastic Exposure

Microplastic disintegration is therefore crucial in the phycosphere, which serves as a reservoir for a unique microbiome assemblage. Microalgae release organic substances that promote microbial processes in the phycosphere. These secretions nourish bacterial communities that can break down plastic materials. They each have the effect of more efficient degradation of microplastics in aquatic environments (Das et al., 2023). The presence of algae makes microplastics susceptible to degradation by microbes, which alters the chemical functionalities present on the surface.

Microalgae release extracellular polymeric substances (EPS), which interact with phycosphere microorganisms, facilitating the adsorption and aggregation process, thus becoming prominent for microplastic reduction (Fan et al., 2024). Exposure to microplastics significantly shifts the phycosphere microbial community composition. Some studies show that microplastics can be a novel platform for colonization (producing plastispheres) or, indirectly, can alter bacterial diversity by changing algal exudate profiles (Zhang et al., 2019). Oxidative stress caused by microplastics may increase the accumulation of superoxide and peroxide radicals within the microalgae, which is not only toxic to the microalgae but also detrimental to the phycosphere's chemical composition in general (Bhattacharya et al., 2010). Excess ROS may lead to the oxidation of the EPS and signalling molecules, so that quorum sensing and symbiosis signaling may be blocked. Furthermore, microplastics can physically block the passage of light to reach cells on algae's surface or inside and, in this manner, impede photosynthesis and lead to a decrease in primary productivity (Sjollema et al., 2016). Under this stress, algae change the composition of the substances they exude. Normally, the release of large, complex polysaccharides decreases, while small and more readily metabolized compounds increase. These shifts in exudate significantly impact which microbes can thrive within the phycosphere and how nutrients are cycled, which in turn alters functional dynamics of this important microenvironment.

11.3 Metagenomics in Microplastic Biodegradation

Microbial communities have been shown to be an effective option for degrading microplastics, and as such, metagenomics has been proposed as an approach for understanding and elucidating the mechanism of microplastic degradation by microbial communities. It has the potential to identify key microbial members and potential novel enzymes involved in microplastic degradation.

11.3.1 Principles and Techniques in Metagenomics

Metagenomics involves the DNA-based genetic analysis of the total genetic material present in a specific natural habitat or environmental sample, such as soil or water. It has several useful applications in medical and environmental microbiology. A major application of metagenomics is profiling the taxonomic and functional microbial diversities within a sample using the rRNA gene marker. Beyond community characterization, it also explores the novel enzymes and genes, even from the unculturable extremophiles, thereby expanding the repertoire of biocatalysts with potential bioremediation applications (Hozzein, 2020; Kumar et al., 2021). In the field of metagenomics, there is a set of core principles where some of the methodologies and applications for guiding are as follows:

(i) *Culture-Independent Analysis*: Enabling the study of uncultured microorganisms by providing the direct extraction and sequencing of DNA from environmental samples.
(ii) *Diversity Assessment*: For the diversity of microbes and their response to environmental perturbations.
(iii) *Gene prediction*: To identify the protein-encoding genes (protein-coding sequences) within a given sequencing dataset and to comprehend the functional capacity of microbial communities.
(iv) *Functional Metagenomics*: This work contributes to the discovery of novel enzymes and biocatalysts from extremophiles (Hozzein, 2020).

This field has evolved significantly, particularly due to advances in high-throughput sequencing technologies, which enable rapid and large data processing. Among these, next-generation sequencing (NGS) allows comprehensive analysis without the need for culture-dependent analysis. In previous research, NGS was used to identify and characterize the bacterial communities capable of degrading PE and PP microplastics in the Qinhuai urban river of China. The results revealed the involvement of core and resuscitated degrader bacteria and also highlighted the role of low-abundance microbial taxa and their association with eutrophication (Niu et al., 2023). Beyond environmental research, NGS has also demonstrated its potential in medical research. In a previous study, NGS was used to detect plastic-degrading genes within the human gut microbiome. This study highlighted the identification of homologous sequences to plastic-degrading enzymes such as PETase, MHERTase, and other hydrolytic enzymes across various gut samples, demonstrating that the human gut microbiota harbors a diverse pool of genes with potential for microplastics degradation (Nugrahapraja et al., 2022). Another powerful technique for analyzing sequenced data and facilitating species identification and abundance estimation is bidirectional Burrows Wheeler Transform (BWT) indexing, which gives an efficient algorithm for taxonomic annotation (Zheng et al., 2023).

11.3.2 Functional Gene Annotations and Metabolic Pathway Mapping

Functional gene annotations and metabolic pathway mapping offer insights into the role of genes in metabolic pathways, thereby facilitating a deeper understanding of biochemical processes. Advancements in methodologies and computational tools have significantly improved the accuracy of these processes. Ruiz-Perez et al. (2021) described MicrobeAnnotator as one of the comprehensive functional annotation pipelines that integrate combinations of reference protein databases for detailed annotation and metabolic reconstructions. Augment the data set and generate sequence embedding for classification using machine learning models in the form of generative adversarial networks (GANs) to predict and discover novel polyethylene terephthalate (PET) degrading enzymes (Jahanshahi et al., 2025). Understanding the genetic and enzymatic mechanisms that enable microorganisms to break down complex plastic polymers into simpler compounds is crucial for metabolic pathway reconstruction. The complete pathways for the degradation of PAHs have recently been reconstructed in *Pseudomonas* sp. and *Deliftia tsuruhetensis* (Wilkes & Aristilde, 2017). Through *in silico techniques*, it was possible to identify novel metabolic pathways for polyhydroxyalkanoates (PHAs) biosynthesis that did not require acetyl-CoA, suggesting alternative routes of plastic degradation (Kalia et al., 2015). In addition, bacterial enzyme cascade reaction systems (BECRS) have been developed to enhance the degradation of native PET by *Escherichia coli* strains, which have been demonstrated to accelerate the rates and efficiency of degradation (Wang et al., 2024a, b). The reconstruction of the metabolic pathway for microplastic-derived compounds (terephthalic acid and ethylene glycol) has been previously studied and demonstrated their processing in microbial cells. From this, it was revealed that some enzymatic steps are required to break down plastic polymers into their constituent monomers, which can, in turn, be utilized as central metabolic intermediates. The pathway analysis can identify bottlenecks, which are enzymatic steps that are rate-limiting due to low expression or high inefficiency. To support these findings, molecular docking simulations were conducted to assess the binding affinity of the predicted enzymes to their target plastic substrates. These simulations provided structural validation of enzyme–substrate affinity, confirming their potential catalytic roles and helping prioritize enzymes for future experimental testing and pathway optimization (Du et al., 2024). Computational methods, such as flux balance analysis and elementary flux modes, are used to model and predict cellular functions based on metabolic networks (Aplop, 2016). Text mining is another technique used to extract metabolic pathway information from vast scientific literature (Kwon et al., 2007). Other strategies involving reference-based reconstruction utilize known enzymatic reactions as a template to identify homologous enzymes in the target organism, whereas de novo methods predict reactions and enzymes from chemical transformations when no known enzymes exist, thereby highlighting their importance in understanding enzyme classification and the structure–function relationship (Kotera & Goto, 2016). An automated framework, such as the use of orthologous and homologous gene groups, facilitates the reconstruction of microbial metabolic pathways. In silico techniques, including phylogenomic and comparative genomics, enable the reconstruction, origin, and evolution of metabolic pathways by analyzing gene interactions (Presta et al., 2015). Apart from automated and *in silico* techniques, some other tissue-specific metabolic reconstruction is also used, such as cost optimization reaction dependency assessment (CORDA), which models genome-scale networks, identifying critical reactions across tissues (Schultz & Qutub, 2016). Using multi-omics approaches, including genome-scale metabolic modeling, it is now possible to map key enzymatic pathways involved in the breakdown of PET, PS, and PE, along with pinpointing specific enzymes and intermediates; however, challenges remain (Barone et al., 2024). The efficiency of these processes can be limited by environmental factors and the inherent resistance of plastics to degradation. Additionally, the diversity of microplastic types and their varying chemical compositions requires tailored approaches for effective degradation. These pathways require further investigation to optimize them and explore the potential of engineered microbial consortia for large-scale applications in environmental remediation.

11.3.3 Comparative Metagenomics for Environmental Samples

The comparative analysis of metagenomes can reveal ecological and metabolic differences between microbial communities, providing insights into their adaptation to specific environmental conditions. In a previous case, the Deepwater Horizon oil spill, one of the largest oil spills in the Gulf of Mexico, the microbial population was analyzed using metagenomic sequencing to understand the responses to the influx of hydrocarbons. Delmont and Eren (2016) suggested that, in oil contamination zones, *Oceanospirillae, Coleiaceae,* and *Cycloclasticus* members were dominant, *while others were suppressed.* These groups are well-known hydrocarbon degraders, particularly the members of *Oceanospirillae*, which are potential alkane degraders, while *Cycloclausticus* is known to degrade PAHs efficiently, and members of *Colelliaceae* thrive in cold marine environments that contribute to dispersed hydrocarbon degradation. Additionally, the study highlighted the enriched genome, which carried genes for nitrogen metabolism and oxidative stress response mechanisms, essential for sustaining hydrocarbon degradation under oil-polluted conditions. In another study, metagenomes from three hydrocarbon-degrading methanogenic microbial cultures were compared to 41 environmental samples. Despite their enrichment from different sources and the various hydrocarbon types, these cultures shared a functionally redundant core, including common genes for hydrocarbon activation (e.g., assA, bssA, and nmsA genes) and methane production, while exhibiting a substrate-driven shift in the dominance of microbial members (Peptococcaceae, Smithella, and Methanolinea) for degradation. However, they differed from lab-derived cultures obtained from natural sources such as oil sands tailing ponds and oil-contaminated marine sediments, suggesting that laboratory-enriched cultures generate distinct functional profiles adapted to their conditions and selection pressures (Tan et al., 2015).

To date, comparative metagenomics has been used in the human microbiome project to analyze and compare microbial communities residing on different body parts in the human body. Taxonomic and functional profiling also enabled the determination of not only the types of microbes present but also the roles they could serve, the biological activities they performed, and the metabolic capabilities they possessed. Using this comprehensive approach, we gained deeper insights into the site-specific composition and function of the microbiome (Maltez Thomas et al., 2018). Traditional light microscopy was compared with metagenomic analysis of microalgal diversity in freshwater ponds. Although using light microscopy, 299 species in 81 genera were identified, whereas the metagenomic approach detected 207 algal genera, 157 of which were unique to this approach. A significant difference is that metagenomics is more sensitive and more resolutive than classical microscopy, allowing the detection of cryptic or hard-to-detect algal taxa that might otherwise go unnoticed. The work demonstrates that metagenomics can offer, at least in some cases, a broader and complementary range of microbial or algal diversity in environmental samples compared to traditional methods (Linne von Berg et al., 2024). This included the use of omics-based techniques (metagenomics, transcriptomics, and proteomics) to study microbial communities that form biofilms in the phycosphere. The microalgal strains were found to support differential microbial populations, such as Chlorella and Scenedesmus, which were highly associated with α-Proteobacteria, and *Micrasterias* was predominantly associated with Bacteroidetes. These microbial associations are specific to host algal species, indicating that microbial communities are selected by the host algal species and may potentially be important for algal growth, nutrient exchange or plant–microbe interactions (Krohn-Molt et al., 2017). Using a high-resolution metagenomic study, the dynamics of the microbes during a phytoplankton bloom cycle were followed in East Sound, Washington, USA. Changes in gene abundance and composition of the microbial community over time, through bloom stages, revealed in detail how bacteria, archaea, and viruses interact with one another and respond. With this time-resolved approach, they were able to reveal successional patterns and functional shifts in the microbial ecosystem, providing valuable insights into the role of microbes in nutrient recycling, bloom modulation, and ecosystem stability during such natural events (Nunn et al., 2024). In a previous study, degraded microplastics (PE, PET, and PVS) from landfill leachate were identified by an integrated metagenomic and biochemical approach. The key plastic-degrading enzymes, such as alkane monooxygenase, cutinase, and novel esterase-like enzymes, were reconstructed using a genome-centric metagenomic approach, and 70 metagenome-assembled genomes (MAGs) were identified. Also, these microbes and in particular the microbes attached to microplastic surfaces, were enriched in degradation genes. Conducting metagenomics provides a powerful way to discover unculturable plastic-degrading microbes and their metabolic pathways in complex environmental samples (Giangeri et al., 2022).

11.4 Meta-Transcriptomics for Unravelling the Functional Activity

11.4.1 RNA Sequencing and Expression Profiling Under Microplastic Exposure

Exposure to microplastics affected microalgae and bacteria, resulting in visible changes in RNA sequencing and gene expression profiles. These alterations are a result of the way in which the microalgae respond to stress or changes in their metabolic activities (including photosynthesis, respiration, and nutrient uptake), and the way in which cells function is changed. Analyzing these expression patterns, it was possible to determine that microplastics can disturb the microbial physiology and interactions between microbes. Understanding these insights is crucial for comprehending the ecological implications of microplastic pollution in aquatic ecosystems, including its potential detrimental effects on primary production, microbial food webs, and overall ecosystem health. Exposure to PS micro- and nanoplastics (PS-MNPs) in *Chlamydomonas reinhardtii* resulted in a size- and concentration-dependent inhibition of growth, as well as an induction of oxidative stress (Li et al., 2024). The more severe the effects, the smaller the particles. PS-MNPs also impair key proteins involved in photosynthesis (proteomic analysis), suggesting a reduction in photosynthetic machinery. Reductions in chlorophyll content and photosystem II efficiency were also observed, more so in smaller PS-MNPs, suggesting that they are toxic to *Catharanthus roseus*. They demonstrate that exposing photosynthetic organisms to PS-MNPs can disrupt core physiological functions, with potential implications for the functioning of aquatic ecosystems (Li et al., 2024). Another example of exposure of the microalga *Isochrysis galbana* to polyethylene nanoplastics (PE-NPs) caused a significant physiological stress, including inhibition of cell growth, reduction in chlorophyll content, carotenoid levels, and concentration of soluble protein. PE-NPs induced downregulation of the TCA cycle and purine metabolism, which serve as central pathways for energy production and nucleic acid synthesis, as determined by transcriptome analysis. The Calvin cycle and fatty acid metabolism were upregulated, likely as a compensatory stress response to sustain basic metabolic functions and cell survival. Such changes suggest PE-NPs have disturbance effects on core metabolic pathways in microalgae and consequently, on their growth and ecological function (Xiao et al., 2023).

11.4.2 Role of Artificial Intelligence and Predictive Modeling for Bioremediation Efficiency

AI and predictive modeling are becoming valuable for developing more effective bioremediation of microplastics using bacteria and microalgae. Environmental datasets can be large and complex; this technology can process them in real-time to monitor conditions, predict degradation efficiency, and optimize pH, temperature, and nutrient levels, thereby enhancing plastic breakdown. The forecasting of bioremediation outcomes by AI systems may enable the systems to design treatment protocols more efficiently, resulting in time, cost, and resource savings. Therefore, researchers and industries, through the integration of AI with biological remediation methods, can come up with smarter and more scalable solutions to tackle the increasing issue of microplastic pollution in ecosystems (Sahu et al., 2023). Microbial remediation integrated with nanotechnology (nanoremediation) represents a novel and promising approach for mitigating microplastic pollution. Plastic-degrading microbes are utilized to engineer ZnO and FeO_2 nanoparticles, which exhibit an enhanced ability to break down microplastics. AI can also be applied to design immobilized microbial nano-enzyme composites, hybrid systems where microbes or enzymes are immobilized on nanomaterials. The use of these composites leverages the high surface area, reactivity, and stability of nanomaterials, resulting in more efficient and targeted degradation of microplastics. The use of these biological, nanotechnological, and AI tools combined is a powerful and scalable solution for environmental remediation (Akintola, 2024). Currently, one

Table 11.3 Characterization of microplastic-degrading microbes using metagenomic and meta-transcriptomic tools

Organism	Type of microplastic degraded	Identification technique	Tools/platforms used	Reference
Ideonella sakaiensis (bacterium)	PET (polyethylene terephthalate)	Whole-genome sequencing (genomic analysis)	Illumina WGS, gene annotation (PETase/ MHETase)	Yoshida et al. (2016)
Bacillus cereus (bacterium)	PE, PET, and PS	16S rRNA gene sequencing (metagenomic amplicon)	PCR, Sanger sequencing, NCBI BLAST, SEM, and FTIR	Auta et al. (2017)
Rhodococcus sp. strain 36 (bacterium)	PP (polypropylene)	16S rRNA gene sequencing	PCR, Sanger sequencing, SEM, and FTIR	Auta et al. (2018)
Exiguobacterium sp. strain YT2 (bacterium)	PS (polystyrene)	16S rRNA sequencing (gut microbiome)	16S sequencing, PS film bioassay, and weight loss measurement	Yang et al. (2015)
Chlorella sp. (microalga)	LDPE (low-density polyethylene)	18S rRNA sequencing and microscopy	Light microscopy, 18S sequencing, SEM, FTIR, and EDX	Govindan et al. (2021)
Spirulina sp. (cyanobacterium/ microalga)	PET and PP	Material degradation analysis	Tensile testing, FTIR, and EDX	Khoironi et al. (2019)
Halomonas sp. (bacterium)	PET and PE	Metagenomic analysis and culture-based isolation	Illumina 16S rRNA sequencing, SEM, and FTIR	Gao and Sun (2021)

of the most successful works is the machine learning models made for the prediction of microplastic biodegradation by bacteria, such as the multi-layer perceptron artificial neural networks (MLPA). The models have also shown high accuracy in simulating degradation processes in aquatic environments, allowing researchers to predict outcomes without the need for lengthy laboratory experimentation. Furthermore, AI and machine learning are driving a transformation in wastewater treatment, enhancing the symbiosis between microalgae and bacteria. In a recent study, a machine learning model (random forest) predicted the enrichment ratio of PE/PP-degrading bacteria in the plastisphere. Similarly, this model also predicted the type of plastic from the community profile (Chen et al., 2025). The characterization of microplastic-degrading microbes using metagenomic and meta-transcriptomic tools is shown in Table 11.3.

11.5 Prospects and Challenges

Metagenomics and meta-transcriptomics have significantly advanced our understanding of microbial communities; however, these approaches are still limited by several technical and methodological challenges. Such limitations directly influence data interpretation, reproducibility, and the reliability of biological insights. Microbial communities are highly dynamic and sensitive to spatial and temporal fluctuations, making consistent analysis difficult. Environmental variability impacts not only taxonomic composition but also functional gene expression, often leading to misinterpretations in meta-transcriptomic studies (Singh et al., 2021). Furthermore, the absence of standardized protocols across laboratories adds to reproducibility issues. Differences in DNA extraction methods, library preparation strategies, sequencing technologies, and bioinformatics workflows all contribute to technical inconsistencies. For example, the choice of DNA extraction method alone can account for 3–16% of variability in microbial community profiles, with the effect being most pronounced in low-biomass samples. Hence, adopting uniform sample preparation protocols across all studies is crucial to minimize such biases (Sui et al., 2020). Algae–bacteria consortia for MP bioremediation also have some limitations in their practical implementation. The features of the plastic molecule and the participating set of microbial species, as well as the environmental conditions in which they react, primarily govern the degradation of MPs. Some MPs, such as PET, enriched with aromatic components, are notably stable and hard to degrade; polyolefins show a low degree of biodegradation due to the presence of heteroatoms in their structure (Song et al., 2024). Although microbial degradation offers a promising route, it can only serve as a complementary method, not a standalone solution, to plastic pollution. The use of GMOs, including engineered cyanobacteria and microalgae, for applications such as bioremediation and photo-biocatalysis needs to be guided by careful ethical and regulatory considerations to ensure safe and responsible use. The selection of microbial species is challenging, as various environmental factors, such as light, pH, humidity, temperature, and oxygen levels, significantly impact their growth and degradation activity, making biodegradation a slow process. These parameters just not only affect microbes but also the chemical structure of plastic surfaces, thereby impacting degradation rates (Chettri et al., 2023). Though algae–bacteria consortia show promising effects in degrading microplastics, they face some significant challenges in scaling these systems for practical applications. Research is still needed to understand their effectiveness under variable environmental factors mentioned above. Advances in genetic engineering and biotechnology might help in process optimization, enhancing the performance of MPs' biodegradation and adaptability of these microbial systems for more efficient bioremediation (Barone et al., 2020).

These approaches also uncover unculturable microbes and support the selection of minimal communities with beneficial traits for designing synthetic microbial consortia (SynComs). Nevertheless, challenges remain in capturing microbial complexity and translating findings into practical applications, highlighting the need for improved computational tools and synthetic biology. A major hurdle lies in managing and processing the vast datasets generated, where the presence of multiple genomes often leads to uneven sequencing coverage and higher error rates. Even with 90% accuracy of gene prediction tools, the small fraction of undetected genes may include novel and potentially valuable ones. Additionally, the multivariate nature of metagenomic data complicates downstream analysis. Discovery of enzymes is also hindered by factors like thermostability, stereoselectivity, and poor expression levels (Wani et al., 2023). The integration of meta-transcriptomics with metagenomics enhances the identification of microbial consortia and their functional genetics; however, difficulties remain in translating these findings into effective bioremediation. In the future, proteomics/metaproteomics-based approaches will help address these limitations through in situ confirmation of expressed functions. The taxonomic diversity and shared genes result in an incorrect assessment of gene expression profiles. These technical errors during data processing can be overcome using ML and AI, but the diversity within microbial communities, the functional dependency of microorganisms, and MP-degrading gene expression on various physical and chemical parameters challenge the building of ML, indicating the need for extensive research (Gambarini et al., 2024). AI offers great potential to improve bioremediation strategies, but overdependence on technological solutions could lead to overlooking traditional methods. For successful environmental management, it is important to strike a balance between modern and conventional technologies. As microbial biodegradation is a slow process and takes months to degrade MPs, advancements in modelling and monitoring technologies are essential for tracking MPs' movement and hotspots, enabling targeted cleanup efforts and development of effective future mitigation strategies.

References

Afonso, V., Borges, R., Rodrigues, B., Barros, R., João Bebianno, M., & Raposo, S. (2024). Are native microalgae consortia able to remove microplastics from wastewater effluents? *Environmental Pollution, 349*, 123931. https://doi.org/10.1016/j.envpol.2024.123931

Akintola, A. A. (2024). AI-driven monitoring systems for bioremediation: Real-time data analysis and predictive modelling. *World Journal of Advanced Research and Reviews, 24*(1), 788–803. https://doi.org/10.30574/wjarr.2024.24.1.3099

Aplop, F. (2016). *Computational approaches to improving the reconstruction of metabolic pathway*. Doctoral dissertation, Concordia University.

Auta, H. S., Emenike, C. U., & Fauziah, S. H. (2017). Screening of *Bacillus* strains isolated from mangrove ecosystems in Peninsular Malaysia for microplastic degradation. *Environmental Pollution, 231*, 1552–1559.

Auta, H. S., Emenike, C. U., Jayanthi, B., & Fauziah, S. H. (2018). Growth kinetics and biodeterioration of polypropylene microplastics by *Bacillus* sp. and *Rhodococcus* sp. isolated from mangrove sediment. *Marine Pollution Bulletin, 127*, 15–21.

Barone, G. D., Ferizović, D., Biundo, A., & Lindblad, P. (2020). Hints at the applicability of microalgae and cyanobacteria for the biodegradation of plastics. *Sustainability, 12*(24), 10449. https://doi.org/10.3390/su122410449

Barone, G. D., Rodríguez-Seijo, A., Parati, M., Johnston, B., Erdem, E., Cernava, T., Zhu, Z., Liu, X., Axmann, I. M., Lindblad, P., & Radecka, I. (2024). Harnessing photosynthetic

microorganisms for enhanced bioremediation of microplastics: A comprehensive review. *Environmental Science and Ecotechnology, 20*, 100407. https://doi.org/10.1016/j.ese.2024.100407
Bhattacharya, P., Lin, S., Turner, J. P., & Ke, P. C. (2010). Physical adsorption of charged plastic nanoparticles affects algal photosynthesis. *The Journal of Physical Chemistry C, 114*(39), 16556–16561. https://doi.org/10.1021/jp1054759
Bubu-Davies, O. A., & Anwuri, P. A. (2022). Microplastics: Potential impacts on aquatic biodiversity. *Tropical Freshwater Biology, 31*(1), Article 1. https://doi.org/10.4314/tfb.v31i1.4
Chandel, M., Sharma, S., Kaur, H., & Raina, M. (2025). Role of microorganisms in biodegradation of microplastics. In *Microplastics and soil microbiome: Recent trends and future prospects* (pp. 247–257). Springer.
Chen, Y., Li, Y., & Niu, L. (2025). Microbial degradation potential of microplastics in urban river sediments: Assessing and predicting the enrichment of PE/PP-degrading bacteria using SourceTracker and machine learning. *Journal of Environmental Management, 386*, 125755.
Chettri, D., Pati, T., & Verma, A. K. (2023). Microbe-mediated biodegradation of microplastics from wastes. *Water and Environment Journal, 37*(4), 671–685. https://doi.org/10.1111/wej.12882
Das, P., Halder, G., & Bal, M. (2023). A critical review on remediation of microplastics using microalgae from aqueous system. *Science of the Total Environment, 898*, 166425. https://doi.org/10.1016/j.scitotenv.2023.166425
Delmont, T. O., & Eren, A. M. (2016). Linking comparative genomics and environmental distribution patterns of microbial populations through metagenomics. *BioRxiv, 058750.*
Du, M., Pu, Q., Xu, Y., Li, Y., & Li, X. (2024). Improved microalgae carbon fixation and microplastic sedimentation in the lake through in silico method. *Science of the Total Environment, 924*, 171623.
Dvořák, P., Nikel, P. I., Damborský, J., & de Lorenzo, V. (2017). Bioremediation 3.0: Engineering pollutant-removing bacteria in the times of systemic biology. *Biotechnology Advances, 35*(7), 845–866. https://doi.org/10.1016/j.biotechadv.2017.08.001
Esmaeili Nasrabadi, A., Eydi, M., & Bonyadi, Z. (2023). Utilizing Chlorella vulgaris algae as an eco-friendly coagulant for efficient removal of polyethylene microplastics from aquatic environments. *Heliyon, 9*(11), e22338. https://doi.org/10.1016/j.heliyon.2023.e22338
Eydi Gabrabad, M., Yari, M., & Bonyadi, Z. (2024). Using Spirulina platensis as a natural biocoagulant for polystyrene removal from aqueous medium: Performance, optimization, and modeling. *Scientific Reports, 14*(1), 2506. https://doi.org/10.1038/s41598-024-53123-y
Fallahi, A., Rezvani, F., Asgharnejad, H., Khorshidi Nazloo, E., Hajinajaf, N., & Higgins, B. (2021). Interactions of microalgae-bacteria consortia for nutrient removal from wastewater: A review. *Chemosphere, 272*, 129878. https://doi.org/10.1016/j.chemosphere.2021.129878
Fan, X., Kong, L., Wang, J., Tan, Y., Xu, X., Li, M., & Zhu, L. (2024). Surface-programmed microbiome assembly in phycosphere to microplastics contamination. *Water Research, 262*, 122064. https://doi.org/10.1016/j.watres.2024.122064
Gambarini, V., Drost, C. J., Kingsbury, J. M., Weaver, L., Pantos, O., Handley, K. M., & Lear, G. (2024). Uncoupled: Investigating the lack of correlation between the transcription of putative plastic-degrading genes in the global ocean microbiome and marine plastic pollution. *Environmental Microbiome, 19*(1), 34. https://doi.org/10.1186/s40793-024-00575-4
Gao, R. R., & Sun, C. M. (2021). A marine bacterial community capable of degrading poly(ethylene terephthalate) and polyethylene. *Journal of Hazardous Materials, 416*, 125928.
Gao, W., Xu, M., Zhao, W., Yang, X., Xin, F., Dong, W., Jia, H., & Wu, X. (2024). Microbial degradation of (micro)plastics: Mechanisms, enhancements, and future directions. *Fermentation, 10*(9), 441. https://doi.org/10.3390/fermentation10090441
Giangeri, G., et al. (2022). Preliminary investigation of microorganisms potentially involved in microplastics degradation using an integrated metagenomic and biochemical approach. *Science of the Total Environment, 843*, 157017.
Govindan, N., Bhuyar, P., Feng, H. X., Nasri, N. S., & Maniam, G. P. (2021). Evaluation of microalgae's plastic biodeterioration property by a consortium of *Chlorella* sp. and

Cyanobacteria sp. *Environmental Research, Engineering and Management, 77*(3), 86–98. https://doi.org/10.5755/j01.erem.77.3.25317

Gowthami, A., Syed Marjuk, M., Santhanam, P., Thirumurugan, R., Muralisankar, T., & Perumal, P. (2025). Marine microalgae – Mediated biodegradation of polystyrene microplastics: Insights from enzymatic and molecular docking studies. *Chemosphere, 370*, 144024. https://doi.org/10.1016/j.chemosphere.2024.144024

Hadiyanto, H., Joelyna, F. A., Khoironi, A., Sudarno, S., Safaat, J. A., Pratama, W. D., & Nur, M. M. A. (2025). Harnessing Chlorella vulgaris – Aspergilus niger interactions for effective microplastic removal in aquatic ecosystems. *Waste and Biomass Valorization*. https://doi.org/10.1007/s12649-025-03062-0

Hozzein, W. N. (2020). Introductory chapter: Metagenomics and metagenomic approaches. In *Metagenomics-basics, methods and applications*. IntechOpen.

Hu, X., Gu, H., Sun, X., Wang, Y., Liu, J., Yu, Z., Li, Y., Jin, J., & Wang, G. (2024). Metagenomic exploration of microbial and enzymatic traits involved in microplastic biodegradation. *Chemosphere, 348*, 140762. https://doi.org/10.1016/j.chemosphere.2023.140762

Jahanshahi, D. A., Barzani, M. R. R., Bahram, M., Ariaeenejad, S., & Kavousi, K. (2025). Metagenomic exploration and computational prediction of novel enzymes for polyethylene terephthalate degradation. *Ecotoxicology and Environmental Safety, 289*, 1176.

Kalia, V. C., Lal, S., Rashmi, Chauhan, A., & Bhattacharyya, G. (2015). In silico reconstitution of novel routes for microbial plastic. *Microbial Factories: Biodiversity, Biopolymers, Bioactive Molecules, 2*, 299–315.

Khoironi, A., Anggoro, S., & Sudarno, S. (2019). Evaluation of the interaction among microalgae Spirulina sp, plastics polyethylene terephthalate and polypropylene in freshwater environment. *Journal of Ecological Engineering, 20*(6), 161–173. https://doi.org/10.12911/22998993/108637

Kotera, M., & Goto, S. (2016). Metabolic pathway reconstruction strategies for central metabolism and natural product biosynthesis. *Biophysics and Physicobiology, 13*, 195–205.

Krohn-Molt, I., Alawi, M., Förstner, K. U., Wiegandt, A., Burkhardt, L., Indenbirken, D., & Streit, W. R. (2017). Insights into microalga and bacteria interactions of selected phycosphere biofilms using metagenomic, transcriptomic, and proteomic approaches. *Frontiers in Microbiology, 8*, 1941.

Kumar, L., Satyam, R., & Bharadvaja, N. (2021). Metagenomics: A powerful lens viewing the microbial world. *Wastewater Treatment Reactors*, 185–218.

Kwon, H. R., Na, J. H., Yoo, J. S., & Cho, W. S. (2007). Text-mining techniques for metabolic pathway reconstruction. *Journal of Korea Society of Industrial Information Systems, 12*(4), 138–147.

León-Vaz, A., Torres-Franco, A. F., García-Encina, P. A., & Muñoz, R. (2025). Developing a microalgal-bacterial consortium for the removal of organic pollutants from petrochemical industry. *Journal of Water Process Engineering, 73*, 107663. https://doi.org/10.1016/j.jwpe.2025.107663

Li, X., Chu, Z., Feng, C., Song, P., Yang, T., Zhou, L., & Tang, H. (2024). Unveiling the molecular mechanisms of size-dependent effect of polystyrene micro/nano-plastics on Chlamydomonas reinhardtii through proteomic profiling. *Chemosphere, 358*, 142220.

Linne von Berg, K. H., Keilholz, L., Küchenmeister, N., Pushkareva, E., & Becker, B. (2024). Microalgal diversity and molecular ecology: A comparative study of classical and metagenomic approaches in ponds of the Eifel National Park, Germany. *Phycology, 4*(3), 414–426.

Liu, W., Zhang, J., Liu, H., Guo, X., Zhang, X., Yao, X., & Zhang, T. (2021). A review of the removal of microplastics in global wastewater treatment plants: Characteristics and mechanisms. *Environment International, 146*, 106277.

Long, M., Moriceau, B., Gallinari, M., Lambert, C., Huvet, A., Raffray, J., & Soudant, P. (2015). Interactions between microplastics and phytoplankton aggregates: Impact on their respective fates. *Marine Chemistry, 175*, 39–46. https://doi.org/10.1016/j.marchem.2015.04.003

Lotfigolsefidi, F., Davoudi, M., Sarkhosh, M., & Bonyadi, Z. (2025). Removal of microplastics by algal biomass from aqueous solutions: Performance, optimization, and modeling. *Scientific Reports, 15*(1), 501. https://doi.org/10.1038/s41598-024-84114-8

Madiraju, S. V. H., Pamula, A. S. P., & Darsi, B. P. (2024). Theoretical review on microplastic pollution: A multifaceted threat to marine ecosystems, human health, and environment. *Igmin Research, 2*(6), 460–468. https://doi.org/10.61927/igmin203

Maltez Thomas, A., Prata Lima, F., Maria Silva Moura, L., Maria da Silva, A., Dias-Neto, E., & Setubal, J. C. (2018). Comparative metagenomics. In *Comparative genomics: Methods and protocols* (pp. 243–260).

Muhonja, C. N., Makonde, H., Magoma, G., & Imbuga, M. (2018). Biodegradability of polyethylene by bacteria and fungi from Dandora dumpsite Nairobi-Kenya. *PLoS One, 13*(7), e0198446. https://doi.org/10.1371/journal.pone.0198446

Nava, V., & Leoni, B. (2021). A critical review of interactions between microplastics, microalgae and aquatic ecosystem function. *Water Research, 188*, 116476. https://doi.org/10.1016/j.watres.2020.116476

Newrick, B. A., Valdés, D., Laca, A., Laca, A., & Díaz, M. (2025). Enhanced biodegradation of high-density polyethylene microplastics: Study of bacterial efficiency and process parameters. *Journal of Hazardous Materials, 485*, 136822. https://doi.org/10.1016/j.jhazmat.2024.136822

Niu, L., Chen, Y., Li, Y., Wang, Y., Shen, J., Wang, L., & Zhao, B. (2023). Diversity, abundance and distribution characteristics of potential polyethylene and polypropylene microplastic degradation bacterial communities in the urban river. *Water Research, 232*, 119704.

Nugrahapraja, H., Sugiyo, P. W. W., Putri, B. Q., Huang, L., Hafza, N., Götz, F., & Luqman, A. (2022). Effects of microplastic on human gut microbiome: detection of plastic-degrading genes in human gut exposed to microplastics – Preliminary study. *Environments, 9*(11), 140.

Nunn, B. L., Timmins-Schiffman, E., Mudge, M. C., Plubell, D. L., Chebli, G., Kubanek, J., & Eloe-Fadrosh, E. A. (2024). Microbial metagenomes across a complete phytoplankton bloom cycle: High-resolution sampling every 4 hours over 22 days. *Scientific Data, 11*(1), 1270.

Presta, L., Fondi, M., Emiliani, G., Fani, R., Presta, L., Fondi, M., & Fani, R. (2015). Protocols and methods for the in silico reconstruction of the origin and evolution of metabolic pathways. In *Molybdenum cofactors and their role in the evolution of metabolic pathways* (pp. 67–75).

Purohit, J., Chattopadhyay, A., & Teli, B. (2020). Metagenomic exploration of plastic degrading microbes for biotechnological application. *Current Genomics, 21*(4), 253–270.

Rambabu, K., Bharath, G., Govarthanan, M., Senthil Kumar, P., Show, P. L., & Banat, F. (2023). Bioprocessing of plastics for sustainable environment: Progress, challenges, and prospects. *Trends in Analytical Chemistry, 166*, 117189. https://doi.org/10.1016/j.trac.2023.117189

Ren, X., Feng, M., Mao, M., Long, X., Pan, J., Tang, Y., & Yang, F. (2025). Cyanobacteria for environmental, energy and biomedical application: A review. *Environmental Chemistry Letters, 23*(2), 491–515.

Rosariastuti, R., Prakosa, M. H. H., Sutami, S., Sumani, S., & Purwanto, P. (2024). Identification and degradation potential of microplastics by indigenous bacteria isolated from Putri Cempo Landfill, Surakarta, Indonesia. *Eurasian Journal of Soil Science (EJSS), 14*(1), 79–86. https://doi.org/10.18393/ejss.1582987

Ruiz-Perez, C. A., Conrad, R. E., & Konstantinidis, K. T. (2021). MicrobeAnnotator: A user-friendly, comprehensive functional annotation pipeline for microbial genomes. *BMC Bioinformatics, 22*, 1–16.

Sahu, S., Kaur, A., Singh, G., & Arya, S. K. (2023). Harnessing the potential of microalgae-bacteria interaction for eco-friendly wastewater treatment: A review on new strategies involving machine learning and artificial intelligence. *Journal of Environmental Management, 346*, 119004.

Sánchez, C. (2020). Fungal potential for the degradation of petroleum-based polymers: An overview of macro- and microplasticsbiodegradation. Biotechnology Advances, 40, 107501. https://doi.org/10.1016/j.biotechadv.2019.107501

Sanniyasi, E., Gopal, R. K., Gunasekar, D. K., & Raj, P. P. (2021). Biodegradation of low-density polyethylene (LDPE) sheet by microalga, Uronema africanum Borge. *Scientific Reports, 11*(1), 17233. https://doi.org/10.1038/s41598-021-96315-6

Schultz, A., & Qutub, A. A. (2016). Reconstruction of tissue-specific metabolic networks using CORDA. *PLoS Computational Biology, 12*(3), e1004808.

Singh, A., Vats, S., & Bhargava, P. (2021). Advances and challenges in metatranscriptomic analysis. In M. Nath, D. Bhatt, P. Bhargava, & D. K. Choudhary (Eds.), *Microbial metatranscriptomics belowground* (pp. 453–469). Springer. https://doi.org/10.1007/978-981-15-9758-9_21

Sjollema, S. B., Redondo-Hasselerharm, P., Leslie, H. A., Kraak, M. H. S., & Vethaak, A. D. (2016). Do plastic particles affect microalgal photosynthesis and growth? *Aquatic Toxicology, 170*, 259–261. https://doi.org/10.1016/j.aquatox.2015.12.002

Song, Q., Zhang, Y., Ju, C., Zhao, T., Meng, Q., & Cong, J. (2024). Microbial strategies for effective microplastics biodegradation: Insights and innovations in environmental remediation. *Environmental Research, 263*, 120046. https://doi.org/10.1016/j.envres.2024.120046

Sponza, D. T., & Öztekin, R. (2023). Removals of Some High- and Low-Density Polyethylene (HDPE and LDPE), Polypropylene (PP) and Polyvinyl Chloride (PVC) microplastics using some microalgae types, energy production and energy recovery. *Molecular Sciences and Applications, 3*, 66–88. https://doi.org/10.37394/232023.2023.3.7

Srikanth, M., Sandeep, T. S. R. S., Sucharitha, K., & Godi, S. (2022). Biodegradation of plastic polymers by fungi: A brief review. *Bioresources and Bioprocessing, 9*(1), 42. https://doi.org/10.1186/s40643-022-00532-4

Sui, H., Weil, A. A., Nuwagira, E., Qadri, F., Ryan, E. T., Mezzari, M. P., Phipatanakul, W., & Lai, P. S. (2020). Impact of DNA extraction method on variation in human and built environment microbial community and functional profiles assessed by shotgun metagenomics sequencing. *Frontiers in Microbiology, 11*. https://doi.org/10.3389/fmicb.2020.00953

Tan, B., Jane Fowler, S., Laban, N. A., Dong, X., Sensen, C. W., Foght, J., & Gieg, L. M. (2015). Comparative analysis of metagenomes from three methanogenic hydrocarbon-degrading enrichment cultures with 41 environmental samples. *The ISME Journal, 9*(9), 2028–2045.

Tareen, A., Saeed, S., Iqbal, A., Batool, R., & Jamil, N. (2022). Biodeterioration of microplastics: a promising step towards plastics waste management. *Polymers, 14*(11), 2275. https://doi.org/10.3390/polym14112275

Thapliyal, C., Priya, A., Singh, S. B., Bahuguna, V., & Daverey, A. (2024). Potential strategies for bioremediation of microplastic contaminated soil. *Environmental Chemistry and Ecotoxicology, 6*, 117–131. https://doi.org/10.1016/j.enceco.2024.05.001

Wang, Q., Hong, L., Wu, K., Li, M., Zhang, J., Li, X., Jin, J., & Liu, B. (2024a). Research progress in microbial degradation of microplastics. *Journal of Physics: Conference Series, 2706*(1), 012043. https://doi.org/10.1088/1742-6596/2706/1/012043

Wang, C., Long, R., Lin, X., Liu, W., Zhu, L., & Jiang, L. (2024b). Development and characterization of a bacterial enzyme cascade reaction system for efficient and stable PET degradation. *Journal of Hazardous Materials, 472*, 134480.

Wani, A. K., Akhtar, N., Naqash, N., Rahayu, F., Djajadi, D., Chopra, C., Singh, R., Mulla, S. I., Sher, F., & Américo-Pinheiro, J. H. P. (2023). Discovering untapped microbial communities through metagenomics for microplastic remediation: Recent advances, challenges, and way forward. *Environmental Science and Pollution Research, 30*(34), 81450–81473. https://doi.org/10.1007/s11356-023-25192-5

Wilkes, R. A., & Aristilde, L. (2017). Degradation and metabolism of synthetic plastics and associated products by Pseudomonas sp.: Capabilities and challenges. *Journal of Applied Microbiology, 123*(3), 582–593.

Xiang, P., Zhang, Y., Zhang, T., Wu, Q., Zhao, C., & Li, Q. (2023). A novel bacterial combination for efficient degradation of polystyrene microplastics. *Journal of Hazardous Materials, 458*, 131856. https://doi.org/10.1016/j.jhazmat.2023.131856

Xiao, X., Li, W., Li, S., Zuo, X., Liu, J., Guo, L., & Zhang, L. (2023). The growth inhibition of polyethylene nanoplastics on the bait-microalgae isochrysis galbana based on the transcriptome analysis. *Microorganisms, 11*(5), 1108.

Yang, Y., Yang, J., Wu, W.-M., Zhao, J., Song, Y., Gao, L., & Jiang, L. (2015). Biodegradation and mineralization of polystyrene by plastic-eating mealworms: Part 2 – Role of gut microorganisms. *Environmental Science & Technology, 49*(20), 12087–12093.

Yin, J., Zhu, T., Li, X., Wang, F., & Xu, G. (2025). Phytoremediation of microplastics by water hyacinth. *Environmental Science and Ecotechnology, 24*, 100540. https://doi.org/10.1016/j.ese.2025.100540

Yoshida, S., Hiraga, K., Takehana, T., Taniguchi, I., Yamaji, H., Maeda, Y., Toyohara, K., Miyamoto, K., Kimura, Y., & Oda, K. (2016). A bacterium that degrades and assimilates poly(ethylene terephthalate). *Science, 351*(6278), 1196–1199. https://doi.org/10.1126/science.aad6359

Zhang, B., Wu, D., Yang, X., Teng, J., Liu, Y., Zhang, C., Zhao, J., Yin, X., You, L., Liu, Y., & Wang, Q. (2019). Microplastic pollution in the surface sediments collected from Sishili Bay, North Yellow Sea, China. *Marine Pollution Bulletin, 141*, 9–15. https://doi.org/10.1016/j.marpolbul.2019.02.021

Zhang, J., Gao, D., Li, Q., Zhao, Y., Li, L., Lin, H., Bi, Q., & Zhao, Y. (2020). Biodegradation of polyethylene microplastic particles by the fungus Aspergillus flavus from the guts of wax moth Galleria mellonella. *Science of the Total Environment, 704*, 135931. https://doi.org/10.1016/j.scitotenv.2019.135931

Zheng, H., Marçais, G., & Kingsford, C. (2023). Creating and using minimizer sketches in computational genomics. *Journal of Computational Biology, 30*(12), 1251–1276.

Multi-Omics-Driven Systems Biology of Microalgal Bioremediation: Mechanisms and Environmental Applications

12

Gurunathan Baskar and M. Ramya

Abstract

The escalating burden of environmental contamination from industry, agriculture, and domestic activities has increased the quest for effective and suitable remediation technologies. Microalgae, with their metabolic versatility and ecological adaptability, have become recognized as one of the promising tools for bioremediation of a broad range of contaminants, including heavy metals, dyes, pesticides, cosmetics and pharmaceuticals. Recent omics technological advancements, including genomics, transcriptomics, proteomics, and metabolomics, have provided pivotal insights into molecular processes. Economic weaponry has identified key genes, regulatory circuits, and transporters involved in pollutant uptake, detoxification, and degradation in microalgae. Transcriptomic studies further support this information by showing how these genes are differentially expressed under various environmental stresses, providing a dynamic understanding of cell responses. Proteomic profiling relates these transcriptional signals to real protein production, post-translational changes, and enzyme activities that transmit adaptive and detoxification processes. Metabolomics complements these dimensions by charting the end-point biochemical pathways, metabolic intermediates, and secondary metabolites engaged in pollutant assimilation. By combining these omics dimensions, scientists can build a systems biology platform that bridges genes to function and metabolites, thereby exposing the coordinated regulation and metabolic fluxes that govern algal bioremediation. This multidimensional strategy not only enriches mechanistic knowledge but also informs directed strain engineering and process optimization of bioremediation. These multi-omics strategies provide an integrated system biology platform to enhance algal bioremediation through targeted strain

G. Baskar (✉) · M. Ramya
Department of Biotechnology, St. Joseph's College of Engineering, Chennai, India

L. Kumar et al. (eds.), *Algal Bioremediation*,
https://doi.org/10.1007/978-981-95-8793-3_12

development, metabolic engineering, and optimized cultivation protocols. This chapter examines the current state of omics studies in algal bioremediation, presents several key case studies, and outlines future directions for integrating omics data into scalable and ecologically efficient remediation technologies.

Keywords

Bioremediation · Multi-Omics integration · Systems biology · Pollutant degradation · Environmental sustainability

12.1 Introduction

The rapid pace of urbanization and industrialization has significantly increased environmental pollution and heavily impacted ecosystem services. Both the generation of solid and liquid waste has reached alarming figures on a global scale, with estimates suggesting an increase in yearly waste production from 2.01 to 3.40 billion metric tons by the year 2050 (Upadhyay et al., 2024). Environmental contaminants, resulting from both human activities and natural phenomena, pose a significant threat to human health. Industrialization, as much as it is needed for growth, has had a great role in releasing deadly contaminants into the human body primarily by inhalation, ingestion, dermal contact, causing acute, and chronic health impacts. Air pollution is caused by vehicle emissions, industrial emissions, power plant emissions, and natural sources such as volcanic eruptions. Sulfur dioxide, carbon monoxide, nitrogen oxides, ozone, heavy metals, and tobacco smoke are some common airborne pollutants that contribute to respiratory diseases, cardiovascular disease, neurological injury, reproductive effects, and cancer. Bacteria and pollen are among the biological agents that exacerbate allergies and respiratory ailments. Soil contamination results from the improper disposal of industrial, agricultural, and household waste. Pesticides, heavy metals, plastics, drugs, and emerging pollutants are introduced into the soil and accumulate, posing a threat to human health through direct contact or ingestion of contaminated crops. Chronic exposure to soil contaminants can cause skin disease, organ impairment, developmental issues, and heightened cancer risk. Water pollution by agricultural runoff, industrial effluent, and poor waste disposal releases dangerous chemicals such as heavy metals, pesticides, and diseases such as cholera, hepatitis, typhoid, and kidney diseases. Natural pollutants, such as arsenic and fluoride, exacerbate the problem. It is difficult to monitor and respond to pollutant exposure with limited data, particularly in low-resource environments. Long-term consequences typically emerge only after years of exposure, making research and intervention efforts cumbersome (Shetty et al., 2023).

Bioremediation is a green and innovative technology that utilizes microorganisms to break down and decontaminate environmental contaminants, thereby reclaiming ecosystems and preventing secondary contamination. It has extensive applications in the remediation of problems such as acid mine drainage, industrial effluents, heavy metals, pesticides, and other toxic substances, utilizing microbial metabolic pathways, predominantly through oxidation–reduction reactions. Bioremediation is a more sustainable, economical, and less disruptive approach compared to traditional methods. Recent developments have involved the application of genetically modified microbes, microbial consortia, and synthetic biology to improve pollutant degradation. Integration with phytoremediation and the adoption of bioinformatics and machine learning have further enhanced its efficiency and effectiveness. Although increasingly successful, challenges persist that prevent wide-scale deployment, necessitating further investigation and technological advancement (Kuppan et al., 2024). This chapter discusses the application of omics technologies to advance bioremediation strategies based on microalgae. The chapter starts with discussing the environmental contamination load from pollutants and the imperative for cleanup processes to be sustainable. Microalgae are introduced as bioremediation agents that are naturally occurring and metabolically diverse, addressing a wide range of pollutants, including heavy metals, dyes, pesticides, and pharmaceuticals. The center of the chapter is on multi-omics platforms—genomics, transcriptomics, proteomics, and metabolomics—and how they all work to understand and improve pollutant degradation pathways in microalgae. Key mechanisms, ranging from gene expression to metabolite formation and data integration through bioinformatics, are explained. Practical applications, presented in the form of real-world case studies, illustrate actual usage. Forthcoming trends, such as CRISPR, synthetic biology, and AI-assisted modeling, are outlined to envision the future of environmental bioremediation.

12.2 Microalgae as Bioremediation Agents

Microalgae are highly versatile, photosynthetic microorganisms with superior metabolic plasticity, which enables them to thrive in various environments and effectively assimilate essential nutrients such as carbon, nitrogen, phosphorus, and sulfur, which are typically pollutants in wastewater. Being able to grow autotrophically, heterotrophically, or mixotrophically allows them to be very efficient in wastewater treatment (WWT), eliminating nutrient loads and greenhouse gases such as nitrous oxide. In addition, microalgae yield beneficial bio-products, thereby increasing their biotechnological value and aligning with the objectives of the circular bioeconomy (Calatrava et al., 2024). Microalgae exhibit very high photosynthetic efficiency and biomass yields, surpassing those of terrestrial vegetation, and can be produced without occupying arable land. While commercially used by only a few species, most have been found to be useful in the treatment of agricultural, industrial, and domestic wastewater. They effectively remove BOD, COD, nutrients (C, N, and P), and heavy metals through natural disinfection and high biosorption ability, thanks to their surface-to-volume ratio and metabolic adaptability.

In contrast to traditional wastewater treatment (WWT) technologies, microalgae offer a cost-efficient and sustainable one-step process with little secondary pollution. They also facilitate CO_2 sequestration and the recovery of high-value bioproducts such as biofuels, pigments, and proteins, complementing circular bioeconomy targets. Their biomass can be used to produce biohydrogen, bioalcohols, and other high-value products. Combining microalgae with WWT not only minimizes environmental footprint but also maximizes resource recovery through biorefinery, thus rendering them an effective weapon for environmental sustainability and pollution management (Abdelfattah et al., 2023). Heavy metals, which are naturally occurring, have become significant environmental pollutants due to accelerated urbanization, industrialization, and agricultural activities. High-density and toxic elements that accumulate in water and soil systems cause harm to ecosystems and human well-being. Traditional methods of remediation often fail because heavy metals are not biodegradable. New developments comprise emerging nanomaterial and sensor technologies for sensing and elimination. Besides, microorganism-based biological processes involving bacteria, fungi, plants, and especially microalgae have been proven to remediate heavy metals.

Microalgae are photosynthetic microorganisms that can fix CO_2 through photosynthesis and are gaining prominence for their potential to treat wastewater by removing nutrients and heavy metals. The last 30 years have seen numerous species exhibit a strong capacity for removing heavy metals. For instance, *Scenedesmus incrassatulus* exhibited efficient removal of Cr(VI), Cd(II), and Cu(II) with up to 78% removal of Cr(VI). *Scenedesmus obliquus* had a greater Zn removal efficiency than *S. quadricauda*. Some other species, such as *Chlorella* sp. and *Porphyridium* sp., removed Pb, Cd, and Cu efficiently, with *Chlorella* sp. removing 90% of Pb. Further, *Picochlorum* strains have also been reported to be highly versatile in removing heavy metals from diverse wastewaters. Dead algal cells or biomass, as well as algal derivatives, have also been found to possess high biosorption capacity. For example, *Chlorella vulgaris* removed more than 95% Cd(II) in both dead and living forms, whereas *Scenedesmus* sp., removed more than 92% of Cr(VI) with the assistance of functional groups, such as carboxyls and amides. *S. obliquus* removed Pb(II) by both biosorption (85.5%) and bioaccumulation (14.5%). These observations highlight the species-specific effectiveness and processes, such as biosorption, bioaccumulation, and algal biochar utilization, that render microalgae a promising candidate for heavy metal bioremediation (Goswami et al., 2022).

12.2.1 Metabolic Flexibility and Ecological Resilience

Microalgae exhibit great metabolic flexibility, allowing them to grow under autotrophic, heterotrophic, photoheterotrophic, and mixotrophic modes. This is crucial for maximizing biomass yield to meet production needs, such as biofuels and wastewater treatment. Autotrophic growth is carried out using light and CO_2, with organisms such as *Chlorella*, *Dunaliella*, and *Nannochloropsis* being cultivated in open raceway ponds or closed photobioreactors. Although cost-saving, light penetration limitations can impact productivity. Heterotrophic cultivation, where organic carbon serves as the source of energy in dark conditions, enables high biomass production and simpler reactor systems. However, only certain species, such as *Chlorella* sp. and *Scenedesmus* sp., can adapt well to this type of cultivation. It restricts light-dependent metabolite synthesis. Phototrophic and mixotrophic cultivation unite light with organic carbon. Mixotrophic organisms, especially, increase growth and biomass yield by reconciling photosynthetic CO_2 fixation with organic carbon assimilation. It also maintains the generation of pigments and lipids and sustains photoprotective functions. Generally, mixotrophic systems provide better efficiency and metabolite yield than other trophic modes (Andrade-Bustamante et al., 2025). Metabolic cross-feeding within microbial communities represents a key cooperative strategy, wherein one species degrades complex compounds into intermediate byproducts that can be further utilized by another species. This interaction facilitates synergistic pathways for pollutant degradation, thereby enhancing the overall efficiency of bioremediation processes. Such tropic interactions contribute significantly to the robustness, resilience, and stability of microbial consortia involved in pollutant removal (Oña et al., 2022).

Phototrophic microorganisms, particularly microalgae and cyanobacteria, also display remarkable metabolic plasticity, enabling them to grow under diverse trophic modes—including autotrophic, heterotrophic, and mixotrophic conditions. This versatility allows them to efficiently remove inorganic nutrients (e.g., nitrogen and phosphorus), heavy metals, and various organic pollutants from industrial effluents and wastewater (Minkina et al., 2023). For example, *Chlorella vulgaris* can thrive under mixotrophic conditions, utilizing both CO_2 and organic carbon sources, thereby enhancing nutrient uptake efficiency and improving tolerance to environmental stressors (Tan et al., 2021). Microalgae are also resilient to oxidative, thermal, and nutrient stress by overexpressing certain enzymes (e.g., superoxide dismutase and catalase), storing protective pigments such as carotenoids, and modifying membrane lipid composition. These help sustain photosynthesis activity and pollutant removal efficiency under varying environmental conditions (Zhao et al., 2024). Omics technologies, including transcriptomics, proteomics, and metabolomics, have enabled the identification of major metabolic switches and stress–responsive pathways that mediate such adaptive responses. These findings facilitate the development of engineered microbial strains with improved tolerance and degradation capacity for given pollutants (Zhao et al., 2024).

12.2.2 Major Classes of Pollutants Addressed by Algae

12.2.2.1 Organic Hydrocarbon

Organic hydrocarbon contaminants, such as polycyclic aromatic hydrocarbons (PAHs), polychlorinated biphenyls (PCBs), phthalates (e.g., DEHP), surfactants, and dioxins (PCDD/PCDF), are hydrophobic and persistent chemicals that tend to accumulate in aquatic sediments and do not readily degrade. These contaminants, which originate mostly from petroleum, enter the aquatic environment through industrial effluent, atmospheric deposition, and river runoff. The stability of these contaminants increases with molecular weight and the number of aromatic rings, lowering biodegradability under aerobic conditions. PAHs, which are carcinogenic and environmentally persistent, are of specific worry. Likewise, phenol, a typical pollutant of petroleum refineries, presents severe ecological hazards at concentrations as low as 5–25 ppm. Conventional removal methods have low efficacy; however, a potential alternative is offered through biological treatment, due to the high removal effectiveness of microbes capable of degrading such substances (Touliabah et al., 2022).

Microalgae and cyanobacteria are receiving increasing attention as new candidates for the remediation of hydrocarbons due to their photoautotrophic efficiency and high biomass productivity. Several species, including *Chlorella vulgaris*, *Nannochloropsis oculata*, and certain marine *Phormidium* strains, have demonstrated the effective removal of petroleum hydrocarbons, achieving up to 98% removal from polluted environments. Although freshwater as well as marine species have shown promise, marine algae possess additional advantages, including the ability to cultivate in saltwater and more efficient solar energy conversion. The processes involved in hydrocarbon degradation are still, to some extent, unclear. Although microalgae adsorb pollutants, mounting evidence suggests that bacterial consortia supported by algal cultures may play a vital role in biodegradation. These bacteria, e.g., *Alcanivorax* and *Marinobacter* spp., gain advantage from photosynthesis by algae (oxygen and organic exudates), as they contribute to algal growth by solubilizing nutrients and producing phtohormones. Algae–bacteria synergistic systems, therefore, provide an environmentally friendly approach for hydrocarbon remediation. Nevertheless, limiting problems, such as poor light penetration in sediments and the need for optimized conditions, persist. Alternatives, such as mixotrophic microalgae, enzymatic extracts, or algae-derived biochar, are being researched, and recent findings have shown promising outcomes for ex situ sediment remediation (Dell' Anno et al., 2021).

12.2.2.2 Synthetic Dyes

Industrialization, particularly from the textile industry, has led to extensive dye pollution, resulting in the release of millions of liters of untreated effluent per day. Synthetic dyes, although economical, are stable pollutants that pose serious environmental and health hazards. Conventional methods for removing dyes are energy-intensive and can form toxic byproducts, making biological methods, such as phycoremediation, the preferred choice. Microalgae have demonstrated effective dye removal capabilities due to their functional groups (such as amino, carboxyl, hydroxyl, and phosphate) and biosorption ability. *Spirulina* and *Oscillatoria* species were found to efficiently biodegrade red and blue dyes by biosorption, enzymatic conversion (such as azoreductase activity), and metabolic assimilation into smaller molecules.

Phycoremediation offers the potential for low cost, high efficacy, and environmental safety, with applications in developing countries. Optimization, however, is essential to improve its scale-up potential and overcome limitations under different wastewater conditions (El-Sheekh et al., 2025). Microalgae, with their high surface area and functional groups, efficiently remove textile wastewater dyes by mechanisms such as biosorption, electrostatic attraction, complexation, and bioconversion. *Spirogyra*, *Caulerpa*, and *Chlorella vulgaris* have been reported to exhibit high dye removal efficiency, and *C. vulgaris* has been reported to remove up to 69% of monoazo dyes by bioconversion to aniline. Several microalgal species, including *N. elepsosporum* and *C. vulgaris*, demonstrated greater than 90% removal of red textile dyes, indicating their effectiveness even in the presence of complex wastewater matrices (Kundu et al., 2024).

12.2.2.3 Pharmaceuticals and Emerging Pollutants

Pharmaceutical drugs (PCs) such as antibiotics, analgesics, and antidepressants are increasingly found in aquatic ecosystems because of their widespread use and longevity. Traditional wastewater treatment plants are not efficient in eliminating these contaminants, which has stimulated interest in the utilization of environmentally friendly alternatives, such as microalgae-based removal. Microalgae present a viable solution due to their high growth rates, photosynthetic utilization of sunlight and CO_2, and potential for biomass valorization. They eliminate pharmaceutical drugs through bioadsorption, bioaccumulation, and biodegradation. Bioadsorption occurs through electrostatic attraction with negatively charged cell walls, while bioaccumulation enables the adsorption and sequestration of PCs into algal cells. Intracellular and extracellular biodegradation hydrolyze complex substances into simpler, less toxic substances using secreted enzymes and extracellular polymeric substances (EPS). Removal efficiencies have varied as a function of microalgal species, polarity of the compound interaction, and operating conditions in studies. *Chlorella vulgaris* and *C. saccharophila* demonstrated greater removal of 19 APIs over 12 days, removing up to 88% of lipophilic compounds. Hydrophilic compounds such as caffeine and carbamazepine were less resistant to degradation. Microalgal remediation is generally compound- and strain-specific, with potential for combined wastewater treatment and biomass-derived bioproduct production (Iakovidou et al., 2024).

12.2.2.4 Pesticide

Pesticides are widely used to enhance crop production by controlling pests and disease vectors; however, their stability and mobility pose significant environmental hazards. Although possessing desirable traits, such as target specificity and degradability, most pesticides pollute soil and water, impacting nontarget animals, including humans. Their lingering nature in soil can also destabilize microbial populations, decrease nitrogen fixation, and reduce soil fertility, thereby increasing fertilizer dependency. Systemic pesticides have the ability to contaminate pollen and nectar, harming pollinators such as bees, which play a vital role in the pollination of crops. The bioaccumulation of pesticide residues affects soil fauna, aquatic ecosystems, and food webs, posing risks to neurological diseases, developmental disorders, and carcinogenesis in humans. Microalgae eliminate pesticides by three primary modes of action: Biosorption, bioaccumulation, and biodegradation. Biosorption is a fast, passive process mediated by cell wall functional groups, including sulfated polysaccharides, amino, and carboxyl groups. Bioaccumulation is an energy-requiring process that entails the active uptake and internalization of contaminants.

Biodegradation is an enzyme-mediated process (e.g., oxygenase, esterase, and cytochrome P450) that degrades pesticides into less toxic, more soluble forms. Although these processes show great potential, further research is needed for a comprehensive understanding of microalgae-mediated remediation of various types of pesticides (Verasoundarapandian et al., 2022).

Microalgae-based remediation of pesticides can be achieved through open systems, such as high-rate algal ponds (HRAPs), or closed systems, like photobioreactors (PBRs). HRAPs facilitate co-cultivation with bacteria, enabling the simultaneous degradation of organic matter and the production of oxygen. PBRs offer greater control over environmental conditions, increased biomass productivity, and a lower risk of contamination, although they involve higher operating costs and energy input compared to open systems. However, PBRs are more efficient in terms of energy consumption compared to membrane bioreactors because microalgal photosynthesis does not require mechanical aeration. Integrated microalgae systems, such as immobilized microalgal–bacterial consortia and microalgal fuel cells, offer enhanced pesticide removal and wastewater treatment. Immobilization within matrices, such as polyurethane foam, enhances cell stability, symbiosis, and efficiency in pollutant degradation, while also facilitating ease of biomass recovery. Microalgal fuel cells with anaerobic and aerobic chambers allow for simultaneous pesticide biodegradation (e.g., imidacloprid and thiaclopprid) and bioelectricity production. Nevertheless, excessive pesticide levels can cause oxidative stress and inhibit the growth of microalgae, making concentration regulation paramount in such systems (Goh et al., 2023).

12.2.2.5 Heavy Metal Pollutant

Heavy metals with specific gravities greater than 5000 kg/m^3 are recalcitrant pollutants that can cause severe health and environmental problems, even at trace levels, due to their toxicity and nonbiodegradability. Typical sources are industrial effluent, agriculture, and natural processes, while traditional treatment options tend to be expensive and produce secondary waste. Microalgae offer an eco-friendly option through biosorption and bioaccumulation, achieving metal removal rates of up to 15 mg/g biomass. Organisms like *C. vulgaris*, *Scenedesmus*, and *Phormidium* are capable of efficiently removing metals like Hg^{2+}, Cd^{2+}, and Pb^{2+} through rapid surface adsorption and subsequent intracellular chelation. *Chlorella vulgaris* converts Cr(VI) to less toxic Cr(III), which is supported by functional groups ($-NH_2$, $-COOH$). *Spirulina platensis* removed 97% in minutes. Furthermore, *Ostreococcus tauri* transforms toxic inorganic arsenic to less toxic organic forms through biomethylation (Kundu et al., 2024).

Native microalgae possess inherent abilities for bioremediating heavy metals through biosorption and bioaccumulation. Nonetheless, metal sensitivity and low tolerance in high-growing strains have evoked interest in synthetic biology to improve these characteristics. Recent advances have enabled the genetic modification of microalgae to enhance biomass productivity, binding affinity, and metal tolerance. The design–build–test–learn (DBTL) platform accommodates synthetic biology applications. During the design process, tactics involve remodeling surface anionic moieties, augmenting extracellular polymeric substance (EPS) production for biofilm development, and adding high-affinity heavy metal transporters. Genetic tools are engineered against metal-binding peptide overexpression (phytochelatins and metallothioneins), transporters, and antioxidant enzymes (e.g., SOD and GPX) to enhance metal uptake and stress defense. During build, omics and NGS facilitate the discovery of new transporter and tolerance genes.

Gene circuits are maximized through promoter/terminator engineering and computational redesigns of proteins to maximize expression and metal binding. Through test-and-learn iterative engineering, system performance is tested, as evidenced by enhanced heavy metal accumulation through surface-anchored synthetic phytochelatins and the co-expression of transporters. Despite regulatory restrictions on GMOs and the limited use of algal genetic components, the continuous development of the field of omics, computational packages, and synthetic pathway design is favoring the increasing role of synthetic biology in scalable and specific microalgal-based bioremediation (Sattayawat et al., 2021). The overall pollutant degradation and the omics platforms utilized are summarized in Table 12.1. This table summarizes representative contaminants, the omics platforms applied, and the key findings derived from transcriptomic, proteomic, metabolomic, and metagenomic studies. These studies collectively demonstrate how multi-omics tools can elucidate the genes, enzymes, and metabolites involved in detoxification, metal resistance, and the breakdown of organic pollutants.

12.2.3 Mechanisms of Contaminant Removal

Chlamydomonas species exhibit excellent potential in bioremediation due to processes like biosorption, bioaccumulation, and biotransformation. This overall process in microalgae is shown in Fig. 12.1. Biosorption is a physical surface-binding process, whereas bioaccumulation is a metabolic activity-based uptake process. Biotransformation is the enzymatic conversion of pollutants, which in some cases produces more toxic intermediates. Several *Chlamydomonas* strains have been demonstrated to effectively remove nitrogen, phosphorus, COD, heavy metals (e.g., Cu, Pb, Cd, and U), and new pollutants such as drugs and microplastics in different types of wastewaters. Their xenobiotic metabolism is facilitated by enzymatic reactions (e.g., CYP450 oxidation and hydrolysis), excretion of laccases, and increased tolerance through genetic alterations. Technologically advanced systems, such as photobioreactors, biofilm reactors, and alginate encapsulation, have proven effective in improving pollutant removal. *C. reinhardtii*, for example, can be genetically engineered to produce plastic-degrading enzymes (such as PETase) and is efficient in CO_2 biofixation, sequestering 1.8 g of CO_2 per gram of biomass. Although promising in pilot-scale and lab experiments, large-scale implementations are restricted. Some of the major research gaps are real-world validation, long-term stability, multispecies interactions, toxicity of byproducts, and optimization of cultivation conditions. These, when addressed, will allow more scalable and

Table 12.1 Summary of omics-based insights into algal and microbial bioremediation of key pollutants

Pollutant type	Representative contaminants	Omics platform used	Key findings	References
Heavy metals	Cu^{2+}, Cd^{2+}, Pb^{2+}	Transcriptomics	Differential gene expression identified ABC transporters and ROS-related genes upregulated under Cu and Cd stress	Ferreira et al. (2023), Seo et al. (2023)
Polycyclic aromatic hydrocarbons (PAHs)	Phenanthrene and naphthalene	Metagenomics + proteomics	Metagenomics mining identified novel dioxygenases and peroxidases; proteomics confirmed enzyme activity in degradation	Nagy et al. (2024)
Pharmaceuticals (NSAIDs)	Diclofenac and ibuprofen	Metabolomics	Review highlights biodegradation pathways of diclofenac and ibuprofen via metabolic profiling and enzyme detection	Ferreira et al. (2023), Silva et al. (2019)
Dyes and pigments	Methylene blue and Congo red	Transcriptomics and proteomics	Differential expression of stress-related and degradative enzymes in dye-exposed organisms	Kumar et al. (2025), Padilla-Garfias et al. (2024)
Microplastics (nanoplastics)	Polystyrene nanoplastics (oral exposure in mice)	Transcriptomics, metabolomics	Disrupted lipid and amino acid metabolism; oxidative stress and immune perturbation	Shi et al. (2024)
Microplastics (reproductive toxicity)	Polystyrene nanoplastics (GC-2spd (ts) spermatocyte cell line)	Transcriptomics and metabolomics	Altered energy and amino acid metabolism; reproductive toxicity mechanisms identified	Han et al. (2024)
Pesticides (field mixture)	Imidacloprid, chlorpyrifos, and glyphosate (*Apis cerana* bees)	Transcriptomics and metabolomics	Combined pesticide exposure impairs flight ability, alters energy, and detox pathways	Ma et al. (2024)
Pesticides (glyphosate based herbicider)	Glyphosate (repeated exposure in mice)	Transcriptomics and metabolomics	Reproductive dysfunction linked to altered metabolic and gene expression pathways	Qi et al. (2023)
Endocrine disruptors (Bisphenol A)	Bisphenol A (BPA) exposure (multi-tissue analysis)	Transcriptomics	Tissue-specific immune pathway activation and T-cell differentiation changes	Park et al. (2024)

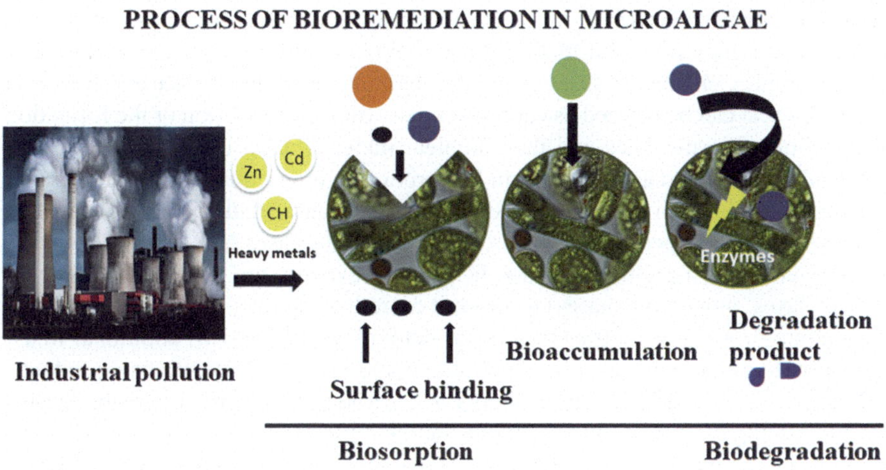

Fig. 12.1 Mechanistic representation of the bioremediation process in microalgae

sustainable applications of *Chlamydomonas* for environmental bioremediation (Bellido-Pedraza et al., 2024).

Conventional wastewater treatment (WWT) processes, such as primary and secondary treatment, are typically expensive, energy-intensive, and generate substantial amounts of sludge that require further treatment. Chemical precipitation with iron or aluminum salts likewise generates unnecessary waste. Microalgae-based bioremediation, on the other hand, presents a cost-efficient, environmentally friendly solution by integrating with existing WWT technologies to minimize waste and generate valuable biomass. Microalgae are fast-growing, can endure extreme wastewater conditions, and occupy a small amount of land. Their cultivation through autotrophic, heterotrophic, or mixotrophic growth enables effective uptake and conversion of CO_2, nitrogen, and phosphorus, as well as the synthesis of lipids, proteins, and other biomolecules. *Ankistrodesmus falcatus, for example, had more than 35% lipid content at moderate light, while Chlorella vulgaris* demonstrated improved lipid productivity using soil extract media. Microalgal integration thus not only enhances WWT efficiency but also facilitates bioresource recovery and minimizes carbon footprint (Abdelfattah et al., 2023).

Microalgae are very efficient at eliminating pesticides owing to their intense biosorption, bioaccumulation, and biodegradation properties. Cell wall carbohydrates in microalgae enhance passive pesticide adsorption, whereas bioaccumulation is primarily based on the lipid composition, which is a function of growth conditions. Research indicates that *Chlorella vulgaris* possesses the potential to intensively biosorb pesticides such as atrazine, carbofuran, and simazine quickly. The efficiency of removal is influenced by the pesticide's structure, the microalgal strain, and the particle size. Microalgae can also utilize contaminants as a source of carbon and nitrogen, making them suitable for treating organic pollutants (Verasoundarapandian et al., 2022).

12.2.3.1 Bioconversion

Bioconversion is a powerful method for removing contaminants from wastewater, where complex chemicals are biodegraded by enzymes into simpler and harmless molecules that can be utilized as carbon sources. Biotransformation or the formation of metabolic intermediates and the complete mineralization to CO_2 and H_2O are involved in biodegradation, but not in biosorption or bioaccumulation. Biodegradation by microalgae can occur either extracellularly or intracellularly, and is catalyzed by enzymes such as peroxidases, azoreductases, and laccases. The pathway consists of three phases: (i) preliminary modification by cytochrome P450 enzymes (e.g., hydroxylases, monooxygenases) to make it more hydrophilic; (ii) conjugation with glutathione or glucose by transferases for detoxification; and (iii) additional transformation by oxidoreductases and hydrolases into less toxic intermediate products. Pollutants serve as both electron donors and carbon sources in co-metabolic processes. Adding carbon sources from outside the cultures, such as glucose, has been found to increase degradation efficiency above 80% for tetracycline, sulfamethoxazole, and bisphenol A. However, excessive carbon can result in catabolite repression. Thus, optimum carbon addition is key to achieving maximal biodegradation efficiency of microalgae in wastewater treatment processes (Liberti et al., 2024).

12.2.3.2 Biosorption

Biosorption is a passive, metabolism-independent phenomenon by which microalgae adsorb contaminants onto their cell surfaces through processes such as ion exchange, surface complexation, and electrostatic attraction. Both live and dead biomass can act as biosorbents because they contain functional groups (such as carboxyl, hydroxyl, sulfate, phosphate, and amino) in their cell walls and extracellular polymeric substances (EPS) that can bind heavy metals. Cell surface characteristics, such as porosity, area, and charge, as well as environmental parameters like pH, temperature, and metal ion concentration, influence the efficiency of biosorption. Maximum biosorption occurs when functional groups coordinate with metals without proton competition (at low pH) or precipitation (at high pH). EPS is capable of facilitating heavy metal removal through complexation, while analytical instruments such as FTIR and NMR are utilized to identify the active binding groups responsible for this process (Abdelfattah et al., 2023).

12.2.3.3 Bioaccumulation and Bio-Uptake

Microalgae actively take up various inorganic and organic contaminants through energy-requiring metabolic processes, distinct from biosorption. While slower, the process supports the uptake of nutrients and contaminants, including heavy metals, nitrates, phosphates, and pharmaceuticals. Uptake of pollutants also becomes possible through passive diffusion following membrane depolarization. Microalgae in wastewater systems also provide carbon sequestration and nutrient removal, particularly when combined with bacterial systems. This synergy enhances the value of nitrogen and phosphorus removal, improves oxygenation through photosynthesis, and reduces the energy required for aeration in wastewater treatment systems. The performance of such processes depends on pH, light, redox potential, temperature, and concentration of the pollutant (Liberti et al., 2024).

12.2.3.4 Biodegradation

Microalgal biodegradation involves enzymatic degradation of contaminants into nontoxic substances such as sugars or CO_2. Some organisms, including *Nannochloropsis oculata*, *Chlorella vulgaris*, and *Phaeodactylum tricornutum*, show selective biodegradation of PAHs and pharmaceuticals with remarkable efficiency. Complex contaminants, however, hinder this process. Adaptive laboratory evolution (ALE) is a solution to this through increased capacity for degradation, evidenced by *Isochrysis galbana* mutants breaking down high levels of phenol. However, ALE strains require further testing for seawater tolerance and variable conditions (Diankristanti & Ng, 2024).

12.2.3.5 Photodegradation

Photodegradation, both direct and indirect, is a crucial abiotic process through which microalgae contribute to the removal of pharmaceutical and personal care contaminants from aquatic systems. Direct photolysis occurs when pollutants absorb a photon and undergo structural breakdown, particularly in chemicals containing aromatic rings, conjugated systems, and heteroatoms, such as fluoroquinolones (e.g., ciprofloxacin) and diclofenac. Hom-Diaz et al. (2022) illustrated that microalgae, including *Chlamydomonas reinhardtii*, *Chlorella sorokiniana*, *Dunaliella tertiolecta*, and *Pseudokirchneriella subcapitata*, removed more than 78% of fluoroquinolones largely through photodegradation, while macrolide antibiotics were removed mostly through a mix of sorption and biodegradation due to their poor photolytic susceptibility. A 2020–2021 systematic review emphasized that the photodegradation efficacy for compounds such as sulfamethazine can be improved by optimizing photoperiods, thereby augmenting removal by up to 28%. Recent experimental trials with *Nannochloropsis oculata* have indicated that approximately 60–100% of drugs, such as Diclofenac and carbamazepine, can be removed under treatment regimes that integrate algal activity and light exposure, during which photodegradation and biodegradation processes occur. Another controlled experiment with microalgal photobioreactors documented that direct photolysis was responsible for only 13–19% removal of priority emerging contaminants (such as caffeine and DEET) after 1–7 days, reaffirming that while photodegradation is important, the dominant removal mechanism is biodegradation facilitated by microalgae and frequently enhanced by bacterial consortia. Together, these results highlight the importance of photodegradation, particularly for light-sensitive drugs such as ciprofloxacin and diclofenac, within microalgal systems. Nonetheless, the efficacy is highly reliant on the structure of the compound, environmental conditions (e.g., pH, light intensity), and system design. Photodegradation, hence, operates in synergistic interaction with sorption and biodegradation to enable efficient contaminant removal within engineered algal treatment systems.

12.2.3.6 Hydrolysis

Depending on the pollutant structure, concentration, temperature, and pH, degradation occurs for some emerging pollutants, but most, particularly pharmaceuticals such as sulfonamides and fluoroquinolones, are resistant. It is more efficient for individual substances, such as β-lactam antibiotics. In algae systems, the rates of hydrolysis can be enhanced with increasing temperatures and fluctuations in pH, leading to daytime promotion of pollutant degradation and nighttime neutral pH degradation of other compounds (Kundu et al., 2024).

Current studies of antibiotic degradation in microalgal photobioreactors have evaluated abiotic degradation under dark-controlled conditions, separating the effects of hydrolysis from photolysis. One report indicated that, at a neutral pH (~7), hydrolysis alone contributed to more than 80% removal of ciprofloxacin (CIP) and ofloxacin (OFL) within 9 days in the dark. Conversely, at acidic pH, hydrolysis of CIP was zero, with photolysis playing a leading role instead. Erythromycin (ERY) and clarithromycin (CLA) showed more than 70% hydrolytic degradation under acidic conditions, but much lower activity in neutral conditions (34–49% based on pH). Although the direct incidence of hydrolysis within microalgal systems is less investigated than photodegradation or biodegradation, these results highlight its conditional function in the degradation of planktonic pollutants. Thus, hydrolysis must also be regarded as a secondary but at times considerable process, contingent upon compound chemistry, environmental pH, and thermal regimes in algal remediation systems. The schematic illustration in Fig. 12.1 shows the sequential steps through which microalgae mitigate industrial pollution. Emissions from industrial sources release heavy metals and organic pollutants such as Zn, Cd, and hydrocarbons (CH) into the environment. These contaminants are initially bound to the algal cell surface via biosorption, followed by intracellular uptake (bioaccumulation). Within the algal cells, enzymatic actions lead to the breakdown of pollutants into simpler, nontoxic degradation products (biodegradation). This integrated process highlights the potential of microalgae as a sustainable tool for eco-remediating contaminated water and air environments.

12.3 Omics Technologies: A Systems Biology Toolbox

12.3.1 Overview of Multi-Omics Platforms

Omics technologies, including metagenomics, transcriptomics, proteomics, and metabolomics, have revolutionized our understanding of the complexity of microbial communities and their role in wastewater bioremediation. The technologies provide in-depth information on the responses of microalgae and bacteria to environmental stressors, such as pollutants and nutrient loads, and facilitate the optimization of microalgae–bacteria consortia (MBC). Metagenomics provides comprehensive insights into microbial diversity and metabolic potential in contaminated environments by analyzing community-level DNA sequences. Transcriptomics complements this by elucidating the differential expression of genes in response to environmental stressors, revealing molecular pathways underlying adaptation and toxicity responses. Together, these omics approaches contribute to understanding the structural and functional dynamics of organisms under exposure to pollutants. Proteomics further expands this understanding by profiling protein expression and post-translational modifications, thereby linking gene expression to actual functional responses. Each omics platform requires specific sample preparation and analytical considerations, and when integrated, they provide a holistic understanding of the structural and functional dynamics of organisms under pollutant exposure. Collectively, these omics strategies provide a system-level understanding of wastewater microbial ecology and are central to the formation of sustainable, high-performance bioremediation strategies (Vo et al., 2024). Omics technologies (genomics, transcriptomics, proteomics, and metabolomics) enable essential information regarding microbial interactions, nutrient uptake, and stress–responses in microalgae consortia. Omics technologies enable the optimization of key parameters, such as carbon-to-nitrogen ratio, light, pH, and temperature, to enhance biomass yield, lipid storage, and pollutant degradation. Co-culture with bacteria, fungi, or yeast increases nutrient recycling and harvesting efficiency. Despite their high complexity and cost, omics-guided systems facilitate precision cultivation, making them valuable tools for developing sustainable bioprocesses (Rasheed et al., 2023).

12.3.2 Integration of Omics with Bioremediation Research

Advancements in omics technologies, including metagenomics, transcriptomics, proteomics, and metabolomics, have significantly enhanced our understanding of environmental microbial communities in contaminated ecosystems. A schematic representation of this process flow is shown in Fig. 12.2. These approaches overcome the limitations of conventional culture-dependent techniques by enabling the direct exploration of genetic diversity, functional genes, and pathways for pollutant degradation. Integration of multi-omics platforms is essential, as no single technology can fully capture the complexity and functional potential of environmental microbiomes (Chandran et al., 2020). Progress in systems biology and computing methods has transformed microbiologists' understanding of the interactions between microorganisms and pollutants, facilitating effective strategies for bioremediation. In silico strategies, including flux balance analysis (FBA), metabolic flux analysis (MFA), and metabolic pathway analysis (MPA), facilitate the modeling and optimization of microbial metabolic networks for pollutant degradation. QSAR and 3D-QSAR tools are utilized to predict microbial–pesticide interactions at the molecular level, including toxicity in diverse ecosystems. Gene-level utilities, such as OptKnock and OptStrain, assist in genome-scale modeling and the incorporation of new biodegradation pathways, while OptReg aids in pathway regulation for optimized bioremediation. These computational frameworks facilitate the design and manipulation of microbial strains, enabling customization for efficient and targeted degradation of environmental contaminants (Jaiswal et al., 2019). A

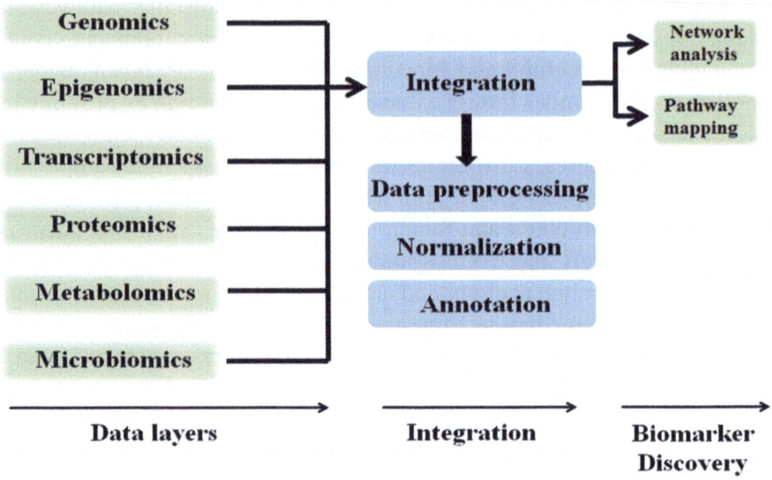

Fig. 12.2 Workflow for multi-omics integration toward biomarker discovery

representation of the overall omics technologies, including their analytical tools and key insights, is provided in Table 12.2. Figure 12.2 illustrates the layered structure and processing steps involved in integrating multi-omics data—namely, genomics, epigenomics, transcriptomics, proteomics, metabolomics, and microbiomics. After collecting omics data across these domains (data layers), integration is carried out using preprocessing steps, including normalization and annotation. The integrated dataset can then be analyzed through network analysis and pathway mapping to identify potential biomarkers, advancing systems biology and personalized medicine applications.

12.4 Genomics: Decoding the Bioremediation Blueprint

Metagenomic tools have been widely applied to identify functional genes responsible for degrading organic pollutants (OPs) and conferring antibiotic resistance in wastewater treatment systems. Functional metagenomics enables the detection of antibiotic resistance genes and degradation pathways, offering strategies to monitor and mitigate the spread of resistance genes. For instance, Wang et al. (2021) identify key microbial families such as Rhizobiaceae, Rhodocyclaceae, and Phycisphaeraceae, which are involved in ciprofloxacin degradation via oxidation reactions, including hydroxylation, defluorination, and dealkylation. Another author described that the biodegradation of sulfamethoxazole by microalgal–bacteria consortia (MBc), wherein the drug was degraded into metabolites such as 4-aminobenzene sulfonic acid and further metabolized to pyruvate. Microbial community composition was altered by stress induced by exposure to sulfamethoxazole, resulting in a decrease in proteobacteria and an increase in Scenedesmaceae, which

Table 12.2 Comparative summary of omics platforms used in algal and microbial bioremediation applications

Omics platform	Key insight provided	Analytical tools	Limitation	Typical application in bioremediation	References
Genomics/ metagenomics	Genome-resolved metagenomic approaches have enabled linking powerful functional predictions to specific taxonomic groups	Shotgun sequencing, metagenome assembly, and BLAST	Gene presence but not expression of enzymatic activity	Discovering pollutant-degrading genes and metabolic pathways	McDaniel et al. (2021)
Transcriptomics	Whole community gene expression surveys permitted direct surveys of community-scale function	RNA-Seq and differential expression profiling (e.g., DESeq2)	mRNA levels may not reflect protein abundance or activity	Identifying stress–response and detoxification gene networks	McDaniel et al. (2021)
Proteomics	Proteomics offers precise functional insights into static and dynamic physiological contexts	LC–MS/MS, Mascot, MaxQuant, and 2-D electrophoresis	Complex sample prep; low-abundance protein hard to detect	Pinpointing active biodegradation enzymes and pathways	Kumar et al. (2025), Ayilara and Babalola (2023)
Metabolomics	Profiling large-scale metabolite changes using GC–MS, LC–MS, NMR workflows	GC–MS, LC–MS, NMR via workflow4metabolomics pipeline	May miss transient or low-abundance compounds; incomplete annotation libraries	Mapping metabolic flux and biodegradation intermediates	Kumar et al. (2025), Gunjal et al. (2023)
Multi-omics	Integrating across DNA, RNA, protein, and metabolite data reveals regulatory networks and genotype-phenotype links	MixOmics, Cytoscape, PaintOmics integration tools	Integration complexity; annotation discrepancies across layers	Systems-level modeling, biomarker discovery, and strain improvement	Kumar et al. (2025), McDaniel et al. (2021)

(continued)

Table 12.2 (continued)

Omics platform	Key insight provided	Analytical tools	Limitation	Typical application in bioremediation	References
Epigenomics	Stress can induce changes in gene expression through hypo- or hyper-methylation of DNA at specific loci adaptive significance	Bisulfite sequencing (WGBS), ChIP-Seq, and MeDIP-seq	Few algal methylome studies; requires high quality genome assemblies	Understanding the regulation of stress defense and adaptive memory	Ferrari et al. (2023), Bacova et al. (2020)
Microbiomics	Microbiome analysis characterizes taxonomic composition and functional potential of microbial consortia in contaminated environments	16S rRNA amplicon sequencing, shotgun metagenomics, and QIIME2	Taxonomy-only resolution missing functional-level insight without complementing other omics	Linking microbial shifts to degradation efficiency in consortia	Gunjal et al. (2023), Dell' Anno et al. (2021)

suggests an upregulation of antioxidant genes such as catalase and superoxide dismutase. Metagenomic sequencing also enables the analysis of shifts in microbial communities. Another author identified dominant phyla in MBCs and purple photosynthetic bacteria from piggery wastewater, primarily cyanobacteria, proteobacteria, and synergistetes. Similarly, another author detected key bacterial taxa such as *E. coli*, *Klebsiella*, and *Pseudomonas*, alongside algal species like *Chlorella*, *Thalassiosira*, and *Synechocystis*, highlighting the diverse microbial ecosystem in wastewater treatment consortia (Vo et al., 2024).

A study conducted with Genome mining of hydrocarbonoclastic bacteria has also revealed a core group of genes (e.g., alkane hydroxylase, cyclohexanol dehydrogenase, ferredoxin reductase) regularly implicated in the degradation of hydrocarbons. Gene presence is not, however, proof of activity; hence, metatranscriptomics and metaproteomics are employed to assess gene expression and protein activity under stress caused by pollutants. These technologies, combined with metagenomics and fluxomics, facilitate a deeper understanding of microbial adaptation responses and interactions in consortia, thereby supporting the optimization of bioremediation techniques. Culture-dependent methods shall. Therefore, remains crucial for successful large-scale bioremediation through isolation of effective strains. Integration with laboratory validation will be crucial in designing efficient, scalable, and eco-friendly remediation strategies for petroleum-contaminated marine sediments. Further efforts should thus focus on microbial interactions, pathways for degradation, and in situ performance to make sustainable interventions for bioremediation feasible (Dell' Anno et al., 2021).

Another research explores the current advances in marine microalgae research, including genetic engineering for augmenting pollutant degradation and valorization. For instance, *Phaeodactylum tricornutum* was modified to produce PHB and degrade PET by expressing bacterial genes. Omics research identified new targets, such as ferroptosis-associated detoxification and genes such as SULTR2, for heavy metal sequestration. CRISPR technologies in marine microalgae, such as Nannochloropsis and Chaetoceros, are being refined through the design of sgRNA and the use of anti-CRISPR tools. To address challenging pollutant situations, microalgal consortia, such as those comprising *Tetraselmis* and *Pelagibacter*, perform better than axenic cultures in terms of biomass and nutrient uptake. Metagenomics can facilitate optimization of such synergistic systems. The incorporation of microalgae into conventional treatment systems like wetlands, membrane systems, or new trends like biohybrid micro/nano-robots and biophotovoltaics provides promising avenues for energy-efficient and multifunctional wastewater treatment. These technologies enable sustainable waste-to-resource strategies and contribute to carbon sequestration (Diankristanti & Ng, 2024).

12.5 Transcriptomics: Exploring Gene Expression Landscapes

Transcriptome analysis provides a comprehensive view of microalgal gene expression patterns, offering insights into stress adaptation, resistance, and metabolite production. Hundreds of annotated transcriptomes from various species are hosted by public databases such as MMETSP and Alganaut. RNA-seq analysis, e.g., in *Chlamydomonas moewusii*, has identified principal anaerobic metabolic pathways that have contributed to biofuel research. Transcriptomic data have also supported genetic engineering activities, e.g., transcriptional overexpression of bZIP TFs in *Nannochloropsis* increases lipid yield. In contrast, novel methylomic studies reveal low but functionally significant levels of DNA methylation in microalgae such as *C. reinhardtii* and *Chlorella* spp. With 6 mA modifications enriched at transcriptional start sites. These epigenetic markers are now more commonly understood to be regulators of gene expression and targets for metabolic increase strategies (Stavridou et al., 2024). Transcriptomics shows how microalgae–bacteria consortia (MBC) adapt to internal (developmental processes and epigenetics) and external (toxins and nutrients) stimuli by modifying gene expression. Research indicates that exposure to sulfamethoxazole and phenol induces genes involved in photosynthesis (Psb, Psa, and Lhca/b), ATP synthesis, and carbon fixation, thereby increasing oxygen release and facilitating pollutant breakdown. In *Desmodesmus* and *Chlorella*, transcriptome changes also impact protein biosynthesis, oxidative phosphorylation, and ribosomal function, thereby favoring growth and metabolic adaptation. In general, transcriptomic tools provide critical information on stress tolerance and pollutant degradation to help optimize algal-based wastewater treatment plants (Vo et al., 2024).

Another study conducted by scientists has investigated the effectiveness of different microalgal strains in removing perfluorooctanoic acid from polluted water, with a thorough examination of the molecular mechanisms underlying the process. The potential of four different microalgal strains in removing perfluorooctanoic acid was screened, and the most effective strains were selected for further investigation. To understand the underlying biological mechanisms that enable perfluorooctanoic acid degradation, a transcriptomic analysis was performed to identify the key functional genes that were upregulated upon exposure to perfluorooctanoic acid. After achieving the removal of perfluorooctanoic acid, the microalgae were harvested and used for transesterification to yield biodiesel, and the quality was assessed. This study not only fills the gap in the requirement for efficient and sustainable technologies for the remediation of perfluorooctanoic acid but also investigates the possible dual advantage of microalgae in both contaminant removal and biofuel generation. Transcriptomic profiling of 5 ppm perfluorooctanoic acid-exposed *S. quadricauda* was performed with Illumina Novaseq™ 6000. Following the extraction of RNA, quality evaluation, and cDNA library construction, sequencing data were de novo assembled using Trinity and clustered into unigenes with CD-HIT-EST. Functional annotation was done against several databases (NCBI, Pfam, GO, UniProt, and EggNOG). And gene expression levels were calculated using RSEM. Differentially expressed genes (DEGs) were detected based on fold-change >1.5 and adjusted *p*-value <0.05 (Ha et al., 2025).

A study examining the transcriptome profiling of *Desmodesmus* sp. under sewage exposure revealed significant changes in gene expression, with 18,872 genes upregulated and 35,871 downregulated. GO and KEGG analyses showed that DEGs were mainly related to oxidative phosphorylation, ribosome biogenesis, ubiquitin-mediated proteolysis, and photosynthesis. These processes are significant for energy metabolism in cells and stress–response, indicating their pivotal role in the adaptation of microalgal cells to sewage environments. Interestingly, ATP biosynthesis genes responsible for oxidative phosphorylation and photosynthesis were upregulated, serving the energy requirements for active transport, biosynthesis, and cellular growth during sewage treatment (Wang et al., 2022).

A study conducted by Ranjbar and Malcata (2022) stated that the phytohormones are also key factors in promoting heavy metal tolerance in microalgae by governing antioxidant mechanisms, metal transport, and stress–responsive pathways. Cytokinin biosynthesis and degradation have been genetically manipulated with enhanced metal tolerance in plants, suggesting potential avenues for microalgae. Gibberellins (GA), abscisic acid (ABA), auxins, and brassinosteroids (BRs) have also been correlated with improved heavy metal biosorption, growth, and alleviation of oxidative stress in various algal species. Yet, microalgae phytochrome biosynthesis genes are relatively uncharacterized and require additional omics studies. Concurrently, microRNAs (miRNAs) are the principal post-transcriptional modulators of heavy metal stress through the regulation of transcriptional factors, metal transport, detoxification mechanisms, and phytohormone signaling. Some metal-responsive miRNAs (e.g., miR395, miR398, and miR319) have been reported in plants, but few studies have been conducted in microalgae. Developing evidence suggests that a sophisticated interplay exists between hormones and miRNAs in modulating heavy metal stress–responses, and further studies should investigate the miRNA networks in microalgae in greater depth (Ranjbar & Malcata, 2022).

12.6 Proteomics: Linking Gene Expression to Function

Proteomics enables the revelation of protein-level alterations in algal–bacterial systems. A study conducted by Shen et al. demonstrated that photosynthetic bacteria regulated microalgal carbon metabolism by modulating protein expression, decreasing RuBisCo levels, and Calvin cycle activity. Another study conducted by Gao et al. found that bicarbonate supplementation enhanced the expression of important calvin cycle and photosystem proteins, as well as magnesium chelatase, thus promoting chlorophyll biosynthesis, biomass yields, and photosynthetic performance (Vo et al., 2024). An author reported on the latest developments in the genetic engineering of microalgae, with a view to enhancing their potential for removing heavy metals and improving selectivity. In addition, candidate genes and possible pathways amenable to manipulate are presented, in efforts toward developing hardy microalgae strains that can transfer sustainable heavy metal removal from wastewater. The proteomic investigation in *Euglena gracilis* under heavy metal stress demonstrated strong upregulation of metal-binding proteins and metal transporters. Of particular note were increases of 5.5-fold in MFs transporters in heavy metal compartmentalization and ~3.6-fold upregulation in P1B-ATPases (HMA2 and HMA3) essential for metal homeostasis. A TrkA transmembrane transporter responsible for potassium and sodium/sulfate transport was upregulated 6.5-fold (Ranjbar & Malcata, 2022). A study conducted by Andrade et al. (2022) investigated the proteomics of *Chlorella protothecoides* under copper stress, identifying major responses related to photosynthesis, protein biosynthesis, and oxidative stress management. Ten most expressed proteins were mainly related to the light-harvesting comples (LHC) and ATP production, which suggests intact photosynthetic activity. Although there was no marked variation in growth rate, copper exposure (0.3–0.9 mg/L) suppressed protein biosynthesis by as much as 16.3%, affecting major enzymes such as dihydroxy-acid dehydratase. The antioxidant enzymes, cytochrome *c* peroxidase and superoxide dismutase (SOD), were induced, indicating the activation of ROS detoxification pathways. Stress proteins Ycf3-interacting isoform X1, RNA polymerase III subunit RPC5, and pre-mRNA-processing factor 19 were found specifically under copper treatment, which indicates their usage as likely biomarkers for copper pollution in microalgal systems (Andrade et al., 2022).

Proteomics gives significant information on microbial processes in bioremediation by examining protein expression, stability, and post-translational modification, which better represent the true physiological condition of cells than transcriptomics. Metaproteomics extends this approach to complex environments, allowing for the identification of proteins involved in contaminant degradation within microbial consortia. Mass spectrometry has been applied in studies to detect hydrocarbon- and xenobiotic-degradation enzymes like dioxygenases, GSTs, catalase–peroxidase, and cytochrome P450s in bacteria and fungi. For example, *Mycobacterium vanbaalenii*, *Sphingobium chungbukense*, and *Achromobacter xylosoxidans* induced dioxygenases following exposure to PAHs. Likewise, fungi such as *Phanerochaete chrysosporium* and *Metarhizium robertsii* exhibited induction of oxidative enzymes in brominated flame-retardant degradation. In all, proteomics unmasks central catabolic routes, stress–response regimes, and metabolic adjustments crucial for microbial detoxification processes (Mishra et al., 2021).

12.7 Metabolomics: Mapping the Chemical Fingerprint

Metabolomics provides insights into metabolic transitions in algal–bacterial consortia during wastewater treatment. A study established that co-cultivation of *Prototheca zopfii* with *P. aeruginosa* and *B. subtilis* transformed carbohydrate and amino acid metabolism to increase tolerance to amoxicillin through enhanced production of glucose-6-phosphate, trehalose, and poly-γ-glutamate. Likewise, another study identified 114 significant metabolite transitions in consortia where bacterial presence increased protein and fatty acid synthesis but repressed phosphate uptake through decreased expression of transporter proteins (Vo et al., 2024). A study conducted by Wang et al. metabolomics analysis revealed more than 500 significantly changed metabolites following sewage treatment. The metabolic pathways for amino acids, fatty acids, and nucleotide metabolism were enriched, including those for alanine, aspartate, glutamate, riboflavin, and arachidonic acid metabolism. The combined analysis of transcriptomic and metabolomics data emphasized the induction of oxidative phosphorylation, photosynthesis, and propanoate metabolism. Notably, the downregulation of toxic intermediates, 2-oxobutanoate and succinate, indicates a metabolic shift favoring improved microalgal resilience and detoxification efficiency. Such metabolic adjustments facilitate the capture of nutrients and energy production, thereby enhancing sewage treatment performance under stress conditions (Wang et al., 2022). A study revealed that the metabolomics profiling of *Chlorella pyrenoidosa* under 100 mg/L phenol and 4-fluorophenol exposure revealed upregulation of important photosynthetic pigments (e.g., chlorophyll a and porphobilinogen) and glycerophospholipids (e.g., phosphatidylcholine, phosphatidylethanolamine, and lysophosphatidylcholine). These shifts in metabolism enhanced photosynthesis, antioxidant activity, and membrane integrity, thereby supporting algal growth under contaminant stress. Similarity in the responses of metabolites to both phenol and 4-fluorophenol suggests a common adaptive mechanism, and this points to *C. pyrenoidosa* as a resilient and efficient microalgal system for the remediation of phenolic pollutants (Li et al., 2023). A study conducted by Salem et al. in the year 2021 studied the metabolomics profiling using 1D and 2D NMR analysis, showing that treatment with azo dyes—malachite green (MG) and crystal violet (CV) has caused changes in the intracellular metabolites of *Chlorella vulgaris* and *Neochloris paludosum* without the appearance of any new compound, indicating that the dye treatment caused quantitative changes in the metabolic pathways but not qualitative changes. The lack of dye accumulation within algal cells, as verified by NMR spectra, also provided evidence that decolorization was not caused by biosorption or bioaccumulation, but rather by enzymatic degradation processes. The results align with previous findings attributing the removal of dye in microalgae to extracellular or cell-surface-bound enzymatic activity and thereby providing evidence for the potential of *C. vulgaris* and *N. paludosum* in metabolomics-facilitated bioremediation of poisonous dyes (Salem et al., 2021).

Sequence-based metagenomics, frequently conducted on platforms such as SOLiD and 454 Roche, circumvents conventional cloning, while function-based metagenomics enables the identification of enzymes like esterases and glycoside hydrolases. Interestingly, devices such as the META thin-layer chromatography system have facilitated the identification of functional enzymes, including glycosyltransferases. Function-driven screens also identified genes for toluene degradation. Notwithstanding its expense and sophistication, metagenomics provides previously unrivaled resolution for taxonomic and functional profiling. For instance, PICRUSt-supported KEGG analysis and 16S rRNA sequencing identified hydrocarbon-degrading gene families in petroleum-contaminated soil, including alkane monooxygenases and dehydrogenases. Third-generation sequencers such as PacBio and Oxford Nanopore enhance metagenomic accuracy through full-length, real-time DNA sequencing. Some research used functional metagenomics to define microbial consortia in contaminated environments. Unveiled unique taxonomic and enzymatic signatures in soil of varying pesticide degradation abilities and isolated microbes like *Burkholderia*, *Bradyrhizobium*, and enzymes like phosphodiesterases. Likewise, authors identified various aromatic-hydrocarbon-degrading genera (e.g., Cellulomonas, Streptomyces, and Kribbella) and genes, such as linA and linB, in indane-contaminated sediments. Studies have reported lower microbial diversity in e-waste-contaminated areas, and aerobic and anaerobic phthalate degraders such as *Rhodococcus*, *Burkholderia*, and *Geobacteracea* with great metabolic potential for toluene and benzene bioremediation (Mishra et al., 2021). Table 12.2 provides a comparative overview of commonly used omics platforms, including genomics, transcriptomics, proteomics, metabolomics, epigenomics, metagenomics, and microbiomics, highlighting the key insights they provide, the tools employed, known limitations, and their relevance in environmental bioremediation workflows. The content was compiled from multiple open-access research and review studies to ensure comprehensive and reliable coverage.

12.8 Integrative Omics: Toward a Holistic Remediation Strategy

Exposome research faces significant challenges, including evaluating multiple life stages, performing repeated measurements of biomarkers, and analyzing intricate biological data using sophisticated statistical and bioinformatics resources. With the imperative to develop mitigation plans for countering climate change and its effects on the environment, the incorporation of omics technologies, such as genomics, metabolomics, transcriptomics, and multi-omics, has become a must. The technologies provide profound knowledge of intricate biological systems, but only with interdisciplinary synergy, especially in the field of bioinformatics, can they harness and decipher large-scale, high-throughput data (Gruszecka-Kosowska et al., 2022).

12.8.1 Systems Biology Approaches to Algal Engineering

The emerging trends in system biology and omics sciences have tremendously helped improve microalgal strains. Genomic resources have enabled the discovery of gene clusters associated with the biosynthesis of high-value metabolites, thanks to massive sequencing initiatives such as ALG-ALL-CODE and 10KP, which have opened access to the genomes of microalgae. Public databases such as JGI PhycoCosm, MCBI Genome, and Ensembl Protists now contains more than 190 algal genomes, facilitating comparative genomics and bioprospecting in industrially important species such as *Chlamydomonas reinhardtii*, *Nannochloropsis* spp., and *Phaeodactylum tricornutum*. Transcriptomics, and most notably RNA-seq, reveals gene expression under various stress conditions, including salinity, nutrient limitation, heavy metal exposure, CO_2, and light fluctuations. Datasets such as

MMETSP and Alganaut provide large transcriptome resources. Epigenomic regulation has also been explored in recent research, with the identification of DNA methylation (e.g., 6 mA and 5 mC) patterns that impact gene expression and stress adaptation. Combining multi-omics data using systems biology enables the reconstruction of metabolic pathways and regulatory networks.

Bioinformatics tools such as COBRApy, OptFlux, Cytoscape, and KEGG Mapper enable the modeling and flux analysis necessary to optimize the production of metabolites and enhance stress tolerance. Genetic engineering strategies, such as CRISPR/Cas9, TALEN, ZFN and RNAi, are now used extensively to improve lipid accumulation, pigment production, and environmental stress tolerance. Software such as CHLAMYLibrary, CRISPOR, and Benchling facilitate the design and verification of experiments, whereas reporter genes (e.g., GFP, luciferase) facilitate the monitoring of transformation. Such approaches have been applied to various microalgae, resulting in enhanced productivity and improvements in specific traits. In total, the integration of omics technologies, systems biology, and precision genome editing is opening up opportunities for stable microalgal strains with specific applications in biofuels, pharmaceuticals, nutraceuticals, cosmetics, and bioremediation (Stavridou et al., 2024).

Additionally, transcriptome-wide association studies (TWAS) and comparative genomics workflows, combined with machine learning, are emerging tools for predicting gene function and prioritizing engineering targets. For instance, transcriptomic studies under stressful conditions (e.g., nitrogen starvation and light stress) in *Phaeodactylum tricornutum* identified regulatory genes for lipid accumulation, which were further confirmed through CRISPR-mediated knockouts (Yang et al., 2022). Together, these computational methods provide a platform to bridge the gap from descriptive omics to predictive design, enabling precision metabolic engineering of microalgae for industrial production.

12.8.2 Bioinformatics and Data Integration Platforms

The current bibliometric evidence (1981–2018) indicates an increasing focus on microalgae bioremediation, driven by environmental issues such as water pollution, resource scarcity, and the need for sustainable wastewater treatment. The research has moved from nutrient removal and bioreactor development to areas such as pharmaceutical degradation, high-rate algal ponds, and biofilm-based cultures. Microalgae exhibit potential in removing nutrients, metals, and emerging pollutants while facilitating the valorization of biomass into high-value bio-products. Despite progress, challenges remain in maximizing cultivation, selecting suitable species, and scaling up technologies. Future research aims to integrate bioremediation with bioeconomy objectives, aligning with global sustainability and circular economy initiatives (Pacheco et al., 2020). The technological advances in bioinformatics and next-generation sequencing (NGS) have revolutionized the field of bioremediation research, enabling researchers to investigate intricate microbial communities and pollutant degradation pathways.

High-throughput sequencing approaches, such as amplicon sequencing, metagenomics, metatranscriptomics, and metaproteomics, have enabled researchers to detect unculturable microorganisms and their functional contributions to the degradation of environmental pollutants. Major tools such as MEGAN, MG-RAST, QIIME2, Metavelvet, and Metacyc facilitate taxonomic classification, functional annotation, and inference of metabolic pathways. Sequencing platforms (e.g., Illumina, Ion Torrent, and Nanopore) combined with robust pipelines facilitate microbial gene expression analysis (e.g., 16S/18S rRNA, and ITS) and evaluation of microbial adaptation under environmental stress. Binning approaches (taxonomy-dependent/independent) and functional profiling based on KEGG, Pfam, and egg-NOG databases provide insights into metabolic capabilities. Metatranscriptomics reveals in situ functional genes and regulatory mechanisms, while metaproteomics facilitates an understanding of microbial function through protein expression. Metabolomics and Metabonomics measure small molecules and metabolic reactions to environmental stresses. Together, multi-omics integration enables a systems-level understanding of the microbial consortia responsible for xenobiotic degradation, allowing for goal-oriented and effective bioremediation strategies (Michealsamy et al., 2021).

The combination of multi-omics data poses substantial computational challenges because of high dimensionality, nonlinear interactions, and heterogeneity across datasets originating from different biological layers and analytical platforms. Successful integration starts with data normalization to achieve comparability, followed by methods like PCA, CCA, Sparse CCA, MFA, and PLSR for dimensionality reduction and correlation analysis. More sophisticated strategies, such as weighted gene co-expression network analysis (WGCNA), fuzzy logic modeling, and regulatory integrative clustering, have been employed in complex datasets, including cancer omics. Common software tools for integrating multi-omics data include both programming-based platforms, such as R (with packages Mixomics, iClusterplus, WGCNA, and MOFA), Python, and Bioconductor, as well as web-based, user-friendly tools like Paintomics, 3Omics, and Galaxy. Tools like Cytoscape and its plugins (e.g., ClueGO and stringAPP) are regularly applied for biological network visualization. Pathway tools, MetaboAnalyst, and ingenuity pathway analysis (IPA) facilitate functional and pathway-based integration. While user-friendly tools reduce technical entry barriers, an effective application requires a basic understanding of underlying statistical models and assumptions to avoid misinterpretation. With the increasing use of multi-omics methods in systems biology and environmental science, developing and applying integrative pipelines that involve AI, machine learning, and domain knowledge is necessary to derive meaningful biological insights from complex datasets (Misra et al., 2019).

12.9 Applications and Case Studies

Despite the large number of compounds reported from marine organisms, drug discovery programs explicitly aimed at marine microalgae have been scarce in the EU's FP7 and Horizon 2020 (H2020) programs. These programs primarily funded the development of sampling cultivation and omics technologies (genomics, transcriptomics, proteomics, and metabolomics) to drive the discovery of bioactive compounds. Some of the key FP7 projects include BAMMBO, GIAVAP, Pharmasea, and SUNBIOPATH, while for H2020, notable projects are EMBRIC, Nomorfilm, and TriforC. Of these, GIAVAP (*Parietochloris incise* and *Haemotococcus pluvialis*) and PharmaSea utilized-omics. PharmaSea documented anti-inflammatory, anticancer, and anti-biofilm activities in a range of diatom species (*Cylindrotheca closterium*, *Odontella mobiliensis*, *Pseudo-nitzschia*, *Pseudodelicatissima*, *Skeletonema marinoi*, *Leptocylindrus aporus*, *L. danicus*), with current research into characterizing the metabolites responsible by transcriptomic analysis. EMBRIC aims to enhance innovation by connecting marine biotechnology stakeholders and advancing metabolic engineering in species such as *Ostreococcus tauri* and *diatoms*. Similarly, GIAVAP provided information on the engineering of carotenoid and PUFA pathways in genetically modified microalgae. The EMBRC infrastructure (European Marine Biological Resource Center) and its consortium ASSEMBLE plus facilitate access to marine biodiversity, omics platforms, and collaborative research opportunities in 16 countries. To address the increasing bioinformatics challenges associated with marine data, ELIXIR unites European bioinformatics infrastructures, providing databases, tools, training, and cloud facilities for marine biotechnology research (Lauritano et al., 2019).

Analogously, in *Phaeodactylum tricornutum*, genome-scale CRISPR-Cas9 editing, guided by transcriptomic and proteomic information, enabled the knockout of carbon flux diversion genes, thereby rerouting metabolism toward improved lipid production, with potential applications in large-scale biofuel production (Yang et al., 2022). Additionally, in the treatment of wastewater, *Chlorella vulgaris* and *Scenedesmus obliquus* strains were optimized by proteomic and transcriptomic knowledge to withstand heavy metals and nutrient-rich effluents. These omics-guided strains were implemented in industrial effluent treatment plants, demonstrating efficient nutrient elimination and biomass valorization for use as feed and fertilizer (Rawat et al., 2011). Wang et al. (2022) demonstrated that exposure to blue light and salicylic acid (SA) triggered intense metabolic reactions, resulting in more than 13,000 differentially expressed genes (DEGs) and several hundred differentially expressed proteins (DEPs) related to carotenoid biosynthesis, fatty acid metabolism, and antioxidant defense. The outcome supports the use of omics-guided stress induction for maximizing Astaxanthin yield for commercial application. In a more recent work, Bian et al. (2023) constructed a high-quality chromosome-level genome of *H. pluvialis* that uncovered six expanded copies of the β-carotene ketolase (bkt) gene. This expansion, validated by transcriptomic profiling under stress, further highlights the genomic potential for large-scale astaxanthin accumulation and provides a basis for metabolic engineering approaches.

Other omics-based case studies have focused on stress modulation for enhanced metabolite productivity. He et al. (2018) conducted transcriptome analysis of *H. pluvialis* under high light with supplemented acetate and Fe^{2+}, and demonstrated that acetate significantly upregulated carotenoid and fatty acid synthesis-related genes. This combined stress strategy is increasingly being investigated in large-scale cultivation platforms to enhance both lipid and pigment productivities. These multi-omics strategies, encompassing genomics, transcriptomics, and proteomics, provide robust blueprints for enhancing production efficiency in photobioreactor and raceway-based systems. These practical applications illustrate how omics data not only discover key biosynthetic genes but also guide cultivation conditions and metabolic interventions. Such data-guided strain optimization has sealed the gap between lab-scale work and industrial-scale production, enabling applications in the nutraceutical sector and paving the way for further research in algal biotechnology.

12.10 Future Directions and Emerging Trends

The incorporation of multi-omics platforms into algal bioremediation studies has significantly enhanced our understanding of the intricate cellular processes involved in pollutant breakdown. Some critical areas need particular emphasis to fully exploit the opportunities of omics-informed environmental remediation. There is an urgent need for the creation of species-specific multi-omics reference databases, particularly for non-model algal strains with bioremediation value, as this will enhance the accuracy of annotation and facilitate more robust comparative analysis. Moreover, the integration of temporal and spatial factors in omics studies will give a better understanding of the dynamic and context-dependent nature of mechanisms involved in pollutant responses. Algal–microbiome interactions are also a promising area, in which metagenomic and microbiomics research can lay bare cooperative detoxification mechanisms and adaptive resilience measures at the community level. Epigenomic processes, such as stress-induced DNA methylation and histone modification, are also relatively underexplored, with the potential to uncover heritable adaptations that may be harnessed for strain improvement. In addition, the convergence of artificial intelligence and machine learning solutions will be necessary to handle and interpret sophisticated, multilayered omics data, facilitating the prediction of pollutant responses and the detection of new biomarkers. Lastly, to unlock laboratory discoveries for real-world applications, field-scale validation of omics-based knowledge under a range of environmental conditions and types of pollutants must be pursued.

12.11 Conclusion

Multi-omics platforms, including genomics, transcriptomics, proteomics, metabolomics, epigenomics, and microbiomics, have revolutionized our understanding of algal bioremediation. These platforms provide tiered information on the molecular machinery activated under pollutant stress, facilitating the identification of crucial genes, pathways, enzymes, and metabolites involved in detoxification and stress tolerance. Integrating omics information offers a systems-level view, allowing the rational design of efficient algal strains and consortia optimized for environmental remediation. Yet, imperfections in reference genomes, data heterogeneity, and lack of field validation constrain translational use. Overcoming these challenges through the development of specifically designed tools, machine learning-enabled data analysis, and enhanced ecological modeling will unlock the full potential of algal-mediated bioremediation. Ultimately, omics-guided interventions offer a sustainable and targeted approach for reducing coupled environmental pollutants and ensuring ecosystem health.

References

Abdelfattah, A., Ali, S. S., Ramadan, H., El-Aswar, E. I., Eltawab, R., Ho, S. H., et al. (2023). Microalgae-based wastewater treatment: Mechanisms, challenges, recent advances, and future prospects. *Environmental Science and Ecotechnology, 13*, 100205. https://doi.org/10.1016/j.ese.2022.100205

Andrade, L. M., Tito, C. A., Mascarenhas, C., Lima, F. A., Dias, M., Andrade, C. J., Mendes, M. A., & Nascimento, C. A. O. (2022). Phycoremediation of copper by Chlorella protothecoides (UTEX 256): Proteomics of protein biosynthesis and stress response. *Biomass, 2*(3), 116–129. https://doi.org/10.3390/biomass2030008

Andrade-Bustamante, G., Martínez-Ruiz, F. E., Ortega-García, J., Renganathan, P., Gaysina, L. A., Mahendhiran, M., & Puente, E. O. R. (2025). Microalgae-based functional foods: A blue-green revolution in sustainable nutrition and health. *Applied Microbiology, 5*(2), 39. https://doi.org/10.3390/applmicrobiol5020039

Ayilara, M. S., & Babalola, O. O. (2023). Bioremediation of environmental wastes: The role of microorganisms. *Frontiers in Agronomy, 5*, 1183691.

Bacova, R., Kolackova, M., Klejdus, B., Adam, V., & Huska, D. (2020). Epigenetic mechanisms leading to genetic flexibility during abiotic stress responses in microalgae: A review. *Algal Research, 50*, 101999.

Bellido-Pedraza, C. M., Torres, M. J., & Llamas, A. (2024). The microalgae Chlamydomonas for bioremediation and bioproduct production. *Cells, 13*(13), 1137. https://doi.org/10.3390/cells13131137

Bian, C., et al. (2023). Chromosome-level genome assembly for the astaxanthin-producing microalga *Haematococcus pluvialis. Scientific Data, 10*(1), 267.

Calatrava, V., Ballester, D. G., & Dubini, A. (2024). Microalgae for bioremediation: Advances, challenges, and public perception on genetic engineering. *BMC Plant Biology, 24*(1), 1261. https://doi.org/10.1186/s12870-024-05995-5

Chandran, H., Meena, M., & Sharma, K. (2020). Microbial biodiversity and bioremediation assessment through omics approaches. *Frontiers in Environmental Chemistry, 1*, 570326. https://doi.org/10.3389/fenvc.2020.570326

Sánchez-Sandoval, D.S., González-Ortega, O., Vazquez-Martínez, J. et al. Diclofenac removal by the microalgae species Chlorella vulgaris, Nannochloropsis oculata, Scenedesmus acutus, and Scenedesmus obliquus. 3 Biotech 12, 210 (2022). https://doi.org/10.1007/s13205-022-03268-2

Dell' Anno, F., Rastelli, E., Sansone, C., Brunet, C., Ianora, A., & Dell' Anno, A. (2021). Bacteria, fungi and microalgae for the bioremediation of marine sediments contaminated by petroleum hydrocarbons in the omics era. *Microorganisms, 9*(8), 1695. https://doi.org/10.3390/microorganisms9081695

Diankristanti, P. A., & Ng, I. S. (2024). Marine microalgae for bioremediation and waste-to-worth valorization: Recent progress and future prospects. *Blue Biotechnology, 1*, 10. https://doi.org/10.1186/s44315-024-00010-w

El-Sheekh, M. M., El-Kassas, H. Y., & Ali, S. S. (2025). Microalgae-based bioremediation of refractory pollutants: An approach towards environmental sustainability. *Microbial Cell Factories, 24*(1), 19. https://doi.org/10.1186/s12934-024-02638-0

Ferrari, M., Muto, A., Bruno, L., & Cozza, R. (2023). DNA methylation in algae and its impact on abiotic stress responses. *Plants, 12*(2), 241. https://doi.org/10.3390/plants12020241

Ferreira, B. L., Ferreira, D. P., Borges, S. F., Ferreira, A. M., Holanda, F. H., Ucella-Filho, J. G., et al. (2023). Diclofenac, ibuprofen, and paracetamol biodegradation: Overconsumed non-steroidal anti-inflammatories drugs at COVID-19 pandemic. *Frontiers in Microbiology, 14*, 1207664.

Goh, P. S., Lau, W. J., Ismail, A. F., Samawati, Z., Liang, Y. Y., & Kanakaraju, D. (2023). Microalgae-enabled wastewater treatment: A sustainable strategy for bioremediation of pesticides. *Water, 15*(1), 70. https://doi.org/10.3390/w15010070

Goswami, R. K., Agrawal, K., Shah, M. P., & Verma, P. (2022). Bioremediation of heavy metals from wastewater: A current perspective on microalgae-based future. *Letters in Applied Microbiology, 75*(4), 701–717. https://doi.org/10.1111/lam.13564

Gruszecka-Kosowska, A., Ampatzoglou, A., & Aguilera, M. (2022). Integration of omics approaches enhances the impact of scientific research in environmental applications. *International Journal of Environmental Research and Public Health, 19*(14), 8758. https://doi.org/10.3390/ijerph19148758

Gunjal, A., Gupta, S., Nweze, J. E., & Nweze, J. A. (2023). Metagenomics in bioremediation: Recent advances, challenges, and perspectives. In *Metagenomics to bioremediation* (pp. 81–102). Academic Press.

Ha, G. S., Sim, M. G., Jeon, B. H., & Baek, G. (2025). Bioremediation of perfluorooctanoic acid using microalgae with a transcriptomic approach. *Journal of Hazardous Materials, 488*, 137508. https://doi.org/10.1016/j.jhazmat.2025.137508

Han, H., Zhang, Z., Li, S., & Liu, X. (2024). Integrated transcriptomic and metabolomic analysis reveals mechanisms for polystyrene nanoplastics reproductive toxicity in GC-2 cells. *Toxicology In Vitro, 100*, 105893. https://doi.org/10.1016/j.tiv.2024.105893

He, B., et al. (2018). Transcriptome analysis in *Haematococcus pluvialis*: Astaxanthin induction by high light with acetate and Fe^{2+}. *International Journal of Molecular Sciences, 19*(1), 175.

Hom-Diaz, A., et al. (2022). Insights into removal of antibiotics by selected microalgae including photodegradation (*Chlamydomonas reinhardtii*, *Chlorella sorokiniana*, *Dunaliella tertiolecta* and *Pseudokirchneriella subcapitata*). *Algal Research, 61*, 102560.

Iakovidou, G., Itziou, A., Tsiotsias, A., Lakioti, E., Samaras, P., Tsanaktsidis, C., & Karayannis, V. (2024). Application of microalgae to wastewater bioremediation, with CO_2 biomitigation, health product and biofuel development, and environmental biomonitoring. *Applied Sciences, 14*(15), 6727. https://doi.org/10.3390/app14156727

Jaiswal, S., Singh, D. K., & Shukla, P. (2019). Gene editing and systems biology tools for pesticide bioremediation: A review. *Frontiers in Microbiology, 10*, 87. https://doi.org/10.3389/fmicb.2019.00087

Kumar, V., Sharma, J. K., Kumar, S., Gulia, J., Singh, N. P., & Santal, A. R. (2025). Metagenomic and proteomic approach for bioremediation of environmental pollutants. In *Development in waste water treatment research and processes* (pp. 635–647). Elsevier.

Kundu, P., Dutta, N., & Bhattacharya, S. (2024). Application of microalgae in wastewater treatment with special reference to emerging contaminants: A step towards sustainability. *Frontiers in Analytical Science, 4*, 1513153. https://doi.org/10.3389/frans.2024.1513153

Kuppan, N., Padman, M., Mahadeva, M., Srinivasan, S., & Devarajan, R. (2024). A comprehensive review of sustainable bioremediation techniques: Eco friendly solutions for waste and pollution management. *Waste Management Bulletin, 2*(3), 154–171. https://doi.org/10.1016/j.wmb.2024.07.005

Lauritano, C., Ferrante, M. I., & Rogato, A. (2019). Marine natural products from microalgae: An-omics overview. *Marine Drugs, 17*(5), 269. https://doi.org/10.3390/md17050269

Li, M., Ma, L., An, Y., Wei, D., Ma, H., Zhu, J., & Wang, C. (2023). Bioremoval efficiency and metabolomic profiles of cellular responses of *Chlorella pyrenoidosa* to phenol and 4-fluorophenol. *Water Reuse, 13*(1), 97–106. https://doi.org/10.2166/wrd.2023.003

Liberti, D., Pinheiro, F., Simões, B., Varela, J., & Barreira, L. (2024). Beyond bioremediation: The untapped potential of microalgae in wastewater treatment. *Water, 16*(19), 2710. https://doi.org/10.3390/w16192710

Ma, C., Shi, X., Chen, S., & Zhang, Y. (2024). Combined pesticides in field doses weaken honey bee (*Apis cerana*) flight ability revealed by transcriptome and metabolome analyses. *Pesticide Biochemistry and Physiology, 201*, 105793. https://doi.org/10.1016/j.pestbp.2024.105793

McDaniel, E. A., Wahl, S. A., Ishii, S. I., Pinto, A., Ziels, R., Nielsen, P. H., et al. (2021). Prospects for multi-omics in the microbial ecology of water engineering. *Water Research, 205*, 117608.

Michealsamy, A., Thangamani, L., Manivel, G., Kumar, P., Sundar, S., Piramanayagam, S., & Natarajan, J. (2021). Current research and applications of meta-omics stratagems in bioremediation: A bird's-eye view. *Journal Of Applied Biotechnology Reports, 8*(2), 109–115. https://doi.org/10.30491/JABR.2020.237662.1248

Minkina, T., et al. (2023). Advanced value-added bioproducts from microalgae. In P. N. L. Lens & A. Khandelwal (Eds.), *Algal systems for resource recovery from waste and wastewater* (Vol. 183). IWA Publishing. https://doi.org/10.2166/9781789063547_0183

Mishra, S., Lin, Z., Pang, S., Zhang, W., Bhatt, P., & Chen, S. (2021). Recent advanced technologies for the characterization of xenobiotic-degrading microorganisms and microbial communities. *Frontiers in Bioengineering and Biotechnology, 9*, 632059. https://doi.org/10.3389/fbioe.2021.632059

Misra, B. B., Langefeld, C., Olivier, M., & Cox, L. A. (2019). Integrated omics: Tools, advances and future approaches. *Journal of Molecular Endocrinology, 62*(1), R21–R45. https://doi.org/10.1530/JME-18-0055

Nagy, K. K., Takács, K., Németh, I., Varga, B., Grolmusz, V., Molnár, M., & Vértessy, B. G. (2024). Novel enzymes for biodegradation of polycyclic aromatic hydrocarbons identified by metagenomics and functional analysis in short-term soil microcosm experiments. *Scientific Reports, 14*(1), 11608.

Oña, L., et al. (2022). Trophic interactions and metabolic cross-feeding in microbial communities. *Ecology Letters, 25*(8), 1760–1773.

Pacheco, D., Rocha, A. C., Pereira, L., & Verdelhos, T. (2020). Microalgae water bioremediation: Trends and hot topics. *Applied Sciences, 10*(5), 1886. https://doi.org/10.3390/app10051886

Padilla-Garfias, F., Araiza-Villanueva, M., Calahorra, M., Sánchez, N. S., & Peña, A. (2024). Advances in the degradation of polycyclic aromatic hydrocarbons by yeasts: A review. *Microorganisms, 12*(12), 2484. https://doi.org/10.3390/microorganisms12122484

Park, Y., Kim, H., & Lee, J. (2024). Integrative transcriptomic profiling reveals immune and tissue responses to bisphenol a exposure. *Environmental Research, 250*, 120145. https://doi.org/10.1016/j.envres.2024.120145

Qi, L., Zhang, Y., Wang, Y., & Liu, J. (2023). Integrated transcriptomics and metabolomics reveal mechanism of glyphosate-based herbicide reproductive toxicity in mice. *Ecotoxicology and Environmental Safety, 254*, 114628. https://doi.org/10.1016/j.ecoenv.2023.114628

Ranjbar, S., & Malcata, F. X. (2022). Is genetic engineering a route to enhance microalgae-mediated bioremediation of heavy metal-containing effluents? *Molecules, 27*(5), 1473. https://doi.org/10.3390/molecules27051473

Rasheed, R. N., Pourbakhtiar, A., Mehdizadeh Allaf, M., Baharlooeian, M., Rafiei, N., Alishah Aratboni, H., et al. (2023). Microalgal co-cultivation-recent methods, trends in omic-studies, applications, and future challenges. *Frontiers in Bioengineering and Biotechnology, 11*, 1193424. https://doi.org/10.3389/fbioe.2023.1193424

Rawat I., Ranjith Kumar R., Mutanda T., Bux F (2011) Dual role of microalgae: Phycoremediation of domestic wastewater and biomass production for sustainable biofuels production Applied Energy 88(10) 3411–3424 https://doi.org/10.1016/j.apenergy.2010.11.025

Salem, O. M., Abdelsalam, A., & Boroujerdi, A. (2021). Bioremediation potential of *Chlorella vulgaris* and *Nostoc paludosum* on azo dyes with analysis of metabolite changes. *Baghdad Science Journal, 18*(3), 12. https://doi.org/10.21123/bsj.2021.18.3.0445

Sattayawat, P., Yunus, I. S., Noirungsee, N., Mukjang, N., Pathom-Aree, W., Pekkoh, J., & Pumas, C. (2021). Synthetic biology-based approaches for microalgal bio-removal of heavy metals from wastewater effluents. *Frontiers in Environmental Science, 9*, 778260. https://doi.org/10.3389/fenvs.2021.778260

Seo, D. Y., Park, M., Park, J. I., Kim, J. K., Yum, S., & Kim, Y. J. (2023). Transcriptomic changes induced by low and high concentrations of heavy metal exposure in *Ulva pertusa*. *Toxics, 11*(7), 549. https://doi.org/10.3390/toxics11070549

Shetty, S. S., Deepthi, D., Harshitha, S., Sonkusare, S., Naik, P. B., & Madhyastha, H. (2023). Environmental pollutants and their effects on human health. *Heliyon, 9*(9), e19496. https://doi.org/10.1016/j.heliyon.2023.e19496

Shi, J., Yu, X., Zhao, J., Zhang, L., & Wang, H. (2024). Integrated transcriptomics and metabolomics reveal the mechanism of polystyrene nanoplastics toxicity to mice. *Ecotoxicology and Environmental Safety, 284*, 116925. https://doi.org/10.1016/j.ecoenv.2024.116925

Silva, A., Delerue-Matos, C., Figueiredo, S. A., & Freitas, O. M. (2019). The use of algae and fungi for removal of pharmaceuticals by bioremediation and biosorption processes: A review. *Water, 11*(8), 1555. https://doi.org/10.3390/w11081555

Stavridou, E., Karapetsi, L., Nteve, G. M., Tsintzou, G., Chatzikonstantinou, M., Tsaousi, M., et al. (2024). Landscape of microalgae omics and metabolic engineering research for strain improvement: An overview. *Aquaculture, 587*, 740803. https://doi.org/10.1016/j.aquaculture.2024.740803

Tan, H. L., Lam, M. K., Cheng, Y. W., Lim, J. W., Tan, I. S., Foo, C. Y. H., & Show, P. L. (2021). Heterotrophic and mixotrophic cultivation of *Chlorella vulgaris* using chicken waste compost as nutrients source for lipid production. In *IOP conference series: Earth and environmental science* (Vol. 721, No. 1, p. 012011). IOP Publishing.

Touliabah, H. E. S., El-Sheekh, M. M., Ismail, M. M., & El-Kassas, H. (2022). A review of microalgae-and cyanobacteria-based biodegradation of organic pollutants. *Molecules, 27*(3), 1141. https://doi.org/10.3390/molecules27031141

Upadhyay, M., Hansa, A., Devi, A., Lajayer, B. A., Price, G. W., & Sharma, R. (2024). Status and future scope of algal biomass-based remediation for various environmental contaminants. *Journal of Water Process Engineering, 65*, 105809. https://doi.org/10.1016/j.jwpe.2024.105809

Verasoundarapandian, G., Lim, Z. S., Radziff, S. B. M., Taufik, S. H., Puasa, N. A., Shaharuddin, N. A., Merican, F., Wong, C.-Y., Lalung, J., & Ahmad, S. A. (2022). Remediation of pesticides by microalgae as feasible approach in agriculture: Bibliometric strategies. *Agronomy, 12*(1), 117. https://doi.org/10.3390/agronomy12010117

Vo, T. P., Danaee, S., Chaiwong, C., Pham, B. T., Kim, M., Kuzhiumparambil, U., et al. (2024). Microalgae-bacteria consortia for organic pollutants remediation from wastewater: A critical review. *Journal of Environmental Chemical Engineering, 12*(6), 114213. https://doi.org/10.1016/j.jece.2024.114213

Wang, X., Meng, C., Zhang, H., Xing, W., Cao, K., Zhu, B., Zhang, C., Sun, F., & Gao, Z. (2022). Transcriptomic and Proteomic Characterizations of the Molecular Response to Blue Light and Salicylic Acid in Haematococcus pluvialis. Marine Drugs, 20(1), 1. https://doi.org/10.3390/md20010001

Wang, J., Zhang, Q., Chen, J., Zhou, J., Li, J., Wei, Y., Regmi, B., & Bu, D. (2022). Combined transcriptome and metabolome analysis of a new species of microalgae from the Tibetan plateau and its response to sewage treatment. *Water, 14*(21), 3391. https://doi.org/10.3390/w14213391

Yang, W., Wang, D., Zhang, X., et al. (2022). *CRISPR-Cas*-mediated targeted mutagenesis reveals key lipid regulatory genes in *Phaeodactylum tricornutum*. *Algal Research, 65*, 102735. https://doi.org/10.1016/j.algal.2022.102735

Zhao, Z., Chen, G., & Zhang, L. (2024). Epigenetic regulation in algae: Implications for growth, development, and stress response. *International Journal of Aquaculture, 14*, 257–265. https://doi.org/10.5376/ija.2024.14.0026

Microalgae–Microbe Consortia for Agricultural Wastewater Remediation and Biofertilizer Valorization: A Circular Bioeconomy Perspective

13

Prabhaharan Renganathan, Muhilan Mahendhiran, Winston Franz Ríos-Ruiz, Lira Gaysina, and Edgar Omar Rueda Puente

Abstract

Agricultural intensification generates substantial volumes of wastewater enriched with nitrogen, phosphorus, agrochemicals, and suspended solids. Conventional treatments often fail to effectively eliminate these complex pollutants, leading to eutrophication, groundwater contamination, and degradation of soil health. This chapter examines the integrated application of microalgae and plant growth-promoting microorganisms (PGPMs) for the remediation of agricultural wastewater and the production of sustainable biofertilizers, in line with circular bioeconomy principles. Microalgal species, such as *Chlorella vulgaris, Scenedesmus obliquus, Chlamydomonas reinhardtii*, and *Nannochloropsis oculata,* have demonstrated excellent potential for recovering nutrients and degrading various organic and inorganic pollutants in wastewater. When co-cultured with PGPMs, including nitrogen-fixing bacteria, phosphate-solubilizing fungi, and IAA-producing endophytes, these consortia enhance pollutant removal, biofilm stability, and biomass productivity. The resulting

P. Renganathan (✉) · L. Gaysina
Department of Bioecology and Biological Education, M. Akmullah Bashkir State Pedagogical University, Ufa, Russia

M. Mahendhiran
Department of Agri Business Management, Faculty of Agriculture, Vivekananda Global University, Jaipur, Rajasthan, India

W. F. Ríos-Ruiz
Laboratorio de Microbiología Agrícola "Raúl Ríos Reátegui", Departamento Académico Agrosilvopastoril, Facultad de Ciencias Agrarias, Universidad Nacional de San Martín, Tarapoto, Peru

E. O. R. Puente
Departamento de Agricultura y Ganadería, Universidad de Sonora, Hermosillo, Sonora, México

L. Kumar et al. (eds.), *Algal Bioremediation*,
https://doi.org/10.1007/978-981-95-8793-3_13

biomass is rich in macronutrients, phytohormones, and bioactive compounds, making it highly suitable as a biofertilizer to improve crop productivity and restore soil fertility. This chapter also discusses the mechanisms of phycoremediation, the performance of algal–microbial systems, and the development of low-cost cultivation strategies, such as bamboo-based biofilm reactors and photo-sequencing batch systems, which are especially suited to the Indian rural context. Further discussions include harvesting technologies, biomass processing, and strain optimization using omics and synthetic biology tools. This chapter also assesses the techno-economic viability, environmental impact, and regulatory frameworks necessary for practical implementation. Field trials of Indian cropping systems provide strong evidence for the feasibility of this approach among small and marginal farmers. In conclusion, the microalgae–PGPM-based strategy offers a regenerative and climate-resilient approach to nutrient recovery and wastewater valorization, thereby promoting sustainable agriculture in the Global South.

Keywords

Phycoremediation mechanisms · Nutrient recycling · Resource recovery · Plant Growth-Promoting Microorganisms (PGPMs) · Multi-Omics and systems biology integration

13.1 Introduction

The circular bioeconomy offers a sustainable alternative to the traditional linear "take-make-use-dispose" model by promoting the efficient use of biological resources, waste recycling, and ecosystem restoration. It aims to close resource loops and reduce environmental impacts by integrating ecological principles such as resource efficiency, biomass reuse, and reduction of chemical inputs (Venkatesh, 2022). Within this framework, biorefineries play a significant role in converting waste biomass and wastewater into valuable products, such as biofuels, biofertilizers, bioplastics, and biochemicals, thereby supporting both environmental sustainability and rural bioeconomies (Ubando et al., 2020). In the Indian context, promoting a circular bioeconomy in agriculture has become an urgent priority. The sector supports the livelihoods of over half the population, yet it faces growing pressures due to the excessive use of synthetic fertilizers, particularly urea and diammonium phosphate (DAP), which have led to soil nutrient imbalance, groundwater contamination, and inefficient utilization of organic waste (Venkata Mohan et al., 2018; Sarangi et al., 2022). Despite the availability of nutrient-rich agricultural and agro-industrial wastewater, it remains largely underutilized or untreated, particularly in rural and peri-urban regions of developing countries. Circular strategies, such as wastewater valorization using microalgae and beneficial microbes, can support nutrient recycling, reduce dependence on chemical fertilizers, and improve ecological balance (Mehta et al., 2021). These technologies offer low-input, nature-based solutions for wastewater treatment while generating biofertilizers, biogas, and other value-added outputs. They also align with India's goals under the UN sustainable development goals (SDGs) by addressing clean water, sustainable agriculture, and climate resilience (Venkata Mohan et al., 2018).

Agricultural wastewater typically contains high levels of nitrogen, phosphorus, potassium, pesticides, antibiotics, heavy metals, and suspended solids. It is also characterized by high chemical and biological oxygen demands (COD and BOD, respectively) (Martínez-Burgos et al., 2021). In many parts of the world, untreated agricultural wastewater is discharged into natural water bodies, leading to eutrophication, algal blooms, and biodiversity loss (Khalid et al., 2018). Furthermore, the reuse of wastewater in agriculture without proper treatment poses risks, including soil contamination, microbial imbalance, and the accumulation of toxic substances in crops, ultimately affecting food safety (Trotta et al., 2024). Heavy metals, such as cadmium, lead, nickel, chromium, and arsenic, present in wastewater, accumulate in soil over time, affecting soil structure, microbial communities, and crop yields (Aydin et al., 2015; Trotta et al., 2024). Studies from the Indo-Gangetic Plains have shown that continuous irrigation with untreated effluents increases soil salinity, electrical conductivity, and sodium adsorption ratio, which adversely affects soil enzymatic activity and plant productivity (Aydin et al., 2015). Conventional treatment systems, such as anaerobic lagoons and activated sludge, are often costly, energy-intensive, and poorly suited for rural applications. Consequently, there is a growing need for biologically integrated, low-cost, and decentralized solutions, especially in Indian villages and semi-urban farming zones. Microalgae and plant growth-promoting microorganisms (PGPMs) offer a promising approach owing to their combined ability to remove pollutants, produce value-added biomass, and enhance soil fertility. When cultivated together, these organisms form synergistic consortia that degrade contaminants, fix atmospheric nitrogen, solubilize phosphates, and release bioactive compounds beneficial for plant growth (Khalid et al., 2018; Renganathan et al., 2024a) (Fig. 13.1).

This chapter aims to provide a mechanistic and application-oriented perspective on the use of microalgae–PGPM systems for agricultural wastewater remediation under the principles of the circular bioeconomy. The key objectives include (1) understanding the nutrient assimilation and pollutant degradation mechanisms in algal–microbial consortia; (2) examining the synergy, bioactivity, and community dynamics of microalgae–PGPM interactions; (3) assessing cultivation techniques and biomass harvesting methods suited to rural settings; (4) discussing formulation strategies for biofertilizers derived from algal–microbial biomass; (5) highlighting omics and synthetic biology approaches for strain improvement and system optimization; and (6) evaluating techno-economic feasibility, environmental impact, and regulatory considerations, particularly in the Indian context. Through this detailed analysis, this chapter positions algal–microbial technologies as vital components of regenerative, resource-efficient, and climate-resilient agricultural systems.

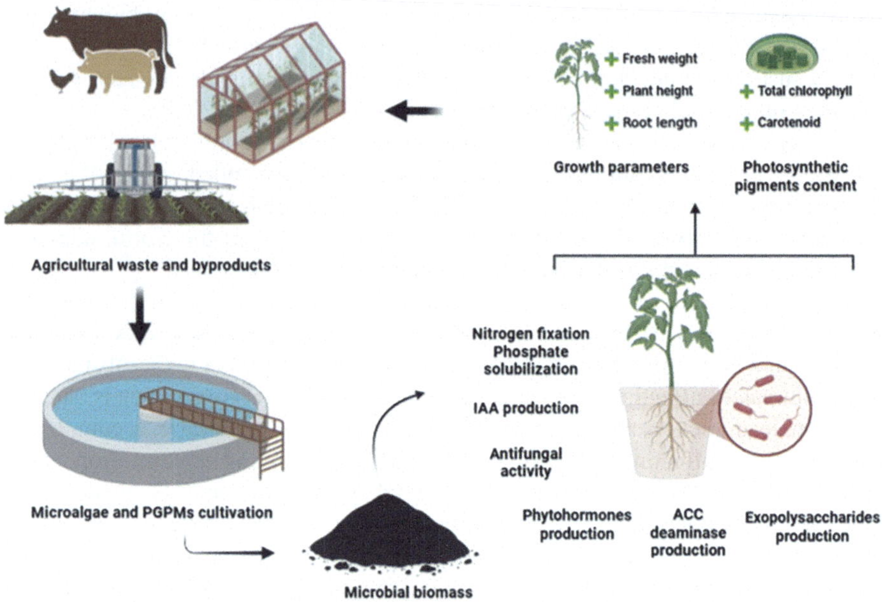

Fig. 13.1 Integrated circular bioeconomy model: Agricultural waste bioremediation using microalgae and PGPMs for sustainable biofertilizer production and enhanced plant growth

13.2 Phycoremediation: Microalgae in Nutrient Recovery

13.2.1 Mechanisms of Nutrient Assimilation and Contaminant Degradation

Microalgae, such as *Chlorella* sp., *Nostoc* sp., *Scendesmus* sp., and *Anabaena* sp., have emerged as model strains for phycoremediation because of their exceptional ability to assimilate nutrients and reduce pollutant loads in complex wastewater effluents, and their cultivated biomass has been utilized in the development of biofertilizers for crop development (Table 13.1). Studies have demonstrated that *Chlorella minutissima* can achieve up to 89% nitrate, 48% ammonium, 67% phosphate, and 66% potassium removal, along with ~80–90% reductions in BOD, COD, TDS, and EC within 15 days of inoculation (Sharma et al., 2020; Sharma et al., 2021). Additionally, its biomass serves as a potent organic substitute for mineral nitrogen fertilizers, yielding spinach and baby corn comparable to or exceeding those obtained with synthetic fertilizers (Sharma et al., 2021). The application of this algal biomass significantly improved soil biochemical properties, including enhanced activities of key enzymes, such as urease, nitrate reductase, and dehydrogenase, alongside reduced nitrate leaching, indicating its efficacy as a soil health enhancer under circular bioeconomic paradigms. The nutrient-rich biomass of *C. minutissima*, laden with nitrogen, phosphorus, and phytohormones, positions it

Table 13.1 Bioremediation efficiencies and plant growth-promoting characteristics of microalgae as a biofertilizer in different types of wastewaters (Renganathan et al., 2024a)

Microalgal species	Wastewater			Biomass		Promoted plant growth parameters and soil properties
	Culture medium	Characteristics	Removal efficiency	Production	Composition	
Chlorella minutissima, *Nostoc muscorum*, *Scendesmus* sp., and *Scendesmus consortium*	Domestic wastewater	EC: 3.14 dS m^{-1}, NH_4^+: 39.5 mg L^{-1}, NO_3^-: 2.38 mg L^{-1}, P: 3.68 mg L^{-1}, COD: 149.75 mg L^{-1}, BOD5: 99.5 mg L^{-1}, and TDS: 2196 mg L^{-1}	NH_4^+: 92%, NO_3^-: 87%, PO_4^{3-}: 85%, COD: 81%, BOD5: 90%, and TDS: 96%	0.14–0.45 g L^{-1}	N: 2–6%, P: 0.5–1%, K: <0.5%, and LP: 11.33–81.23 mg L^{-1}	–
C. minutissima	Domestic wastewater	EC: 3.52 dS m^{-1}, NH_4^+: 5.60 mg L^{-1}, NO_3^-: 3.06 mg L^{-1}, P: 3.54 mg L^{-1}, K: 5.50 mg L^{-1}, COD: 157 mg L^{-1}, BOD5: 114 mg L^{-1}, DO: 3.50 mg L^{-1}, and TDS: 2416 mg L^{-1}	EC: 92.9%, NH_4^+: 48.2%, NO_3^-: 88.9%, P: 67.5%, K: 66.4%, COD: 80.5%, BOD5: 93.2%, and TDS: 94.4%	1.26 ± 0.07 g L^{-1} FW and 0.44 ± 0.04 g L^{-1} DW	N: 6.0%, P: 1.0%, and K: 0.48%	Leaf length, leaf and root biomass in spinach Yields with and without husk and cob length in baby corn Soil organic carbon, nitrogen, and phosphorus Dehydrogenase, urease, and nitrate reductase activity
Chlorella sp., *Scendesmus* sp., and	Domestic wastewater	TN: 61.47 mg L^{-1}, NH_4^+: 37.64 mg L^{-1}, NO_3^-: 16.58 mg L^{-1}, P: 7.42 mg L^{-1}, COD:	TN: 85–94%, NH_4^+: 95–98%, NO_3^-: 84–96%, P:	1.78 g L^{-1}	N: 7.21–7.81%, P: 1.55–1.72%, K: 0.75–1.06%, Ca: 0.21–0.28%, Na:	Shoot and root length, fresh and dry weight, and yields of tomato

(continued)

Table 13.1 (continued)

Microalgal species	Wastewater			Biomass		Promoted plant growth parameters and soil properties
	Culture medium	Characteristics	Removal efficiency	Production	Composition	
Scendesmus consortium		446.25 mg L^{-1}, and TOC: 208.15 mg L^{-1}	89–95%, COD: 78–88%, and TOC: 81–86%		1.08–1.18%, Mg: 0.11–0.17%, S: 0.21–0.27%, Fe: 0.30–0.36%, chlorophyll: 27.03 μg mL^{-1}, protein: 175 μg mL^{-1}, and lipid: 34.83% dry cell weight	Increased macro (N, P, K, and Ca) and micronutrients (Mg and Fe) of tomato
Scenedesmus sp.	Domestic wastewater	NH_4^+: 38.6 mg L^{-1}, NO_3^-: 17.1 mg L^{-1}, PO_4^{3-}: 9.24 mg L^{-1}, and COD: 142.2 mg L^{-1}	–	0.68 g L^{-1}	N: 7.45%, P: 1.6%, K: 0.7%, S: 0.3%, Na: 1.41%, Ca: 0.14%, Mg: 0.12%, Fe: 0.3%, Mn: 210 ppm, Cu: 6.8 ppm, Zn: 34 ppm, and lipid: 24.1%	Plant height, root weight, and yields in rice Increased NPK content in the grain and straw of rice
Chlorella sp., *Scenedesmus* sp., *Chlorococcum* sp., and	Domestic wastewater	–	–	–	–	Plant fresh and dry weight, root length, spike and grain weight, and nutrient contents (NPK)

Chroococcus sp.						of wheat. Increased soil nutrients NPK Higher acetylene-reducing activity
Phormidium sp., *Anabaena* sp., *Westiellopsis* sp., *Fischerella* sp., *Spirogyra* sp., *Scenedesmus* sp.; and *Chlorella vulgaris*	Dairy cattle wastewater	TOC: 623.3 mg L^{-1}, DOC: 361.7 mg L^{-1}, NH_3: 141.8 mg L^{-1}, TKN: 174 mg L^{-1}, TP: 1144.1 mg L^{-1}, SP: 629.4 mg L^{-1}, VSS: 623.9 mg L^{-1}, TSS: 729.9 mg L^{-1}, tCOD: 3106.3 mg L^{-1}, and sCOD: 1015 mg L^{-1}	TOC: 83.9%, DOC: 82.4%, NH_3^-: 99.8%, TKN: 78.4%, TP: 53.2%, SP: 66.9%, VSS: 57.4%, TSS: 55.7%, tCOD: 35.4%, and sCOD: 55.7%	7.1 g^{-2} d^{-1}	TP: 1992 mg L^{-1}, TKN: 1657.4 mg L^{-1}, Cu: 0.53 mg L^{-1}, B: 0.55 mg L^{-1}, Mo: <0.05 mg L^{-1}, and Zn: 0.005 mg L^{-1}	Pasture yield, dry matter, ash, and nutrients (P, Ca, Zn, Mn, and B)
Chlorella pyrenoidosa	Paddy-soaked rice mill wastewater	NH_4^+: 147–154 mg L^{-1}, PO_4: 67–70 mg L^{-1}, S:30–38 mg L^{-1}, C: 640–760 mg L^{-1}, TS: 4554–4640 mg L^{-1}, SS: 106–160 mg L^{-1}, DS: 4448–4480 mg L^{-1}, COD: 960–1280 mg L^{-1}, and BOD: 680–851 mg L^{-1}	NH_4^+: 69.39% and PO_4: 64.76%	0.11 g L^{-1} d^{-1}	Carbohydrate: 8.84%, lipid: 32.12%, and protein: 34.15%	Seed germination, chlorophyll, fresh shoot and root weight, dry shoot and root weight, and root-to-shoot biomass ratio of okra

as a dual-function agent for pollutant removal and sustainable fertilization (Sharma et al., 2020, 2021). This integrated approach addresses environmental pollution and contributes to resource conservation, as well as the sustainable production of crops.

13.2.2 Phycoremediation Performance of Microalgal Species

Comparative studies among key microalgal taxa, particularly *Scenedesmus dimorphus, Scenedesmus quadricauda,* and *C. vulgaris,* have shown significant species-specific differences in nutrient removal efficiency, pollutant tolerance, and biomass productivity in agro-industrial wastewater. Under controlled cylindrical photobioreactors, *S. dimorphus* achieved ammonia–nitrogen removal rates of 92–96% and phosphorus removal up to 89%, whereas *C. vulgaris* showed total nitrogen and orthophosphate removal efficiencies of 85–94 % and 90–95 %, respectively, reflecting different enzymatic affinities for nitrogen assimilation (Hu et al., 2021; Scarponi et al., 2024). In co-culture systems, these species displayed a 15–25% increase in overall pollutant removal and biomass yield, with total dry biomass production ranging between 1.5 and 2.0 g L^{-1}, compared with 1.0–1.2 g L^{-1} in monocultures (Asmare et al., 2014). *S. dimorphus* exhibited higher lipid accumulation (30–40% DCW) and tolerance to elevated ammonia (up to 150 mg L^{-1}) and COD levels (>400 mg L^{-1}), making it suitable for energy valorization routes, whereas *C. vulgaris* demonstrated superior chlorophyll content (12–18 μg mL^{-1}) and higher orthophosphate uptake under moderate nutrient loads, favoring its application as a biofertilizer. Reactor geometry also influenced performance; flat-panel configurations enhanced light utilization for *C. vulgaris*, increasing nitrogen uptake by 10–12%, whereas tubular reactors favored *Scenedesmus* sp. due to higher mixing and mass-transfer rates. These results confirm that *Scenedesmus* excels in ammonium and organic load removal, while *Chlorella* contributes to greater total nitrogen and phosphorus recovery with richer pigment and protein yields. The strategic co-cultivation of these taxa within biofilms or photo-sequencing batch systems can therefore maximize nutrient capture, reduce treatment time by 20–30%, and generate biomass suitable for dual valorization as a bioenergy feedstock and high-nutrient biofertilizer, integral to the circular bioeconomy framework for rural wastewater management (Hu et al., 2021; Asmare et al., 2014; Scarponi et al., 2024).

13.2.3 Cultivation Systems for Rural Contexts

Low-cost decentralized phycoremediation systems are crucial for rural and peri-urban farming communities, where access to centralized wastewater treatment is limited. Innovations such as the bamboo-based algal–bacterial biofilm reactor developed in India have demonstrated resource-efficient designs engineered for local conditions, supporting efficient algal and bacterial consortia year-round (Anusuyadevi et al., 2023; Kumar et al., 2024). These systems effectively treat agricultural wastewater while generating valuable biomass that can be used for biogas, cattle feed, and biofertilizers, aligning with the principles of the circular bioeconomy (Anusuyadevi et al., 2023; Kumar et al., 2024). Pilot studies have demonstrated high nutrient removal efficiencies and substantial biomass productivity in both batch and continuous operation modes, making this technology adaptable and scalable for diverse rural settings (Anusuyadevi et al., 2023; Kumar et al., 2024). The simplicity and low operational costs of such systems, combined with their ability to valorize waste into multiple coproducts, make them especially promising for sustainable agri-environmental management (Anusuyadevi et al., 2023; Kumar et al., 2024). Additionally, integrating phycoremediation with other decentralized renewable energy solutions, such as biogas-based hybrid systems, can further enhance resource recovery and rural resilience (Pal & Bhattacharjee, 2020).

13.3 Microalgae–Microorganism Consortia: Synergy and Bioactivity

13.3.1 Synergistic Interactions: Microalgae and Bacteria

Microalgae–bacterial consortia (MBCs) are increasingly recognized for their mutualistic interactions, which significantly enhance nutrient removal, organic pollutant degradation, and biomass productivity compared to monocultures (Nagarajan et al., 2022). Bacteria in these systems supply essential metabolites, such as vitamins, carbon substrates, siderophores, and growth promoters that stimulate algal growth. Microalgae provide oxygen through photosynthesis and release organic exudates that fuel bacterial metabolism (Dai & Wang, 2024). Meta-analyses and comprehensive reviews have reported that MBCs can achieve up to 15% higher removal efficiencies and significantly lower treatment times than pure algal systems, with biogranulation further improving biomass recovery and simplifying downstream processing (Oviedo et al., 2022). In the context of textile wastewater, MBCs have demonstrated rapid dye decolorization, effective heavy metal removal, reduced COD, and improved valorization of biomass for pigments and other valuable products, supporting both environmental remediation and circular economic goals (Vo et al., 2024). The adaptability and stability of MBCs, along with their ability to recover resources such as biofertilizers and biofuels, make them especially promising for sustainable wastewater treatment and biorefinery applications (Dai & Wang, 2024). These systems also benefit from advances in reactor design, omics-based optimization, and integration with artificial intelligence for process control, which further enhances their efficiency and scalability (Nagarajan et al., 2022).

13.3.2 Plant Growth-Promoting Microorganisms

Plant growth-promoting microorganisms (PGPMs), including rhizobacteria and cyanobacteria, play a vital role in enhancing the bioactivity of algal consortia by solubilizing phosphate, producing phytohormones such as indole acetic acid (IAA), fixing atmospheric nitrogen, solubilizing phosphates, and enhancing tolerance to heavy metals (Renganathan et al., 2025). When integrated into algal consortia, these beneficial microbes stimulate algal growth and metabolite production through mutualistic interactions and provide essential nutrients and growth factors to the host. Microalgae contribute oxygen and organic exudates that support bacterial metabolism (Renganathan et al., 2024b). For example, rhizospheric and endophytic bacteria isolated from fields irrigated with agro-industrial wastewater have shown strong IAA production, phosphate solubilization, and Cd tolerance, making them promising plant growth-promoting rhizobacteria (PGPR) strains for use as algal-derived biofertilizers (Renganathan et al., 2018, 2024a; Prabhaharan et al., 2019). Studies have indicated that such consortia can improve crop yields and soil health, as the combined action of PGPR and microalgae enhances nutrient availability, stress tolerance, and biocontrol properties. The co-application of algal hydrolysates and PGPR strains has also been shown to promote plant growth more effectively than either component alone, highlighting the synergistic potential of these microbial partnerships (Renganathan et al., 2024b). As research in this area expands, the integration of PGPR into algal consortia is gaining attention for its ability to deliver sustainable agricultural benefits and support circular bioeconomic strategies (Renganathan et al., 2024a).

13.3.3 Biofilm Formation and Phototrophic Biofilms

Phototrophic biofilm complexes, multilayered microbial mats composed of cyanobacteria, microalgae, heterotrophic bacteria, and fungi, serve as highly effective platforms for nutrient capture and environmental resilience, including storm events. These biofilms leverage natural processes; photosynthetic activity during daylight elevates oxygen and pH, which in turn precipitates soluble phosphates and reduces coliform bacteria, thereby enhancing effluent safety (Li et al., 2023). Extracellular polymeric substances (EPS) produced by the biofilm matrix play a crucial role in the biosorption and immobilization of heavy metals, with efficiency modulated by factors such as pH, light, and biofilm density (Tenore et al., 2021; Li et al., 2023). Biosorption and bioaccumulation processes enable metals to bind to extracellular sites and are gradually taken up by biofilms, limiting their mobility and environmental impact (Tenore et al., 2021). Research in paddy fields and aquatic systems has shown that phototrophic biofilms can intercept and immobilize both phosphorus and nitrogen, and their effectiveness is influenced by the organic carbon and nutrient ratios in the environment (Liu et al., 2019). Additionally, modeling and pilot studies have confirmed that the structural and functional integrity provided by EPS not only enhances metal precipitation and microbial aggregation but also supports robust nutrient cycling and resilience to environmental fluctuations (Tenore et al., 2021). These properties make phototrophic biofilms valuable for bioremediation, wastewater treatment, and improving soil and water quality in both natural and engineered systems (Li et al., 2023).

13.4 Biomass Harvesting and Biofertilizer Formulation

13.4.1 Harvesting Techniques

The separation of microalgae–bacterial biomass from treated wastewater is a critical and costly step, often accounting for 20–30% of downstream processing costs. Several techniques are available, each with specific advantages and limitations. Filtration methods (micro-, ultra-, and macro-filtration) are effective but prone to membrane fouling, require frequent maintenance, and provide rapid, high-purity dewatering at the expense of high energy consumption, making them less suitable for decentralized or rural applications (Singh & Patidar, 2018). Flocculation using chemical, physical, or biological agents is the most practical approach for wastewater treatment. Chemical flocculants, such as ferric chloride or aluminum sulfate, can achieve over 90% harvesting efficiency at optimal pH but may leave residual metals unless replaced with organic alternatives, such as chitosan or natural tannins, which maintain biomass purity and reduce environmental risks (Singh & Patidar, 2018; Perales-Pérez et al., 2023). Bioflocculation, driven by extracellular polymeric substances from bacteria or fungi, enables the formation of dense microalgal–bacterial flocs that settle by gravity without added chemicals, significantly lowering energy requirements, although large-scale adoption is still in its infancy (Alam et al., 2016). Flotation, especially when combined with flocculation, is suitable for low-density cultures and low-energy operations, whereas gravity sedimentation, although slow, is often enhanced by prior flocculation (Singh & Patidar, 2018; Perales-Pérez et al., 2023). In rural or resource-limited settings, biofilm-based or immobilized systems allow for simple biomass scraping or harvesting from carriers, offering low mechanical input and ease of recovery (Alam et al., 2016). The choice of separation method depends on the specific operational context, balancing the cost, efficiency, and intended use of the harvested biomass (Alam et al., 2016; Singh & Patidar, 2018).

13.4.2 Forms of Fertilizer and Nutrient Content

Harvested algal–microbial biomass is a potent biofertilizer rich in essential macronutrients, such as N, P, and K; micronutrients, such as Cu, Fe, and Zn; and bioactive compounds, such as phytohormones, amino acids, and extracellular polymeric substances (EPS) (Renganathan et al., 2024a; Wichaphian et al., 2025). Field trials with *C. minutissima* demonstrated that applying its powdered biomass could fully substitute conventional nitrogen fertilizers while also enhancing soil enzyme activities, including urease, nitrate reductase, and dehydrogenase, and surpassing the effects of mineral fertilizers on spinach and baby corn yields (Sharma et al., 2021). These treatments lead to improved soil microbial activity, higher organic carbon content, and better nutrient retention, indicating a positive impact on soil health and fertility (Sharma et al., 2021; Wichaphian et al., 2025; Renuka et al., 2016). Studies on various crops, including lettuce, wheat, and cucumber, have confirmed that

Table 13.2 Algal-based products for plant growth promotion and soil health improvement

Microalgae	Type and application	Major bioactive components	Plant growth-promoting effects	Reference
Chlorella vulgaris and Scenedesmus quadricauda biomass/ hydrolysate	Biofertilizer or biostimulant (seed/soil application)	Proteins, amino acids, IAA, vitamins, and polysaccharides	Improves germination, shoot biomass, and nutrient uptake in spinach, lettuce, baby corn, and tomato	Renuka et al. (2016) and Sharma et al. (2021)
Scenedesmus obliquus and *S. quadricauda*	Microalgal biomass (biofertilizer)	NPK-rich macronutrients, carotenoids, and enzymes	Stimulates root growth, chlorophyll content, and soil enzymatic activity	Renuka et al. (2016)
Arthrospira platensis	Dried powder/ extract (foliar feed)	Amino acids, vitamins B_{12}, antioxidants, and polyunsaturated fatty acids	Enhances photosynthetic rate and protein accumulation in maize and lettuce	Renganathan et al. (2025)
Nostoc muscorum, Anabaena sp.	Cyanobacterial inoculant	Nitrogenase enzymes, EPS, and IAA	Biological N-fixation, phosphate solubilization, and improved soil aggregation	Renganathan et al. (2025)
Chlamydomonas reinhardtii	Research-grade extract	IAA, gibberellins, and polyamines	Promotes seedling vigor and stress tolerance under salinity	Dai and Wang (2024)

microalgal biofertilizers boost plant growth, nutrient uptake, and soil microbial diversity while promoting beneficial bacteria and fungi in the rhizosphere (Renuka et al., 2016; Wichaphian et al., 2025). Rapid nutrient release from algal biomass, combined with gradual mineralization of processed residues, supports both immediate and sustained plant nutrition (Renganathan et al., 2024a; Wichaphian et al., 2025). Additionally, microalgal biofertilizers and biostimulants can enhance crop resilience to stress, improve yield quality, and reduce reliance on synthetic fertilizers, aligning with circular economy and sustainable agriculture principles (Renganathan et al., 2024a). In recent years, several microalgal and seaweed-based formulations have been developed and commercialized as biofertilizers and biostimulants. These products vary in terms of source taxa, bioactive composition, and plant growth promotion mechanisms. Table 13.2 provides an overview of representative commercial and experimental algal-derived products, their functional components, and their associated agronomic benefits.

13.4.3 Effects on Crop Performance and Soil Health

Sewage-derived microalgae-based biofertilizers, whether applied alone or in combination with biosolids, have been shown to significantly enhance crop growth and physiological performance. In studies on *Amaranthus cruentus*, dry microalgae treatments yielded the highest shoot biomass and resulted in substantial increases in leaf nutrient concentrations, particularly sodium, zinc, iron, and copper (Ferreira et al., 2023). These amendments also improved growth rates, chlorophyll content, and photosynthetic efficiency, with dry microalgae and biosolid applications outperforming wet microalgae and supplemented control (Ferreira et al., 2023). Although wet microalgae resulted in lower early stage photosynthetic pigments, they still promoted greater biomass than the controls, highlighting the overall benefits of microalgal amendments (Ferreira et al., 2023). The superior performance of dry microalgae underscores the importance of drying and concentrating biomass for optimal formulation and nutrient delivery (Ferreira et al., 2023, 2025). In addition to serving as nutrient carriers, these biofertilizers act as bioactive amendments that enhance soil fertility, enzyme activity, and plant physiological functions (Ferreira et al., 2023, 2025).

13.5 Omics and Genetic Optimization of Strains

13.5.1 Multi-Omics for Mechanistic Insights

Recent advancements in multi-omics platforms, including genomics, transcriptomics, proteomics, and metabolomics, have transformed our understanding of microalgal physiology, particularly under wastewater stress and in consortia (Fig. 13.2). High-throughput sequencing and bioinformatics have enabled the functional characterization of genes, reconstruction of metabolic pathways, and detailed profiling of stress responses, accelerating the development of microalgal strains with improved nutrient uptake, pollutant tolerance, and biochemical productivity (Kuo et al., 2022; Nagarajan et al., 2022; Stavridou et al., 2024). Integrative omics approaches reveal how microalgae and their bacterial partners dynamically express detoxification genes, nutrient transporters, and secondary metabolites in response to wastewater-derived pollutants. In contrast, metagenomics tracks shifts in microbial community composition during phycoremediation, informing the rational design of consortia (Nagarajan et al., 2022). The synergy of metabolomics with other omics layers overcomes the limitations of individual datasets, providing a comprehensive phenotype-level view of metabolic flux and pathway bottlenecks (Kuo et al., 2022; Stavridou et al., 2024). This holistic perspective enables predictive strain improvement, targeted manipulation of enzymatic steps, and identification of genes associated with salinity tolerance, xenobiotic degradation, and lipid biosynthesis (Stavridou et al., 2024). Consequently, multi-omics platforms are now central to both fundamental research and applied metabolic engineering of microalgae for

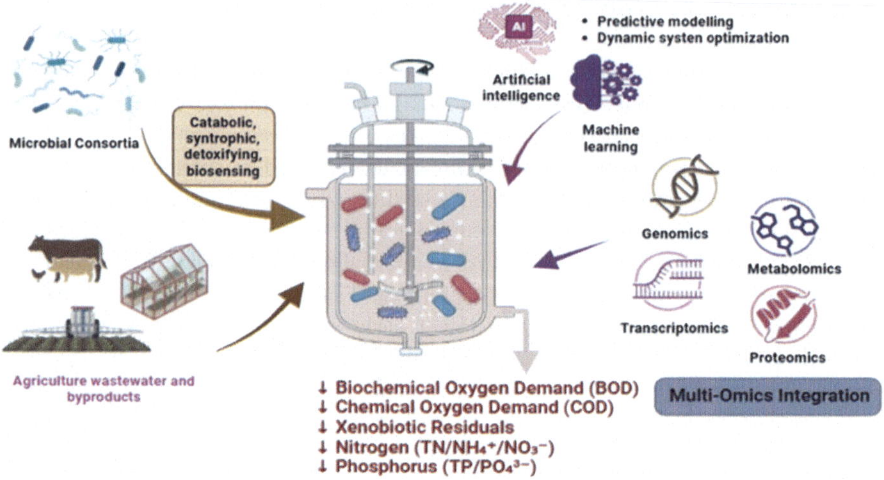

Fig. 13.2 Synergistic role of microbial consortia, multi-omics integration, and AI in agricultural wastewater bioremediation

sustainable wastewater treatment, nutrient recovery, and bioproduct generation (Nagarajan et al., 2022; Stavridou et al., 2024).

13.5.2 Controlled Consortium Engineering

The dynamic control of algal–bacterial consortia in bioreactor systems represents a cutting-edge approach to maximizing biomass yield and ecosystem functions. Recent modeling and control theory research has shown that dynamically allocating resources between bacterial partners and using time-varying, "bang–bang" strategies can significantly outperform static, fixed-allocation regimes in continuous bioreactor operations, leading to cyclic control inputs that synchronize nutrient supply with algal demand and boost net biomass production (Asswad et al., 2024). This approach aligns with chemostat-based reactor principles, where careful tuning of dilution rates, nutrient feeds, and metabolic outputs maintains stable culture conditions and allows engineers to direct microbial behaviors, such as growth rate, metabolite secretion, and EPS production, for both pollutant removal and biomass enrichment (Liu et al., 2017; Yang et al., 2020; Asswad et al., 2024). Integrating multi-omics feedback further enables near-real-time adaptation of system parameters and optimization of performance under fluctuating wastewater conditions by tracking community shifts and metabolic responses (Yang et al., 2020). Studies have also highlighted the importance of operational strategies, such as light regime management and control of selection pressure, in shaping the consortium structure, stability, and productivity. Dynamic or cyclic inputs often provide advantages in both yield and system resilience (Liu et al., 2017). Therefore, controlled consortium engineering, supported by advanced modeling and real-time feedback, offers a powerful framework for enhancing the efficiency and robustness of algal–bacterial bioreactor systems (Yang et al., 2020; Asswad et al., 2024).

13.6 Technoeconomic, Regulatory, and Environmental Considerations

13.6.1 Energy and Resource Efficiency

The photo-sequencing batch reactor (PSBR) represents a major innovation in energy-efficient wastewater treatment, integrating microalgae and bacteria into a single system. In this approach, microalgae generate oxygen through photosynthesis, which is then utilized by nitrifying bacteria to oxidize ammonium to nitrate. This process is followed by denitrification under anoxic conditions, thereby eliminating the need for external aeration and significantly reducing energy consumption (Ye et al., 2018). Studies have shown that PSBR systems can achieve energy savings of up to 91% compared to conventional oxygenation-based methods, while maintaining high removal efficiencies for COD, ammonium, total nitrogen, and phosphorus (Ye et al., 2018; Clagnan et al., 2024). The PSBR also supports stable nitrification and denitrification, enhances pathogen removal, and increases the abundance of beneficial photosynthetic and denitrifying microorganisms while reducing greenhouse gas emissions and operational costs (Clagnan et al., 2024). Maintaining an optimal balance between microalgae and bacteria is crucial for system stability and performance because excessive microalgal concentrations can inhibit certain bacterial groups (Ye et al., 2018). Additionally, PSBRs have demonstrated effective removal of persistent pollutants, such as antibiotics, and a reduction in antibiotic resistance genes, further highlighting their environmental benefits (Liu et al., 2022). Therefore, the PSBR exemplifies how biological oxygen generation and process integration can dramatically improve the sustainability and cost-effectiveness of decentralized wastewater treatment systems (Ye et al., 2018; Clagnan et al., 2024).

13.6.2 Cost–Benefit Analysis and Scalability

Scalable hybrid reactor architectures, such as photobioreactors, algal biofilm reactors, and integrated biorefinery models, offer promising solutions for rural wastewater treatment and the valorization of circular nutrients. In a field study by Mathur et al. (2024), an algal–bacterial biofilm reactor constructed from low-cost bamboo and fiber materials achieved high removal efficiencies for phosphate (up to 88%), ammoniacal nitrogen (83%), COD (81%), and total coliforms (100%) in rural Indian graywater, while nearly doubling the biomass productivity compared with conventional polypropylene supports. These biofilm-based systems are notable for their minimal energy requirements, use of locally available substrates, and compatibility with downstream biomass valorization, such as biofertilizer or biogas production, which enhances economic viability and sustainability (de Assis et al., 2020; Liu et al., 2023). Reviews and field studies have further highlighted that hybrid systems combining biofilm reactors with high-rate algal ponds or moving bed biofilm reactors can optimize pollutant removal, biomass harvesting, and microbial community stability, even under variable rural conditions (de Assis et al., 2020). Innovations such as wind-solar hybrid-powered reactors and multi-compartment ecological filter beds further reduce operational costs and environmental impacts, making these systems particularly suitable for decentralized, resource-limited settings (Liu et al., 2023). These hybrid reactor models support rural adoption by integrating efficient treatment, local resource use, and circular economy principles, while delivering robust environmental and economic benefits (de Assis et al., 2020; Liu et al., 2023).

The global biofertilizer market is expanding rapidly, driven by sustainable agricultural policies, increasing demand for organic farming, and the transition toward carbon-neutral nutrient management. According to Global Market Insights (2024), the global biofertilizer market was valued at approximately USD 2.5 billion in 2023 and is projected to reach USD 5.6 billion by 2034, registering a compound annual growth rate (CAGR) of approximately 8.6%. (Global Market Insights, Inc., 2025). Within India, the biofertilizer market was estimated at USD 142.97 million in 2024 and is projected to grow to USD 399.67 million by 2033, exhibiting a CAGR of approximately 11.5% (IMARC Group, 2025). Algal-based biofertilizers, including formulations of microalgae and cyanobacteria, represent an emerging high-value segment due to their multifunctional roles in nutrient enrichment, soil microbiome restoration, and mitigation of abiotic stress. Recent techno-economic analyses suggest that phycoremediated algal biomass can be produced at a cost of as low as USD 120–180 per ton, significantly below the cost of conventional chemical nitrogen fertilizers (Sharma et al., 2021; Wichaphian et al., 2025). In the Indian context, given the government's sustained focus via initiatives such as the National Mission on Sustainable Agriculture (NMSA) and the Pradhan Mantri Krishi Sinchayee Yojana (PMKSY), the algal biofertilizer segment could feasibly capture 5–8% of India's organic-fertilizer market within the next decade, thus creating decentralized rural bioindustries aligned with the circular bioeconomy and "Atmanirbhar Krishi" frameworks (Government of India, 2024).

13.6.3 Regulatory, Safety, and Environmental Considerations

The implementation of large-scale microalgae–microbial remediation and biofertilizer production in India requires strict adherence to the national regulatory frameworks, safety protocols, and environmental safeguards. Biofertilizer products must comply with the Fertilizer Control Order (FCO) and Bureau of Indian Standards (BIS) norms, which set permissible limits for heavy metals, pathogens, and residual agrochemicals to ensure agricultural and environmental safety (Arjjumend & Koutouki, 2020; Patil et al., 2021). Rigorous monitoring of emerging contaminants, such as pesticides, antibiotics, and heavy metals, is essential to prevent their bioaccumulation in harvested biomass or soils. Post-harvest treatments, including composting or pasteurization, are mandated for pathogen sanitization and toxin removal. Regulatory clarity is particularly important for genetically optimized strains or engineered consortia, which fall under India's biosafety and genetically modified organism (GMO) legislation, requiring additional approval and risk assessment (Arjjumend & Koutouki, 2020). Quality compliance and monitoring remain challenges, with calls for more efficient government oversight and industry accountability to ensure product safety and efficacy (Arjjumend & Koutouki, 2020; Patil et al., 2021). Environmental safety must be harmonized with farmer education and on-farm validation trials to build trust and facilitate adoption, especially as these technologies transition from pilot to rural deployment (Arjjumend & Koutouki, 2020). These coordinated approaches, which combine regulatory compliance, robust contaminant testing, biosafety oversight, and stakeholder engagement, are vital for the safe, effective, and socially accepted scale-up of microalgae–microbial biofertilizer systems in India (Patil et al., 2021).

The practical viability of integrating wastewater remediation with algal biofertilizer production has been validated through several field-scale demonstrations across Asia and Europe. In southern India, the ICAR–CSIR collaborative pilot at Coimbatore successfully employed *a C. vulgaris–Azospirillum consortia for treating dairy wastewater, recovering 92% of the ammonium and 88% of the phosphate, and generating nutrient-rich biomass that increased baby corn yield by 23%* (Sharma et al., 2021). In Spain's Murcia region, *S. obliquus* was integrated with biogas digestate treatment, producing 1.7 g L^{-1} of algal biomass that was reused in tomato cultivation, enhancing chlorophyll and fruit yield by 18% (Renuka et al., 2016). Similarly, a Vietnamese demonstration in Hau Giang Province utilized *Arthrospira platensis* and indigenous nitrifying bacteria to treat rice effluent, achieving 82% COD removal and improving rice productivity by 20% (Wichaphian et al., 2025). These case studies highlight the environmental, agronomic, and economic co-benefits of circular bioeconomy models that integrate wastewater remediation with algal biofertilizer valorization.

13.7 Future Perspectives and Knowledge Gaps

13.7.1 Scaling-Up and Process Integration

Despite the strong potential of microalgae–microbial consortia for agricultural wastewater valorization, a major limitation is the scarcity of long-duration, demonstration-scale systems that capture the real-world variability of wastewater composition, climate, and user practice. Most pilot studies have shown robust nutrient removal and biomass productivity under controlled or semi-controlled conditions. However, a clear gap exists in comprehensive techno-economic analyses (TEA) and life cycle assessments (LCA), particularly in the Indian context (Morillas-España et al., 2022; Nagarajan et al., 2022). Field-scale integration across diverse agroecological zones is urgently needed to assess seasonal performance, energy balances, and labor requirements, as system efficiency can vary by up to 25% depending on factors such as irradiance and wastewater dilution (Bhatia et al., 2022; Morillas-España et al., 2022). Modular and circular process designs that combine wastewater treatment, biomass valorization into biofertilizers, and coproducts, such as biogas or aquafeed, are recommended to ensure compatibility with rural infrastructure and climatic diversity (Morillas-España et al., 2022). Reviews emphasize that while microalgae–bacteria consortia offer adaptability and stability, upscaling to reactors larger than 100 m^2 is necessary to predict their industrial relevance and optimize both nutrient recovery and biomass yield (Bhatia et al., 2022; Morillas-España et al., 2022). Additionally, the integration of multi-omics and advanced monitoring can help tailor consortia to local conditions; however, real-world demonstration projects are required to validate these approaches (Nagarajan et al., 2022). Ultimately, addressing these gaps through long-term field-based studies and holistic system assessments is essential for the widespread and sustainable adoption of microalgae–microorganism consortia in rural wastewater valorization (Morillas-España et al., 2022; Nagarajan et al., 2022).

13.7.2 Strain Improvement and Tailored Consortia

Optimizing algal and microbial strains in Indian agricultural effluents is crucial for achieving resilient and efficient wastewater remediation, as commonly used strains, such as Chlorella vulgaris and *Scenedesmus* obliquus, may not always tolerate or thrive in effluents rich in agrochemical residues, antibiotics, or heavy metals. Recent studies have highlighted the value of isolating and systematically adapting local strains, such as *Chlorella pyrenoidosa*, from Indian fertilizer industry effluent, which demonstrated exceptional ammonium tolerance and removal capacity of up to 700 ppm, far exceeding typical literature values (Ahmed et al., 2017). Similarly, screening and optimization of indigenous microalgae, such as *Desmodesmus* sp. SNN1 has been shown to yield strains with high nutrient removal and biomass productivity under local wastewater conditions (Wang et al., 2023). Fungal pretreatment using locally isolated strains, such as *Trichoderma* spp. and *Lichtheimia ornata*, can further enhance algal growth and nutrient removal by reducing the color and toxicity of high-strength effluents (Qian et al., 2022). Advanced approaches, including genomic and phenomic screening, metagenomic assembly, and synthetic ecology, are recommended for engineering stable, high-performance consortia tailored to specific effluent profiles (Wood et al., 2025). Functional traits, such as upregulated nitrogen assimilation genes under urea-rich conditions, improved lipid yields via CRISPR/Cas9 modifications, and enhanced biofilm or EPS production, should be prioritized for both remediation and value addition. Ultimately, leveraging local biodiversity and modern molecular tools will enable the development of robust, efficient, and context-specific algal–microbial systems for valorizing Indian agricultural wastewater (Ahmed et al., 2017).

13.7.3 Policy Alignment and Rural Adoption

The widespread adoption of microalgae–microbe technologies in rural India depends on coherent policy frameworks, robust community engagement, and strengthened institutional capacities. Although national programs such as Paramparagat Krishi Vikas Yojana (PKVY), Rashtriya Krishi Vikas Yojana (RKVY), and Jal Shakti Abhiyan promote sustainable agriculture and water management, there is a notable gap in the institutional mechanisms supporting the integration of biological wastewater treatment with on-farm biofertilizer production (Hemaiswarya et al., 2012). Policy reforms should prioritize subsidies or tax incentives for decentralized treatment units, the inclusion of microalgal biofertilizers in FCO standards, and streamlined approval of novel bioinputs to foster innovation and uptake (Hemaiswarya et al., 2012; Renganathan et al., 2024a). Building local capacity is essential; evidence from community-owned energy projects shows that early and meaningful community involvement, clear governance structures, and targeted training for farmers and technicians are critical for long-term sustainability and satisfaction (Katre et al., 2019). Extension services can leverage ICT tools, mobile applications, and field demonstrations to enhance knowledge transfer and trust. In contrast, socioeconomic research must address barriers such as landholding size, gender equity, and cost perceptions to ensure inclusivity (Katre et al., 2019). Ultimately, aligning policy incentives, community participation, and institutional support will be key to scaling microalgae–microbe solutions for rural wastewater valorization and circular agriculture in India (Katre et al., 2019; Hemaiswarya et al., 2012; Renganathan et al., 2024a).

13.8 Conclusion

Microalgae–microbe consortia represent an ecologically sound and economically feasible strategy for transforming agricultural wastewater into valuable biofertilizers, thereby closing nutrient loops within the circular bioeconomy. Among the studied species, *C. vulgaris*, *S. dimorphus*, and *A. platensis* exhibited superior capabilities for nitrogen and phosphorus assimilation, biomass yield, and stress resilience. Integrating such systems with plant growth-promoting microorganisms accelerates nutrient conversion, improves biomass quality, and minimizes secondary pollution levels. The recovered algal biomass functions as a nutrient-rich biofertilizer and plant biostimulant containing amino acids, phytohormones, and polysaccharides that enhance soil fertility and crop productivity. The techno-economic feasibility demonstrated by case studies in India, Spain, and Vietnam validates the scalability of these systems under diverse agro-climatic conditions. Furthermore, compliance with established biosafety and fertilizer regulations (FCO 2021; EU 2019/1009) affirms the environmental compatibility of these products. Advancing this technology requires an integrated life cycle assessment, regulatory harmonization, and industrial partnerships to facilitate rural bioindustrialization. The convergence of circular bioeconomy principles with algal biotechnology holds significant promise for sustainable nutrient recovery, reduced chemical fertilizer dependency, and enhanced agricultural resilience in the face of climate change scenarios.

References

Ahmed, A., Jyothi, N., & Ramesh, A. (2017). Improved ammonium removal from industrial wastewater through systematic adaptation of wild type *Chlorella pyrenoidosa*. *Water Science and Technology, 75*(1), 182–188. https://doi.org/10.2166/wst.2016.504

Alam, M. A., Vandamme, D., Chun, W., Zhao, X., Foubert, I., Wang, Z., Muylaert, K., & Yuan, Z. (2016). Bioflocculation as an innovative harvesting strategy for microalgae. *Reviews in Environmental Science and Bio/Technology, 15*(4), 573–583. https://doi.org/10.1007/s11157-016-9408-8

Anusuyadevi, P. R., Kumar, D. J., Jyothi, A. O., Patwardhan, N. S. V. J., & Mol, A. (2023). Towards viable eco-friendly local treatment of blackwater in sparsely populated regions. *Water, 15*(3), 542. https://doi.org/10.3390/w15030542

Arjjumend, H., & Koutouki, K. (2020). Legal barriers and quality compliance in the business of biofertilizers and biopesticides in India. *Journal of Legal Studies, 26*(40), 81–101.

Asmare, A. M., Demessie, B. A., & Murthy, G. S. (2014). Investigation of microalgae co-cultures for nutrient recovery and algal biomass production from dairy manure. *Applied Engineering in Agriculture, 30*(2), 335–342. https://doi.org/10.13031/aea.30.10261

Asswad, R., Djema, W., Bernard, O., Gouzé, J. L., & Cinquemani, E. (2024). Optimization of microalgae biosynthesis via controlled algal-bacterial symbiosis. In *2024 IEEE 63rd Conference on Decision and Control (CDC)* (pp. 589–594). IEEE. https://doi.org/10.1109/CDC49753.2024.10217452

Aydin, M., Aydın, S., Beduk, F., Tor, A., Tekinay, A., Kolb, M., & Bahadir, M. (2015). Effects of long-term irrigation with untreated municipal wastewater on soil properties and crop quality. *Environmental Science and Pollution Research, 22*, 19203–19212. https://doi.org/10.1007/s11356-015-5074-6

Bhatia, S. K., Ahuja, V., Chandel, N., Mehariya, S., Kumar, P., Vinayak, V., Saratale, G. D., Raj, T., Kim, S. H., & Yang, Y. H. (2022). An overview on microalgal-bacterial granular consortia for resource recovery and wastewater treatment. *Bioresource Technology, 351*, 127028. https://doi.org/10.1016/j.biortech.2022.127028

Clagnan, E., Petrini, S., Pioli, S., Piergiacomo, F., Chowdhury, A. A., Brusetti, L., & Foladori, P. (2024). Conventional activated sludge vs. photo-sequencing batch reactor for enhanced nitrogen removal in municipal wastewater: Microalgal-bacterial consortium and pathogenic load insights. *Bioresource Technology, 401*, 130735. https://doi.org/10.1016/j.biortech.2024.130735

Dai, C., & Wang, F. (2024). Potential applications of microalgae–bacteria consortia in wastewater treatment and biorefinery. *Bioresource Technology, 393*, 130019. https://doi.org/10.1016/j.biortech.2023.130019

de Assis, L. R., Calijuri, M. L., Assemany, P. P., Silva, T. A., & Teixeira, J. S. (2020). Innovative hybrid system for wastewater treatment: High-rate algal ponds for effluent treatment and biofilm reactor for biomass production and harvesting. *Journal of Environmental Management, 274*, 111183. https://doi.org/10.1016/j.jenvman.2020.111183

Ferreira, E. T., Barrochelo, S. C., de Melo, S. D. P., Araujo, T., Xavier, A. C. C., Cechin, I., & Da Silva, G. H. R. (2023). Biofertilizers from wastewater treatment as a potential source of mineral nutrients for growth of amaranth plants. *PLoS One, 18*(12), e0295624. https://doi.org/10.1371/journal.pone.0295624

Ferreira, E. T., Caetano, L. E. S., Candido, J. M. B., Cechin, I., & da Silva, G. H. R. (2025). Enhancing plant growth and photosynthesis with biofertilizers from sewage treatment. *Agronomy, 15*(3), 610. https://doi.org/10.3390/agronomy15030610

Global Market Insights, Inc. (2025). *Biofertilizers Market Size, Share & Growth Report, 2032*. Available at: https://www.gminsights.com/industry-analysis/biofertilizers-market. Accessed 20 Oct 2025.

Government of India. (2024). *Answer to Starred Question No. 85 on promotion of organic fertilizers and biofertilizers*. Ministry of Agriculture and Farmers Welfare. Available at: https://sansad.in/getFile/annex/265/AS85_ektSRe.pdf?source=pqars. Accessed 20 Oct 2025

Hemaiswarya, S., Raja, R., Carvalho, I. S., Ravikumar, R., Zambare, V., & Barh, D. (2012). An Indian scenario on renewable and sustainable energy sources with emphasis on algae. *Applied Microbiology and Biotechnology, 96*(5), 1125–1135. https://doi.org/10.1007/s00253-012-4440-4

Hu, D., Zhang, J., Chu, R., Yin, Z., Hu, J., Nugroho, Y. K., Li, Z., & Zhu, L. (2021). *Chlorella vulgaris* and *Scenedesmus dimorphus* co-cultivation with landfill leachate for pollutant removal and lipid production. *Bioresource Technology, 342*, 126003. https://doi.org/10.1016/j.biortech.2021.126003

IMARC Group. (2025). India biofertilizer market size, share, trends and forecast 2025–2033. Available at: https://www.imarcgroup.com/india-biofertilizer-market. Accessed 20 Oct 2025.

Katre, A., Tozzi, A., & Bhattacharyya, S. (2019). Sustainability of community-owned mini-grids: Evidence from India. *Energy, Sustainability and Society, 9*(1), 1–17. https://doi.org/10.1186/s13705-019-0216-0

Khalid, S., Shahid, M., Natasha, B. I., Sarwar, T., Shah, A. H., & Niazi, N. K. (2018). A review of environmental contamination and health risk assessment of wastewater use for crop irrigation with a focus on low and high-income countries. *International Journal of Environmental Research and Public Health, 15*(5), 895. https://doi.org/10.3390/ijerph15050895

Kumar, R., Kundu, D., Kormoker, T., Joshi, S., Rose, P. K., Kumar, S., Sahoo, P. K., Sharma, P., & Lamba, J. (2024). Phycoremediation of potentially toxic elements for agricultural and industrial wastewater treatment: Recent advances, challenges, and future prospects. *Desalination and Water Treatment, 319*, 100505. https://doi.org/10.5004/dwt.2024.100505

Kuo, E., Yang, R., Chin, Y., Chien, Y., Chen, Y., Wei, C., Kao, L., Chang, Y., Li, Y., Chen, T., & Lee, T. (2022). Multiomics approaches and genetic engineering of metabolism for improved biorefinery and wastewater treatment in microalgae. *Biotechnology Journal, 17*(11), e2100359. https://doi.org/10.1002/biot.202100359

Li, H. Y., Xu, R., Liu, T. F., & Hu, Z. X. (2023). The pretreatment of micro-polluted source water through phototrophic biofilms under variant light conditions. *Water, 15*(4), 621. https://doi.org/10.3390/w15040621

Liu, L., Fan, H., Liu, Y., Liu, C., & Huang, X. (2017). Development of algae-bacteria granular consortia in photo-sequencing batch reactor. *Bioresource Technology, 232*, 64–71. https://doi.org/10.1016/j.biortech.2017.02.008

Liu, J., Sun, P., Sun, R., Wang, S., Gao, B., Tang, J., Wu, Y., & Dolfing, J. (2019). Carbon-nutrient stoichiometry drives phosphorus immobilization in phototrophic biofilms at the soil–water interface in paddy fields. *Water Research, 167*, 115129. https://doi.org/10.1016/j.watres.2019.115129

Liu, H., Yao, Y., Ye, W., Qian, R., Chen, H., Liang, J., & Ye, J. (2022). Enhanced removal of antibiotics and decreased antibiotic resistance genes in the photo-sequencing batch reactor during the aquaculture wastewater treatment. *Environmental Technology, 43*(23), 3608–3619. https://doi.org/10.1080/09593330.2021.1942697

Liu, J., Wei, Z., Xu, S., & Tian, H. (2023). A novel enhanced bio-ecological combined reactor for rural wastewater treatment: Operational performance and microbial communities. *Biochemical Engineering Journal, 198*, 108991. https://doi.org/10.1016/j.bej.2023.108991

Martínez-Burgos, W., Sydney, E., Medeiros, A., Magalhães, A., De Carvalho, J., Karp, S., De Souza Vandenberghe, L., Letti, L., Soccol, T., De Melo Pereira, G., Rodrigues, C., Woiciechowski, A., & Soccol, C. (2021). Agro-industrial wastewater in a circular economy: Characteristics, impacts and applications for bioenergy and biochemicals. *Bioresource Technology, 341*, 125795. https://doi.org/10.1016/j.biortech.2021.125795

Mathur, M., Choudhary, P., Sujathan, S., Naaz, F., & Malik, A. (2024). A biologically driven model for rural wastewater management: Feasibility and efficiency of algal-bacterial biofilm reactors for combined treatment and algae farming. *Frontiers in Water, 6*, 1430900. https://doi.org/10.3389/frwa.2024.1430900

Mehta, N., Shah, K. J., Lin, Y. I., Sun, Y., & Pan, S. Y. (2021). Advances in circular bioeconomy technologies: From agricultural wastewater to value-added resources. *Environments, 8*(3), 20. https://doi.org/10.3390/environments8030020

Morillas-España, A., Lafarga, T., Sánchez-Zurano, A., Acién-Fernández, F. G., & González-López, C. (2022). Microalgae-based wastewater treatment coupled to the production of high-value agricultural products: Current needs and challenges. *Chemosphere, 291*, 132968. https://doi.org/10.1016/j.chemosphere.2021.132968

Nagarajan, D., Lee, D. J., Varjani, S., Lam, S. S., Allakhverdiev, S. I., & Chang, J. S. (2022). Microalgae-based wastewater treatment–Microalgae-bacteria consortia, multi-omics approaches and algal stress response. *Science of the Total Environment, 845*, 157110. https://doi.org/10.1016/j.scitotenv.2022.157110

Oviedo, J. A., Muñoz, R., Donoso-Bravo, A., Bernard, O., Casagli, F., & Jeison, D. (2022). A half-century of research on microalgae-bacteria for wastewater treatment. *Algal Research, 67*, 102828. https://doi.org/10.1016/j.algal.2022.102828

Pal, A., & Bhattacharjee, S. (2020). Effectuation of biogas-based hybrid energy system for cost-effective decentralized application in small rural community. *Energy, 203*, 117819. https://doi.org/10.1016/j.energy.2020.117819

Patil, C. R., Navi, V., & Santosh, G. P. (2021). Microbial agents as biopesticides for nutrients: Management in organic agriculture. In *Biopesticides in organic farming* (pp. 49–52). CRC Press. https://doi.org/10.1201/9781003139705-6

Perales-Pérez, Á., Macías-Sánchez, M. D., Ruiz, J., Perales, J. A., & Garrido-Pérez, C. (2023). Process for nutrient recycling from intensive aquaculture through microalgae-bacteria consortium. *Science of the Total Environment, 901*, 165848. https://doi.org/10.1016/j.scitotenv.2023.165848

Prabhaharan, R., Borboa-Flores, J., Rosas-Burgos, E. C., Cárdenas-López, J. L., Ortega-García, J., & Rueda-Puente, E. O. (2019). *Phaseolus acutifolius* associated with *Bacillus amyloliquefaciens* and *Azospirillum halopraeferens* under salinity conditions. *Biotecnia, 21*(1), 127–132. https://doi.org/10.18633/biotecnia.v21i1.807

Qian, J., Zhang, J., Jin, Z., Cheng, J., Li, J., Song, H., Lu, Q., Li, H., Wan, T., Fu, S., & Li, J. (2022). Enhancing algal yield and nutrient removal from anaerobic digestion piggery effluent by an integrated process-optimization strategy of fungal decolorization and microalgae cultivation. *Applied Sciences, 12*(9), 4741. https://doi.org/10.3390/app12094741

Renganathan, P., Borboa-Flores, J., Rosas-Burgos, E. C., Cárdenas-López, J. L., Murillo-Amador, B., Ortega-García, J., & Rueda-Puente, E. O. (2018). Inoculation of nitrogen-fixing halobacteria in the contribution to tolerance to salt stress in bean tepary. *Revista Mexicana de Ciencias Agrícolas, 9*(SPE20), 4289–4300.

Renganathan, P., Gaysina, L. A., Holguín-Peña, R. J., Sainz-Hernández, J. C., Ortega-García, J., & Rueda-Puente, E. O. (2024a). Phycoremediated microalgae and cyanobacteria biomass as biofertilizer for sustainable agriculture: A holistic biorefinery approach to promote circular bioeconomy. *Biomass, 4*(4), 1047–1077. https://doi.org/10.3390/biomass4040060

Renganathan, P., Puente, E. O., Sukhanova, N. V., & Gaysina, L. A. (2024b). Hydroponics with microalgae and cyanobacteria: Emerging trends and opportunities in modern agriculture. *BioTech, 13*(3), 27. https://doi.org/10.3390/biotech13030027

Renganathan, P., Astorga-Eló, M., Gaysina, L. A., Puente, E. O., & Sainz-Hernández, J. C. (2025). Nitrogen fixation by diazotrophs: A sustainable alternative to synthetic fertilizers in hydroponic cultivation. *Sustainability, 17*(13), 5922. https://doi.org/10.3390/su17135922

Renuka, N., Prasanna, R., Sood, A., Ahluwalia, A. S., Bansal, R., Babu, S., Singh, R., Shivay, Y. S., & Nain, L. (2016). Exploring the efficacy of wastewater-grown microalgal biomass as a biofertilizer for wheat. *Environmental Science and Pollution Research, 23*(7), 6608–6620. https://doi.org/10.1007/s11356-015-5877-9

Sarangi, P., Subudhi, S., Bhatia, L., Saha, K., Mudgil, D., Shadangi, K., Srivastava, R., Pattnaik, B., & Arya, R. (2022). Utilization of agricultural waste biomass and recycling toward circular bioeconomy. *Environmental Science and Pollution Research, 30*, 8526–8539. https://doi.org/10.1007/s11356-022-24339-5

Scarponi, P., Frongia, F., Cramarossa, M. R., Roncaglia, F., Arru, L., & Forti, L. (2024). Bioremediation of basil pesto sauce-manufactured wastewater by the microalgae *Chlorella vulgaris* Beij. and *Scenedesmus* sp. *AgriEngineering, 6*(2), 1674–1682. https://doi.org/10.3390/agriengineering6020097

Sharma, G. K., Khan, S. A., Shrivastava, M., Gupta, N., Kumar, S., Malav, L. C., Nogiya, M., & Dubey, S. K. (2020). Bioremediation of sewage wastewater through microalgae (*Chlorella minutissima*). *Indian Journal of Agricultural Sciences, 90*(10), 2024–2028.

Sharma, G. K., Khan, S. A., Shrivastava, M., Bhattacharyya, R., Sharma, A., Gupta, D. K., Kishore, P., & Gupta, N. (2021). Circular economy fertilization: Phycoremediated algal biomass as biofertilizers for sustainable crop production. *Journal of Environmental Management, 287*, 112295. https://doi.org/10.1016/j.jenvman.2021.112295

Singh, G., & Patidar, S. K. (2018). Microalgae harvesting techniques: A review. *Journal of Environmental Management, 217*, 499–508. https://doi.org/10.1016/j.jenvman.2018.04.010

Stavridou, E., Karapetsi, L., Nteve, G. M., Tsintzou, G., Chatzikonstantinou, M., Tsaousi, M., Martinez, A., Flores, P., Merino, M., Dobrovic, L., & Mullor, J. L. (2024). Landscape of microalgae omics and metabolic engineering research for strain improvement: An overview. *Aquaculture, 587*, 740803. https://doi.org/10.1016/j.aquaculture.2024.740803

Tenore, A., Mattei, M. R., & Frunzo, L. (2021). Modelling the ecology of phototrophic–heterotrophic biofilms. *Communications in Nonlinear Science and Numerical Simulation, 94*, 105577. https://doi.org/10.1016/j.cnsns.2020.105577

Trotta, V., Baaloudj, O., & Brienza, M. (2024). Risks associated with wastewater reuse in agriculture: Investigating the effects of contaminants in soil, plants, and insects. *Frontiers in Environmental Science, 12*, 1358842. https://doi.org/10.3389/fenvs.2024.1358842

Ubando, A. T., Felix, C. B., & Chen, W. H. (2020). Biorefineries in circular bioeconomy: A comprehensive review. *Bioresource Technology, 299*, 122585. https://doi.org/10.1016/j.biortech.2019.122585

Venkata Mohan, S., Chiranjeevi, P., Dahiya, S., & Kumar, N. (2018). Waste-derived bioeconomy in India: A perspective. *New Biotechnology, 40*, 60–69. https://doi.org/10.1016/j.nbt.2017.06.010

Venkatesh, G. (2022). Circular bio-economy – Paradigm for the future: Systematic review of scientific journal publications from 2015 to 2021. *Circular Economy and Sustainability, 2*(1), 231–279. https://doi.org/10.1007/s43615-021-00042-2

Vo, T. P., Danaee, S., Chaiwong, C., Pham, B. T., Kim, M., Kuzhiumparambil, U., Songsomboon, C., Pernice, M., Ngo, H. H., Ralph, P. J., & Vo, P. H. (2024). Microalgae-bacteria consortia for organic pollutants remediation from wastewater: A critical review. *Journal of Environmental Chemical Engineering, 12*(6), 114213. https://doi.org/10.1016/j.jece.2024.114213

Wang, P., Shao, Y., Geng, Y., Mushtaq, R., Yang, W., Li, M., Sun, X., Wang, H., & Chen, G. (2023). Advanced treatment of secondary effluent from wastewater treatment plant by a newly isolated microalga *Desmodesmus* sp. SNN1. *Frontiers in Microbiology, 14*, 1111468. https://doi.org/10.3389/fmicb.2023.1111468

Wichaphian, A., Kamngoen, A., Pathom-Aree, W., Maneechote, W., Khuendee, T., Chromkaew, Y., Cheirsilp, B., Shyu, D. J., & Srinuanpan, S. (2025). Integrating microalgal *Chlorella* biomass and biorefinery residues into sustainable agriculture and food production: Insights from lettuce cultivation. *Foods, 14*(5), 808. https://doi.org/10.3390/foods14050808

Wood, E., Edvardsen, B., Skjånes, K., & Šupraha, L. (2025). Phycosphere of an algal co-culture phycoremediation system: Stability of bacterial communities in an *Oedogonium–Stigeoclonium* co-culture during cultivation in microbially rich wastewater. *Journal of Applied Phycology, 37*(2), 837–853. https://doi.org/10.1007/s10811-024-03072-z

Yang, J., Li, Z., Lu, L., Fang, F., Guo, J., & Ma, H. (2020). Model-based evaluation of algal-bacterial systems for sewage treatment. *Journal of Water Process Engineering, 38*, 101568. https://doi.org/10.1016/j.jwpe.2020.101568

Ye, J., Liang, J., Wang, L., Markou, G., & Jia, Q. (2018). Operation optimization of a photo-sequencing batch reactor for wastewater treatment: Study on influencing factors and impact on symbiotic microbial ecology. *Bioresource Technology, 252*, 7–13. https://doi.org/10.1016/j.biortech.2018.01.091

A Green Solution for Waste: Microalgal Bioremediation for Wastewater Treatment in Food and Agro-Food Industries

14

Arnab Sau, Bikash Kumar Mondal, Jayabrata Dhar, Edita Baltrėnaitė-Gedienė, Kartik Chandra Ghanta, and Susmita Dutta

Abstract

Food processing and agro-food industries generate wastewater rich in organic matter, heavy metals, and surplus nutrients, such as nitrogen and phosphorus. When this effluent enters rivers or lakes without proper treatment, it decreases the dissolved oxygen (DO) level of the water bodies, while parameters such as chemical oxygen demand (COD) and biochemical oxygen demand (BOD) increase, endangering fish and other aquatic life. Microalgae offer an efficient solution for this problem. They absorb heavy metals, feed on excess nutrients, and break down organic pollutants as they grow. Algal biomass can later be used for various purposes, such as producing bioactive compounds in pharmaceuticals, animal feed, or converted into biofuels. This chapter highlights key microalgal strains that excel at cleaning up the effluents of food processing and agro-food industries. It also examines the factors influencing the efficiency of bioremediation and the challenges associated with scaling up the technology. Microalgal bioremediation simultaneously treats wastewater and converts waste into a valuable biomass, advancing both circular economy goals and environmental sustainability.

A. Sau · B. K. Mondal · K. C. Ghanta · S. Dutta (✉)
Department of Chemical Engineering, National Institute of Technology Durgapur, Durgapur, India
e-mail: sdutta.che@nitdgp.ac.in

J. Dhar
Department of Mechanical Engineering, National Institute of Technology Durgapur, Durgapur, India

E. Baltrėnaitė-Gedienė
Institute of Environmental Protection, Vilnius Gediminas Technical University, VILNIUS TECH, Vilnius, Lithuania

L. Kumar et al. (eds.), *Algal Bioremediation*,
https://doi.org/10.1007/978-981-95-8793-3_14

Keywords

Phycoremediation · Microalgae · Agro-food industries · Bioaccumulation of pollutants · Value-added products

14.1 Introduction

The safe disposal of wastewater has become a significant environmental challenge worldwide. Untreated wastewater discharge pollutes natural water bodies, harming the ecosystem and posing a threat to biodiversity. Different sectors, like industrial, domestic, and agricultural, generate about 2.2 million m^3 of wastewater worldwide each year (Abedi et al., 2019). The food processing and agro-food industries are one of the primary contributors to environmental pollution because the wastewater released from such industries contains a variety of pollutants, such as organic pollutants, oils and greases, heavy metals, volatile organic compounds (VOCs), and nutrients (Kumar et al., 2024). Owing to having elevated organic content, the wastewater from this sector, if not properly treated, is harmful to the receiving water bodies by reducing dissolved oxygen levels and ultimately threatening aquatic life (Valiela et al., 2016). There are various physicochemical and biological techniques for treating such wastewater. Physicochemical techniques such as membrane filtration, ion exchange, electrochemical processes, reverse osmosis, chemical precipitation, and evaporation are used commercially. These commercial processes frequently face challenges with high operational costs and limited environmental compatibility (Kumar et al., 2024). These conventional physicochemical processes can quickly mitigate pollutants, but they also produce secondary pollutants that pose another risk to the environment. This has led to a search for sustainable, cost-effective, and eco-friendly integrated treatment technologies (Crini & Lichtfouse, 2019; Rani et al., 2019).

In recent years, the biological treatment has increasingly been recognized as a sustainable option compared to conventional physicochemical methods. On the other hand, biological processes, particularly bioremediation, offer an environmental friendly and economical solution for wastewater treatment. Bioremediation utilizes microorganisms, including bacteria, fungi, and microalgae, to break down pollutants in wastewater. While bioremediation with bacteria has limitations like requirements for nutrients, susceptibility problems at high pollutant loads, inefficiency in meeting standard discharge limits, and generation of solid sludge, the biomitigation of pollutants using fungi depends on specific nutrients, the risk of foam formation, overgrowth, and the generation of additional solid sludge. Besides, many fungal strains are pathogenic to human health (Shahid et al., 2020). Now, nutrient-rich wastewater offers an opportunity for microalgae cultivation, as algae utilize these nutrients for growth and biomass production. Three fundamental mechanisms, like biosorption, bioaccumulation, and biodegradation, are responsible for microalgal removal of pollutants. During the biosorption process, pollutants attach to microalgal cell walls through passive binding. In contrast, bioaccumulation involves the active transport of pollutants from the outer microenvironment into the cell. The breaking down process of complex pollutants, leading to simpler, non-harmful chemical products through enzymatic action, is another way of biomitigation of pollutants (Abdelfattah et al., 2023). Microalgae assimilate pollutants through their metabolic pathways. Furthermore, microalgae absorb CO_2 and release O_2 during photosynthesis, making the environment oxygen-rich. Moreover, microalgae require minimal energy and chemical inputs for treating different types of wastewaters in an eco-friendly manner, making it a practical and environmentally benign solution for wastewater treatment. In addition to the bioremediation capabilities, microalgae have the potential to generate a variety of value-added compounds.

High-value compounds as obtained from microalgae include carotenoids, phycobiliproteins, polysaccharides, polyunsaturated fatty acids, and UV-screening agents (Zhuang et al., 2022). Scientists showed microalgae as a potential biofuel feedstock for the production of biodiesel and bioethanol that substitute traditional petroleum-based fuels (Pérez et al., 2021). Hence, the cultivation of algae for wastewater treatment, commonly known as phycoremediation, makes the treatment method both environmentally and economically beneficial.

Research has now increasingly focused on microalgae-based wastewater treatment as a sustainable and efficient treatment solution. Figure 14.1 shows the research studies on the treatment of wastewater from agro-food and food processing industries using microalgae from 2015 to April 2025. The figure illustrates that research studies on phycoremediation for treating agro-food and food-processing wastewater have increased steadily over the past decade. Figure 14.1a depicts an increase of relevant studies on agro-food processing wastewater treatment, gradually, from essentially none in 2015 to almost 600 by April 2025. Figure 14.1b illustrates a growing scholarly interest in food processing wastewater treatment using phycoremediation, which has expanded from over 4,000 papers in 2015 to nearly 18,000 by 2025. Overall, these numbers demonstrate the applicability of phycoremediation as a valuable, environmentally benign, sustainable treatment option. The application of microalgae in treating wastewater from agro-food industries, such as palm oil production, rice mills, and cassava starch production, is reviewed here. The consumption of freshwater by these industries is not only quite high, but the generation of nutrient-rich wastewater is also huge (Ummalyma et al., 2021). Again, food production stands as one of the most water-intensive industrial sectors because it includes animal-based products among its extensive product catalog. About 1.0 g of protein produced from meat, milk, and eggs needs 112 L, 31 L, and 29 L of water, respectively (Amit et al., 2021).

The organic material, along with nitrogen, phosphorus, and chlorides, is a common pollutant present in food processing wastewater. Consequently, such wastewater streams contain vital nutrients that can support microalgal growth by providing the necessary ingredients. Remediation of pollutants from various food processing industrial wastewater using microalgae, and its application in different fields, is illustrated in Fig. 14.2. The figure illustrates that microalgae thrive on nutrient-rich wastewater coming from food and agro-food industries. They consume macronutrients (carbohydrates, proteins, and lipids) and micronutrients (various

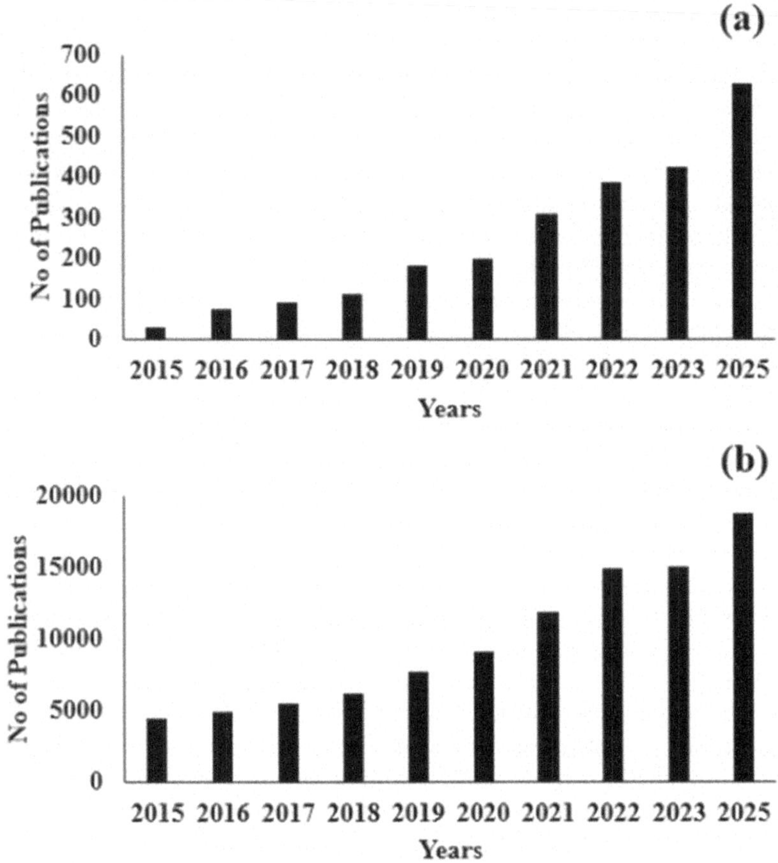

Fig. 14.1 Number of studies on the treatment of wastewater from (**a**) agro-food processing, (**b**) food-processing industries using phycoremediation, till April 2025. (Data collected from Google Scholar)

salts and minerals) to purify the wastewater and produce valuable biomass. Algal biomass can produce a range of useful products, including biofuels (such as biodiesel, biohydrogen, biomethane, and bioalcohol), pigments, nutraceuticals, medicines, and biofertilizers. This chapter focuses on exploring strategies for treating food and agro-food processing wastewater within the framework of a circular economy. It discusses key aspects, such as the characterization of wastewater from these industries, the selection of efficient microalgal species for bioremediation, and the recovery of high-value bioactive compounds.

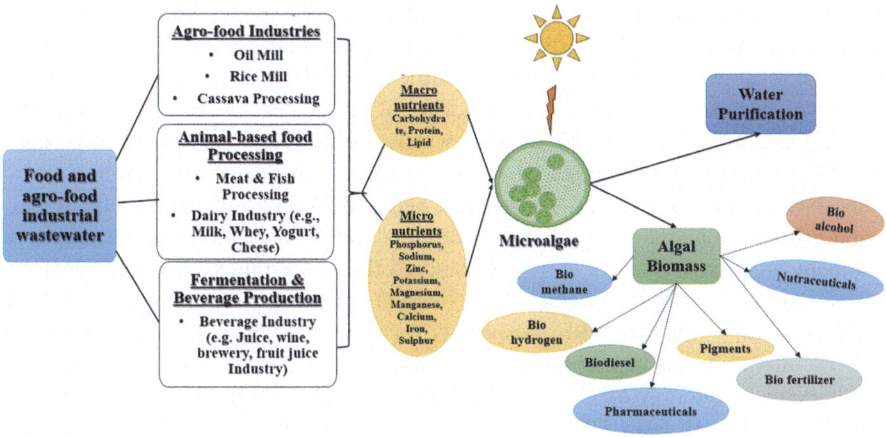

Fig. 14.2 Overview of food-processing wastewater treatment using microalgae and its conversion into high-value products (Amit et al., 2021)

14.2 Wastewater Treatment Through Phycoremediation

The release of untreated or improperly treated food and agro-food industrial wastewater to the environment poses a serious threat to human health and aquatic life. Phycoremediation represents a viable and environmentally sustainable method for reducing pollutants from such industrial effluents. The microalgal species, such as *Chlorella vulgaris*, *Scenedesmus dimorphus*, *Nannochloropsis* sp., *Chlamydomonas* sp., and *Dunaliella salina,* have been the subject of scientific research on phycoremediation of pollutants from food and agro-food industrial wastewater.

14.2.1 Agro-Food Industries Wastewater

The agro-food industrial sector is one of the largest consumers of freshwater and also generates a substantial amount of wastewater. Every stage of food processing, starting from washing to heating, cooling, and packaging, generates a huge volume of spent water. In fact, the industry as a whole withdraws roughly 4×10^{12} m^3 of water annually (Walsh et al., 2016). Although agro-food effluents differ in composition and concentrations depending on the products, such as palm oil, rice, and cassava starch, they share some common pollutants. Though they are typically rich in a substantial amount of suspended solids and biodegradable organics, they seldom carry toxic chemicals (Sehar & Nasser, 2019). Nitrogen compounds, fats and oils, phosphorus, and chlorides also appear in appreciable concentrations. Wastewater from the agro-food industry may be as concentrated as the discharges from meat processing industries, or it can be as diluted as streams like dairy wash water (Kolev Slavov, 2017). Such nutrient and carbon-rich wastewater provides an opportunity for phycoremediation process through cultivation of microalgae, while spent algal biomass can further be processed to get valuable by-products meeting the goal of the circular economy. The palm oil mill effluent (POME) generation rate reaches a high level because it requires 5 to 7.5 tons of water per ton of crude palm oil, resulting in a substantial amount of wastewater. The conventional treatment process of POME requires three sequential stages, starting with acidification, followed by anaerobic digestion for biogas production, and concluding with aerobic treatment, despite the effluent remaining rich in nutrients and organic carbon after all these treatment processes. Shah et al. (2016) studied the possibilities of using POME as cultivation media of *Nannochloropsis oculata* and *Tetraselmis suecica*, which readily consume nitrogen and phosphorus for their growth and lipid production. POME cultivation has been optimized to produce high amounts of lipid along with simultaneous reduction of chemical oxygen demand (COD) (95%), biochemical oxygen demand (BOD) (97%), total organic carbon (TOC) (75%), total nitrogen (TN) (91%), and oil and grease (95%) (Shah et al., 2016). In another study, Ummalyma et al. (2021) demonstrated that the microalgal strains—*N. oculata* and *Chlorella* sp. could significantly remove COD (95–98%), BOD (90–98%), TOC (80–86%), and TN (80%) from POME (Ummalyma et al., 2021).

Rice mills are another polluting industry because they consume a huge amount of water and yield an equally large amount of wastewater. Simply soaking paddy before milling produces about 1.0–1.2 L of wastewater for every kilogram of grain processed. In India alone, the annual production of 105 million tonnes of parboiled rice requires roughly 136 billion litres of water, all of which returns as effluent (Challa et al., 2024). Such wastewater carries very high loads of organic matter, including starch, proteins, and other biodegradable compounds, resulting in elevated levels of COD, BOD, nitrogen, and phosphorus, along with an offensive odor. Umamaheswari and Shanthakumar (2020) investigated the efficiency of algal species, such as *Chlorella vulgaris, Scenedesmus obliquus,* and *Chlorella pyrenoidosa*, for treating rice mill wastewater. They showed more than 80% removal of ammoniacal-N and phosphorus from this wastewater with a maximum dry biomass content of 831 mg/L (Umamaheswari & Shanthakumar, 2020). Roy et al. (2024) tested the efficacy of *Scenedesmus obliquus* in treatment of rice bran oil processing wastewater and showed that *Scenedesmus obliquus* could grow in the 75% rice bran oil processing wastewater and could reduce COD (85.04 $\pm$ 0.05%), nitrate (95.18 $\pm$ 0.36%), total dissolved solid (TDS) (79.78 $\pm$ 0.07%), and total suspended solid (TSS) (64.07 $\pm$ 2.55) (Roy et al., 2024). Cassava processing wastewater, commonly known as Manipueira, contains very high levels of organic materials and nutrients. Microalgae efficiently removed 85.5–86.2% COD and total solids of cassava starch wastewater in a horizontal fixed-bed anaerobic reactor as reported by Watthier et al. (2019) (Watthier et al., 2019). The use of various microalgal strains like *Scenedesmus* sp. (Romaidi et al., 2018), *Chlorella sorokiniana* (Gonçalves, 2021), and *Spirulina platensis* (Hadiyanto et al., 2023) for the treatment of cassava processing wastewater by efficiently reducing COD, nitrate, phosphate, and other chemical pollutants has been reported in the literature.

14.2.2 Dairy Wastewater

Effluents from dairy plants are heavily loaded with easily biodegradable organic compounds; therefore, thorough treatment of such wastewater is necessary before release. The bulk of the effluent originates from the extensive rinsing and sanitation carried out during milk-processing operations, and its volume typically reaches approximately 2.5 times the quantity of milk processed. As a result, India's dairy sector is estimated to generate nearly 200 million tonnes of wastewater each year (Agrawal et al., 2023). A greenish-yellow liquid (cheese whey), a byproduct of the cheese-making process, is being produced at a ratio of 9 kg per 1 kg of cheese (Remón et al., 2016). About 2.9 million m^3 of whey is being produced each year in Mexico alone during the production of 332,251 tons of cheese, and only 50% of this whey is recycled. Therefore, it is clear that more than 1.495 billion litres are dumped into waterways, adding to pollution (Osorio-González et al., 2018). The content of cheese whey varies according to the type of cheese and processing steps; however, it is rich in lactose, proteins, lipids, and salts. COD values between 50,000 and 80,000 mg/L and BOD levels between 40,000 and 60,000 mg/L clearly show the elevated organic loading (Zandona et al., 2021). Its environmental impact includes eutrophication, acidification, salinization, and odor problems due to the direct dumping of such wastewater into water bodies. Literature showed that the dairy industry wastewater provides a nutrient-rich environment for the cultivation of *Ascochloris* sp., which may remove up to 95% of COD and produce a moderate amount of algal biomass (Kumar et al., 2019) (Zhu et al., 2019). *Ascochloris* sp. showed an 89.7% reduction of COD within 8 days and complete removal of total nitrogen, including nitrite and ammonia, within 6 days when the strain was cultured in non-sterilized dairy farm wastewater. In another study, Talapatra et al. (2023) reported that, in contrast to the axenic microalgal culture, the symbiotic growth of *Tetraselmis indica* and *Pseudomonas aeruginosa* in dairy wastewater produced 1454.88 mg/L of biomass, a 38.80% increase over that which would be obtained with pure culture. Such a consortium demonstrated removal efficiencies of 87.49%, 83.76%, and 79.83% for COD, TN, and TP, respectively. These results underscore the potential of the consortium for improved biomass growth, nutrient removal, and biofuel applications (Talapatra et al., 2023).

14.2.3 Fish and Meat Processing Wastewater

The wastewater generated from fish and meat processing, particularly in slaughterhouses, poses significant environmental problems because of the high levels of organic matter, nutrients, and pollutants such as total phosphorus (TP), total nitrogen (TN), and COD. For such effluents, phycoremediation has become a viable and efficient treatment technique. This biological process improves the economic viability by facilitating resource recovery in addition to assisting in the removal of nutrients (Kothari et al., 2024). Microalgae like *Botryococcus* sp. have shown great efficacy in eliminating nutrients such as phosphate (PO_4^{3-}) and ammonium (NH_4^+) with removal efficiency as high as 89.7% for NH_4^+ from meat processing wastewater. The research on the kinetic model has offered important insights into the particular pollutant removal rate (Abirama et al., 2021). Hassan et al. (2024) studied the efficacy of both *Chlorella vulgaris* and *Chlorogonium* species in the treatment of poultry slaughterhouse wastewater. The scientists reported that a significant amount of nitrate, phosphate, total dissolved solids (TDS), and BOD were removed from poultry slaughterhouse wastewater within a 21-day treatment period (Hassan et al., 2024). In another study, scientists used a 15% inoculum concentration to treat chicken slaughterhouse wastewater with *Chlorella vulgaris* Beijerinck. It was observed that TOC and BOD_5 were removed completely (100%) within 14 days, and COD, ammoniacal-N, and phosphate were removed $98.69 \pm 1.30\%$, $87.32 \pm 0.63\%$, and $88.81 \pm 0.56\%$, respectively, for the same time period (Sau et al., 2024).

14.2.4 Beverage Wastewater

The characterization of brewery wastewater has been reported to have a high moisture content and high organic strength, resulting in high COD and BOD values. The major organic components are sugars, solubilized starch, ethanol, and volatile fatty acids. Depending on the use of cleaning products containing caustic soda, phosphoric acid, and nitric acid, pH of the wastewater swings. Nitrogen (N) and phosphorus (P) concentrations are influenced by raw material handling and yeast content in the effluents (Amenorfenyo et al., 2019). Microalgae are highly effective for wastewater treatment processes because they have the capacity for high nutrient absorption and conversion into biomass. Microalgae can easily adsorb N, P, and some other nutritive elements during the treatment of brewery wastewater, which is favorable to the growth of microalgae and effectively diminishes contaminant concentration. Microalgae produce oxygen through photosynthesis, thereby facilitating the activity of bacteria in decomposing organic matter. Microalgae and cyanobacteria have demonstrated their potential in treating distillery wastewater (DWW). A notable example is *Chlamydomonas reinhardtii*, which was cultivated in anaerobically digested vinasse. Under these conditions, the culture eliminated approximately 84% of the residual contaminants, while the harvested biomass delivered an ethanol conversion yield of about 68%. Exposure to elevated chloride further triggered the alga to secrete extracellular polysaccharides (~120 mg L^{-1}), adding a valuable coproduct to the remediation process (Tasic et al., 2021). The concentration of carbon and nitrogen in vinasse strongly influences the microalgal remediation process. When *Geitlerinema* sp. was cultivated at a C/N ratio of 5%, the culture removed 71% of the total carbon in the wastewater, achieving a carbon-removal rate constant of around 0.045 h^{-1}, demonstrating efficient remediation alongside biomass production (Ravikumar et al., 2021). In another study, the efficiencies of the native bacterial composition in different microalgal strains (*C. reinhardtii, C. vulgaris*, and *S. obliquus*) were investigated for treating brewery wastewater. This algal–bacterial consortium achieved an 85% removal of COD,

More than 94% removal of total nitrogen, and above 80% removal of total phosphorus from the brewery wastewater (Su et al., 2022). The treatment of distillery or brewery wastewater using different microalgal or cyanobacterial strains, such as *Scenedesmus dimorphus*, *Nannochloropsis oceanica*, *Auxenochlorella pyrenoidosa*, *Arthrospira platensis*, *Schizochytrium limacinum* (Duan et al., 2018), *Ulva prolifera*, *Saccharina japonica*, *Zostera Marina,* and *Chlorella vulgaris,* was studied by various researchers (Amenorfenyo et al., 2019). They showed that the removal of COD, BOD, TN, TP, and other organic pollutants is taken by these microalgae, and later, this algal biomass can be processed into biofuel and other useful products (Amenorfenyo et al., 2019).

14.3 Effective Microalgal Strains for Treatment of Food and Agro-Food Processing Wastewater

The application of phycoremediation for treating food processing wastewaters is an emerging area. Dairy whey water, brewery effluent, fruit and vegetable wash water, starch liquors, and distillery vinasse are among such wastewater. Microalgal species that have shown consistently high removal efficiencies include *Chlorella* sp., *Scenedesmus* sp., *Chlamydomonas* sp., *Spirulina* sp., etc. When cultivated in such effluents, these microalgae can effectively remove COD, TN, and total phosphorus. They also fix CO_2 through photosynthesis and produce value-added products, such as proteins, pigments, and lipids. The approach, therefore, supports both environmental compliance and circular-economy objectives by converting pollutants into marketable algal products. However, other microalgal or cyanobacterial species rich in high-value bioactive compounds have also demonstrated strong capacities for wastewater treatment, making them equally promising candidates for integrated biorefinery applications. Some recent studies on microalgae-based treatment of food and agro-food processing effluents are shown in Table 14.1.

14.3.1 Application of *Chlorella* sp. for Treatment of Food and Agro-Food Processing Wastewater

Chlorella sp. has been found to be a promising agent for treating various effluents, including nejayote (wastewater generated during conventional methods for producing corn tortilla flour), cheese whey, and vinasse. Research on the bioremediation capabilities of the species underscores the importance of medium composition. In a study, the combination of 25% nejayote, 25% swine wastewater, and 50% water showed removal of 90% nitrogen, 80% phosphorus, and 96% COD by *Chlorella vulgaris* (López-Pacheco et al., 2019). For the treatment of chicken-slaughterhouse wastewater, a phycoremediation strategy using *Chlorella vulgaris* resulted in almost complete elimination of total organic carbon and BOD_5, as well as a very high reduction in COD, ammoniacal nitrogen, and phosphate. Such results demonstrate that microalgal treatment can provide an exceptionally effective, single-step

Table 14.1 Recent studies on microalgae-based treatment of food and agro-food processing effluents

Wastewater	Microalgal strain	Pollutant removal (%)			Reference
		COD	N	P	
Vinasse	*Chlorella vulgaris*	–	66.33 ± 3.32	93.77 ± 4.69	Jasmin Nivetha et al. (2019)
Glucose recovered from enzymatic hydrolysis of food waste	*Chlorella* sp.	–	–	–	Wang et al. (2020)
Piggery wastewater	C. *vulgaris*	–	100	100	Molinuevo-Salces et al. (2016)
Tequila vinasses	*Chlorella* sp.	74 ± 4.9	97.8 ± 1.3	35.6 ± 7.4	Choix et al. (2021)
Tequila vinasses	*Chlorella vulgaris* U162	–	–	–	Choix et al. (2018)
Dairy wastewater	*Chlorella vulgaris* Beijerinck	59.7 ± 1.23	55.4 ± 0.49	69.6 ± 2.69	Zaky et al. (2019)
Swine Wastewater	*Chlorella vulgaris*	96	91	85	López-Pacheco et al. (2019)
Aquaculture wastewater	*Scenedesmus obliquus*	42	88.7	100	Ansari et al. (2017)
Molasses wastewater	*Scenedesmus* sp. Z-4	87.2	90.5	88.6	Ma et al. (2017)
Diary Effluent	*Scenedesmus* sp. ASK22	90.5	100	91.24	Pandey et al. (2019)
Municipal wastewater	*Scenedesmus obliquus*	71.2 ± 3.5	100	94.1 ± 4.7	Ansari et al. (2019)
Diary wastewater	*Chlamydomonas debaryana* IITRIND3	78.57	87.56	82.17	Arora et al. (2016)
Palm oil mill effluent	*Chlamydomonas* sp. UKM 6	29.13	72.9	63.53	Ding et al. (2016)
Paper and pulp mill effluent	*Chlamydomonas reinhardtii*	93	86	88	Sasi et al. (2020)
Tequila vinasses	*Chlamydomonas* sp.	69 ± 4.80	98.1 ± 0.5	38.8 ± 2.60	Choix et al. (2021)
Brewery effluent	*Spirulina* sp.	75.2	78.3	97.4	Lu et al. (2017)
10% nejayote + 90% water	*Spirulina maxima*	81	88	–	López-Pacheco et al. (2019)
25% nejayote + 25% swine wastewater + 50% water	*Spirulina maxima*	84	87	75	López-Pacheco et al. (2019)
5% cheese whey + 95% Zarrouk medium	*Spirulina platensis*	–	–	–	Pereira et al. (2019)
Soy sauce wastewater	*Spirulina maxima*	84.08	81.76		Han et al. (2021)
Aquaculture wastewater	*Spirulina* sp. LEB 18	90	–	93.84	Cardoso et al. (2021)

approach for polishing high-strength abattoir effluents (Sau et al., 2024). Despite its effectiveness, the challenge of cultivating microalgae solely in untreated effluents persists. However, studies showed that treatment of whey (50%, diluted with tap water) using *Chlorella vulgaris* promotes an increased production of biomass, as well as a higher level of chlorophyll a and lipid content (Zaky et al., 2019). This implies that optimization of effluent concentration is another critical factor for upscaling bioremediation procedures while conserving freshwater resources. For the treatment of food-processing effluents using C. *vulgaris*, pre-treatment enhances outcomes highly. For example, the use of filtered vinasse was observed to increase biomass yield, CO_2 uptake level, and accumulation of carbohydrates and proteins as compared to the synthetic media (Choix et al., 2018). This emphasizes the need for effluent conditioning to ensure that the microalgae have a maximum remedial potential.

14.3.2 Application of *Scenedesmus* sp. for Treatment of Food and Agro-Food Processing Wastewater

Scenedesmus sp. has demonstrated significant potential for treating highly polluted effluents, such as dairy wastewater and vinasse. When *Scenedesmus* sp. was cultivated in pretreated vinasse under a mixotrophic environment with constant light, it became highly efficient for removing nitrogen (N), phosphorus (P), and COD (Choix et al., 2021). In comparison to heterotrophic cultures, this method enhances biomass yield while increasing protein content and improving nutrient removal efficiency. Ansari et al., (2017) showed that *Scenedesmus obliquus* grew well in aquaculture effluent and effectively removed contaminants like ammonia, nitrate, phosphate, and COD. Supplementing with sodium nitrate could maximize biomass production and enhance nutrient absorption, thereby increasing protein, carbohydrate, and lipid productivity to levels comparable to those achieved in synthetic media. This procedure made *Scenedesmus obliquus* an ideal biological agent for both wastewater treatment and resource recovery, since it enhanced pollutant removal while promoting sustainable biomass production (Ansari et al., 2017). With its ability to effectively absorb nutrients and reduce pollutants from various industrial effluents, Scenedesmus sp. remains a promising choice for wastewater treatment. The operating parameters could be optimized for large-scale treatment by enhancing culture conditions and reducing freshwater dependency.

14.3.3 Application of *Chlamydomonas* sp. for Treatment of Food and Agro-Food Processing Wastewater

Chlamydomonas sp. has emerged as a multipurpose species that produces useful metabolites while simultaneously polishing nutrient-rich wastewaters. Mixotrophic cultures demonstrated endurance in tough agro-industrial effluent by removing 98% of nitrogen, 69% of COD, and 38% of phosphorus while attaining cell densities above 4 × 10^7 cells mL^{-1} in tequila-vinasse effluents (Choix et al., 2021). Application of *Chlamydomonas* sp. is positioned as an effective, low-energy polishing step because comparative studies with municipal and food-processing effluents showed ~90% BOD reduction and a significant decrease in COD and total nitrogen (Bellido-Pedraza et al., 2024). Another study with *Chlamydomonas debaryana* IITRIND3 highlighted its capacity to clean multiple effluent streams, such as, domestic, municipal sewage, paper-mill, and dairy. Biomass was used for lipid extraction for biodiesel production. Cultivation of such a strain in dairy wastewater proved most favorable, yielding a lipid productivity of 87.5 ± 2.3 mg L^{-1} day^{-1} while simultaneously removing 87.56% of total nitrogen, 82.17% of total phosphorus, 78.57% of COD, and 85.97% of total organic carbon. These results confirmed the credibility of *Chlamydomonas* sp. as a strong candidate for integrated wastewater remediation and biofuel generation (Arora et al., 2016).

14.3.4 Application of *Spirulina* sp. for Treatment of Food and Agro-Food Processing Wastewater

Spirulina sp., a versatile cyanobacterium with a high protein content, is already used in the production of various products in the cosmetic, food supplement, and pharmaceutical industries. Beyond these commercial uses, *Spirulina* sp. is highly efficient in treating wastewater from the food processing sector. In a study, *Spirulina platensis* was grown on Zarrouk medium supplemented with 0–10% cheese whey. The highest biomass (2.98 g L^{-1}) and carbohydrate fraction (40.83%) were obtained with a 5% addition of whey (Pereira et al., 2019). High COD indicates a high organic load in wastewater generated during the conversion of cassava to tapioca. The direct cultivation of *Spirulina platensis* in this effluent provides a useful polishing step, as this strain absorbs nutrients and soluble organics, resulting in a significant removal of COD from the produced tapioca wastewater while producing biomass (55.4 ± 6.4 mg L^{-1} day^{-1}) simultaneously. The findings highlighted *S. platensis* as a useful biological agent for lowering organic pollution in effluents from cassava processing industry (Hadiyanto et al., 2023). As culture media for *Spirulina maxima*, López-Pacheco et al. (2019) studied various dilutions of swine wastewater and nejayote (a corn-processing effluent). By day 12, the formulation with 10% nejayote diluted with 90% tap water had the fastest and highest biomass, with around 3.2 × 10^5 cells mL^{-1}. Only after 18 days did they do a second blend, consisting of 25% swine effluent, 25% nejayote, and 50% water. Although *Spirulina* sp. removed more phosphorus (75%) and achieved the highest removal in COD (84%) from the swine–nejayote mixture, the 10% nejayote broth was superior for nitrogen abatement, where around 88% of total nitrogen was removed (López-Pacheco et al., 2019). These microalgal species have demonstrated efficacy in eliminating pollutants from wastewater from the food and agro-food processing sector. Their ability to absorb excess nutrients and other contaminants enables them to flourish in a variety of effluent compositions, thereby lowering key pollutant parameters, including COD, nitrogen, and phosphorus, while producing valuable algal biomass. They are flexible options for large-scale treatment systems due to their ability to withstand changes in pH, salinity, and organic load. However, further research on long-term stability, ideal working conditions, and integration with existing treatment infrastructure is still needed. A comparative table (Table 14.2) summarizes the growth conditions and biomass yield under standard conditions for different microalgal strains used for the treatment of food and agro-food processing wastewater.

14.4 Value-Added Metabolites from Microalgal Biomass

Microalgae are rich in high-value chemicals that have a wide range of applications in different industries. They generate bioactive metabolites that are used in food items, medicines, cosmetics, and nutraceuticals, including carotenoids (lutein, β-carotene, and astaxanthin), polyunsaturated fatty acids, mycosporine-like amino acids, phycobiliproteins (like phycocyanin), and exopolysaccharides. To support sustainable energy solutions, microalgae can also be utilized to produce green energy sources, such as biodiesel and bioethanol. These qualities make microalgae attractive options for achieving a circular bioeconomy. Phycobiliproteins are water-soluble light-harvesting pigment proteins present in phycobilisomes of cyanobacteria and red algae. Phycocyanin, a blue phycobiliprotein, absorbs green and orange light, aiding in photosynthesis, offering antioxidant and nutraceutical value, and serving as a fluorescent food and cosmetic colorant. Phycocyanin has several health advantages, such as anticancer, anti-inflammatory, antidiabetic, antioxidant, and immunoregulatory (Wan et al., 2021). *Spirulina maxima* and *Spirulina platensis* can be effectively produced on an industrial scale to produce phycobiliproteins. Lower light intensities can increase the production of phycobiliproteins because microalgae need more of these substances to efficiently capture light (Chaiklahan et al., 2022).

Carotenoids are lipid-soluble pigments that are produced by photosynthetic organisms and have two functions. They help them to absorb light and protect themselves from it. Because of their oxygen concentration, they are structurally classified as more polar xanthophylls and nonpolar carotenes (Sun et al., 2020). Among the economically significant carotenoids, fucoxanthin contributes special bioactive properties, astaxanthin acts as a red antioxidant barrier against UV rays, and β-carotene, an orange pigment, is a vital vitamin A precursor that is commonly produced by microalgae. H. *pluvialis* is the main microalgal source for the production of astaxanthin (Ma et al., 2020). The genera like *Scenedesmus* and *Haematococcus* are important industrial sources in the *Chlorophyceae* (Casella Patrizia et al., 2019). Under high-light stress, lutein, a yellow xanthophyll, builds up to aid microalgae in adjusting to changing lighting conditions (Zheng et al., 2022). The researchers demonstrated that microalgal or cyanobacterial species like as *C. vulgaris*, *S. platensis*, *S. maxima*, *Chlamydomonas* sp., *Scenedesmus* sp., and *H. pluvialis* can efficiently synthesize carotenoids from their biomass. Numerous health benefits are associated with these carotenoids, including antioxidant,

Table 14.2 Summary of growth parameters and biomass yield of microalgae used for food and agro-food processing wastewater treatment

Microalgal strain	Growth conditions	Amount of biomass (in growth medium)	Wastewater	Amount of biomass (in wastewater)	Reference
Chlorella vulgaris	At 23 ± 2 °C temperature for 15 days	4.16 ± 0.21 g/L	Vinasse	6.85 ± 0.34 g/L	Jasmin Nivetha et al. (2019)
Chlorella sp. GY-H4	At 21 ± 0.5 °C temperature, illumination was provided at 120μmol photons m^{-2} s^{-1} with a light:dark cycle of 12 h:12 h		Glucose recovered from enzymatic hydrolysis of food waste	6.9 g/L	Wang et al. (2020)
Chlorella vulgaris U162	At 27 ± 2 °C, 200μmol photons m^{-2} s^{-1}, with stirring at 120 rpm for 14 days		Tequila vinasses	2.22 ± 0.26 g/L	Choix et al. (2018)
Chlorella vulgaris Beijerinck	At 25 ± 2 °C and 40.5μE m^{-2} S^{-1} for 14 days	406.10 ± 18.75 mg/L	Dairy wastewater	405.23 ± 7.12 mg/L	Zaky et al. (2019)
Scenedesmus obliquus	At 25 °C with Illumination conditions at 120μmol photons m^{-2} S^{-1} with a light: dark cycle of 16 h:8 h	1.30 ± 0.05 g/L	Aquaculture wastewater	0.88 ± 0.04 g/L	Ansari et al. (2019)
Scenedesmus sp. Z-4	At 25 °C under white fluorescent light with 3000 lux with a light:dark cycle of 12 h:12 h	3.4 g/L	Molasses wastewater	2.9 g/L	Ma et al. (2017)
Scenedesmus obliquus U169	At 27 ± 2 °C, 200μmol photons m^{-2} S^{-1}, with stirring at 120 rpm for 14 days		Tequila vinasses	1.84 ± 0.07 g/L	Choix et al. (2018)
Chlamydomonas debaryana IITRIND3	At 27 °C and 140 rpm with L/D cycle of 16:8-h white light illumination (200 mmol m^{-1} S^{-1})		Diary wastewater	3.66 ± 0.21 g/L	Arora et al. (2016)

Chlamydomonas sp. UKM 6	At 25 ± 1 °C with illumination at 4000 lux (light/dark period: 12:12) and 0.5 vvm of air sparging		Palm oil mill effluent	0.917 ± 0.026 g/L	Ding et al. (2016)
Spirulina sp.	At 28 °C with a rotating speed of 200 rpm and with continuous fluorescent light (300µmol photon m^{-2} S^{-1})		Brewery effluent	0.925 g/L	Lu et al. (2017)
Spirulina maxima	at 30 ± 1 °C with 50µmol photons m^{-2} S^{-1}	2.451 g/L	Soy sauce wastewater	1.984 g/L	Han et al. (2021)

pro-vitamin A, anticancer, cardiovascular disease prevention, decreased metabolic syndrome, and immunomodulatory properties (Yuan et al., 2021; Akepach et al., 2022).

Polyunsaturated fatty acids (PUFAs) have more than two carbon–carbon double bonds and accumulate as lipid droplets in microalgae, protecting metabolic energy during environmental stressors such as intense UV, nutrient starvation, or extreme temperatures. The omega-3 series is a well-known PUFA subgroup, with its last double bond located three carbons away from the methyl terminus. Eicosapentaenoic acid (EPA) and docosahexaenoic acid (DHA) are two examples of omega-3 members that are biologically valuable. These EPA and DHA contribute to different health benefits in the human body, development of retina, brain, and nervous system, prevention of cardiovascular problems, anti-inflammatory, anticancer, etc. (Djuricic & Calder, 2021). *Scenedesmus* sp. are known for producing a high concentration of EPA, subsequently most microalgae and even *Haematococcus pluvialis* (Batista et al., 2013). Traditionally, DHA is obtained from fish, but can also be extracted directly from microalgae; for example, the cyanobacteria *Spirulina platensis* can accumulate up to 44.47 mg g^{1} of DHA, providing a sustainable substitute source (El-Sheekh et al., 2024).

Biodiesel, which is mainly fatty acid methyl esters (FAME), is produced from the trans-esterification of triglycerides (TAG). Microalgae store TAG in specialized lipid bodies, and when exposed to stressors like intense light, nitrogen starvation, high salinity, or extremely high temperatures, some green strains, including *Chlorella vulgaris*, *Haematococcus pluvialis*, and *Chlamydomonas* sp., can channel over 50% of their biomass into TAG. These circumstances are due to lipid buildup that can subsequently be transformed into FAME by slowing cell division. The main components of biodiesel, a nontoxic, biodegradable fuel with performance comparable to petroleum diesel and applications requiring little engine modification, are fatty acid methyl esters (FAMEs) (Suastes-Rivas et al., 2020). Saleh (2022) showed the high potential of *Chlorella sorokiniana* in the treatment of secondary-treated slaughterhouse effluent and for the production of biodiesel feedstock. After the incubation period, the culture exhibited high lipid productivity of 48.36 mg L^{1}, evidencing benefits both for environmental remediation as well as renewable energy production (Saleh, 2022). Esters made from palmitic, oleic, linoleic, and stearic acids are particularly prized due to their resistance to oxidative degradation, which ensures stable, high-quality biodiesel. Microalgae provide FAMEs by trans-esterifying their stored triglycerides (Pérez et al., 2021). Glycogen (a glucose reserve), cellulose (a cell-wall structural polysaccharide), and microalgal starch are valuable sources of bioethanol. Species like *Chlorella*, *Chlamydomonas*, and *Scenedesmus* are excellent candidates for carbohydrate-driven biofuel production because they can devote up to 50% of their dry weight to these carbohydrates when cultivated in conditions of high light, mesophilic temperatures, and nitrogen starvation (De Farias Silva & Bertucco, 2016). Table 14.3 illustrates the production of different value-added products using microalgal species when they were used for the treatment of food and agro-food processing industries' wastewater.

14.5 Life Cycle and Environmental Impact for Microalgae Bioremediation

A vast amount of wastewater is produced by industrial processes, and the release of untreated wastewater into water bodies can cause significant damage to the aquatic ecosystem. The majority of nations have rigorous policies requiring industries to treat their wastewater before disposing of it. In the past, the industry has adopted various procedures, including adsorption, ion exchange, chemical precipitation, oxidation, reverse osmosis, and electrochemical processes. Although successful, these techniques are expensive, especially when activated carbon is used in adsorption, and in cases of chemical oxidation, resistant intermediates are produced (Crini et al., 2019). In life cycle terms, wastewater treatment using microalgal strains offers significant ecological and operational benefits compared to conventional technologies (Table 14.4). It has lower energy demand, produces no sludge, and has some apparent reliance on chemical supplements, resulting in lower overhead expenses and subsequent environmental benefits. Moreover, nutrient recovery is naturally coupled to CO_2 fixing by microalgal cultivation, where nitrogen and phosphorus-rich effluents are converted into biofuel, pigments, proteins, and other value-added products (Rahman et al., 2020). This type of integration aligns well with the principles of the circular bioeconomy, as outlined in Table 14.1, by cultivating *Chlorella vulgaris* with 100% of food and beverage-manufacturing effluents, including nejayote, cheese whey, and tequila vinasses, without the need for freshwater dilution. Some systems achieve total removal of nitrogen and phosphorus. Together, these properties make the microalgal-based wastewater treatment process a viable option that is both environmentally sustainable and economically perceptible, and can meet the objectives of both environmental water quality and resource recovery in terms of food and agro-food industry wastewater treatment.

14.6 Challenges in Microalgal Bioremediation of Food and Agro-Food Processing Wastewater

Microalgae-assisted bioremediation offers numerous benefits; however, various bottlenecks must be addressed to make the phycoremediation process a viable treatment option. One of the major constraints of this bioremediation is that effluents from food and agro-food processing industries often contain significant levels of complex organic load. Microalgae struggle to metabolize that complex organic load, which results in lower growth of microalgae and bioremediation efficiency. Microalgal growth in this complex wastewater can be improved by the acclimatization method. In this method, microalgal strains are gradually adapted to increasing effluent concentrations, hence improving growth and biomass quality. Another method is co-culturing microalgae with bacteria or fungi, which promotes synergistic exchanges, where oxygen from microalgae supports heterotrophs. This increases biomass yield and nutrient removal efficiency in food and agro-food wastewater treatment (Abdelfattah et al., 2023). Another constraint of this

Table 14.3 Summary of value-added products obtained during phycotreatment of food and agro-food processing industries wastewater

Microalgal strain	Food and agro-food processing industries wastewater	Value-added products	Amount of value added products	Reference
Chlorella sp. GY-H4	Glucose recovered from the enzymatic hydrolysis of food waste.	Lutein	63 (mg/L)	Wang et al. (2020)
		Lipid	1.8 (mg/L)	
Chlorella vulgaris Beijerinck	Dairy wastewater	Lipid	80.90 ± 1.83 (mg/L)	Zaky et al. (2019)
Chlorella sorokiniana	Slaughterhouse wastewater	Lipid	48.37 ± 5.44 (mg/L)	
		Carotenoid	5.32 (mg/dry weight)	
		Chlorophyll-a	10.35 (mg/dry weight)	
		Chlorophyll-b	12.29 (mg/dry weight)	
Scenedesmus sp. Z-4	Molasses wastewater	Lipid	92.3 (mg/L)	Ma et al. (2017)
Chlamydomonas debaryana IITRIND3	Diary wastewater	FAME profile		Arora et al. (2016)
		Palmitic acid	15.36 ± 0.05 (%)	
		7,10-Hexadecadienoic acid methyl ester	2.78 ± 0.14 (%)	
		Stearic acid	6.37 ± 0.03 (%)	
		Oleic acid	37.11 ± 1.7 (%)	
		Linoleic acid	12.86 ± 0.6 (%)	
Spirulina maxima	Soy sauce wastewater	Protein	50.92 ± 1.09 (%)	Han et al. (2021)
		Chlorophyll-a	10.99 ± 0.60 (mg/g)	
		Carotenoid	3.11 ± 0.22 (mg/g)	
Spirulina (Arthrospira) platensis	Aquaculture wastewater	Phycobiliproteins (Phycocyanin)	101.95 ± 1.49 (mg/g)	Kumari et al. (2023)

Table 14.4 Ecological/operational benefits of using microalgae-based wastewater treatment technique

Aspect	Microalgae-based wastewater treatment	Conventional wastewater treatment	Ecological/operational benefit of microalgae-based wastewater treatment
Energy demand	Low (light-driven and passive aeration possible)	High (aeration and mechanical processes)	Reduced operational costs and carbon footprint
Sludge generation	Minimal	High	Lower sludge disposal cost and environmental burden
Chemical usage	Low or none	High (coagulants, flocculants, disinfectants)	Avoids secondary pollution and chemical procurement
CO_2 management	Direct fixation during growth	No CO_2 capture	Mitigates greenhouse gas emissions
Nutrient recovery	Converts N and P into biomass	Nutrients are removed as waste.	Enables resource recovery and circular economy integration
Biomass valorization	Biofuels, pigments, proteins, and bioactive compounds	Limited or no biomass utilization	Generates additional revenue streams
Scalability & adaptability	Enhanced via acclimatization, UV mutagenesis, and immobilized systems	Often rigid to influent variability	Stable performance under variable wastewater composition

wastewater treatment is that the effluent of various industries is dark in color, which inhibits light penetration and reduces photosynthesis and growth of the microalgae. This is a common issue in food and agro-food processing effluents, where microalgal growth is reduced due to excessive color intensity and suspended particles. Some targeted pre-treatments, such as filtration and adsorption with activated charcoal, can address these barriers without the need for dilution. These techniques improve light availability, microalgal growth, and the overall efficiency of the treatment of wastewater (Choix et al., 2021). Harvesting of microalgal biomass is another challenge in this treatment method. After wastewater treatment, the efficient separation and purification of harvested algal biomass are generally expensive and energy-intensive processes. Integration of a multiproduct biorefinery within a circular economy framework offers a solution to this challenge. It enables the entire biomass to be converted into various value-added products, including food, cosmetics, and medicinal purposes, as well as biofuels. This technique can balance operational costs, improve economic feasibility, and transform wastewater treatment into a long-term, value-generating process (Ahmed et al., 2022). Another important challenge for scaling up this microalgal bioremediation is the strong influence of environmental variables on the growth of the microalgae, pollutant removal, and productivity of biomass. Sometimes, laboratory research yields positive and feasible outcomes, but real-world systems encounter hurdles due to temperature and light changes. Low temperatures and insufficient light can impede the metabolic activity of microalgae, slowing growth rates, nutrient intake, and the production of value-added components. These consequences are particularly significant in regions where the weather fluctuates seasonally or daily. A detailed understanding of these parameters and making strategies to stabilize them is essential for increasing biomass yield. It also ensures consistent and efficient wastewater treatment (Abdelfattah et al., 2023).

14.7 Conclusion and Future Perspectives

The treatment of wastewater from food and agro-food industries using microalgae-based biorefineries represents a highly promising approach when integrated into a circular bioeconomy framework. Although they may be promising, there are several challenging factors that hinder their widespread application. One of their greatest drawbacks is the necessity to dilute wastewater with freshwater or synthetic media to provide enough conditions for microalgae to grow. Besides raising the cost of operating, it also uses large amounts of freshwater, which is already in short supply in most areas. To sustain the scale-up of this technology, it is thus critical to mitigate the requirement for dilution. Various strategies, such as UV mutagenesis or acclimatization, can produce microalgal strains that can survive in higher pollutant concentrations and more severe physicochemical conditions. Mutation breeding programs have yielded high-performance strains of *Chlorella* with enhanced resistance to salinity and nutrient shock, enabling them to grow in industrial effluents without dilution. Suitable combinations have also been demonstrated to improve tolerance and nutrient removal by co-culturing, i.e., microalgae with bacteria or fungi co-culture systems. In addition, the immobilized algal growth technology, such as the one where cells are embedded in matrices, i.e., alginate beads, offers operational robustness, enhanced biomass harvesting, and the ability to grow cells at higher cell densities in wastewater with low nutrient content. Such immobilized systems are being tested on a pilot scale in industrial effluents. It has been demonstrated to perform with encouraging efficiency in nutrient removal and has been noted to exhibit stability under various operating conditions. The recovery of the value-added compounds from algal biomass using downstream processing is equally important. The conventional processes of extraction typically use organic solvents, which have environmental impact and safety concerns, and this compromises the sustainability of the operation. Green extraction methods, such as microwave-assisted extraction, ultrasound-assisted extraction (UAE), pulsed electric fields (PEF), supercritical fluid extraction (SFE), and high-pressure homogenization, offer eco-friendly alternatives to achieve the target extraction levels. Lastly, the multifunctional version of mixed-culture systems, in which several species of microalgae, bacteria, or fungi are cultured together, provides the possibility of enhanced performance in pollutant removal as well as a broader range of product offerings. It means that each organism can provide a different metabolic capacity, allowing the synthesis of a wide range of value-added compounds, such as pigments, lipids, proteins, and bioactive molecules, in higher amounts. By integrating strong cultivation strategies, genomic breeding, environmentally friendly downstream processing, and mixed-species cultivation, microalgae biorefineries have the potential to become sustainable and economically feasible alternatives to the large-scale treatment of wastewater from the food and agro-food industries.

References

Abdelfattah, A., Ali, S. S., Ramadan, H., El-Aswar, E. I., Eltawab, R., Ho, S.-H., Elsamahy, T., Li, S., El-Sheekh, M. M., Schagerl, M., Kornaros, M., & Sun, J. (2023). Microalgae-based wastewater treatment: Mechanisms, challenges, recent advances, and future prospects. *Environmental Science and Ecotechnology, 13*, 100205. https://doi.org/10.1016/j.ese.2022.100205

Abedi, S., Astaraei, F. R., Ghobadian, B., Tavakoli, O., Jalili, H., Greenwell, H. C., Cummins, I., & Chivasa, S. (2019). Decoupling a novel Trichormus variabilis-Synechocystis sp. Interaction to boost phycoremediation. *Scientific Reports, 9*(1), 2511. https://doi.org/10.1038/s41598-019-38997-7

Abirama, V., Mohamed, R. M. S. R., Al-Gheethi, A., Abdul Malek, M., & Kassim, A. H. M. (2021). Meat processing wastewater Phycoremediation by *Botryococcus* sp.: A biokinetic study and a techno-economic analysis. *Separation Science and Technology, 56*(3), 577–591. https://doi.org/10.1080/01496395.2020.1718708

Agrawal, V., Achari, M., Kharade, S., Vadaliya, K., Karkar, M., & Sarode, D. (2023). Understanding the operations of the indian dairy industry – A case study. *Bhartiya Krishi Anusandhan Patrika*. https://doi.org/10.18805/BKAP619

Ahmed, S. F., Mofijur, M., Parisa, T. A., Islam, N., Kusumo, F., Inayat, A., Le, V. G., Badruddin, I. A., Khan, T. M. Y., & Ong, H. C. (2022). Progress and challenges of contaminate removal from wastewater using microalgae biomass. *Chemosphere, 286*, 131656. https://doi.org/10.1016/j.chemosphere.2021.131656

Akepach, P., Ribeiro-Filho, N., Wattanakul, J., Darwish, R., Gedi, M. A., & Gray, D. A. (2022). Bioaccessibility of carotenoids (β-carotene and lutein) from intact and disrupted microalgae (Chlamydomonas reinhardtii). *LWT, 160*, 113292. https://doi.org/10.1016/j.lwt.2022.113292

Amenorfenyo, D. K., Huang, X., Zhang, Y., Zeng, Q., Zhang, N., Ren, J., & Huang, Q. (2019). Microalgae brewery wastewater treatment: Potentials, benefits and the challenges. *International Journal of Environmental Research and Public Health, 16*(11), 1910. https://doi.org/10.3390/ijerph16111910

Amit, D., Ghosh, U. K., Nigam, P. S., & Jaiswal, A. K. (2021). Food industries wastewater recycling for biodiesel production through microalgal remediation. *Sustainability, 13*(15), 8267. https://doi.org/10.3390/su13158267

Ansari, F. A., Singh, P., Guldhe, A., & Bux, F. (2017). Microalgal cultivation using aquaculture wastewater: Integrated biomass generation and nutrient remediation. *Algal Research, 21*, 169–177. https://doi.org/10.1016/j.algal.2016.11.015

Ansari, F. A., Ravindran, B., Gupta, S. K., Nasr, M., Rawat, I., & Bux, F. (2019). Techno-economic estimation of wastewater phycoremediation and environmental benefits using Scenedesmus obliquus microalgae. *Journal of Environmental Management, 240*, 293–302. https://doi.org/10.1016/j.jenvman.2019.03.123

Arora, N., Patel, A., Sartaj, K., Pruthi, P. A., & Pruthi, V. (2016). Bioremediation of domestic and industrial wastewaters integrated with enhanced biodiesel production using novel oleaginous microalgae. *Environmental Science and Pollution Research, 23*(20), 20997–21007. https://doi.org/10.1007/s11356-016-7320-y

Batista, A. P., Gouveia, L., Bandarra, N. M., Franco, J. M., & Raymundo, A. (2013). Comparison of microalgal biomass profiles as novel functional ingredient for food products. *Algal Research, 2*(2), 164–173. https://doi.org/10.1016/j.algal.2013.01.004

Bellido-Pedraza, C. M., Torres, M. J., & Llamas, A. (2024). The microalgae Chlamydomonas for bioremediation and bioproduct production. *Cells, 13*(13), 1137. https://doi.org/10.3390/cells13131137

Cardoso, L. G., Duarte, J. H., Costa, J. A. V., De Jesus Assis, D., Lemos, P. V. F., Druzian, J. I., De Souza, C. O., Nunes, I. L., & Chinalia, F. A. (2021). Spirulina sp. as a bioremediation agent for aquaculture wastewater: Production of high added value compounds and estimation of theoretical biodiesel. *BioEnergy Research, 14*(1), 254–264. https://doi.org/10.1007/s12155-020-10153-4

Chaiklahan, R., Chirasuwan, N., Srinorasing, T., Attasat, S., Nopharatana, A., & Bunnag, B. (2022). Enhanced biomass and phycocyanin production of Arthrospira (Spirulina) platensis by a cultivation management strategy: Light intensity and cell concentration. *Bioresource Technology, 343*, 126077. https://doi.org/10.1016/j.biortech.2021.126077

Challa, M., Dash, R. R., & Behera, M. (2024). A review on treatment of rice mill wastewater with emphasis on biological technologies. *International Biodeterioration & Biodegradation, 195*, 105895. https://doi.org/10.1016/j.ibiod.2024.105895

Choix, F. J., Ochoa-Becerra, M. A., Hsieh-Lo, M., Mondragón-Cortez, P., & Méndez-Acosta, H. O. (2018). High biomass production and CO2 fixation from biogas by Chlorella and Scenedesmus microalgae using tequila vinasses as culture medium. *Journal of Applied Phycology, 30*(4), 2247–2258. https://doi.org/10.1007/s10811-018-1433-2.

Choix, F. J., Ramos-Ibarra, J. R., Mondragón-Cortez, P., Lara-González, M. A., Juárez-Carrillo, E., Becerril-Espinosa, A., Ocampo-Alvarez, H., & Torres, J. R. (2021). Mixotrophic growth regime as a strategy to develop microalgal bioprocess from nutrimental composition of tequila vinasses. *Bioprocess and Biosystems Engineering, 44*(6), 1155–1166. https://doi.org/10.1007/s00449-021-02512-y

Crini, G., & Lichtfouse, E. (2019). Advantages and disadvantages of techniques used for wastewater treatment. *Environmental Chemistry Letters, 17*(1), 145–155. https://doi.org/10.1007/s10311-018-0785-9

De Farias Silva, C. E., & Bertucco, A. (2016). Bioethanol from microalgae and cyanobacteria: A review and technological outlook. *Process Biochemistry, 51*(11), 1833–1842. https://doi.org/10.1016/j.procbio.2016.02.016

Ding, G. T., Yaakob, Z., Takriff, M. S., Salihon, J., & Abd Rahaman, M. S. (2016). Biomass production and nutrients removal by a newly-isolated microalgal strain Chlamydomonas sp in palm oil mill effluent (POME). *International Journal of Hydrogen Energy, 41*(8), 4888–4895. https://doi.org/10.1016/j.ijhydene.2015.12.010

Djuricic, I., & Calder, P. C. (2021). Beneficial outcomes of Omega-6 and Omega-3 polyunsaturated fatty acids on human health: An update for 2021. *Nutrients, 13*(7), 2421. https://doi.org/10.3390/nu13072421

Duan, P.-G., Yang, S.-K., Xu, Y.-P., Wang, F., Zhao, D., Weng, Y.-J., & Shi, X.-L. (2018). Integration of hydrothermal liquefaction and supercritical water gasification for improvement of energy recovery from algal biomass. *Energy, 155*, 734–745. https://doi.org/10.1016/j.energy.2018.05.044

El-Sheekh, M. M., Salman, J. M., Grmasha, R. A., Abdul-Adel, E., Saleh, M. M., & Al-sareji, O. J. (2024). Influence of Fe+2 on the biomass, pigments, and essential fatty acids of Arthrospira platensis. *Biomass Conversion and Biorefinery, 14*(1), 621–629. https://doi.org/10.1007/s13399-022-02470-9

Gonçalves, B. (2021). Análise de viabilidade da produção de biomassa microalgal utilizando diferentes efluentes como meio de cultivo.

Hadiyanto, H., Christwardana, M., & Da Costa, C. (2023). Electrogenic and biomass production capabilities of a Microalgae–Microbial fuel cell (MMFC) system using tapioca wastewater and *Spirulina platensis* for COD reduction. *Energy Sources, Part A: Recovery, Utilization, and Environmental Effects, 45*(2), 3409–3420. https://doi.org/10.1080/15567036.2019.1668085

Han, P., Lu, Q., Zhong, H., Xie, J., Leng, L., Li, J., Fan, L., Li, J., Chen, P., Yan, Y., Wei, F., & Zhou, W. (2021). Recycling nutrients from soy sauce wastewater to culture value-added Spirulina maxima. *Algal Research, 53*, 102157. https://doi.org/10.1016/j.algal.2020.102157

Hassan, M. A., Adamu, N., Moi, I. M., Mohammad, A., & Abubakar, B. M. (2024). *Phycoremediation efficacy of different microalgae species in treating poultry slaughterhouse wastewater in Bauchi Local Government Area, Bauchi State, Nigeria.*

Jasmin Nivetha, B., Bhakyalakshmi, S. V., Dinesh Kumar, S., Santhanam, P., Vijayalakshmi, D., Divya, M., & Krishnaveni, N. (2019). Utilization of sugarcane industry effluent for high value biomass and photosynthetic pigments production of Chlorella vulgaris (PSBDU06). *Bioresource Technology Reports, 7*, 100260. https://doi.org/10.1016/j.biteb.2019.100260

Kolev Slavov, A. (2017). Dairy wastewaters – General characteristics and treatment possibilities – A review. *Food Technology and Biotechnology, 55*(1). https://doi.org/10.17113/ftb.55.01.17.4520

Kothari, R., Azam, R., Bharti, A., Goria, K., Allen, T., Ashokkumar, V., Pathania, D., Singh, R. P., & Tyagi, V. V. (2024). Biobased treatment and resource recovery from slaughterhouse wastewater via reutilization and recycling for sustainable waste approach. *Journal of Water Process Engineering, 58*, 104712. https://doi.org/10.1016/j.jwpe.2023.104712

Kumar, A. K., Sharma, S., Shah, E., Parikh, B. S., Patel, A., Dixit, G., Gupta, S., & Divecha, J. M. (2019). Cultivation of Ascochloris sp. ADW007-enriched microalga in raw dairy wastewater for enhanced biomass and lipid productivity. *International Journal of Environmental Science and Technology, 16*(2), 943–954. https://doi.org/10.1007/s13762-018-1712-0

Kumar, R., Kundu, D., Kormoker, T., Joshi, S., Rose, P. K., Kumar, S., Sahoo, P. K., Sharma, P., & Lamba, J. (2024). Phycoremediation of potentially toxic elements for agricultural and industrial wastewater treatment: Recent advances, challenges, and future prospects. *Desalination and Water Treatment, 319*, 100505. https://doi.org/10.1016/j.dwt.2024.100505

Kumari, P., Shukla, S. P., Rathi Bhuvaneswari, G., Kumar, S., Xavier, M., & Kumar, M. (2023). High value pigment production and carbon sequestration through wastewater grown Spirulina (Arthrospira) platensis: A green technology for wastewater utilization. *Waste Management Bulletin, 1*(3), 1–10. https://doi.org/10.1016/j.wmb.2023.06.003

López-Pacheco, I. Y., Carrillo-Nieves, D., Salinas-Salazar, C., Silva-Núñez, A., Arévalo-Gallegos, A., Barceló, D., Afewerki, S., Iqbal, H. M. N., & Parra-Saldívar, R. (2019). Combination of nejayote and swine wastewater as a medium for Arthrospira maxima and Chlorella vulgaris production and wastewater treatment. *Science of the Total Environment, 676*, 356–367. https://doi.org/10.1016/j.scitotenv.2019.04.278

Lu, Q., Liu, H., Liu, W., Zhong, Y., Ming, C., Qian, W., Wang, Q., & Liu, J. (2017). Pretreatment of brewery effluent to cultivate Spirulina sp. For nutrients removal and biomass production. *Water Science and Technology, 76*(7), 1852–1866. https://doi.org/10.2166/wst.2017.363

Ma, C., Wen, H., Xing, D., Pei, X., Zhu, J., Ren, N., & Liu, B. (2017). Molasses wastewater treatment and lipid production at low temperature conditions by a microalgal mutant Scenedesmus sp. Z-4. *Biotechnology for Biofuels, 10*(1), 111. https://doi.org/10.1186/s13068-017-0797-x

Ma, R., Zhao, X., Ho, S.-H., Shi, X., Liu, L., Xie, Y., Chen, J., & Lu, Y. (2020). Co-production of lutein and fatty acid in microalga Chlamydomonas sp. JSC4 in response to different temperatures with gene expression profiles. *Algal Research, 47*, 101821. https://doi.org/10.1016/j.algal.2020.101821

Molinuevo-Salces, B., Mahdy, A., Ballesteros, M., & González-Fernández, C. (2016). From piggery wastewater nutrients to biogas: Microalgae biomass revalorization through anaerobic digestion. *Renewable Energy, 96*, 1103–1110. https://doi.org/10.1016/j.renene.2016.01.090

Osorio-González, C. S., Sandoval-Salas, F., Hernández-Rosas, F., Hidalgo-Contreras, J. V., Gómez-Merino, F. C., & Ávalos de la Cruz, D. A. (2018). Potential for the use of cheese whey in Mexico.

Pandey, A., Srivastava, S., & Kumar, S. (2019). Sequential optimization of essential nutrients addition in simulated dairy effluent for improved *Scenedesmus* sp ASK22 growth, lipid production and nutrients removal. *Biomass and Bioenergy, 128*, 105319. https://doi.org/10.1016/j.biombioe.2019.105319

Patrizia, C., Juri, R., Angela, I., Sanjeet, M., Dino, M., & Antonio, M. (2019). Characterization of extracts from Heamatococcus pluvialis red phase by using accelerated solvent extraction. *Chemical Engineering Transactions, 74*, 1417–1422. https://doi.org/10.3303/CET1974237

Pereira, M. I. B., Chagas, B. M. E., Sassi, R., Medeiros, G. F., Aguiar, E. M., Borba, L. H. F., Silva, E. P. E., Neto, J. C. A., & Rangel, A. H. N. (2019). Mixotrophic cultivation of Spirulina platensis in dairy wastewater: Effects on the production of biomass, biochemical composition and antioxidant capacity. *PLoS One, 14*(10), e0224294. https://doi.org/10.1371/journal.pone.0224294

Pérez, J. P., Muñoz, A. A., Figueroa, C. P., & Agurto-Muñoz, C. (2021). Current analytical techniques for the characterization of lipophilic bioactive compounds from microalgae extracts. *Biomass and Bioenergy, 149*, 106078. https://doi.org/10.1016/j.biombioe.2021.106078

Rahman, A., Agrawal, S., Nawaz, T., Pan, S., & Selvaratnam, T. (2020). A review of algae-based produced water treatment for biomass and biofuel production. *Water, 12*(9), 2351. https://doi.org/10.3390/w12092351

Rani, N., Sangwan, P., Joshi, M., Sagar, A., & Bala, K. (2019). Microbes. In *Microbial wastewater treatment* (pp. 83–102). Elsevier. https://doi.org/10.1016/B978-0-12-816809-7.00005-1

Ravikumar, Y., Razack, S. A., Yun, J., Zhang, G., Zabed, H. M., & Qi, X. (2021). Recent advances in Microalgae-based distillery wastewater treatment. *Environmental Technology & Innovation, 24*, 101839. https://doi.org/10.1016/j.eti.2021.101839

Remón, J., Ruiz, J., Oliva, M., García, L., & Arauzo, J. (2016). Cheese whey valorisation: Production of valuable gaseous and liquid chemicals from lactose by aqueous phase reforming. Energy Conversion and Management, 124, 453–469. https://doi.org/10.1016/j.enconman.2016.07.044

Romaidi, Hasanudin, M., Kholifah, K., Maulidiyah, A., Putro, S. P., Kikuchi, A., & Sakaguchi, T. (2018). Lipid production from tapioca wastewater by culture of Scenedesmus sp. With simultaneous BOD, COD and nitrogen removal. Journal of Physics: Conference Series, 1025, 012075. https://doi.org/10.1088/1742-6596/1025/1/012075

Roy, H. P., Eldiehy, K. S. H., & Deka, D. (2024). Phycoremediation of rice bran oil processing wastewater and biodiesel production using green microalgae, Scenedesmus obliquus: A green approach to environmental protection and remediation. *Environmental Science and Pollution Research, 31*(57), 65288–65301. https://doi.org/10.1007/s11356-024-35599-3

Saleh, D. (2022). Phycoremediation of slaughterhouse wastewater using microalgae for nutrient recovery and biodiesel production. *Egyptian Journal of Chemistry, 65*(13), 1283–1289. https://doi.org/10.21608/ejchem.2022.138609.6094

Sasi, P. K. C., Mechery, J., Thomas, M., Jacob, J. P., & Paulose, S. V. (2020). Phycoremediation of paper and pulp mill effluent using Planktochlorella nurekis and Chlamydomonas reinhardtii – A comparative study, *8*(2).

Sau, A., Ghosh, S., Kandar, B., Ghanta, K. C., Baltrėnaitė-Gedienė, E., & Dutta, S. (2024). Enhanced slaughterhouse wastewater treatment: A comparative approach with phycoremediation and adsorption. *Journal of the Indian Chemical Society, 101*(12), 101499. https://doi.org/10.1016/j.jics.2024.101499

Sehar, S., & Nasser, H. A. A. (2019). Wastewater treatment of food industries through constructed wetland: A review. *International Journal of Environmental Science and Technology, 16*(10), 6453–6472. https://doi.org/10.1007/s13762-019-02472-7

Shah, S. M. U., Ahmad, A., Othman, M. F., & Abdullah, M. A. (2016). Effects of palm oil mill effluent media on cell growth and lipid content of *Nannochloropsis oculata* and *Tetraselmis suecica*. *International Journal of Green Energy, 13*(2), 200–207. https://doi.org/10.1080/15435075.2014.938340

Shahid, M. J., AL-Surhanee, A. A., Kouadri, F., Ali, S., Nawaz, N., Afzal, M., Rizwan, M., Ali, B., & Soliman, M. H. (2020). Role of microorganisms in the remediation of wastewater in floating treatment wetlands: A review. *Sustainability, 12*(14), 5559. https://doi.org/10.3390/su12145559

Su, Y., Zhu, X., Zou, R., & Zhang, Y. (2022). The interactions between microalgae and wastewater indigenous bacteria for treatment and valorization of brewery wastewater. *Resources, Conservation and Recycling, 182*, 106341. https://doi.org/10.1016/j.resconrec.2022.106341

Suastes-Rivas, J. K., Hernández-Altamirano, R., Mena-Cervantes, V. Y., Barrios Gómez, E. J., & Chairez, I. (2020). Biodiesel production, through intensification and profitable distribution of fatty acid methyl esters by a microalgae-yeast co-culture, isolated from wastewater as a function of the nutrients' composition of the culture media. Fuel, 280, 118633. https://doi.org/10.1016/j.fuel.2020.118633

Sun, Y., Zhang, N., Zhou, J., Dong, S., Zhang, X., Guo, L., & Guo, G. (2020). Distribution, contents, and types of Mycosporine-Like Amino Acids (MAAs) in marine macroalgae and a database for MAAs based on these characteristics. *Marine Drugs, 18*(1), 43. https://doi.org/10.3390/md18010043

Talapatra, N., Gautam, R., Mittal, V., & Ghosh, U. K. (2023). A comparative study of the growth of microalgae-bacteria symbiotic consortium with the axenic culture of microalgae in dairy wastewater through extraction and quantification of chlorophyll. *Materials Today: Proceedings, 80*, 2268–2273. https://doi.org/10.1016/j.matpr.2021.06.227

Tasic, M. B., Bonon, A. D. J., Rocha Barbosa Schiavon, M. I., Colling Klein, B., Veljković, V. B., & Maciel Filho, R. (2021). Cultivation of *Chlamydomonas reinhardtii* in anaerobically digested vinasse for bioethanol production. *Waste and Biomass Valorization, 12*(2), 857–865. https://doi.org/10.1007/s12649-020-01034-0

Umamaheswari, J., & Shanthakumar, S. (2020). Optimization of temperature and inoculum size for phycoremediation of paddy-soaked rice mill wastewater. *Journal of Environmental Engineering, 146*(1), 04019091. https://doi.org/10.1061/(ASCE)EE.1943-7870.0001612

Ummalyma, S. B., Sahoo, D., & Pandey, A. (2021). Resource recovery through bioremediation of wastewaters and waste carbon by microalgae: A circular bioeconomy approach. *Environmental Science and Pollution Research, 28*(42), 58837–58856. https://doi.org/10.1007/s11356-020-11645-8

Valiela, I., Owens, C., Elmstrom, E., & Lloret, J. (2016). Eutrophication of Cape Cod estuaries: Effect of decadal changes in global-driven atmospheric and local-scale wastewater nutrient loads. *Marine Pollution Bulletin, 110*(1), 309–315. https://doi.org/10.1016/j.marpolbul.2016.06.047

Walsh, B. P., Cusack, D. O., & O'Sullivan, D. T. J. (2016). An industrial water management value system framework development. *Sustainable Production and Consumption, 5*, 82–93. https://doi.org/10.1016/j.spc.2015.11.004

Wan, M., Zhao, H., Guo, J., Yan, L., Zhang, D., Bai, W., & Li, Y. (2021). Comparison of C-phycocyanin from extremophilic *Galdieria sulphuraria* and *Spirulina platensis* on stability and antioxidant capacity. *Algal Research, 58*, 102391. https://doi.org/10.1016/j.algal.2021.102391

Wang, X., Zhang, M.-M., Sun, Z., Liu, S.-F., Qin, Z.-H., Mou, J.-H., Zhou, Z.-G., & Lin, C. S. K. (2020). Sustainable lipid and lutein production from Chlorella mixotrophic fermentation by food waste hydrolysate. *Journal of Hazardous Materials, 400*, 123258. https://doi.org/10.1016/j.jhazmat.2020.123258

Watthier, E., Andreani, C. L., Torres, D. G. B., Kuczman, O., Tavares, M. H. F., Lopes, D. D., & Gomes, S. D. (2019). Cassava wastewater treatment in fixed-bed reactors: Organic matter removal and biogas production. *Frontiers in Sustainable Food Systems, 3*, 6. https://doi.org/10.3389/fsufs.2019.00006

Yuan, S., Ye, S., Yang, S., & Luo, G. (2021). Purification of potato wastewater and production of byproducts using microalgae Scenedesmus and Desmodesmus. *Journal of Water Process Engineering, 43*, 102237. https://doi.org/10.1016/j.jwpe.2021.102237

Zaky, F., Shabana, E., & Shalaby, H. (2019). Feasibility of microalgae culturing on Dairy waste for biodiesel production. *The Egyptian Journal of Experimental Biology (Botany), 0*, 1. https://doi.org/10.5455/egyjebb.20190804100423

Zandona, E., Blažić, M., & Režek Jambrak, A. (2021). Whey utilisation: Sustainable uses and environmental approach. *Food Technology and Biotechnology, 59*(2), 147–161. https://doi.org/10.17113/ftb.59.02.21.6968

Zheng, H., Wang, Y., Li, S., Nagarajan, D., Varjani, S., Lee, D.-J., & Chang, J.-S. (2022). Recent advances in lutein production from microalgae. *Renewable and Sustainable Energy Reviews, 153*, 111795. https://doi.org/10.1016/j.rser.2021.111795

Zhu, S., Feng, S., Xu, Z., Qin, L., Shang, C., Feng, P., Wang, Z., & Yuan, Z. (2019). Cultivation of *Chlorella vulgaris* on unsterilized dairy-derived liquid digestate for simultaneous biofuels feedstock production and pollutant removal. *Bioresource Technology, 285*, 121353. https://doi.org/10.1016/j.biortech.2019.121353

Zhuang, D., He, N., Khoo, K. S., Ng, E.-P., Chew, K. W., & Ling, T. C. (2022). Application progress of bioactive compounds in microalgae on pharmaceutical and cosmetics. *Chemosphere, 291*, 132932. https://doi.org/10.1016/j.chemosphere.2021.132932

Algal-Based Biostimulants and Biofertilizers: Bridging Bioremediation and Sustainable Agriculture

15

Katarzyna Chojnacka, Dawid Skrzypczak, and Rafał Taf

Abstract

Algae-based biostimulants and biofertilizers support crop performance and environmental remediation. Seaweeds and microalgae supply small amounts of growth-promoting compounds, including phytohormones, amino acids, osmoprotectants, and anionic polysaccharides. These compounds stimulate root development and improve nutrient use efficiency. They also help plants tolerate abiotic stress, which includes drought, salinity, and heat. Nitrogen-fixing cyanobacteria contribute biologically available nitrogen and release molecules that facilitate micronutrient delivery to the rhizosphere. Algal biomass contributes to bioremediation. It binds heavy metals, captures phosphate and promotes microbial degradation of pesticide residues. These effects can reduce leaching and runoff. Field applications often deliver higher yields or allow fertilizer savings while lowering nitrate loss and metal uptake. Harmonized regulations in the European Union are streamlining market entry for algae-based biostimulants. Key challenges remain. Seasonal changes in biomass composition affect product consistency. Liquid extracts show limited shelf life in warm supply chains. Decision-support tools for optimizing dose and timing are not yet widely available. Advances in controlled cultivation and strain selection can stabilize biomass quality. Improved formulation technologies, including microencapsulation for stability and controlled release, can extend shelf life and facilitate field application. Integrated algal biorefineries can increase profitability and align production with circular and climate-smart agriculture. The aim of this chapter is to present the potential of algae as biostimulants and fertilizers, as well as

K. Chojnacka (✉) · D. Skrzypczak · R. Taf
Department of Advanced Material Technologies, Wroclaw University of Science and Technology, Wroclaw, Lower Silesia, Poland
e-mail: katarzyna.chojnacka@pwr.edu.pl

L. Kumar et al. (eds.), *Algal Bioremediation*,
https://doi.org/10.1007/978-981-95-8793-3_15

agents supporting bioremediation. The chapter discusses the biochemical profile of algae in the context of their importance in plant–soil systems and the mechanisms of action of algae-based biofertilizers and biostimulants, as well as the use of algae in bioremediation, presenting examples of successful research and commercialization. The chapter addresses legal issues in marketing algae-based products, with particular emphasis on the European Union compared to the USA and Asia.

Keywords

Algal biostimulants and biofertilizers · Circular bioeconomy · Heavy-metal immobilization · Nutrient-use efficiency · Seaweed extracts · Stress tolerance

15.1 Introduction

In the face of increasing food production needs and simultaneous environmental requirements, solutions are being sought to replace conventional agrochemicals (Ghorai & Ghosh, 2022; Kumar et al., 2022). Algae, both macroalgae (multicellular seaweeds) and microalgae (unicellular fresh- or saltwater algae), are promising sources of sustainable bioproducts for agriculture (Miranda et al., 2024). Algal products can provide nutrients to the soil and simultaneously stimulate plant growth through biologically active molecules such as plant hormones, polysaccharides, or amino acids (Morillas-España et al., 2022) and restore soil fertility (Ronga et al., 2019). As a result, algal biostimulants and biofertilizers are seen as an innovative and environmentally friendly alternative to synthetic fertilizers. The use of algae in agriculture also promotes a circular economy. Algae biomass can be produced using waste (e.g., wastewater or industrial gases) and then returned to the fields as a soil improver, reducing production dependence on limited raw materials, such as phosphate rocks and natural gas (Miranda et al., 2024).

The terms biostimulator and biofertilizer are often confused, although they denote different classes of products. Biofertilizers are preparations containing live microorganisms or natural substances capable of improving soil fertility by increasing nutrient availability and stimulating plant growth (Shahzad et al., 2025; Sun et al., 2025). The action of biofertilizers is based, among other things, on the fixation of atmospheric nitrogen, the decomposition of organic matter, or the dissolution of hard-to-access forms of phosphorus in the soil. Biostimulants, on the other hand, are defined as products of organic origin (plant, algal, and microbial) that, when applied in small doses, stimulate the natural physiological processes of plants, improving the efficiency of nutrient utilization, tolerance to abiotic stress, and yield quality (Del Buono, 2021; EBIC, 2025; Tolisano & Del Buono, 2023). The important thing is that a biostimulant works independently of direct fertilization. It does not provide large doses of NPK but enhances the ability of plants to take up and use them (EBIC, 2025). In simple terms, biofertilizers enrich the soil with missing nutrients, while biostimulants promote the metabolism of plants and the soil microbiome. Despite these differences, both groups complement or replace agrochemicals, contributing to more sustainable agriculture (Drobek et al., 2019). It is worth mentioning that the terminology has been standardized in European Union law. According to Regulation (EU) 2019/1009, a plant biostimulant is a product that stimulates the nutritional processes of plants regardless of its nutritional value, with the sole purpose of improving nutrient use efficiency, tolerance to abiotic stresses, yield quality traits, or availability of nutrients in the soil/rhizosphere (EBIC, 2025; European Union, 2019). In other regions of the world, biostimulants are also defined in legislative acts. Such a comparison is particularly important in the context of implementing products and introducing them to the international market, as it is necessary to meet the conditions set by relevant regulations. In the USA, the definition of a biostimulant was presented in the 2018 Farm Bill (Agriculture Improvement Act of 2018), which states that a plant biostimulant is "a substance or micro-organism that, when applied to seeds, plants, or the rhizosphere, stimulates natural processes to enhance or benefit nutrient uptake, nutrient efficiency, tolerance to abiotic stress, or crop quality and yield" (115th Congress, 2018).

In India, the definition of a biostimulant is set out in the Fertilizer Control Order (FCO), 1985, as amended in 2021, which defines a biostimulant as "a substance or micro-organism or a combination of both whose primary function when applied to plants, seeds or rhizosphere is to stimulate physiological processes in plants and to enhance its nutrient uptake, growth, yield, nutrition efficiency, crop quality and tolerance to stress, regardless of its nutrient content, but does not include pesticides or plant growth regulators which are regulated under Insecticides Act, 1968" (Ministry of Agriculture & Farmers Welfare, 2025). In other Asian countries, such as Japan and China, the definition of a biostimulant is not included in legislation, and such products are usually considered as other fertilizer products. The lack of a clear definition of a biostimulant in some Asian countries causes difficulties in their classification and registration process, which may limit international trade and the introduction of innovative preparations to the market. As a result, manufacturers must individually adapt the composition and labeling of their products to meet the requirements of each country, which prolongs the approval process and generates additional costs. Differences in legal definitions also hinder the development of uniform methods for assessing the efficacy and safety of biostimulants. The lack of a common standard leads to discrepancies in the quality criteria applied by national supervisory authorities and thus constitutes one of the main challenges in the process of standardizing the quality control of biostimulants, including algae-based preparations.

This chapter discusses the potential of algae as components of biofertilizers and biostimulants in green agriculture. The biochemical composition of macro- and microalgae relevant to their effects on plants and soil, the mechanisms of action of these preparations (from hormonal effects to improved nutrition and stress resistance), and their role in bioremediation (binding of contaminants and prevention of nutrient losses) are presented. Regulations related to the use of algal formulations in agriculture are also presented and discussed. Finally, the main technological limitations, such as the cost of biomass production and the sustainability of the products, are presented, and directions for further research are identified, which are necessary for the successful integration of algae use in bioremediation and sustainable agriculture practices.

15.2 Biochemical Profiles of Algae Relevant to Plant–Soil Systems

15.2.1 Macroalgae vs. Microalgae: Cell Wall Composition

Macroalgae are characterized by a distinct cell wall structure compared to unicellular microalgae, which determines their properties as a biostimulatory raw material. In addition to cellulose, the cell walls of macroalgae contain significant amounts of unique polysaccharides (El-Beltagi et al., 2022). A comparison of the composition of macroalgae and microalgae cell walls is presented Table 15.1.

Brown algae, for example, are rich in alginates and fucoidan, which promote soil stability and water retention (Ye et al., 2024). Red algae contain the galactan sulfate polysaccharides agar and carrageenan, which influence increased water retention and bonding with phosphorus and trace elements (Rupert et al., 2022). Green seaweeds have cellulose and the unique polysaccharide ulvan in their walls, among others, and their tissues are often less sclerotized and decompose quickly (Ali et al., 2024).

Table 15.1 Differences in the structure of microalgae and macroalgae cell walls and their impact on soil-related properties

Group	Cell wall composition	Characteristic polysaccharides and structures	Soil-related properties
Brown algae	Cellulose, alginates, and fucoidan	Alginates and fucoidan	Promoting soil stability and water retention.
Green algae	Cellulose and ulvan	Ulvan	Providing easily decomposable organic matter and bioactive compounds.
Red algae	Cellulose, galactan sulfate polysaccharides, and carrageenan	Galactan sulfate polysaccharides and carrageenan	Increasing water retention, binding phosphorus, and trace elements
Eukaryotic microalgae	Cellulose or cellulose–pectin, sometimes reinforced with sporopollenin or $CaCO_3$	Exopolysaccharides	Increasing water retention and resistance to erosion
Diatoms	Silica frustule	Silica	Increasing water retention and resistance to erosion
Cyanobacteria	Gram-negative wall with peptidoglycan and polysaccharide sheath	Thick mucilaginous sheath	Reducing soil erosion and water evaporation

These structural polysaccharides give seaweeds a high capacity to absorb water and ions. For example, alginate from brown algae swells and binds heavy metals, while carrageenan from kelp retains water in the soil, acting like a natural hydrogel. Thus, the composition of the cell walls translates into action in the soil: The brown algae bring colloids that improve aggregate structure and water retention, the red algae bring protective and ion chelating substances, while the green algae bring easily decomposable organic matter and bioactive compounds (Yasmeen et al., 2025).

The cell walls of microalgae are more diverse depending on the taxonomic group. Photosynthetic eukaryotic microalgae (e.g., unicellular green algae such as *Chlorella*, *Scenedesmus*) have cellulose or cellulose–pectin walls, sometimes reinforced with sporopollenin or calcium carbonate, while diatoms are distinguished by a frustule composed of silica (Pipitone et al., 2025). In general, microalgae have a thinner wall than seaweeds but secrete significant amounts of extracellular polysaccharides (EPS—exopolysaccharides), forming a mucilaginous sheath (Alvarez et al., 2021). Even small concentrations of such exopolysaccharides from microalgae can improve the physicochemical properties of the soil—they promote the aggregation of soil particles and the formation of structure, making the soil better able to store water and more resistant to erosion (Alvarez et al., 2021). The walls of cyanobacteria (cyanobacteria), which are classified as prokaryotic microalgae, are structured differently. The cell wall of cyanobacteria has a Gram-negative structure (a thin layer of peptidoglycan), often surrounded by a thick mucilaginous polysaccharide sheath. The mucilaginous colonies of cyanobacteria can bind soil particles and form a living crust on the surface, which reduces soil erosion and water evaporation (Cantón et al., 2020; Malešević et al., 2020).

15.2.2 Secondary Metabolites and Nutrients in Algae that Support Plant Growth

In addition to the structural components of the cell wall, algae are a source of many metabolites that have a beneficial biostimulating effect when introduced into the soil or applied to plants. The most important of these are phytohormones, polysaccharides, amino acids, and minerals.

15.2.2.1 Algal Phytohormones

Both macroalgae and microalgae synthesize compounds analogous to plant hormones, such as auxins, cytokinins, gibberellins, abscisic acid (ABA), ethylene, and even brassinosteroids (Stirk et al., 2013a, b). The content of endogenous hormones in algae is generally low, but sufficient to exert an effect when the extract is applied in low concentrations. For example, the brown algae *Ascophyllum nodosum* and *Ecklonia maxima* contain significant amounts of cytokinin-like compounds, while *Spirulina* (*Arthrospira platensis*, microalgae) and green algae *Scenedesmus* are rich in compounds with auxin activity (Plaza et al., 2018; Ronga et al., 2019). Studies have shown that microalgae extracts containing natural phytohormones can stimulate plant growth (Lu & Xu, 2015). Cyanobacteria can release indoleacetic acid (IAA—auxin) into the environment, as well as amino acids and other compounds that stimulate the growth of plant root systems (Ronga et al., 2019; Singh & Trehan, 1973). The presence of hormones in algae preparations translates into their effects: For example, treating seeds or seedlings with algae extract accelerates germination and stimulates root development, while foliar spraying can delay leaf aging and stimulate branching. Seaweed also contains hormone precursors and signaling compounds (e.g., polyamines) that synergistically influence plant development (Papenfus et al., 2013; Ronga et al., 2019). In summary, algal biostimulants provide plants with a "hormone package" that can naturally modify signaling pathways and the expression of genes related to growth and response to environmental stresses.

15.2.2.2 Bioactive Polysaccharides and Oligosaccharides

In addition to their structural function, algal polysaccharides have biostimulating and protective properties. Long-chain polysaccharides, such as alginate or carrageenan, act as fertility enhancers in the soil, increasing its water and sorption capacity, limiting the leaching of nutrients, and providing a source of carbon for beneficial soil microorganisms (Biradar et al., 2025; Martínez-Cano et al., 2022; Torres et al., 2019). Furthermore, partial hydrolysates of these polysaccharides (e.g., algal oligosaccharides formed during extraction) can act as components that increase plant resistance. Research indicates that oligosaccharides from brown algae and red algae can induce defense mechanisms in plants similar to those triggered by pathogen attacks, resulting in increased resistance (so-called induced systemic resistance) (Yasmeen et al., 2025). In addition, algae have the ability to sorb heavy metals and bind toxins, so adding algae to the soil can immobilize certain pollutants (Raize et al., 2004). It is also worth mentioning exopolysaccharides (EPS) produced by microalgae. These soluble or mucilaginous sugars secreted into the medium are a component of many biostimulant formulations—for example, *Spirulina*—and *Chlorella*-based products contain natural EPS rich in rhamnose and arabinose, which improve the adhesion of the preparation to leaves and nourish the rhizosphere microbiome (Koçer et al., 2021; Laroche, 2022). Algal polysaccharides have a multifaceted effect: They improve the physicochemical properties of soil, directly stimulate growth, and indirectly induce plant defense mechanisms.

15.2.2.3 Amino Acids and Other Organic Metabolites

Algae, both macroalgae and microalgae, contain a wide range of amino acids and their derivatives, including proline, glycine betaine, and glutamic acid, which act as important osmoprotectants. Under conditions of salt stress or drought, many microalgae accumulate significant amounts of proline and glycine betaine, which promote osmoregulation, membrane stabilization, and enzyme activity. These mechanisms can be transferred to crops through the use of algal extracts or hydrolysates, helping them maintain water potential and protect proteins from denaturation (Jiménez-Arias et al., 2021; Kumar et al., 2024). Sulfur amino acids, such as methionine and cysteine, are often found in algae in small amounts or as limited protein components, but they are part of endogenous antioxidants, such as glutathione, which strengthens the resistance of plants to oxidative and metallic stress (Bleakley & Hayes, 2017; Kakinuma et al., 2001). Histidine, present in moderate concentrations, can act as a metal-chelating amino acid, reducing the toxicity of elements in the rhizosphere environment (Kumar et al., 2019). Ready-made algae preparations, especially those based on hydrolysates, are often enriched with free amino acids and peptides derived from enzymatic or chemical hydrolysis of algae biomass (Solorzano-Chavez et al., 2019). Such bioactive hydrolysates are easily absorbed by plants and can stimulate their metabolism, photosynthesis, nutrient uptake, and stress tolerance, regardless of the presence of phytohormones. Algae are also a source of vitamins (A, B_1, B_2, B_6, B_{12}, C, and E) (Wu et al., 2023) and pigments with antioxidant properties (carotenoids, phycocyanin, and polyphenols) (Wu et al., 2010). For example, phycocyanin from *Spirulina* has strong antioxidant and anti-inflammatory properties—its presence in a biostimulant may help plants neutralize free radicals generated during oxidative stress (Fernández-Rojas et al., 2014; Varia et al., 2022). Alginic acid and laminaran, on the other hand, provide carbon and energy to beneficial soil microorganisms, stimulating their activity and, as a result, improving the decomposition of organic matter and the release of nutrients in the rhizosphere (Mattner et al., 2013; Singh et al., 2025).

15.2.2.4 Macro- and Microelements

Algal biomass contains many microelements essential for plants, including iron (Fe), zinc, copper, and manganese (Circuncisão et al., 2018; Peñalver et al., 2020). Furthermore, boron and molybdenum, which are important for plant nutrition, have also been found in algae extracts (Soares et al., 2020). Marine macroalgae accumulate significant amounts of macronutrients, especially potassium and calcium, and are characterized by a uniquely high iodine content (Circuncisão et al., 2018; Peñalver et al., 2020). The use of powdered seaweed or algae extracts, therefore, provides plants with deficient macro- and microelements (Ostrowski et al., 2024; Ronga et al., 2019). Research indicates that microalgae extracts applied foliar can partially replace conventional micronutrient fertilizers, acting complementarily to nitrogen fertilization by providing plants with easily assimilable micronutrients and increasing the uptake of macronutrients (e.g., phosphorus and potassium) from the soil (Ronga et al., 2019). Thanks to their chelating ability, algae can also neutralize toxic excess heavy metals in the environment, while providing plants with the necessary micronutrients in the form of safe complexes (Davis et al., 2003). For example, brown algae, thanks to the presence of fucoidan, can bind Fe (III) cations, forming natural chelates that are absorbable by plants, while the alginate polysaccharide contained in their cell walls complexes Ca(II) and Mg (II) ions (Abka-Khajouei et al., 2022; Davis et al., 2003). Algal biopreparations therefore have a multifaceted effect: They supplement micronutrient deficiencies in plants, increase the availability of nutrients in the soil (through chelation of metal ions and acidification of the rhizosphere by algal metabolites), and improve the ability of plants to take up and utilize these nutrients by stimulating root system development and the activity of enzymes that transport minerals.

15.2.2.5 Humic and Fulvic Fractions Derived from Algal Biomass

Cold-processed Ascophyllum nodosum extracts contain humic-like polyphenolic chains rich in carboxyl and phenolic groups. These fractions bind iron and zinc and stimulate H^+-ATPase activity in maize roots, enhancing nutrient acquisition (Ali et al., 2021). Comparable signals emerge in greenhouse studies where kelp extracts increased root length and shoot biomass beyond the response obtained with peat-derived humic material of equal carbon dose (Shukla et al., 2019). Noncalcified kelps and wracks store more than 15% recalcitrant aromatic carbon that gradually oxidizes and polymerizes after incorporation into soil, contributing to the native humic pool (Fiset et al., 2019). Microalgal cultures add further input. Under nutrient sufficiency, *Spirulina* and *Chlorella* release polycarboxylated metabolites that condense abiotically to humic-like substances. Field tests with algal hydrolysate blended into chitosan carriers improved phosphorus and iron uptake in vegetable crops, indicating a chelation role for the resulting fulvate fraction (Parmar et al., 2023). These observations suggest that algal amendments not only supply labile carbon but also reinforce the long-term humus reservoir, with positive effects on cation retention and microbial activity. In summary, the rich chemical profile of algae, ranging from phytohormones and polysaccharides to amino acids and minerals, makes them versatile biofactories of substances that have a positive effect on plant growth and health as well as soil fertility.

15.3 Mechanisms of Action of Biostimulants and Algal Biofertilizers

15.3.1 The Influence of Algal Phytohormones on Plant Physiology

One of the keyways in which algae preparations stimulate plant growth is through their effect on hormonal signaling pathways. The natural phytohormones present in algae modulate plant development in a manner similar to endogenous growth regulators. Auxins present in algae extracts directly stimulate cell division and root elongation (Ali et al., 2021). In practice, this results in better rooting of seedlings and more efficient uptake of water and nutrients from the soil (Tuhy et al., 2020). Algal cytokinins, in turn, stimulate cell division in shoots and leaves, delay their aging, and increase photosynthetic activity.

Brown algae are known for their high content of cytokinin-active compounds. Analyses of commercial *Ascophyllum nodosum* extracts have shown that cytokinins and "cytokinin-like" compounds are the most abundant class of growth regulators in these extracts. Foliar application of such extracts to cereals and vegetables often results in more luxuriant foliage (greater number and surface area of leaves) and a greater number of shoots or yield-producing shoots (Khan et al., 2012; Wally et al., 2013). Additionally, high concentrations of cytokinin in plant tissues delay the aging process. For example, the application of *A. nodosum* extract inhibited signs of leaf senescence by increasing endogenous cytokinin levels and limiting the expression of aging genes (Wally et al., 2013).

Plants treated with algae retain their green leaves longer, which is partly attributed to the presence of betaines in algae that delay chlorophyll degradation. As a result, many crops sprayed with algae extracts show increased chlorophyll content (Al-Ghamdi & Elansary, 2018). Gibberellins present in some algae (especially brown algae) can accelerate seed germination and shoot elongation. However, their role in biostimulant preparations is less significant than that of auxins and cytokinins. Analyses of the hormonal composition of *A. nodosum* extracts have shown that they contain virtually all major classes of phytohormones (including gibberellic acid), but auxin-like and cytokinin-like effects dominate in the observed activity (Olaetxea et al., 2024). It has been reported that extracts contain almost all key phytohormones and other bioactive compounds, including indoleacetic acid, cytokinins, salicylic acid, and abscisic acid (Olaetxea et al., 2024).

Some researchers indicate that the action of algal extracts in plants occurs through the stimulation of the biosynthesis of major phytohormones and the activation of relevant signaling pathways regulated by them (Ali et al., 2021; Khan et al., 2009; Wally et al., 2013). In the context of phytohormone-like effects observed in plants treated with *A. nodosum*, the most commonly reported activities are similar to those of cytokinin and reactions typical of auxin action (Ali et al., 2021; Kumari et al., 2011). However, there are reports of the influence of *A. nodosum* on many different hormonal pathways, including gibberellins, abscisic acid, ethylene, salicylic acid, and jasmonic acid (Ali et al., 2021; Khan et al., 2009). Although cytokinins and indoleacetic acid play a key role as regulators of plant growth and development, and salicylic acid is mainly involved in defense reactions against pathogens, recent studies on the links between growth and defense mechanisms indicate the existence of mutual interactions between auxin, cytokinins, and salicylic acid, which together influence both plant development and resistance (Naseem et al., 2015). The effects of the hormonal action of algal biostimulants are clearly evident in plant growth and yield parameters.

15.3.2 Improvement of Plant Nutrition and Nutrient Uptake

The second keyway in which algae products work is by improving the mineral nutrition of plants, both by directly supplying additional nutrients and by increasing their availability from the soil (Fig. 15.1). Algae used as biofertilizers release macro- and microelements into the soil environment (Rupawalla et al., 2021). In the soil, it undergoes gradual mineralization, providing plants with easily accessible forms of ammonium nitrogen, phosphates, and potassium. Furthermore, cyanobacteria can bind molecular nitrogen from the air thanks to the presence of the nitrogenase enzyme in specialized cells. The introduction of such nitrogen biofertilizers into the soil results in the biological fixation of N_2 and the enrichment of the substrate with nitrogen that is available to plants (Hossain et al., 2023). It has been documented that cyanobacteria can provide an average of 20–30 kg of nitrogen per hectare through the natural fixation of atmospheric N_2 (Issa, 2014). Soil microalgae can also help make phosphorus available in bioavailable forms to plants.

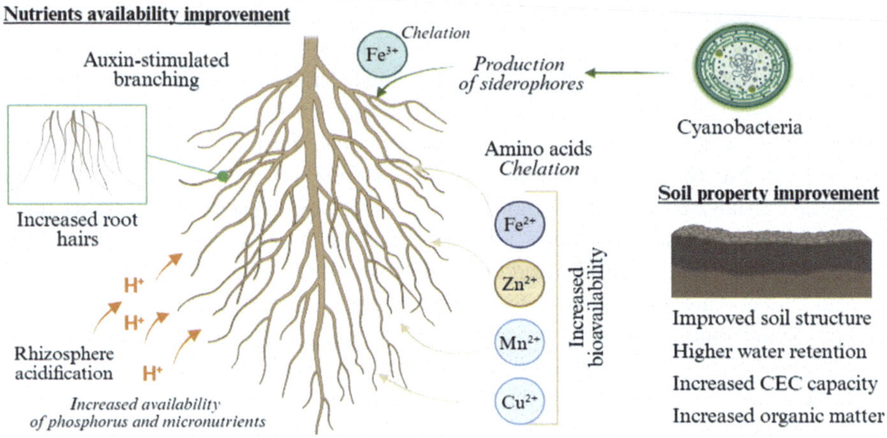

Fig. 15.1 Role of algae in enhancing plant nutrition and soil properties

Some species secrete acids into the rhizosphere that dissolve phosphorus compounds from soil minerals and make them available to roots (Abinandan et al., 2019; Naveed et al., 2017).

Another mechanism is the production of siderophores, i.e., iron-chelating compounds. It has been reported that some cyanobacteria and green algae produce siderophores capable of binding Fe^{3+} and forming complexes that can then be absorbed by plants as a source of iron (Brick et al., 2025). This type of indirect micronutrient supply can be crucial in soils with high pH, where iron is poorly absorbed. Cyanobacterial siderophores can act as an ecological alternative to synthetic chelates. It has been shown that the siderophore secreted by *Synechococcus mundulus* significantly increased iron uptake and the growth rate of corn seedlings (Brick et al., 2025).

Improved nutrient uptake by plants is also associated with improved sorption properties of the soil itself. Algal polysaccharides (e.g., alginates) increase cation exchange capacity (CEC) and the substrate's ability to retain nutrients, reducing their loss through leaching (Baćmaga et al., 2024). In sandy soils, the addition of algae acts as a natural fertilizer store, releasing them gradually according to plant demand. This mechanism is explained by the ability of alginates to retain moisture and ions in the soil (Akbar et al., 2024). Algae also provide substances that increase the solubility of hard-to-access forms of elements. The aforementioned organic acids secreted by microalgae can locally lower the pH and dissolve phosphorus from insoluble iron and calcium phosphates, releasing it into the soil solution (Hossain et al., 2023).

It is worth emphasizing the synergy between algae preparations and traditional mineral fertilizers. Algae biostimulants do not completely replace NPK fertilizers, but they enable plants to utilize them more effectively, increasing the so-called fertilizer utilization efficiency. An example confirming this phenomenon is an experiment conducted on corn (*Zea mays*), where the effects of juices from

Kappaphycus alvarezii (K-sap) and *Gracilaria edulis* (G-sap) algae were tested. The application of 5% G-sap or 7.5% K-sap in combination with a full dose of mineral fertilizers (100%) contributed to an increase in grain yield of 21.4%–29.8% compared to the control. A significant increase in phosphorus (35.5%) and potassium (14.4%) content in corn kernels was also observed, indicating better nutrient utilization. Additionally, thanks to biostimulation, it was possible to reduce the carbon and phosphate footprint while maintaining high productivity, making such solutions more environmentally sustainable (Singh et al., 2016). From a practical point of view, the use of algae reduces fertilizer losses—most of the applied nutrients end up in the crop, and less is lost through volatilization or leaching into the environment (Coppens et al., 2016; Sasaki et al., 2020). For this reason, algae products contribute to increased efficiency and sustainability of fertilization. In summary, the nutritional mechanisms of algae include (1) biological binding and release of additional amounts of nitrogen, (2) chelation and increased availability of unavailable forms of nutrients, (3) improvement of soil sorption and moisture properties, (4) stimulation of root growth and activity in water and ion uptake. All this results in better plant nutrition, higher mineral content in their tissues, and often the possibility of reducing chemical fertilizer doses without compromising yields.

15.3.3 The Role of Algae in Increasing Plant Resistance to Abiotic Stress

15.3.3.1 Osmoprotection and Water Management

During drought or salinity, plants accumulate so-called osmoprotectants (e.g., betaine, proline, and soluble sugars) in their cells, which protect cell structures from dehydration (Ma et al., 2020). Algae produce large amounts of such substances; for example, brown algae contain significant amounts of glycine betaine (Jiménez-Arias et al., 2021). Their application can increase the level of osmoprotectants in plant tissues.

It has been shown that the use of algae extracts increases endogenous concentrations of proline, phenols, and other stress-protective compounds (Table 15.2). In an experiment with wheat, it was shown that treating seeds with an aqueous extract of *Spirulina platensis* significantly improved growth, leaf physiology, and plant yield both under optimal conditions and in the absence of irrigation. Plants treated with the extract showed a higher rate of photosynthesis, which increased by 53.4% compared to the control. An increase in the number of ears by 76.5% and a 190% increase in grain yield under irrigation conditions, and a 153% increase under drought conditions, were also observed. The extract also had a positive effect on leaf morphology, photosynthetic pigment content, gas exchange parameters, and carbohydrate levels, confirming its effectiveness in mitigating the negative effects of drought on wheat plants (Elnajar et al., 2024). Similar effects were observed when using *Ascophyllum nodosum* brown algae extract in the cultivation of *Paspalum vaginatum* grass during prolonged irrigation breaks and increased soil salinity. Regular spraying with the extract (5 and 7 ml per liter

Table 15.2 Impact of algae on plant adaptation to stress conditions (CF—conventional fertilizers and SB—synthetic biostimulants)

Mechanism	Description	Plants effect	Comparison (CF/SB)	References
Osmoprotection and water regulation	Algae provide betaine, proline, and sugars; support osmoregulation and water retention	Better drought tolerance, less dehydration, and higher yield	CF—supply nutrients but lack osmoprotectants and do not improve water retention; SB—typically a single osmolyte; algae are multicomponent and include EPS/alginates that enhance soil moisture retention	Fozi et al. (2024)
Root growth stimulation	Auxins and cytokinins promote root development	Deeper and more extensive root system and better access to water.	CF—do not contain phytohormones—no direct root stimulation; SB—typically single regulators; algae provide a multi-hormonal cocktail with synergistic action	Yasmeen et al. (2014)
Improvement of soil structure	Polysaccharides (alginates) retain water in the root zone	Longer retention of moisture for plants	CF—do not improve soil structure or water-holding capacity; SB—rarely delivers soil-structuring polysaccharides or extracellular polymeric substances; algal products provide these, increasing aggregate stability, and plant-available water	Singh et al. (2016)
Activation of antioxidant enzymes	Extracts increase enzyme activity and induce the expression of defense genes	Protection against oxidative stress and reduction of cellular damage.	CF—do not induce antioxidant priming; SB—typically act via a single signaling pathway; and algal extracts activate multiple pathways and upregulate antioxidant enzymes	Ziaei and Pazoki (2022)

(continued)

Table 15.2 (continued)

Mechanism	Description	Plants effect	Comparison (CF/SB)	References
Supply of antioxidant compounds	Bioactive compounds (carotenoids and vitamins C and E) neutralize free radicals	Limiting damage caused by reactive oxygen species	CF—do not supply antioxidants; SB—typically single molecules; algal extracts deliver a broad spectrum of antioxidants.	Hejna et al. (2024)
Increased activity of soil microorganisms	Extracts support beneficial microbiomes in the rhizosphere	Better nutrient uptake, improved soil structure, and indirect resistance	CF—do not supply labile carbon to the soil microbiome; when used alone can reduce microbial activity and diversity; SB—do not serve as microbial substrates; algal products supply organic carbon and EPS, increasing microbial activity and diversity.	Alam et al. (2013)
Induction of systemic immunity	Laminarin and other oligosaccharides act as signaling molecules recognized by plants	Activation of defense responses, production of pathogenesis-related proteins and increased immunity	CF—do not induce plant immunity; SB—synthetic elicitors are usually narrow-spectrum; algal extracts supply a mixture of oligosaccharides that naturally prime plant defenses and PR—protein responses	Kumar et al. (2024)
Effect on hormone balance	Regulation of hormonal pathways	Better adaptation to environmental stresses	CF—do not directly modulate phytohormone signaling; SB—typically target a single hormone; algal extracts gently modulate multiple hormone pathways simultaneously	Olaetxea et al. (2024)

every 6 days) improved turf quality, photosynthesis, root system development, and the content of carbohydrates, potassium, calcium, and proline. The plants also showed higher antioxidant enzyme activity and lower levels of oxidative damage. The best results were obtained at a dose of 7 ml per liter. The study indicates that the extract supports plant resistance to stress by improving water management, osmotic regulation, and strengthening defense mechanisms (Elansary et al., 2017).

Another beneficial effect is the development of the root system. Algae extracts contain auxins and cytokinins, which stimulate root growth, allowing the plant to reach deeper, moister soil layers during drought. Studies conducted on several strawberry varieties have shown that the use of soluble *Ascophyllum nodosum* extract significantly increased root system development. Regular applications of the extract at doses of 1 and 2 g/L led to more intensive growth of both roots and aboveground parts, as well as higher yields. The strongest root response was observed in the "Chandler" variety. Importantly, this extract also affected soil microorganisms, increasing their abundance and metabolic activity, especially in the rhizosphere (Alam et al., 2013). Similar results were obtained in field trials using extracts from the algae *Duvillaea potatorum* and *Ascophyllum nodosum* in strawberry cultivation. In nurseries, a 22% increase in lateral root density was observed, while in fruit crops, root length per soil volume increased by 38%. A stronger root system was closely associated with higher commercial fruit yields, confirming that algal extracts can effectively support root development and increase the ability of plants to absorb water and nutrients from the soil (Mattner et al., 2018). In addition, algal polysaccharides (e.g., alginates from brown algae and ulvans from green algae) retain water in the substrate, which allows the soil to keep moisture available to plants for longer (Yasmeen et al., 2014).

15.3.3.2 Activation of Antioxidant Enzymes

Algal biostimulants can stimulate the antioxidant system of plants both by providing their own antioxidants and by inducing greater activity of defense enzymes (Jacomassi et al., 2022). Marine algae contain many compounds with strong antioxidant properties. For example, brown algae are exceptionally rich in polyphenols called phlorotannins (Shibata et al., 2004). Red and green algae have a much lower polyphenol content but produce a lot of carotenoids (such as β-carotene, lutein, and zeaxanthin) and vitamins, including vitamin C (Yanshin et al., 2021). When applied as an extract (either foliar or soil), these compounds can act as direct antioxidants, for example, neutralizing hydroxyl radicals before they cause damage to plant cells. More importantly, however, the signals contained in algae extracts activate genes encoding defense enzymes in plants.

In experiments on common beans (*Phaseolus vulgaris* L.), which tested the effect of foliar application of seaweed extract (at doses of 2 and 4 l ha^{-1}) on plant resistance to drought stress, significant decreases in yield, chlorophyll content, relative water content (RWC), and protein content were observed in the untreated groups, along with an increase in soluble sugar levels and SOD and CAT enzyme activity. In contrast, plants treated with algal extract, especially at the higher dose (4 l ha^{-1}), showed a significant improvement in these parameters compared to control plants, despite ongoing water stress. Increased antioxidant enzyme activity and maintenance of higher chlorophyll and protein levels explain higher biological and seed productivity even under limited irrigation conditions (Ziaei & Pazoki, 2022). A similar anti-stress effect was demonstrated in an experiment with *Arabidopsis thaliana*, where *Ascophyllum nodosum* brown algae extract was used under drought conditions. Before stress, the spray caused partial closure of the stomata and changes in the expression of genes related to abscisic acid response pathways and the antioxidant system. Among others, there was an increase in the expression of genes encoding enzymes such as superoxide dismutase, catalase, and ascorbate peroxidase, which are responsible for neutralizing reactive oxygen species. Thanks to the early activation of these mechanisms, the treated plants maintained higher photosynthetic efficiency during dehydration, exhibited better dissipation of excess energy in the photosystem II reaction centers, and showed higher water use efficiency and mesophyll conductance. As a result, the extract effectively increased drought tolerance and protected the photosynthetic apparatus from permanent damage (Santaniello et al., 2017). It has also been shown that certain oligosaccharides from algae (e.g., laminarin from brown algae) are recognized by plants in a similar way to pathogen molecules, thereby increasing the production of antioxidant enzymes and antibacterial compounds (Asimakis et al., 2022). Laminarin, a linear β-1,3-glucan from brown algae, induces the expression of PR proteins and other immunity markers in various species (de Borba et al., 2022). In summary, algal biostimulants play a crucial role in mitigating oxidative stress in plants through both direct and indirect mechanisms. Compounds present in algae, such as phlorotannins, carotenoids, and vitamins C and E, act as natural antioxidants, limiting damage caused by reactive oxygen species. At the same time, algal extracts activate the expression of genes encoding defense enzymes, including superoxide dismutase, catalase, and ascorbate peroxidase, thereby strengthening the plant's internal antioxidant system.

15.3.4 Detoxification of Heavy Metals and Toxins

A special type of abiotic stress is the presence of toxic heavy metals (Cd, Pb, Hg, and As) or xenobiotics (e.g., pesticides and polycyclic aromatic hydrocarbons) in the environment. Algal preparations can reduce the phytotoxicity of these substances in two ways: by immobilizing/binding toxins in the soil and by increasing the internal tolerance of plants to toxins. In the first case, algae added to the substrate act as a biosorbent, and their sulfate polysaccharides and carboxyl groups capture heavy metal cations, forming stable complexes with them and reducing their availability to roots (He & Chen, 2014; Kumar Gupta et al., 2015). In the second case, antioxidant and chelating mechanisms within the plant are crucial. Under the influence of the algal extract, the plant can increase the production of phytochelatins, peptides that bind heavy metals into nontoxic complexes and deposit them in vacuoles.

It was found that barley (*Hordeum vulgare* L.) treated with an aqueous extract of algal wrack (accumulated algae washed up on the beach) tolerated toxic concentrations of copper better. Plants treated with the extract (7.5 g l^{-1}) showed a 34% increase in leaf length compared to seedlings exposed only to Cu, indicating effective detoxification and protection of the photosynthetic apparatus. In addition, despite its low sugar and photosynthetic pigment content, the algal wrack extract was rich in phenolic compounds and flavonoids, natural antioxidants that were most likely responsible for reducing oxidative stress and supporting the plants' defense mechanisms. In the absence of heavy metals, this preparation stimulated the growth of root biomass (by 63%) and leaf area (up to 45%), confirming its potential as a sustainable biostimulant with protective and growth-promoting effects (Sousa et al., 2022). Studies have also shown that extracts from *the brown algae Ascophyllum nodosum* can modulate key pathways of plant stress–responses, including those related to abscisic acid and reactive oxygen species. Of particular importance, pretreatment of plants with *Ascophyllum nodosum* extract was associated with improved water use efficiency, increased antioxidant enzyme activity, and partial closure of stomata under drought conditions (Shukla et al., 2019). Research also confirms that extracts from *the brown algae Ascophyllum nodosum can be effectively used in phytoextraction strategies for removing* heavy metals from contaminated soils. In the experiment conducted on sorghum (*Sorghum bicolor*) aimed at increasing the removal of cadmium (Cd) and lead (Pb) from the soil, it was shown that the use of *Ascophyllum nodosum* extract significantly increased the aboveground and root biomass of plants, thereby intensifying the uptake of heavy metals. After 12 weeks of sorghum cultivation in the presence of the algae extract, an increase in root biomass of 40.7%, 40%, and 100%, respectively, and in shoots of 22.4%, 33.6%, and 31.8%, respectively, was observed, depending on the level of contamination, compared to the control without the extract. Importantly, *Ascophyllum nodosum* enhanced plant growth even at the highest metal concentrations, indicating its role not only as a growth stimulator but also as an aid in detoxifying and transporting toxic elements from the soil to plant tissues. The use of a biostimulant derived from Ascophyllum nodosum increased the total accumulation of metals in the plant, confirming its usefulness as a sustainable tool for the remediation of heavy metal-contaminated soils (Rostami et al., 2023).

Another example confirming the potential of algae in alleviating metal stress is a study on the effect of *Ulva lactuca* extract on sorghum plants growing in cadmium-contaminated conditions. The use of this green algae preparation reduced oxidative stress by lowering the levels of malondialdehyde and superoxide anion radicals and also modified the activity of enzymes involved in carbon and nitrogen metabolism. Importantly, *Ulva* extract increased cadmium accumulation in aboveground parts, while the presence of the mycorrhizal fungus *Glomus intraradices* reduced its transport to the leaves, indicating complementary mechanisms of metal detoxification. The use of both biostimulants improved the plants' tolerance to stress and supported their physiological adaptation to polluted environmental conditions (Kchikich et al., 2024). Numerous studies confirm the effectiveness of algae extracts as natural agents that support the detoxification of heavy metals and toxins in the soil environment. These preparations work by both immobilizing metals in the soil and activating defense mechanisms in plants, such as increased antioxidant enzyme activity. Their use can support the remediation of contaminated soils and increase the resistance and productivity of crops under environmental stress.

15.3.5 Molecular Level Evidence of Algal Biostimulant Action and Stress Tolerance Induction

The mechanisms of action of algae as fertilizers and biostimulants have been presented with particular emphasis on their effects on plant growth under both optimal and stress conditions. To fully understand these processes, analysis at the molecular level is necessary to better understand how algae affect plant metabolism. Such an approach could enable more targeted design of algae-based fertilizer formulations, allowing for products tailored to specific crops.

Numerous transcriptomic and metabolomic studies have confirmed the effects of algal-derived biostimulants at the molecular level. RNA sequencing of tomato plants treated with a commercial preparation of *A. nodosum* revealed that 456 genes were downregulated and 635 were upregulated. These differentially expressed genes were involved in a wide range of biological processes, cellular components, and molecular functions. The extract strongly influenced the expression of genes involved in carbon fixation, secondary metabolism, MAPK (mitogen-activated protein kinase) signaling, hormone signal transduction, the metabolism of glutathione, phenylpropanoids, and stilbenoids. As a result, defense enzyme activity increased, and antioxidant mechanisms were activated, leading to improved plant resistance and metabolic efficiency (Ali et al., 2021).

Similar effects were observed after applying alkaline extracts from *Sargassum vulgare* and *Acanthophora spicifera* to tomato and pepper plants. RNA sequencing showed an increase in the expression of genes related to carbon and nitrogen metabolism, plant hormone signal transduction, secondary metabolism, MAPK signaling, and amino acid biosynthesis. Peroxidase genes were particularly strongly induced (e.g., peroxidase 64 involved in plant defense). Other upregulated genes included cytochrome *c* oxidase subunit 6a (a component of the mitochondrial electron transport chain) and caffeoyl-CoA *O*-methyltransferase. The latter enzyme methylates flavonoids, alkaloids, and phenylpropanoids, thereby increasing the plant's resistance to abiotic stress and disease. Expression of a GDSL esterase/lipase gene increased in tomatoes but decreased in peppers, indicating species-specific responses. Additionally, increased expression of the PTI5 gene, along with upregulation of stilbenoid, diarylheptanoid, and gingerol biosynthetic pathways, confirmed activation of systemic immunity and enhanced antioxidant capacity in the plants (Ali et al., 2021).

Sweet corn treated with the *A. nodosum*-based biostimulant "Yi nuo", showed a significant yield increase and accumulated higher levels of metabolites associated with growth, development, and stress resistance (e.g., glutathione, proline, glutamate, and gibberellin A3). Expression of several development- and stress-responsive genes also increased, including *ABCG40*, *GST34*, *HCT*, *CAD*, *Psb28*, and *CYP709B1*. These genes are involved in metabolite transport, detoxification, and the regulation of photosynthesis. Upregulation of *CHN3*, *UGT79*, *MLO9*, and *XTH15* indicated activation of adaptive mechanisms to both biotic and abiotic stresses (Shi et al., 2024).

In turn, metabolomic and transcriptomic studies confirm that algal extracts strongly reprogram the energy and defense metabolism of plants. In *Arabidopsis thaliana*, application of extracts from *Durvillaea potatorum* and *A. nodosum* increased levels of Krebs cycle metabolites (e.g., citric acid and malate), amino acids (e.g., glutamine and proline), and defense metabolites (e.g., glucosinolate derivatives). It also altered lis changes in lipid metabolism and a decrease in auxin levels (Tran et al., 2023). In tomato plants, brown algae extracts applied before cold stress triggered dynamic changes in the expression of flavonoid biosynthesis genes (*CHS1*, *CHS2*, *CHI1*, *CHI3*, and *ANS*) and upregulated the defense-related *PR1* gene. Treated plants suffered less damage alting in less damage and better photosynthetic functioning (Borella et al., 2023).

A. nodosum extracts have been shown to improve tomato tolerance to both drought and salinity. Under drought stress, genes related to ascorbate, glutathione, and flavanol biosynthesis were induced, while senescence-associated genes in the ethylene pathway were repressed (Kanojia et al., 2024). Under salt stress, these preparations maintained a favorable K^+/Na^+ ratio through overexpression of the *NHX4* and *HKT1;2* genes and regulation of the *PIP2.1* and *TIP2.1* aquaporins, which helped maintain cellular water balance (Ikuyinminu et al., 2023).

Numerous transcriptomic and metabolomic studies demonstrate that algal-derived biostimulants have complex, multi-level effects on plant metabolism. These biostimulants modulate the expression of hundreds of genes related to photosynthesis, carbon and nitrogen metabolism, amino acid biosynthesis, and secondary metabolism, all while activating plant defense pathways. The induction of defense genes, coupled with increased levels of energy-related and antioxidant metabolites, leads to enhanced immunity, improved photosynthetic efficiency, and better adaptation to environmental stresses. The outcome of this regulation is not only greater tolerance to drought, cold, and salinity, but also increased crop productivity and quality. Algal biostimulants, therefore, do not act as mere nutrient sources; rather, they function as activators of the molecular mechanisms of plant growth and immunity.

15.3.6 Practical Validation and Successful Implementation of Algae-Based Products

The beneficial effects of algae-based preparations on plant growth and increased plant resistance to stress mean that these biological products are attracting growing interest, primarily among scientists and fertilizer manufacturers, but also gradually among farmers. This is due to their natural origin, high availability of raw materials, and documented and scientifically proven effectiveness. The beneficial effects of using algae preparations in agriculture are presented in numerous field studies. Staykov et al. (2025) conducted a 2-year field study to evaluate the effectiveness of an *A. nodosum*-based biostimulant on the yield of peppers (*Capsicum annuum*) and eggplants (*Solanum melongena*). The extracts were applied foliar in the early stages of flowering. It was shown that the use of the biostimulant resulted in an increase in total fruit yield (increase in the number of fruits per plant). In the first year of the study, the increase in pepper and eggplant yields compared to the group not treated with the extract was 28% and 81%, respectively, while in the second year, yields increased by 46% and 108%, respectively (Staykov et al., 2025). Another study involved 2 years of field trials to assess the effectiveness of biostimulants in organic strawberry cultivation (*Fragaria ananassa*). The experiment used seaweed extract in combination with a microbiological biostimulant. The preparations were applied foliar during the intensive growth phase of the plants. It was demonstrated that the use of a mixture of seaweed extract and a microbiological biostimulant resulted in a 23% average increase in marketable fruit yield and a 20% increase in total yield compared to the control. When single biostimulants were used, the effects were less stable and dependent on the season (Li et al., 2024).

There are also many studies analyzing commercially available algae-based preparations. One of them tested the effect of the Kelpak® biostimulant on spinach (*Spinacia oleracea*) cultivation in greenhouse conditions and exposure to salinity stress. The application of a 5% solution at a rate of 50 ml per week resulted in a significant improvement in growth, expressed, among other things, by dry and fresh plant mass, relative water content, and chlorophyll content (Sogoni et al., 2024). Another example is research conducted on the commercial biostimulant Expando® in apricot tree cultivation. The preparation was applied foliar in doses of 2.5 l/ha, 4.0 l/ha, and 5.0 l/ha when the fruit reached approximately 40% of its size. The use of the biostimulant increased the content of bioactive compounds, and the dose of 5.0 l/ha resulted in better harvest uniformity (Gatti et al., 2024). Łangowski et al. (2021) conducted field trials in Canada and Brazil to evaluate the commercial biostimulant Sealicit™ (Ascophyllum nodosum extract) in soybean cultivation. In Canada, Sealicit™ was foliar-applied at 1.5 L/ha at the V2–V3 vegetative stage, whereas in Brazil it was tested at 0.75, 1.5, and 3.0 L/ha on the pod shatter-susceptible cultivar UFUS 6901 and the shatter-resistant cultivar UFUS 7415. In UFUS 6901, the lowest dose reduced pod shattering nearly fivefold and increased yield by 6.6% relative to the control, while in UFUS 7415 the greatest yield increase, 17.9%, was observed at 1.5 L/ha (Łangowski et al., 2021).

The research conducted clearly confirms the high effectiveness of algae-based biostimulants in improving plant growth and yield. Numerous studies have shown that products based on algae extracts not only increase yields but also improve the quality and resistance of plants to stress factors. The results of field studies and experiments with commercial algal biostimulants demonstrate that they can be successfully applied to various crop species, including vegetables, fruit trees, and agricultural plants. Their effectiveness, natural origin, and compliance with the principles of sustainable agriculture make them an important element of modern cultivation technologies.

15.4 Algal Bioremediation in Agricultural Ecosystems

Algae play a crucial role at the intersection of agriculture and bioremediation, as they have the ability to bind and detoxify soil contaminants (Fig. 15.2). This applies to heavy metals, as well as pesticide residues and excess nutrients, which cause water eutrophication. Natural algal biopreparations can immobilize toxic metals, break down harmful organic compounds, and reduce nitrogen and phosphorus losses from farmland, thereby supporting environmental protection and sustainable agriculture (Ankit et al., 2022; Hammed et al., 2016; Kundu et al., 2024).

One of the best-known applications of algae is the sorption and neutralization of heavy metals. Metals such as lead (Pb), cadmium (Cd), mercury (Hg), and arsenic (As) pose a serious threat to soils contaminated by industrial and agricultural activities (Machado et al., 2024). Conventional remediation methods are costly and destructive to the soil, which is why biological solutions are being sought.

Marine macroalgae have long been known for their effective biosorption of metals. For example, alginate and fucoidan present in brown algae contain numerous carboxyl and sulfonic groups that strongly complex metal cations (Davis et al., 2003). The mechanism of metal binding by these polysaccharides is based on both ion exchange and the formation of stable complexes, which explains the high selectivity and sorption capacity of brown algae for heavy metals (Foday et al., 2021; Romera et al., 2007; Sanjay et al., 2020).

Microalgae and cyanobacteria also play a crucial role in bioremediation, although they are more often studied in the context of water purification than soil remediation. Microalgae (e.g., *Spirulina* sp.) are highly effective in biosorbing heavy metals, including chromium, cadmium, and copper ions. (Chojnacka et al., 2005). The studies have shown that biosorption occurs mainly through chemisorption, and the

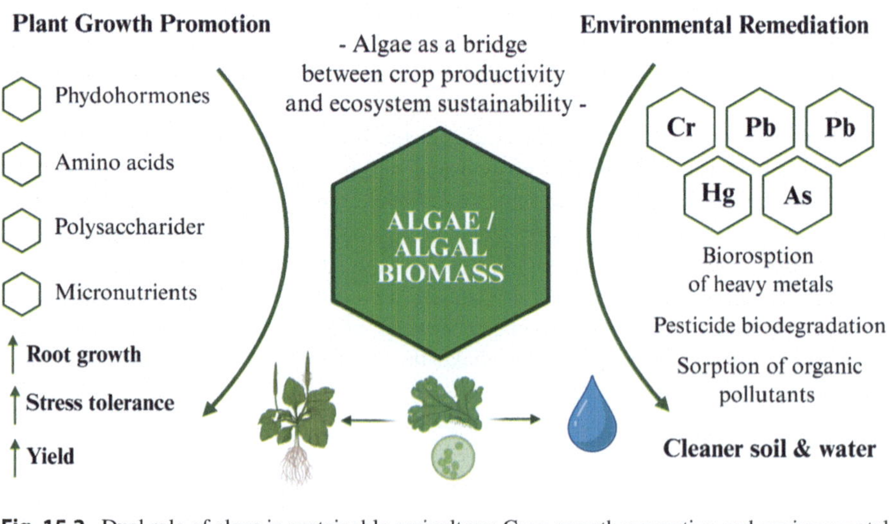

Fig. 15.2 Dual role of algae in sustainable agriculture: Crop growth promotion and environmental remediation

process itself is strongly dependent on pH, reaching equilibrium in less than 10 minutes. These results confirm that the active functional groups present on the cell walls of algae are crucial for the effective binding of metal cations (Chojnacka et al., 2005).

Another method of removing heavy metals is bioaccumulation, which, unlike biosorption, also involves the active transport of ions into cells. Chojnacka (2007) describe the bioaccumulation of Cr(III) ions by Spirulina sp. as a two-phase process, involving a rapid passive stage, similar to biosorption, and a slower stage of active accumulation that requires cellular metabolic activity. The process is significantly longer than biosorption alone, and equilibrium is achieved after approximately 30 hours. The bioaccumulation capacity was reported to be higher than in the case of biosorption alone (Chojnacka, 2007).

Some microalgae, such as *Chlorella vulgaris*, also demonstrate the ability to reduce toxic forms of metals, including Cr(VI), through photochemical processes. In a study conducted under halogen lamp irradiation ($\lambda = 365$ nm, 250 W), it was found that the presence of *C. vulgaris* significantly accelerated the reduction of Cr(VI) to the less toxic form Cr(III), especially in an acidic environment (pH 4). Furthermore, the study noted that the reduction efficiency increased with higher algae concentrations, but when the pH rose to 6, the reaction almost completely stopped, confirming the key role of acidic conditions and the photosynthetic activity of algae in this mechanism (Deng et al., 2006).

Previous studies have shown that microalgae, such as *Chlorella vulgaris*, have the ability not only to accumulate metals and metalloids, but also to transform and excrete them. In experiments conducted in the presence of arsenic (As(III)), it was found that these algae accumulated arsenic at a level of up to 610 mg As g^{-1} dry mass, with the dominant intracellular form being arsenate (As(V)), formed as a result of biooxidation. The formation of methylated arsenic derivatives, including trimethyl arsenic compounds (TMA), was also observed, indicating the ability of *C. vulgaris* to biomethylate arsenic. Arsenic metabolites were actively excreted by the cells, especially under conditions unfavorable for growth, confirming the potential of these algae for biological detoxification of the environment (Suhendrayatna et al., 1999).

The presence of algae also affects the chemical forms of metals in the soil. Thanks to the release of organic compounds and acids, metals are complexed and become less mobile and toxic to plants (Abd-Elhady & El-Zabalawy, 2014). In a pot experiment conducted at an experimental farm in Cairo, the effect of seaweed (*Ulva* sp. and *Gelidium* sp.) on the remediation of soil contaminated with heavy metals (Zn, Pb, Mn, and Cu) and on the growth and accumulation of metals in red radish plants (*Raphanus sativus L.*) was assessed. The application of algae in various doses had a beneficial effect on the physical and chemical properties of the soil, reducing its bulk density and increasing its porosity, organic matter content, and micronutrient availability. An increase in the aboveground and root biomass of radishes was also noted. At the same time, it was observed that the biosorption of heavy metals in the soil by seaweed reduced the concentrations of bioaccumulated metals in the roots of radishes and/or translocated to their shoots. (Abd-Elhady & El-Zabalawy, 2014).

The second area is the biodegradation of pesticides and the sorption of organic pollutants (Raymond Sunday, 2018). The effectiveness of pesticide removal by microalgae largely depends on the chemical structure of the pesticide and the strain of microalgae used. It has been demonstrated that some species of microalgae can use pesticide molecules as a source of carbon or nitrogen (Sutherland & Ralph, 2019; Verasoundarapandian et al., 2022). The mechanisms of pesticide biodegradation by algae include typical detoxification reactions found in higher organisms: oxidation (often involving cytochrome P450 enzymes), reduction, hydrolysis, or conjugation of the xenobiotic with other molecules in the cell (Xu & Huang, 2017).

An example of pesticide biodegradation by microalgae is *Coccomyxa subellipsoidea*, which breaks down organophosphates such as paraoxon, malathion, and diazinon in freshwater. This process occurs through the formation of reactive oxygen species, which is consistent with typical detoxification mechanisms in other organisms. Studies have shown that as a result of decomposition, the concentration of organophosphates drops to 0.1 mg/ml or less within 8–10 days. These studies confirm the potential of microalgae, especially in the bioremediation of pesticide-contaminated waters, offering an ecological solution to the problem of pesticides in the environment (Nicodemus et al., 2020). Similar results were obtained in studies on the microalga *Chlorella sorokiniana*, which showed high effectiveness in removing chlorpyrifos, an organophosphate pesticide. In an experiment conducted under controlled conditions, these microalgae achieved a removal efficiency of 99.85% for 300 ppm of chlorpyrifos after 120 hours of contact. At lower concentrations, i.e., 100 ppm and 500 ppm, the efficiency was 99.18% and 97.86%, respectively. The results confirmed that *Chlorella sorokiniana* can also be an effective bioremediation agent in the purification of water from organophosphate pesticides (Habibah et al., 2020).

It has also been observed that the presence of algae, providing easily degradable organic matter and oxygen, stimulates the growth of pesticide-degrading bacteria in the soil, creating a synergistic degradation system (Yadav et al., 2025). In addition to pesticides, microalgae can remove other harmful organic substances from soil and water, such as pharmaceuticals (e.g., antibiotics and hormones) and petroleum compounds. The mechanisms are analogous: biosorption (physical binding of molecules to the cell surface) and biochemical transformation within cells. For example, it has been reported that algae can accumulate antibiotics and gradually break them down into less active forms, which reduces the risk of these substances entering the food chain (Xiong et al., 2021). In the context of agricultural soils, greater attention is paid to veterinary drug residues, and algae can act as a biofilter, capturing and neutralizing these compounds before they contaminate groundwater.

Algae play a very important role in soil and water bioremediation, effectively removing pollutants such as heavy metals, pesticides, and pharmaceuticals. Their ability to biosorb and biotransform enables the reduction of toxic substances to less harmful forms, contributing to improved environmental quality. The use of algae in pollution management, both in the context of water purification and soil remediation, offers an environmental friendly and cost-effective solution that can support sustainable agriculture and environmental protection.

15.5 Regulation (EU) 2019/1009: Legal Framework for Biostimulants

Introduction of algae products into mainline agriculture requires not only research and implementation, but also an appropriate legal framework. For a long time, plant biostimulants (including those based on algae) operated in a legal gap. This caused difficulties in registering and trading these products on the international market (Ficosterra, 2025). The situation in the European Union was clarified by Regulation (EU) 2019/1009 on fertilizer products, adopted in 2019 (fully applicable from July 2022). This act introduced for the first time an official definition and a separate category for "plant biostimulants" in EU law (European Union, 2019; Ficosterra, 2025). According to the definition, a biostimulant is a product that stimulates plant nutrition processes regardless of nutrient content, with the sole purpose of improving at least one of the following characteristics of the plant or rhizosphere: nutrient use efficiency, abiotic stress tolerance, crop quality characteristics, or the availability of immobilized nutrients in the soil or rhizosphere (European Union, 2019). This is precisely the function performed by algae preparations. Regulation 2019/1009 classifies biostimulants as broadly understood fertilizer products and distinguishes a separate group for them—PFC 6 (Plant Biostimulant). Within PFC 6, the following subgroups are distinguished: PFC 6 (A) microbiological biostimulants and PFC6 (B) non-microbiological biostimulants, which formally included, among others, algae extract as recognized fertilizer products (previously, under the repealed Regulation 2003/2003, EU regulations mainly concerned mineral fertilizers) (European Union, 2019; Ficosterra, 2025). From 2022, biostimulants that meet the requirements of the regulation are eligible for CE marking and can be freely marketed in the EU single market without the need for separate registration in each Member State (Ficosterra, 2025).

The new regulations impose several requirements on biostimulant manufacturers regarding product safety and efficacy. Biostimulants must not pose a threat to human health, animals, or the environment. In practice, this means strictly limited levels of contaminants (heavy metals and pathogens) and a ban on the addition of ingredients considered hazardous (European Commission, 2022). The regulation specifies the maximum permissible concentrations of several potentially toxic elements in the product (Cd, Pb, Hg, Ni, and As) (Table 15.3). In addition, there are also limits on the content of metals that can potentially be accumulated by algae, such as copper up to 600 mg/kg and zinc up to 1500 mg/kg dry mass (European Union, 2019). Microbiological limits have also been introduced for biostimulants (for PFC 6(B): no *Salmonella* in 25 g, *Escherichia coli* or *Enterococcaceae* in 1000 in 1 g or 1 ml). The product must not contain any hazardous substances, such as prohibited active pesticides. The regulation provides that if a given compound would function as a plant protection product, the product cannot be placed on the market as a fertilizer product (European Union, 2019).

Regulation 2019/1009 also emphasizes the importance of documenting the biostimulation effect of the product. The producer is *obliged to conduct tests* demonstrating that the preparation in question actually produces the declared effects.

Table 15.3 Key provisions of Regulation (EU) 2019/1009 on plant biostimulants, with particular emphasis on algal products

Aspect	Requirements of Regulation (EU) 2019/1009 for plant biostimulants
Functional category (PFC)	PFC 6: Plant biostimulants—a new category of fertilizer products alongside fertilizers, liming agents, soil improvers, etc. biostimulants are divided into PFC 6(A) microbiological and PFC 6 (B) non-microbiological. PFC 6(A) covers only preparations containing authorized microorganisms (the list is specified in CMC 7), while PFC 6 (B) covers other biostimulants (e.g., plant extracts, including algae).
Permitted components (CMC)	Algae (macro- and microalgae) are treated as plant material—their extracts fall under CMC 2 (plant extracts, not chemically processed). Cyanobacteria are excluded from the definition of plants and are not permitted as an ingredient (even as an admixture). The only microorganisms (CMC 7) permitted in biostimulants are: *Azotobacter* spp., *Azospirillum* spp., *Rhizobium* spp., and mycorrhizal fungi.
Product safety	Contaminant limits have been set: e.g., Cd $\leq$1.5 mg/kg dry weight, Pb $\leq$120 mg/kg dry weight, as (inorganic) $\leq$40 mg/kg, Cr(VI) $\leq$2 mg/kg. Additionally, Cu $\leq$600 mg/kg and Zn $\leq$1500 mg/kg. Microbial and nonmicrobial biostimulants must be free of pathogens (e.g., *Salmonella* absent in 25 g, *Escherichia coli* or *Enterococcaceae* <1000 in 1 g or 1 ml). The use of hazardous substances, e.g., active pesticides (the product must not have a plant protection function) or phosphonates (prohibited from being added intentionally), is prohibited. The manufacturer must demonstrate that even possible trace contaminants do not compromise the product's safety.
Demonstration of efficacy	Obligation to prove the declared effects—the producer must provide test results confirming that the biostimulant works as stated on the label. Tests (e.g., field trials) should demonstrate a statistically significant improvement in the specified parameters (e.g., increased nutrient uptake, higher yield, and improved drought resistance). This condition prevents the marketing of preparations with untested or questionable effectiveness and raises the quality bar for all suppliers.
Certification and marketing	A biostimulant that meets the criteria can obtain CE marking. A CE-certified product benefits from the EU single market and can be sold in all member states without requiring separate national registration.

The results of such tests must be statistically significant and included in the technical documentation required for CE marking. This is to protect farmers and gardeners from products of dubious effectiveness. The law, therefore, enforces the professionalization of the industry, obliging companies developing biostimulants (including algae-based ones) to invest in R&D and reliable efficacy testing comparable to the requirements for plant protection products (Ficosterra, 2025).

The regulation defines in detail the categories of materials from which fertilizer products may be manufactured (CMC—component material categories, listed in Annex II of the regulation). In the case of algal biostimulants, two categories are key: CMC 2—"plant materials and their extracts" and CMC 7—"microorganisms." Both macroalgae and microalgae have been classified as plant materials (European Commission, 2022). This opens the way for the use of algae extracts in biostimulants in accordance with legal requirements. However, it is important to note that the regulation excludes cyanobacteria from the definition of permitted materials. (European Commission, 2022). In the case of microbial biostimulants (PFC 6(A)), the regulation initially allowed only four groups of microorganisms in CMC 7: bacteria of the genera *Azotobacter, Azospirillum*, and *Rhizobium*, and mycorrhizal fungi (European Union, 2019). Only these microorganisms can be used as components of microbiological biostimulants marketed in the EU. Only after additional organisms are added to CMC 7 will it be possible to place biostimulants containing other living microorganisms (e.g., *Trichoderma* and *Bacillus*) or potentially cyanobacteria/microalgae in living form on the EU market.

This new law has significantly accelerated the biostimulant industry in Europe. Having a common market and clear rules makes investors and companies in the biostimulant business feel more confident. As a result, a bunch of companies (even ones outside the EU) are getting ready to bring algae-based biostimulants to the European market. There has also been an increase in patent activity. Companies are trying to protect their unique formulas and methods of obtaining components from algae in the face of growing competition. Regulation 2019/1009 indirectly supports innovation by creating preferences for biostimulants that use the principles of the circular economy.

15.6 Challenges and Future Perspectives

Algae play a dual role in agriculture: On the one hand, they stimulate plant growth as biostimulants, and on the other, they support environmental bioremediation by binding pollutants in soil and water (Miranda et al., 2024). However, overcoming many challenges is necessary to realize their full potential. One of these challenges is the seasonal variability in the composition of algal biomass, which is influenced by environmental conditions. The chemical composition of seaweed varies significantly depending on the species, location, and time of harvest (James et al., 2025), which makes it difficult to standardize preparations and may cause heterogeneity in their effects. The remedial strategy involves cultivating algae under controlled conditions, resulting in biomass with a more stable and predictable composition throughout the year. Such a cultivation system reduces in vivo variability and may even increase the level of desirable bioactive compounds by optimizing growth conditions (El et al., 2020; Zollmann et al., 2019). The selection or modification of algae strains rich in specific metabolites is also important, as this further improves the repeatability of the effects of the preparations.

Another challenge is optimizing the dosage and application techniques for algal biostimulants. There is still a lack of tools to support farmers in selecting the right dosage and timing of application, which translates into variability in the results obtained (El et al., 2020). It is necessary to develop good practices for use, precise guidelines on dosage, frequency, and method of application in order to increase the predictability of the effects of algae preparations (El et al., 2020). At the same time, standardizing the active ingredients of algae extracts remains a challenge. The complexity of the mixture of bioactive compounds makes it difficult to identify which components are responsible for specific effects, which limits the possibility of unequivocally confirming the effectiveness of such products (Kapoore et al., 2021; Loconsole et al., 2023). Future research must therefore focus on identifying and quantifying key molecules so that biostimulant formulations can be standardized and reliable.

The forms and formulations of algae products also need improvement. Liquid algae extract often has a limited shelf life, making them challenging to store and transport. Advances in formulation technology, such as microencapsulation of ingredients, extend the shelf life of preparations, facilitate field application, and ensure controlled release of active substances (Magnabosco et al., 2023). Encapsulation of bioactive components in biodegradable polymers protects them from degradation and stabilizes the product during storage, increasing the effectiveness and convenience of using algal biostimulants (Nkurunziza et al., 2025; Zabot et al., 2022).

In terms of implementation prospects, commercialization and market regulation barriers are significant. The high costs of obtaining algal biomass and the complex processes involved in its processing limit the competitiveness of such products. At the same time, producers must meet new legal requirements, such as EU regulations imposing an obligation to prove the declared functions of a biostimulant (European Union, 2019; Ricci et al., 2019). Despite these difficulties, harmonization of regulations brings order to the market and increases confidence in algal biopreparations. The key strategy for improving profitability is the concept of an algal biorefinery, which utilizes biomass comprehensively. A single algae crop can be used to produce biostimulants, feed, and energy raw materials in parallel (Kaur & Singh, 2024; Olguín et al., 2022; Ruales et al., 2025), which increases the economic value of the entire process. The transition from wild harvesting to controlled cultivation, combined with the cascading production of multiple products, will reduce both the problem of variable raw material quality and the unit costs of the product (El et al., 2020). In addition, algae cultivation on cheap waste substrates (e.g., sewage) simultaneously reduces costs and performs the function of environmental bioremediation, fitting into the circular economy model (Álvarez-González et al., 2023; Iakovidou et al., 2024). In summary, overcoming the above barriers and implementing innovative solutions should strengthen the dual role of algae in agriculture. Advances in standardization, formulation, and cultivation technologies will translate into more predictable performance of algal biostimulants, facilitating their wider use. Algae as biostimulants and biofertilizers can become an important element of sustainable crop intensification, combining yield improvement with environmental protection.

15.7 Conclusion

Biostimulants and biofertilizers derived from algae offer a solution that combines effective crop management with minimizing the negative environmental impact of agriculture. Due to their natural content of substances such as phytohormones, amino acids, and polysaccharides, algae-based preparations stimulate the development of plant root systems, enhance the utilization of soil nutrients, and increase crop resistance to stress factors. As a result, their use leads to healthier and more productive plants. The use of algae-based biopreparations reduces nitrate emissions into the environment and decreases the accumulation of heavy metals in plant tissues, which improves the quality and safety of crops. The introduction of algae biomass into soil or water systems results in the binding and immobilization of heavy metals, the precipitation of excess phosphates, and the acceleration of the biodegradation of pesticide residues. Such bioremediation reduces the risk of groundwater and surface runoff contamination, contributing to a cleaner ecosystem around agricultural fields. Algal biostimulants and biofertilizers, therefore, not only enhance plant growth but also help protect soil and water from the negative effects of intensive agriculture. Standardized regulations facilitate the introduction of algae-based biostimulants onto the market, promoting their wider use in agricultural practice. The use of wastewater or other waste as a medium for microalgae cultivation, combined with energy-efficient methods of low-temperature biomass dewatering and the recovery of by-products, makes the production of algae-based biostimulants more cost-effective and associated with a smaller carbon footprint. This approach is in line with the idea of a circular economy, where resources are used repeatedly, and waste is minimized. Despite their many advantages, algal biostimulants and biofertilizers still face some challenges in their use. One of them is the seasonal changes in the composition and quality of algal biomass, which can affect the uniformity of the products' performance. Another problem is the limited shelf life of liquid algae extracts, especially at higher temperatures, which significantly hinders the transport and storage of these preparations in warm climates. In some cases, there is still a lack of comprehensive decision support tools for farmers that would allow them to precisely select the optimal dose and application date of the biostimulant for specific field conditions. All these factors mean that the effectiveness of algal products can be variable. Intensive research and development work is focused on improving algal preparations and eliminating these limitations. The selection and modification of algal strains allow for the production of biomass with a more predictable composition and a higher content of desirable active compounds. Simultaneously, formulation technologies such as nutrient encapsulation are being improved, extending product shelf life, facilitating application, and ensuring controlled release of active substances. More importantly, the development of integrated biorefineries enables the full potential of algae biomass to be exploited: A single crop can yield various valuable products (e.g., biostimulants, feed, and biofuels), thereby improving the economic viability of the entire process. In summary, these innovations are expected to contribute to strengthening the role of algae in modern agriculture in the years to come. Algal biostimulants and biofertilizers are becoming an important element of practices promoting the sustainable intensification of plant production, and their wider implementation aligns with the concept of precision agriculture.

References

Abd-Elhady, E. S. E., & El-Zabalawy, K. M. (2014). Remediation of a soil contaminated with heavy metals using some seaweeds. *Journal of Soil Sciences and Agricultural Engineering, 5*, 1623–1633. https://doi.org/10.21608/JSSAE.2014.49817

Abinandan, S., Subashchandrabose, S. R., Venkateswarlu, K., & Megharaj, M. (2019). Soil microalgae and cyanobacteria: The biotechnological potential in the maintenance of soil fertility and health. *Critical Reviews in Biotechnology, 39*, 981–998. https://doi.org/10.1080/07388551.2019.1654972

Abka-khajouei, R., Tounsi, L., Shahabi, N., Patel, A. K., Abdelkafi, S., & Michaud, P. (2022). Structures, properties and applications of alginates. *Marine Drugs, 20*, 364. https://doi.org/10.3390/MD20060364

Akbar, W. A., Rahim, H. U., & Rutigliano, F. A. (2024). Microbial- and seaweed-based biopolymers: Sources, extractions and implications for soil quality improvement and environmental sustainability – A review. *Journal of Environmental Management, 359*, 120964. https://doi.org/10.1016/J.JENVMAN.2024.120964

Alam, M. Z., Braun, G., Norrie, J., & Hodges, D. M. (2013). Effect of Ascophyllum extract application on plant growth, fruit yield and soil microbial communities of strawberry. *Canadian Journal of Plant Science, 93*, 23–36. https://doi.org/10.4141/CJPS2011-260/ASSET/IMAGES/LARGE/CJPS2011-260F9.JPEG

Al-Ghamdi, A. A., & Elansary, H. O. (2018). Synergetic effects of 5-aminolevulinic acid and *Ascophyllum nodosum* seaweed extracts on *Asparagus phenolics* and stress related genes under saline irrigation. *Plant Physiology and Biochemistry, 129*, 273–284. https://doi.org/10.1016/J.PLAPHY.2018.06.008

Ali, O., Ramsubhag, A., & Jayaraman, J. (2021). Biostimulant properties of seaweed extracts in plants: Implications towards sustainable crop production. *Plants, 2021*(10), 531. https://doi.org/10.3390/PLANTS10030531

Ali, M. Q., Azhar, M. A., Munaim, M. S. A., Ruslan, N. F., Alsubhi, L. M., Ahmad, N., & Noman, A. E. (2024). Seaweed organic compounds source of hydrocolloids and sustainable food packaging: Properties, application, and future direction. *Discover Food, 2024*(4), 1–28. https://doi.org/10.1007/S44187-024-00173-W

Alvarez, A. L., Weyers, S. L., Goemann, H. M., Peyton, B. M., & Gardner, R. D. (2021). Microalgae, soil and plants: A critical review of microalgae as renewable resources for agriculture. *Algal Research, 54*, 102200. https://doi.org/10.1016/J.ALGAL.2021.102200

Álvarez-González, A., Greque de Morais, E., Planas-Carbonell, A., & Uggetti, E. (2023). Enhancing sustainability through microalgae cultivation in urban wastewater for biostimulant production and nutrient recovery. *Science of the Total Environment, 904*, 166878. https://doi.org/10.1016/J.SCITOTENV.2023.166878

Ankit, Bauddh, K., & Korstad, J. (2022). Phycoremediation: Use of algae to sequester heavy metals. *Hydrobiology, 2022*(1), 288–303. https://doi.org/10.3390/HYDROBIOLOGY1030021

Asimakis, E., Shehata, A. A., Eisenreich, W., Acheuk, F., Lasram, S., Basiouni, S., Emekci, M., Ntougias, S., Taner, G., May-Simera, H., Yilmaz, M., & Tsiamis, G. (2022). Algae and their metabolites as potential bio-pesticides. *Microorganisms, 10*, 307. https://doi.org/10.3390/MICROORGANISMS10020307

Baćmaga, M., Wyszkowska, J., & Kucharski, J. (2024). The role of sodium alginate hydrogel in maintaining soil homeostasis exposed to Sulcotrione. *Agriculture (Switzerland), 14*, 2081. https://doi.org/10.3390/AGRICULTURE14112081/S1

Biradar, S., Phule, M., & Vidyapeeth, K. (2025). *Seaweed extract: Nectar for plant and soil improvement*. https://doi.org/10.13140/RG.2.2.14812.77448

Bleakley, S., & Hayes, M. (2017). Algal proteins: Extraction, application, and challenges concerning production. *Food, 6*, 33. https://doi.org/10.3390/FOODS6050033

Borella, M., Baghdadi, A., Bertoldo, G., Della Lucia, M. C., Chiodi, C., Celletti, S., Deb, S., Baglieri, A., Zegada-Lizarazu, W., Pagani, E., Monti, A., Mangione, F., Magro, F., Hermans, C., Stevanato, P., & Nardi, S. (2023). Transcriptomic and physiological approaches to decipher cold stress mitigation exerted by brown-seaweed extract application in tomato. *Frontiers in Plant Science, 14*, 1232421. https://doi.org/10.3389/fpls.2023.1232421

Brick, M. B., Hussein, M. H., Mowafy, A. M., Hamouda, R. A., Ayyad, A. M., & Refaay, D. A. (2025). Significance of siderophore-producing cyanobacteria on enhancing iron uptake potentiality of maize plants grown under iron-deficiency. *Microbial Cell Factories, 24*, 1–18. https://doi.org/10.1186/S12934-024-02618-4/TABLES/8

Cantón, Y., Chamizo, S., Rodriguez-Caballero, E., Lázaro, R., Roncero-Ramos, B., Román, J. R., & Solé-Benet, A. (2020). Water regulation in cyanobacterial biocrusts from drylands: Negative impacts of anthropogenic disturbance. *Water, 12*, 720. https://doi.org/10.3390/W12030720

Chojnacka, K. (2007). Bioaccumulation of Cr(III) ions by blue-green alga spirulina sp. Part I. A comparison with biosorption. *American Journal of Agricultural and Biological Sciences, 2*, 218–223.

Chojnacka, K., Chojnacki, A., & Górecka, H. (2005). Biosorption of Cr3+, Cd2+ and Cu2+ ions by blue-green algae spirulina sp.: Kinetics, equilibrium and the mechanism of the process. *Chemosphere, 59*, 75–84. https://doi.org/10.1016/j.chemosphere.2004.10.005

Circuncisão, A. R., Catarino, M. D., Cardoso, S. M., & Silva, A. M. S. (2018). Minerals from macroalgae origin: Health benefits and risks for consumers. *Marine Drugs, 16*, 400. https://doi.org/10.3390/MD16110400

Coppens, J., Grunert, O., Van Den Hende, S., Vanhoutte, I., Boon, N., Haesaert, G., & De Gelder, L. (2016). The use of microalgae as a high-value organic slow-release fertilizer results in tomatoes with increased carotenoid and sugar levels. *Journal of Applied Phycology, 28*, 2367–2377. https://doi.org/10.1007/S10811-015-0775-2/FIGURES/6

Davis, T. A., Volesky, B., & Mucci, A. (2003). A review of the biochemistry of heavy metal biosorption by brown algae. *Water Research, 37*, 4311–4330. https://doi.org/10.1016/S0043-1354(03)00293-8

de Borba, M. C., Velho, A. C., de Freitas, M. B., Holvoet, M., Maia-Grondard, A., Baltenweck, R., Magnin-Robert, M., Randoux, B., Hilbert, J. L., Reignault, P., Hugueney, P., Siah, A., & Stadnik, M. J. (2022). A Laminarin-based formulation protects wheat against Zymoseptoria tritici via direct antifungal activity and elicitation of host defense-related genes. *Plant Disease, 106*, 1408–1418. https://doi.org/10.1094/PDIS-08-21-1675-RE/ASSET/IMAGES/LARGE/PDIS-08-21-1675-REF7-1650633317477.JPEG

Del Buono, D. (2021). Can biostimulants be used to mitigate the effect of anthropogenic climate change on agriculture? It is time to respond. *Science of the Total Environment, 751*, 141763. https://doi.org/10.1016/J.SCITOTENV.2020.141763

Deng, L., Wang, H., & Deng, N. (2006). Photoreduction of chromium(VI) in the presence of algae, Chlorella vulgaris. *Journal of Hazardous Materials, 138*, 288–292. https://doi.org/10.1016/J.JHAZMAT.2006.04.062

Drobek, M., Frąc, M., & Cybulska, J. (2019). Plant biostimulants: Importance of the quality and yield of horticultural crops and the improvement of plant tolerance to abiotic stress—A review. *Agronomy, 9*, 335. https://doi.org/10.3390/AGRONOMY9060335

EBIC. (2025). Plant Biostimulants [WWW Document]. https://biostimulants.eu/plant-biostimulants/. Accessed 7.29.25.

El, M., El Boukhari, M., Barakate, M., Bouhia, Y., & Lyamlouli, K. (2020). Trends in seaweed extract based biostimulants: Manufacturing process and beneficial effect on soil-plant systems. *Plants, 9*, 359. https://doi.org/10.3390/PLANTS9030359

Elansary, H. O., Yessoufou, K., Abdel-Hamid, A. M. E., El-Esawi, M. A., Ali, H., & Elshikh, M. S. (2017). Seaweed extracts enhance salam turfgrass performance during prolonged irrigation intervals and saline shock. *Frontiers in Plant Science, 8*, 264359. https://doi.org/10.3389/FPLS.2017.00830/BIBTEX

El-Beltagi, H. S., Mohamed, A. A., Mohamed, H. I., Ramadan, K. M. A., Barqawi, A. A., & Mansour, A. T. (2022). Phytochemical and potential properties of seaweeds and their recent applications: A review. *Marine Drugs, 20*, 342. https://doi.org/10.3390/MD20060342

Elnajar, M., Aldesuquy, H., Abdelmoteleb, M., & Eltanahy, E. (2024). Mitigating drought stress in wheat plants (*Triticum Aestivum* L.) through grain priming in aqueous extract of spirulina platensis. *BMC Plant Biology, 24*, 1–27. https://doi.org/10.1186/S12870-024-04905-Z

European Commission. (2022). *Regulation (EU) 2019/1009—The Fertilising products regulation frequently asked questions*.

European Union. (2019). *Regulation (EU) 2019/1009 of the European Parliament and of the Council*. Official Journal of the European Union.

Fernández-Rojas, B., Hernández-Juárez, J., & Pedraza-Chaverri, J. (2014). Nutraceutical properties of phycocyanin. *Journal of Functional Foods, 11*, 375–392. https://doi.org/10.1016/J.JFF.2014.10.011

Ficosterra. (2025). Seaweed-Based Biostimulants: A Growing Industry – [WWW Document]. https://www.ficosterra.com/en/bioestimulantes-de-algas-marinas-una-industria-en-crecimiento/. Accessed 7.30.25.

Fiset, C., Irwin, A. J., & Finkel, Z. V. (2019). The macromolecular composition of noncalcified marine macroalgae. *Journal of Phycology, 55*, 1361–1369. https://doi.org/10.1111/JPY.12913; CTYPE:STRING:JOURNAL

Foday, E. H., Bo, B., Xu, X., Núñez-Delgado, A., Zhang, Z., Bontempi, E., Coccia, M., Race, M., Zhou, Y., & Rosen, M. A. (2021). *Sustainability removal of toxic heavy metals from contaminated aqueous solutions using seaweeds: A review*. https://doi.org/10.3390/su132112311

Fozi, V., Esmaeili, H., Alizadeh, A., Eghlima, G., & Mirjalili, M. H. (2024). The interaction effect of water deficit stress and seaweed extract on phytochemical characteristics and antioxidant activity of licorice (Glycyrrhiza glabra L.). *Frontiers in Plant SciencePlant Science, 15*, 1474399. https://doi.org/10.3389/FPLS.2024.1474399/FULL

Gatti, N., Maghrebi, M., Serio, G., Gentile, C., Bunea, V. V., Vigliante, I., Boitte, C., Garabello, C., Contartese, V., Bertea, C. M., & Mannino, G. (2024). Seaweed and yeast extracts as sustainable phytostimulant to boost secondary metabolism of apricot fruits. *Frontiers in Plant Science, 15*, 1455156. https://doi.org/10.3389/fpls.2024.1455156

Ghorai, P., & Ghosh, D. (2022). Ameliorating the performance of NPK biofertilizers to attain sustainable agriculture with special emphasis on bioengineering. *Bioresource Technology Reports, 19*, 101117. https://doi.org/10.1016/J.BITEB.2022.101117

Habibah, R., Iswanto, B., & Rinanti, A. (2020). The significance of tropical microalgae chlorella Sorokiniana as a remediate of polluted water caused by Chlorpyrifos. *International Journal of Scientific & Technology Research, 9*, 1. https://doi.org/10.1016/j.etap.2016.05.032

Hammed, A. M., Prajapati, S. K., Simsek, S., & Simsek, H. (2016). Growth regime and environmental remediation of microalgae. *Algae, 31*, 189–204. https://doi.org/10.4490/ALGAE.2016.31.8.28

He, J., & Chen, J. P. (2014). A comprehensive review on biosorption of heavy metals by algal biomass: Materials, performances, chemistry, and modeling simulation tools. *Bioresource Technology, 160*, 67–78. https://doi.org/10.1016/J.BIORTECH.2014.01.068

Hejna, M., Dell'Anno, M., Liu, Y., Rossi, L., Aksmann, A., Pogorzelski, G., & Jóźwik, A. (2024). Assessment of the antibacterial and antioxidant activities of seaweed-derived extracts. *Scientific Reports, 14*, 1–15. https://doi.org/10.1038/S41598-024-71961-8

Hossain, M. S., Islam, A. S. M. Z., Islam, M. G., Kumar, D., Mahmud, M. H., & Mahato, D. K. (2023). Effects of cyanobacteria on soil properties in forest and cultivated lands of Madhupur tract 2023. *Bangladesh Journal of Agriculture, 48*, 112–122. https://doi.org/10.3329/bjagri.v48i1.66769

Iakovidou, G., Itziou, A., Tsiotsias, A., Lakioti, E., Samaras, P., Tsanaktsidis, C., & Karayannis, V. (2024). Application of microalgae to wastewater bioremediation, with CO2 biomitigation, health product and biofuel development, and environmental biomonitoring. *Applied Sciences, 14*, 6727. https://doi.org/10.3390/APP14156727

Ikuyinminu, E., Goñi, O., Łangowski, Ł., & O'Connell, S. (2023). Transcriptome, biochemical and phenotypic analysis of the effects of a precision engineered biostimulant for inducing salinity stress tolerance in tomato. *International Journal of Molecular Sciences, 24*(8). https://doi.org/10.3390/ijms24086988

Issa, A., Hemida, M., Ohyam, T., 2014. Nitrogen fixing cyanobacteria: Future prospect. Advances in biology and ecology of nitrogen fixation. https://doi.org/10.5772/56995.

Jacomassi, L. M., de Viveiros, J. O., Oliveira, M. P., Momesso, L., de Siqueira, G. F., & Crusciol, C. A. C. (2022). A seaweed extract-based biostimulant mitigates drought stress in sugarcane. *Frontiers in Plant Science, 13*, 865291. https://doi.org/10.3389/FPLS.2022.865291/ENDNOTE

James, V. C. X., Thiraviam, A. G. P., Al-Dosary, M. A., Hatamleh, A. A., Bukhari, N. A., Arokiyaraj, S., & Kalaiyarasi, M. (2025). Evaluation of nutrient composition and biostimulant properties of seaweeds for improving soil microbial population and tomato plant growth. *BioResources, 20*, 1431–1451. https://doi.org/10.15376/BIORES.20.1.1431-1451

Jiménez-Arias, D., García-Machado, F. J., Morales-Sierra, S., García-García, A. L., Herrera, A. J., Valdés, F., Luis, J. C., & Borges, A. A. (2021). A beginner's guide to Osmoprotection by biostimulants. *Plants, 10*, 363. https://doi.org/10.3390/PLANTS10020363

Kakinuma, M., Park, C. S., & Amano, H. (2001). Distribution of free L-cysteine and glutathione in seaweeds. *Fisheries Science, 67*, 194–196. https://doi.org/10.1046/J.1444-2906.2001.00223.X

Kanojia, A., Lyall, R., Sujeeth, N., Alseekh, S., Martínez-Rivas, F. J., Fernie, A. R., Gechev, T. S., & Petrov, V. (2024). Physiological and molecular insights into the effect of a seaweed biostimulant on enhancing fruit yield and drought tolerance in tomato. *Plant Stress, 14*(12), 100692. https://doi.org/10.1016/j.stress.2024.100692

Kapoore, R. V., Wood, E. E., & Llewellyn, C. A. (2021). Algae biostimulants: A critical look at microalgal biostimulants for sustainable agricultural practices. *Biotechnology Advances, 49*, 107754. https://doi.org/10.1016/J.BIOTECHADV.2021.107754

Kaur, S., & Singh, R. (2024). Algae-based biorefineries for animal feed and aquaculture applications. In *Value added products from bioalgae based biorefineries: Opportunities and challenges* (pp. 365–381). https://doi.org/10.1007/978-981-97-1662-3_15

Kchikich, A., Roussi, Z., Krid, A., Nhhala, N., Ennoury, A., Benmrid, B., Kounnoun, A., El Maadoudi, M., Nhiri, N., & Mohamed, N. (2024). Effects of mycorrhizal symbiosis and Ulva lactuca seaweed extract on growth, carbon/nitrogen metabolism, and antioxidant response in cadmium-stressed sorghum plant. *Physiology and Molecular Biology of Plants, 30*, 605–618. https://doi.org/10.1007/S12298-024-01446-5

Khan, W., Rayirath, U. P., Subramanian, S., Jithesh, M. N., Rayorath, P., Hodges, D. M., Critchley, A. T., Craigie, J. S., Norrie, J., & Prithiviraj, B. (2009). Seaweed extracts as biostimulants of plant growth and development. *Journal of Plant Growth Regulation, 28*, 386–399. https://doi.org/10.1007/S00344-009-9103-X/FIGURES/2

Khan, W., Zhai, R., Souleimanov, A., Critchley, A. T., Smith, D. L., & Prithiviraj, B. (2012). Commercial extract of Ascophyllum nodosum improves root colonization of alfalfa by its bacterial symbiont Sinorhizobium meliloti. *Communications in Soil Science and Plant Analysis, 43*, 2425–2436. https://doi.org/10.1080/00103624.2012.708079;PAGE:STRING:ARTICLE/CHAPTER

Koçer, A. T., İnan, B., Kaptan Usul, S., Özçimen, D., Yılmaz, M. T., & Işıldak, İ. (2021). Exopolysaccharides from microalgae: Production, characterization, optimization and techno-economic assessment. *Brazilian Journal of Microbiology, 52*, 1779. https://doi.org/10.1007/S42770-021-00575-3

Kumar Gupta, V., Nayak, A., & Agarwal, S. (2015). Bioadsorbents for remediation of heavy metals: Current status and their future prospects. *Environmental Engineering Research, 20*, 1–18. https://doi.org/10.4491/eer.2015.018

Kumar, J., Khan, S., Mandotra, S. K., Dhar, P., Tayade, A. B., Verma, S., Toppo, K., Arora, R., Upreti, D. K., & Chaurasia, O. P. (2019). Nutraceutical profile and evidence of alleviation of oxidative stress by Spirogyra porticalis (Muell.) Cleve inhabiting the high altitude Trans-Himalayan Region. *Scientific Reports, 9*, 1–13. https://doi.org/10.1038/S41598-018-35595-X

Kumar, S., Diksha, Sindhu, S. S., & Kumar, R. (2022). Biofertilizers: An ecofriendly technology for nutrient recycling and environmental sustainability. *Current Research in Microbial Sciences, 3*, 100094. https://doi.org/10.1016/J.CRMICR.2021.100094

Kumar, G., Nanda, S., Singh, S. K., Kumar, S., Singh, D., Singh, B. N., & Mukherjee, A. (2024). Seaweed extracts: Enhancing plant resilience to biotic and abiotic stresses. *Frontiers in Marine Science, 11*, 1457500. https://doi.org/10.3389/FMARS.2024.1457500/XML

Kumari, R., Kaur, I., & Bhatnagar, A. K. (2011). Effect of aqueous extract of Sargassum johnstonii Setchell & Gardner on growth, yield and quality of Lycopersicon esculentum Mill. *Journal of Applied Phycology, 23*, 623–633. https://doi.org/10.1007/S10811-011-9651-X/FIGURES/4

Kundu, P., Dutta, N., & Bhattacharya, S. (2024). Application of microalgae in wastewater treatment with special reference to emerging contaminants: A step towards sustainability. *Frontiers in Analytical Science, 4*, 1513153. https://doi.org/10.3389/FRANS.2024.1513153/XML

Łangowski, Ł., Goñi, O., Marques, F. S., Hamawaki, O. T., da Silva, C. O., Nogueira, A. P. O., Teixeira, M. A. J., Glasenapp, J. S., Pereira, M., & O'Connell, S. (2021). Ascophyllum nodosum extract (SealicitTM) boosts soybean yield through reduction of pod shattering-related seed loss and enhanced seed production. *Frontiers in Plant Science, 12*, 631768. https://doi.org/10.3389/fpls.2021.631768

Laroche, C. (2022). Exopolysaccharides from microalgae and cyanobacteria: Diversity of strains, production strategies, and applications. *Marine Drugs, 20*, 336. https://doi.org/10.3390/MD20050336

Li, J., Brecht, J. K., Kim, J., Bailey, L. S., Kamat, M. N., Basso, K. B., Colee, J. C., Zhao, X., Li, J., Brecht, J. K., Kim, J., Bailey, L. S., Kamat, M. N., Basso, K. B., Colee, J. C., & Zhao, X. (2024). Seaweed extract and microbial biostimulants show synergistic effects on improving organic strawberry production. *HortScience, 59*(8), 1114–1126. https://doi.org/10.21273/HORTSCI17647-23

Loconsole, D., Cristiano, G., & De Lucia, B. (2023). Biostimulant application, under reduced nutrient supply, enhances quality and sustainability of ornamental containerized transplants. *Agronomy, 13*, 765. https://doi.org/10.3390/AGRONOMY13030765

Lu, Y., & Xu, J. (2015). Phytohormones in microalgae: A new opportunity for microalgal biotechnology? *Trends in Plant Science, 20*, 273–282. https://doi.org/10.1016/J.TPLANTS.2015.01.006/ATTACHMENT/407CC75D-244B-46EF-8B25-10612054CA8B/MMC1.DOCX

Ma, Y., Dias, M. C., & Freitas, H. (2020). Drought and salinity stress responses and microbe-induced tolerance in plants. *Frontiers in Plant Science, 11*, 591911. https://doi.org/10.3389/FPLS.2020.591911/XML

Machado, A. A., Valiaparampil, J. G., & Lavanya, M. (2024). Unlocking the potential of algae for heavy metal remediation. *Water, Air, and Soil Pollution, 235*, 1–13. https://doi.org/10.1007/S11270-024-07436-3/TABLES/1

Magnabosco, P., Masi, A., Shukla, R., Bansal, V., & Carletti, P. (2023). Advancing the impact of plant biostimulants to sustainable agriculture through nanotechnologies chemical and biological technologies in agriculture. *Chemical and Biological Technologies in Agriculture, 10*, 117. https://doi.org/10.1186/s40538-023-00491-8

Malešević, T. P., Dulić, T., Obreht, I., Trivunović, Z., Marković, R., Kostić, B., Važić, T., Meriluoto, J., & Svirčev, Z. (2020). Cyanobacterial potential for restoration of loess surfaces through artificially induced biocrusts. *Applied Sciences, 11*, 66. https://doi.org/10.3390/APP11010066

Martínez-Cano, B., Mendoza-Meneses, C. J., García-Trejo, J. F., Macías-Bobadilla, G., Aguirre-Becerra, H., Soto-Zarazúa, G. M., & Feregrino-Pérez, A. A. (2022). Review and perspectives of the use of alginate as a polymer matrix for microorganisms applied in agro-industry. *Molecules, 27*, 4248. https://doi.org/10.3390/MOLECULES27134248

Mattner, S. W., Wite, D., Riches, D. A., Porter, I. J., & Arioli, T. (2013). The effect of kelp extract on seedling establishment of broccoli on contrasting soil types in southern Victoria, Australia. *Biological Agriculture & Horticulture, 29*, 258–270. https://doi.org/10.1080/01448765.2013.830276

Mattner, S. W., Milinkovic, M., & Arioli, T. (2018). Increased growth response of strawberry roots to a commercial extract from Durvillaea potatorum and Ascophyllum nodosum. *Journal of Applied Phycology, 30*, 2943–2951. https://doi.org/10.1007/S10811-017-1387-9/TABLES/8

Ministry of Agriculture & Farmers Welfare. (2025). Regulation of biostimulant products under Fertilizer Control Order (FCO), 1985. Press Information Bureau, Government of India. https://www.pib.gov.in/PressReleasePage.aspx?PRID=2165081

Miranda, A. M., Hernandez-Tenorio, F., Villalta, F., Vargas, G. J., & Sáez, A. A. (2024). Advances in the development of biofertilizers and biostimulants from microalgae. *Biology-Basel, 13*, 199. https://doi.org/10.3390/BIOLOGY13030199

Morillas-España, A., Ruiz-Nieto, Á., Lafarga, T., Acién, G., Arbib, Z., & González-López, C. V. (2022). Biostimulant capacity of chlorella and Chlamydopodium species produced using wastewater and Centrate. *Biology, 11*, 1086. https://doi.org/10.3390/BIOLOGY11071086

Naseem, M., Kaltdorf, M., & Dandekar, T. (2015). The nexus between growth and defence signalling: Auxin and cytokinin modulate plant immune response pathways. *Journal of Experimental Botany, 66*, 4885–4896. https://doi.org/10.1093/JXB/ERV297

Naveed, S., Dong, B., Zhang, C., & Ge, Y. (2017). Microalgae and their effects on metal bioavailability in paddy fields. *Journal of Soils and Sediments, 18*, 936–945. https://doi.org/10.1007/S11368-017-1881-3

Nicodemus, T. J., DiRusso, C. C., Wilson, M., & Black, P. N. (2020). Reactive Oxygen Species (ROS) mediated degradation of organophosphate pesticides by the green microalgae Coccomyxa subellipsoidea. *Bioresource Technology Reports, 11*, 100461. https://doi.org/10.1016/J.BITEB.2020.100461

Nkurunziza, D., Coad, B. R., & Bulone, V. (2025). A review on integrated biorefining of brown algae focusing on bioactive compounds and holistic biomass valorisation. *Journal of Industrial and Engineering Chemistry, 151*, 200–215. https://doi.org/10.1016/J.JIEC.2025.03.047

Olaetxea, M., Garnica, M., Erro, J., Sanz, J., Monreal, G., Zamarreño, A. M., & García-Mina, J. M. (2024). The plant growth-promoting effect of an Ascophyllum nodosum (L.) extract derives from the interaction of its components and involves salicylic-, auxin- and cytokinin-signaling pathways. *Chemical and Biological Technologies in Agriculture, 11*, 1–16. https://doi.org/10.1186/S40538-024-00707-5/FIGURES/12

Olguín, E. J., Sánchez-Galván, G., Arias-Olguín, I. I., Melo, F. J., González-Portela, R. E., Cruz, L., De Philippis, R., & Adessi, A. (2022). Microalgae-based biorefineries: Challenges and future trends to produce carbohydrate enriched biomass, high-added value products and bioactive compounds. *Biology, 11*, 1146. https://doi.org/10.3390/BIOLOGY11081146

Ostrowski, J., Drozd, A., Olchowski, R., Chałabis-Mazurek, A., Sienkiewicz, A., Kierys, A., Morlo, K., & Dobrowolski, R. (2024). The removal of arsenic and its inorganic forms from marine algae—A base for inexpensive and efficient fertilizers. *Molecules, 29*, 1348. https://doi.org/10.3390/MOLECULES29061348/S1

Papenfus, H. B., Kulkarni, M. G., Stirk, W. A., Finnie, J. F., & Van Staden, J. (2013). Effect of a commercial seaweed extract (Kelpak®) and polyamines on nutrient-deprived (N, P and K) okra seedlings. *Scientia Horticulturae, 151*, 142–146. https://doi.org/10.1016/J.SCIENTA.2012.12.022

Parmar, P., Kumar, R., Neha, Y., & Srivatsan, V. (2023). Microalgae as next generation plant growth additives: Functions, applications, challenges and circular bioeconomy based solutions. *Frontiers in Plant Science, 14*, 1073546. https://doi.org/10.3389/FPLS.2023.1073546/XML

Peñalver, R., Lorenzo, J. M., Ros, G., Amarowicz, R., Pateiro, M., & Nieto, G. (2020). Seaweeds as a functional ingredient for a healthy diet. *Marine Drugs, 18*, 301. https://doi.org/10.3390/MD18060301

Pipitone, G., Monteverde, A., Pataro, G., Eslami, E., Pignataro, F., & Procentese, A. (2025). Downstream processes in a microalgae biorefinery: Cascaded enzymatic hydrolysis and pulsed electric field as green solution. *Processes, 13*, 1629. https://doi.org/10.3390/PR13061629

Plaza, B. M., Gómez-Serrano, C., Acién-Fernández, F. G., & Jimenez-Becker, S. (2018). Effect of microalgae hydrolysate foliar application (*Arthrospira platensis* and *Scenedesmus* sp.) on Petunia x hybrida growth. *Journal of Applied Phycology, 30*, 2359–2365. https://doi.org/10.1007/S10811-018-1427-0/FIGURES/9

Raize, O., Argaman, Y., & Yannai, S. (2004). Mechanisms of biosorption of different heavy metals by brown marine macroalgae. *Biotechnology and Bioengineering, 87*, 451–458. https://doi.org/10.1002/BIT.20136

Raymond Sunday, E. (2018). Phycoremediation: An eco-solution to environmental protection and sustainable remediation. *Journal of Chemical, Environmental and Biological Engineering, 2*, 5. https://doi.org/10.11648/J.JCEBE.20180201.12

Ricci, M., Tilbury, L., Daridon, B., & Sukalac, K. (2019). General principles to justify plant biostimulant claims. *Frontiers in Plant Science, 10*, 444124. https://doi.org/10.3389/FPLS.2019.00494/BIBTEX

Romera, E., González, F., Ballester, A., Blázquez, M. L., & Muñoz, J. A. (2007). Comparative study of biosorption of heavy metals using different types of algae. *Bioresource Technology, 98*, 3344–3353. https://doi.org/10.1016/J.BIORTECH.2006.09.026

Ronga, D., Biazzi, E., Parati, K., Carminati, D., Carminati, E., & Tava, A. (2019). Microalgal biostimulants and Biofertilisers in crop productions. *Agronomy, 9*, 192. https://doi.org/10.3390/AGRONOMY9040192

Rostami, S., Akbari, H., Adibzadeh, A., & Akbari, H. (2023). Effects of *Ascophyllum nodosum*-based biostimulants on improving Phytoextraction of cadmium and lead in contaminated soils. *Environmental Processes, 10*. https://doi.org/10.1007/S40710-023-00643-W

Ruales, E., Gómez-Serrano, C., Morillas-España, A., Garfí, M., González-López, C. V., & Ferrer, I. (2025). Microalgae-based biorefinery for biostimulant and biogas production: An integrated approach for resource recovery. *Algal Research, 91*, 104323. https://doi.org/10.1016/J.ALGAL.2025.104323

Rupawalla, Z., Robinson, N., Schmidt, S., Li, S., Carruthers, S., Buisset, E., Roles, J., Hankamer, B., & Wolf, J. (2021). Algae biofertilisers promote sustainable food production and a circular nutrient economy—An integrated empirical-modelling study. *Science of the Total Environment, 796*. https://doi.org/10.1016/J.SCITOTENV.2021.148913

Rupert, R., Rodrigues, K. F., Thien, V. Y., & Yong, W. T. L. (2022). Carrageenan from Kappaphycus alvarezii (Rhodophyta, Solieriaceae): Metabolism, structure, production, and application. *Frontiers in Plant Science, 13*, 859635. https://doi.org/10.3389/FPLS.2022.859635/XML

Sanjay, M. S., Sudarsanam, D., Raj, G. A., & Baskar, K. (2020). Isolation and identification of chromium reducing bacteria from tannery effluent. *Journal of King Saud University, Science, 32*, 265–271. https://doi.org/10.1016/J.JKSUS.2018.05.001

Santaniello, A., Scartazza, A., Gresta, F., Loreti, E., Biasone, A., Di Tommaso, D., Piaggesi, A., & Perata, P. (2017). Ascophyllum nodosum seaweed extract alleviates drought stress in Arabidopsis by affecting photosynthetic performance and related gene expression. *Frontiers in Plant Science, 8*, 275332. https://doi.org/10.3389/FPLS.2017.01362/XML

Sasaki, M., Takagi, A., Ota, S., Kawano, S., Sasaki, D., & Asayama, M. (2020). Coproduction of lipids and extracellular polysaccharides from the novel green alga *Parachlorella* sp. BX1.5 depending on cultivation conditions. *Biotechnology Reports, 25*, e00392. https://doi.org/10.1016/J.BTRE.2019.E00392

Shahzad, M., Hayat, R., Mujtaba, G., Rehman, W. U., & Nadeem, M. (2025). Biofertilizers in sustainable agriculture: Mechanisms, applications, and future prospects. *Discover Agriculture, 3*, 1–29. https://doi.org/10.1007/S44279-025-00318-0

Shi, J., Zhao, B., Zhao, L., Zha, Y., Yu, X., Yu, B., Luo, L., Wu, J., & Yue, E. (2024). Facilitating growth of maize (Zea mays L.) by biostimulants: A perspective from the interaction between root transcriptome and rhizosphere microbiome. *Journal of Agricultural and Food Chemistry, 72*(7), 3415–3426. https://doi.org/10.1021/acs.jafc.3c09062

Shibata, T., Kawaguchi, S., Hama, Y., Inagaki, M., Yamaguchi, K., & Nakamura, T. (2004). Local and chemical distribution of phlorotannins in brown algae. *Journal of Applied Phycology, 16*, 291–296. https://doi.org/10.1023/B:JAPH.0000047781.24993.0A

Shukla, P. S., Mantin, E. G., Adil, M., Bajpai, S., Critchley, A. T., & Prithiviraj, B. (2019). Ascophyllum nodosum-based biostimulants: Sustainable applications in agriculture for the stimulation of plant growth, stress tolerance, and disease management. *Frontiers in Plant Science, 10*, 462648. https://doi.org/10.3389/FPLS.2019.00655/XML

Singh, V. P., & Trehan, K. (1973). Effect of extracellular products of Aulosira fertilissima on the growth of rice seedlings. *Plant and Soil, 38*, 457–464. https://doi.org/10.1007/BF00779027/METRICS

Singh, S., Singh, M. K., Pal, S. K., Trivedi, K., Yesuraj, D., Singh, C. S., Anand, K. G. V., Chandramohan, M., Patidar, R., Kubavat, D., Zodape, S. T., & Ghosh, A. (2016). Sustainable enhancement in yield and quality of rain-fed maize through Gracilaria edulis and Kappaphycus alvarezii seaweed sap. *Journal of Applied Phycology, 28*, 2099–2112. https://doi.org/10.1007/S10811-015-0680-8/FIGURES/2

Singh, A., Sharma, K., Chahal, H. S., Kaur, H., & Hasanain, M. (2025). Seaweed-derived plant boosters: Revolutionizing sustainable farming and soil health. *Frontiers in Soil Science, 5*, 1504045. https://doi.org/10.3389/FSOIL.2025.1504045/BIBTEX

Soares, C., Švarc-Gajić, J., Oliva-Teles, M. T., Pinto, E., Nastić, N., Savić, S., Almeida, A., & Delerue-Matos, C. (2020). Mineral composition of subcritical water extracts of Saccorhiza Polyschides, a Brown seaweed used as fertilizer in the North of Portugal. *Journal of Marine Science and Engineering, 8*, 244. https://doi.org/10.3390/JMSE8040244

Sogoni, A., Ngcobo, B. L., Jimoh, M. O., Kambizi, L., & Laubscher, C. P. (2024). Seaweed-derived Bio-Stimulant (Kelpak®) Enhanced the Morphophysiological, Biochemical, and Nutritional Quality of Salt-Stressed Spinach (Spinacia oleracea L.). *Horticulturae 10*(12). https://doi.org/10.3390/horticulturae10121340

Solorzano-Chavez, E. G., Paz-Cedeno, F. R., Ezequiel de Oliveira, L., Gelli, V. C., Monti, R., Conceição de Oliveira, S., & Masarin, F. (2019). Evaluation of the Kappaphycus alvarezii growth under different environmental conditions and efficiency of the enzymatic hydrolysis of the residue generated in the carrageenan processing. *Biomass Bioenergy, 127*, 105254. https://doi.org/10.1016/J.BIOMBIOE.2019.105254

Sousa, F., Martins, M., Sousa, B., Soares, C., Azenha, M., Pereira, R., & Fidalgo, F. (2022). The potential of beach wrack as plant biostimulant to mitigate metal toxicity: Mineral composition, antioxidant properties and effects against Cu-induced stress. *Journal of Applied Phycology, 34*, 667–678. https://doi.org/10.1007/S10811-021-02636-4/FIGURES/3

Staykov, N., Kanojia, A., Lyall, R., Ivanova, V., Alseekh, S., Petrov, V., & Gechev, T. (2025). Sustainable agriculture through seaweed biostimulants: a two-year study demonstrates yield enhancement in pepper and eggplant. *Frontiers in Plant Science, 16*, 1655340. https://doi.org/10.3389/fpls.2025.1655340

Stirk, W. A., Bálint, P., Tarkowská, D., Novák, O., Strnad, M., Ördög, V., & van Staden, J. (2013a). Hormone profiles in microalgae: Gibberellins and brassinosteroids. *Plant Physiology and Biochemistry, 70*, 348–353. https://doi.org/10.1016/J.PLAPHY.2013.05.037

Stirk, W. A., Ördög, V., Novák, O., Rolčík, J., Strnad, M., Bálint, P., & van Staden, J. (2013b). Auxin and cytokinin relationships in 24 microalgal strains1. *Journal of Phycology, 49*, 459–467. https://doi.org/10.1111/JPY.12061;PAGEGROUP:STRING:PUBLICATION

Suhendrayatna, Ohki, A., Kuroiwa, T., & Maeda, S. (1999). Arsenic compounds in the freshwater green microalga *Chlorella vulgaris* after exposure to arsenite. *Applied Organometallic Chemistry, 13*, 127–133. https://doi.org/10.1002/(SICI)1099-0739(199902)13:2<127::AID-AOC810>3.0.CO;2-K

Sun, X., Xu, Z., Zhang, N., Miao, Y., Zhang, C., Ma, X., Shen, Q., & Zhang, R. (2025). Biofertilizer industry and research developments in China: A mini-review. *Microbial Biotechnology, 18*, e70163. https://doi.org/10.1111/1751-7915.70163;JOURNAL:JOURNAL:17517915;

WEBSITE:WEBSITE:SFAMJOURNALS;REQUESTEDJOURNAL:JOURNAL:17517915; WGROUP:STRING:PUBLICATION

Sutherland, D. L., & Ralph, P. J. (2019). Microalgal bioremediation of emerging contaminants – Opportunities and challenges. *Water Research, 164*, 114921. https://doi.org/10.1016/J.WATRES.2019.114921

Tolisano, C., & Del Buono, D. (2023). Biobased: Biostimulants and biogenic nanoparticles enter the scene. *Science of the Total Environment, 885*, 163912. https://doi.org/10.1016/J.SCITOTENV.2023.163912

Torres, M. D., Flórez-Fernández, N., & Domínguez, H. (2019). Integral utilization of red seaweed for bioactive production. *Marine Drugs, 17*, 314. https://doi.org/10.3390/MD17060314

Tran, T. L. C., Callahan, D. L., Islam, M. T., Wang, Y., Arioli, T., & Cahill, D. (2023). Comparative metabolomic profiling of Arabidopsis thaliana roots and leaves reveals complex response mechanisms induced by a seaweed extract. *Frontiers in Plant Science, 14*. https://doi.org/10.3389/fpls.2023.1114172

Tuhy, L., Saeid, A., & Chojnacka, K. (2020). Algae fertilizers. In *Encyclopedia of marine biotechnology* (pp. 105–119). https://doi.org/10.1002/9781119143802.CH5;CTYPE:STRING:BOOK

Varia, J., Kamaleson, C., & Lerer, L. (2022). Biostimulation with phycocyanin-rich spirulina extract in hydroponic vertical farming. *Scientia Horticulturae, 299*, 111042. https://doi.org/10.1016/J.SCIENTA.2022.111042

Verasoundarapandian, G., Lim, Z. S., Radziff, S. B. M., Taufik, S. H., Puasa, N. A., Shaharuddin, N. A., Merican, F., Wong, C. Y., Lalung, J., & Ahmad, S. A. (2022). Remediation of pesticides by microalgae as feasible approach in agriculture: Bibliometric strategies. *Agronomy, 12*, 117. https://doi.org/10.3390/AGRONOMY12010117

Wally, O. S. D., Critchley, A. T., Hiltz, D., Craigie, J. S., Han, X., Zaharia, L. I., Abrams, S. R., & Prithiviraj, B. (2013). Regulation of Phytohormone biosynthesis and accumulation in Arabidopsis following treatment with commercial extract from the marine macroalga Ascophyllum nodosum. *Journal of Plant Growth Regulation, 32*, 324–339. https://doi.org/10.1007/S00344-012-9301-9/FIGURES/10

Wu, S. C., Wang, F. J., & Pan, C. L. (2010). The comparison of Antioxidative properties of seaweed oligosaccharides fermented by two lactic acid bacteria. *Journal of Marine Science and Technology, 18*, 8. https://doi.org/10.51400/2709-6998.1908

Wu, J. Y., Tso, R., Teo, H. S., & Haldar, S. (2023). The utility of algae as sources of high value nutritional ingredients, particularly for alternative/complementary proteins to improve human health. *Frontiers in Nutrition, 10*, 1277343. https://doi.org/10.3389/FNUT.2023.1277343/FULL

Xiong, Q., Hu, L. X., Liu, Y. S., Zhao, J. L., He, L. Y., & Ying, G. G. (2021). Microalgae-based technology for antibiotics removal: From mechanisms to application of innovational hybrid systems. *Environment International, 155*, 106594. https://doi.org/10.1016/J.ENVINT.2021.106594

Xu, P., & Huang, L. (2017). Stereoselective bioaccumulation, transformation, and toxicity of triadimefon in Scenedesmus obliquus. *Chirality, 29*, 61–69. https://doi.org/10.1002/CHIR.22671

Yadav, S., Srivastava, R., Singh, N., Kanda, T., Verma, E., Choudhary, P., Yadav, S., & Atri, N. (2025). Cyanobacteria-pesticide interactions and their implications for sustainable rice agroecosystems. *International Journal of Microbiology, 2025*, 7265036. https://doi.org/10.1155/IJM/7265036

Yanshin, N., Kushnareva, A., Lemesheva, V., Birkemeyer, C., & Tarakhovskaya, E. (2021). Chemical composition and potential practical application of 15 red algal species from the White Sea Coast (the Arctic Ocean). *Molecules, 26*, 2489. https://doi.org/10.3390/MOLECULES26092489

Yasmeen, T., Ali, Q., Islam, F., Noman, A., Akram, M. S., & Javed, M. T. (2014). Biologically treated wastewater fertigation induced growth and yield enhancement effects in *Vigna radiata* L. *Agricultural Water Management, 146*, 124–130. https://doi.org/10.1016/j.agwat.2014.07.025

Yasmeen, A. R., Maharajan, T., Rameshkumar, R., Sindhamani, S., Banumathi, B., Prabakaran, M., Atchaya, S., & Rathinapriya, P. (2025). Role of seaweeds for improving soil fertility and crop development to address global food insecurity. *Crops, 5*, 29. https://doi.org/10.3390/CROPS5030029

Ye, S., Xie, C., Agar, O. T., Barrow, C. J., Dunshea, F. R., & Suleria, H. A. R. (2024). Alginates from Brown seaweeds as a promising natural source: A review of its properties and health benefits. *Food Reviews International, 40*, 2682–2710. https://doi.org/10.1080/87559129.2023.2279583

Zabot, G. L., Schaefer Rodrigues, F., Polano Ody, L., Vinícius Tres, M., Herrera, E., Palacin, H., Córdova-Ramos, J. S., Best, I., & Olivera-Montenegro, L. (2022). Encapsulation of bioactive compounds for food and agricultural applications. *Polymers (Basel), 14*, 4194. https://doi.org/10.3390/POLYM14194194

Ziaei, M., & Pazoki, A. (2022). Foliar-applied seaweed extract improves yield of common bean (*Phaseolus vulgaris* L.) cultivars through changes in biochemical and Fatty acid profile under irrigation regimes. *Journal of Soil Science and Plant Nutrition*. https://doi.org/10.1007/S42729-022-00860-6

Zollmann, M., Robin, A., Prabhu, M., Polikovsky, M., Gillis, A., Greiserman, S., & Golberg, A. (2019). Green technology in green macroalgal biorefineries. *Phycologia, 58*, 516–534. https://doi.org/10.1080/00318884.2019.1640516;SUBPAGE:STRING:FULL

The manufacturer's authorised representative in the EU is Springer Nature Customer Service Centre GmbH, Europaplatz 3, 69115 Heidelberg, Germany. If you have any concerns regarding our products, please contact ProductSafety@springernature.com

Printed and bound by CPI Group (UK) Ltd, Croydon, CR0 4YY
21/09/2026
02219991-0016